Tumors
of the
Mammary Gland

Atlas
of
Tumor Pathology

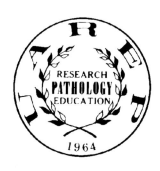

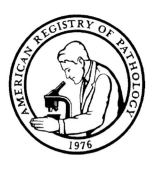

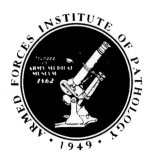

ATLAS OF TUMOR PATHOLOGY

Third Series
Fascicle 7

TUMORS OF THE
MAMMARY GLAND

by

PAUL PETER ROSEN, M.D.
Attending Pathologist and Member
Memorial Sloan-Kettering Cancer Center
1275 York Avenue, New York, New York 10021
Professor of Pathology
Cornell University Medical College

and

HAROLD A. OBERMAN, M.D.
Professor of Pathology
University of Michigan School of Medicine
1500 East Medical Center Drive
Ann Arbor, Michigan 48109

Published by the
ARMED FORCES INSTITUTE OF PATHOLOGY
Washington, D.C.

Under the Auspices of
UNIVERSITIES ASSOCIATED FOR RESEARCH AND EDUCATION IN PATHOLOGY, INC.
Bethesda, Maryland
1993

Accepted for Publication
1992

———————————————

Available from the American Registry of Pathology
Armed Forces Institute of Pathology
Washington, D.C. 20306-600
ISSN 0160-6344
ISBN 1-881041-07-7

ATLAS OF TUMOR PATHOLOGY

EDITOR
JUAN ROSAI, M.D.
Department of Pathology
Memorial Sloan-Kettering Cancer Center
New York, New York 10021-6007

ASSOCIATE EDITOR
LESLIE H. SOBIN, M.D.
Armed Forces Institute of Pathology
Washington, D.C. 20306-6000

EDITORS' NOTE

The Atlas of Tumor Pathology has a long and distinguished history. It was first conceived at a Cancer Research Meeting held in St. Louis in September 1947 as an attempt to standardize the nomenclature of neoplastic diseases. The first series was sponsored by the National Academy of Sciences-National Research Council. The organization of this Sisyphean effort was entrusted to the Subcommittee on Oncology of the Committee on Pathology, and Dr. Arthur Purdy Stout was the first editor-in-chief. Many of the illustrations were provided by the Medical Illustration Service of the Armed Forces Institute of Pathology, the type was set by the Government Printing Office, and the final printing was done at the Armed Forces Institute of Pathology (hence the colloquial appellation "AFIP Fascicles"). The American Registry of Pathology purchased the Fascicles from the Government Printing Office and sold them virtually at cost. Over a period of 20 years, approximately 15,000 copies each of nearly 40 Fascicles were produced. The worldwide impact that these publications have had over the years has largely surpassed the original goal. They quickly became among the most influential publications on tumor pathology ever written, primarily because of their overall high quality but also because their low cost made them easily accessible to pathologists and other students of oncology the world over.

Upon completion of the first series, the National Academy of Sciences-National Research Council handed further pursuit of the project over to the newly created Universities Associated for Research and Education in Pathology (UAREP). A second series was started, generously supported by grants from the AFIP, the National Cancer Institute, and the American Cancer Society. Dr. Harlan I. Firminger became the editor-in-chief and was succeeded by Dr. William H. Hartmann. The second series Fascicles were produced as bound volumes instead of loose leaflets. They featured a more comprehensive coverage of the subjects, to the extent that the Fascicles could no longer be regarded as "atlases" but rather as monographs describing and illustrating in detail the tumors and tumor-like conditions of the various organs and systems.

Once the second series was completed, with a success that matched that of the first, UAREP and AFIP decided to embark on a third series. A new editor-in-chief and an associate editor were selected, and a distinguished editorial board was appointed. The mandate for the third series remains the same as for the previous ones, i.e., to oversee the production of an eminently practical publication with surgical pathologists as its primary audience, but also aimed at other workers in oncology. The main purposes of this series are to promote a consistent, unified, and biologically sound nomenclature; to guide the surgical pathologist in the diagnosis of the various tumors and tumor-like lesions; and to provide relevant histogenetic, pathogenetic, and clinicopathologic information on these entities. Just as the second series included data obtained from ultrastructural (and, in the more recent Fascicles, immunohistochemical) examination, the third series will, in addition, incorporate pertinent information obtained with the newer molecular biology techniques. As in the past, a continuous attempt will be made to correlate, whenever possible, the nomenclature used in the Fascicles with that proposed by the World Health Organization's International Histological Classification of Tumors. The format of the third series has been changed in order to incorporate additional items and to ensure a consistency of style throughout. This includes the dropping of the 's possessive in eponymic terms, in accordance with the WHO and the International Nomenclature of Diseases. Close cooperation between the various authors and their respective liaisons from the editorial board will be emphasized to minimize unnecessary repetition and discrepancies in the text and illustrations.

To its everlasting credit, the participation and commitment of the AFIP to this venture is even more substantial and encompassing than in previous series. It now extends to virtually all scientific, technical, and financial aspects of the production.

The task confronting the organizations and individuals involved in the third series is even more daunting than in the preceding efforts because of the ever-increasing complexity of the matter at hand. It is hoped that this combined effort—of which, needless to say, that represented by the authors is first and foremost—will result in a series worthy of its two illustrious predecessors and will be a suitable introduction to the tumor pathology of the twenty-first century.

Juan Rosai, M.D.
Leslie H. Sobin, M.D.

ACKNOWLEDGMENTS

The authors are responsible for the content of this book but it could not have been prepared without the support and assistance of many individuals. We wish to acknowledge the innumerable patients from whom we have learned about the diseases described in this volume. Many pathology residents, fellows, and faculty associates at Memorial Hospital and at the University of Michigan invested a great deal of time and effort working up specimens that provided some of the material selected for photography. Other illustrations were obtained from cases submitted for diagnostic consultation over several decades by a large number of pathologists. We are especially grateful to these colleagues for their continued support, encouragement, and interest in seeking a better understanding of clinical and pathologic aspects of breast disease. The goal of these efforts is the optimal diagnosis and treatment of breast disease and, ultimately, the development of measures for its prevention. We also wish to acknowledge a number of individuals who made important and direct contributions to the preparation of this Fascicle. Ellen Cohen and Milicent Cranor, of Memorial Sloan-Kettering Cancer Center, and Ann Miller, of the University of Michigan, were responsible for typing and editing as well as for bibliographic work. Kin Kong, chief photographer, and Lisa Hollis, assistant photographer, of Memorial Sloan-Kettering Cancer Center, and Craig Biddle and Mark Deming, photographers in the Department of Pathology of the University of Michigan, developed and printed outstanding photographs from which a modest number were selected for use in this book. Electron photomicrographs were generously supplied by Dr. Robert A. Erlandson, of Memorial Sloan-Kettering Cancer Center.

We also wish to acknowledge the following individuals who provided case material specifically for inclusion in this Fascicle: Dr. Ron Neafie, of the Armed Forces Institute of Pathology, Dr. Juan Rosai, of Memorial Sloan-Kettering Cancer Center, Dr. Jeffrey Searle, of the Royal Brisbane Hospital in Brisbane, Australia, and Dr. Sami Shousha, of the Charing Cross Hospital in London, U.K.

Dr. Frances Pitlick, Beverly Lea, Dian Thomas, Paul Clifford, and Audrey Kahn of the UAREP were extremely helpful during the preparation of the manuscript and production of this book. We also appreciate the helpful comments of the Editor-in-Chief and of the Editorial Advisory Board of the Third Series of the Fascicles, and we are particularly grateful to the anonymous reviewers of the initial draft of the book for many constructive suggestions.

The patient support and assistance of Dr. Carolyn Mies and Dr. Marylen Oberman were crucial to the preparation and completion of this volume.

Paul Peter Rosen, M.D.
Harold A. Oberman, M.D.

Permission to use copyrighted illustrations has been granted by:

American Medical Association:
  Arch Pathol Lab Med 115:141–5, 1991. For figure 377.

American Society of Clinical Pathologists:
  Tumors of the Breast. Proceedings of the 53rd Annual Anatomic Pathology Slide
    Seminar of the American Society of Clinical Pathologists, 1987. For figures 258,
    417, 506, 516, 526, and 530.

Appleton & Lange:
  Pathol Annu 18(Pt 2):215–32, 1983. For figures 251 and 252.
  Pathol Annu 19(Pt 1):195–219, 1984. For figures 345–7.
  Pathol Annu 24(Pt 2):237–54, 1989. For figures 370 and 372.

JB Lippincott Company:
  Am J Clin Pathol 94:371–7, 1990. For figure 393.
  Ann Surg 204:612–3, 1986. For figures 592 and 593.
  Breast Diseases. 2nd ed. 1991. For figures 245, 246, 248, 268, 280–2, 295, 310, 342,
    343, 351, 356, 369, 375, 385, and 583.
  Cancer 59:1927–30, 1987. For figures 127 and 129.
  Cancer 61:1611–20, 1988. For figure 392.
  Cancer 63:1363–9, 1989. For figure 490.

Raven Press:
  Am J Surg Pathol 2:225–51, 1978. For figure 187.
  Am J Surg Pathol 4:241–6, 1980. For figures 203 and 204.
  Am J Surg Pathol 5:629–42, 1981. For figures 505, 507, 508, and 520.
  Am J Surg Pathol 7:739–45, 1983. For figures 122–5.
  Am J Surg Pathol 8:31–41, 1984. For figure 380.
  Am J Surg Pathol 8:907–15, 1984. For figures 562, 566, and 567.
  Am J Surg Pathol 9:491–503, 1985. For figures 456 and 463.
  Am J Surg Pathol 9:659–65, 1985. For figures 471–4.
  Am J Surg Pathol 9:723–9, 1985. For figures 476 and 477.
  Am J Surg Pathol 10:87–101, 1986. For figures 101–3, 108, 113, 116, 118, 119, and 121.
  Am J Surg Pathol 10:464–9, 1986. For figures 296 and 297.
  Am J Surg Pathol 11:351–8, 1987. For figure 329.
  Am J Surg Pathol 14:12–23, 1990. For figure 260.

WB Saunders Company:
  Hum Pathol 17:185–91, 1986. For figures 480–3.
  Hum Pathol 18:1232–7, 1987. For figures 133, 135, 142, and 143.

Williams & Wilkins Company:
  Mod Pathol 1:98–103, 1988. For figures 501 and 503.

TUMORS OF THE MAMMARY GLAND

Contents

TUMORS OF THE MAMMARY GLAND

INTRODUCTION

Like the frames of a motion picture film, the Fascicles of the Armed Forces Institute of Pathology constitute chapters in the history of tumor pathology. This third edition of Tumors of the Mammary Gland is built upon the contributions of its predecessors. Its expanded size and scope reflect the explosive growth of information relating to breast disease that has occurred during the past two decades.

The first Fascicle on Tumors of the Breast, written by Fred W. Stewart, was published in 1950 (6). The 114 pages, 68 figures, and 32 references were designed "to describe and illustrate the pathology of cancer of the human breast" and provide a catalog of tumorous conditions of the breast. Descriptions of benign lesions were brief, "except where the latter are of such pattern that less experienced pathologists often confuse them with mammary cancer." The six major categories (Paget disease, carcinoma, malignant variants of fibroadenoma and cystosarcoma phyllodes, miscellaneous sarcomas, lesions simulating tumors, and benign tumors) were further subdivided into approximately 30 specific diagnoses. As a result, the classification of benign and malignant lesions developed by Ewing and Stewart in the preceding decades was established as an international standard. With the exception of a few histochemical tests, such as the mucicarmine and trichrome stains, the authors relied entirely on hematoxylin- and eosin-stained sections.

The clinical evaluation of patients at that time was limited to physical examination, occasionally assisted by transillumination to detect cysts. The only widely accepted diagnostic procedure was surgical biopsy, although needle aspiration biopsy was practiced in a few centers. Radical mastectomy, sometimes supplemented with local irradiation, was the standard treatment for malignant neoplasms. Introductory comments in the first Fascicle, dealing with "precancerous" lesions, classification, and prognosis contained many observations which are as relevant today as they were then.

Stewart's skeptical views on the concept of a "precancerous" state in the breast were indicated by the following comments:

> ...a progressive change into cancer can be found in duct hyperplasias and papillomas, something that to the unbiased observer means only that cancer can develop in an epithelium that possesses more than the average impetus toward proliferative alteration. But unfortunately, in the same breast one may find cancer without any evidence whatever that it has arisen in such an area. One is apt to be overly impressed by seeing the beginnings in a previously abnormal structure and neglect its origin in another area where the prior abnormality is at least not apparent.... The cancer actually develops in what happens to be in the breast. Even the innocuous old hyalinized fibroadenoma exceedingly rarely develops a cancer.

> ...Really I do not know what "precancerous" means. Is it something upon which cancer is engrafted more often than upon something else, or than upon areas revealing no abnormality one can detect? ...Sometimes I think the word "precancerous" is the most abused expression in the whole cancer field....

Regarding the classification of breast carcinoma, Stewart offered the following observation:

> Although the exacting histologist may find comfort and may derive prestige from the employment of many names in the diagnosis of cancer of the breast, it is my impression that surgeon, patient and pathologist could get along with very few.

Thus, it was clear that Stewart was a "lumper" rather than a "splitter" in his approach to classification; terminology had to be clinically meaningful and not simply descriptive. This conservative approach has guided the expansion of the Stewart classification in the present volume.

The most important prognostic variables cited by Stewart were the presence or absence of invasion, the extent of invasion (localized or diffuse), the presence or absence of true lymphatic invasion, and the presence or absence (and extent) of axillary lymph node metastases. "All these things exceed in prognostic importance the mere looking at cells and assigning names and grades ...." This view of prognostic factors giving primary importance to stage, has largely withstood the test of time. In retrospect, Stewart may have underestimated the prognostic importance of some histologic subtypes, although they account for a minority of tumors and are themselves also subject to the effect of stage.

Nearly 25 years passed before the second Fascicle on Tumors of the Breast, authored by Robert W. McDivitt, Fred W. Stewart, and John W. Berg was published in 1968 (3). This book consisted of 156 pages with 120 figures and 81 references. The classification was virtually unchanged from the prior edition. Electron microscopy offered a new view of the structure of many lesions but few studies were done on breast pathology and there were no ultrastructural photographs. Cytologic examination of needle aspirates and nipple secretion had become a diagnostic procedure in a few medical centers, but was still not widely employed. The diagnostic armamentarium available to pathologists had not appreciably enlarged in the quarter century between the first and second Fascicles.

There was one important clinical advance, however. Mammography, developed and refined as a clinical tool for the diagnosis of palpable breast lesions, increasingly led to the discovery of nonpalpable lesions, thereby expanding the range of diagnostic problems. As a consequence, the distinction between hyperplasia and in situ carcinoma was a major concern, occupying about one third of the text and illustrations of the second Fascicle.

Having concluded that the first Fascicle had contributed to "...a substantial decline in overdiagnosis of breast cancer" and that "...the level of diagnosis is much improved," the authors stated that "the orientation of the new Fascicle is somewhat different...placing emphasis on 'early' lesions." The importance of detecting early lesions was stressed because "lacking something new on the horizon for the treatment of the patient with breast cancer, improvement in end results would seem to rest on increasingly early pathologic diagnosis." Early was defined as "...cancer that is confined to ducts or lobules, or both, and nowhere is seen to be infiltrative," that is, in situ carcinoma.

McDivitt, Stewart, and Berg drew attention to problems engendered by the effort to diagnose in situ carcinoma:

> This search has resulted in the tendency on the part of pathologists to recognize earlier and earlier changes on which a diagnosis of cancer may be made, a tendency which is both useful and dangerous owing to overenthusiasm. In these breast lesions we have said that "early" means they are cytologically cancerous but still within the area of origin, that is, intraductal or intralobular. How long such a situation may be maintained is unknown, but it is highly probable that it may last for years or even decades.

It is interesting to note that the discussion of early (in situ) carcinoma in the Introduction to the second edition was completely separate from, and preceded, comments on "Precancerous Lesions." The latter section was concerned mainly with "the proliferative cystic disease complex and subsequent breast cancer."

Employing several illustrative examples, the authors suggested that the "precancerous" properties of "cystic disease" might be attributable to the presence of unrecognized in situ carcinoma in the breast. This might occur through failure to diagnose in situ carcinoma in a biopsy sample or because the lesion, present elsewhere in the breast, was not included in the tissue removed. They acknowledged, however, that components of "the cystic proliferative complex" might also prove to be precancerous and concluded that to identify such changes

> ...requires segregation of various significant and insignificant patterns.... Much more study of "borderline" lesions is needed, especially with description at the cytologic level rather than merely diagnosis by outdated cliches which do not analyze. Most of all, we need the test of time and we do not even know how much time.... If we must wait an indeterminate time for behaviour patterns in cancer already present, then how long must we wait to judge the capabilities of a "precancerous" lesion?

Implicit in the foregoing discussion of early, precancerous, and borderline lesions is the concept that they are associated with an increased risk of subsequent carcinoma. However, the authors appreciated the substantial difficulties inherent in such a conclusion:

> One cannot remove a section of breast, find an *in situ* carcinoma, and be certain that the infiltrative cancer found elsewhere in the same breast years later was there in an *in situ* form at the time of the initial excision. The mere fact that disease of this type is extremely apt to be multifocal gives support of course to the belief that it was there and has taken years to evolve.... Of course, one could speculate that the carcinogenic stimulus might reach the breast on more than a single occasion; thus, not all foci of *in situ* carcinoma need have existed simultaneously, or for that matter have developed at the same rate.

The diagnosis and treatment of breast carcinoma is far different today than it was in 1967. No longer is the surgeon confronted largely with palpable lesions, and no longer is the treatment of carcinoma restricted to mastectomy. The increased use of mammography has heightened recognition of nonpalpable neoplasia, and fine-needle aspiration cytology has accelerated the diagnosis of carcinoma. Probably the most significant development is the advent of breast conservation therapy. The pathologist's role has expanded beyond distinguishing between a benign and a malignant lesion. Issues related to the feasibility of breast conservation and the extent of the procedure, including multicentricity of the neoplasm, the type and distribution of intraductal carcinoma, and the presence of neoplasm at the margins of surgical excision, have grown in importance during the last decade.

The present Fascicle addresses clinical issues that are increasingly integral responsibilities of the pathologist. Mammography must be utilized to correlate specimen radiography with biopsy specimens; interpretation of fine-needle aspiration cytologic specimens brings patient and pathologist together; and biopsy of nonpalpable lesions necessitates recognition of earlier manifestations of intraductal epithelial proliferation.

The pathologist has become involved in treatment decisions and assessment of the prognostic implication of various neoplasms. Immunohisto-chemical procedures have expanded our ability to detect hormonal receptors in lesions too small for biochemical analysis or in cytologic specimens from lesions not readily accessible to surgical biopsy. A diverse menu of studies for the prognostic appraisal of malignant neoplasms can be utilized, including assessment of the proliferative rate of the tumor, oncogene amplification studies, and flow cytometric determination of the ploidy status of the neoplasm. Many of these studies are new, and their utility has yet to be confirmed.

The pathologist must be aware of benign lesions that can simulate carcinoma, and these are described to a greater extent in this Fascicle than in previous editions. Patterns of mammary neoplasia are sharply distinguished to permit better distinction of their prognostic significance. Most important, there is continued and renewed emphasis on the assessment of "borderline" intraductal epithelial proliferative lesions. This was a central focus of both previous Fascicles, and it continues to be the source of greatest consternation in the pathologic assessment of breast biopsies.

Dr. Joseph Colt Bloodgood, a protégé of Halstead early in this century, was one of a small group of American surgeons who appreciated the crucial role of microscopic pathological studies in the diagnosis and treatment of breast diseases. He advocated early detection as a means of reducing breast cancer mortality decades in advance of mammography, by urging that clinical abnormalities be biopsied before they became obviously malignant. In 1916 he commented "...that the relative proportion of benign lesions of the breast is steadily changing and that the percentage of benign lesions is on the increase" (2). In addition to practicing surgery, Bloodgood was a skilled microscopist. His histopathologic examination of clinically inconspicuous proliferative lesions illuminated the interpretive difficulties that could be presented by microscopic pathologic alterations that did not cause palpable tumors. He used the term "borderline" for lesions about which "both the surgeon and pathologist are in doubt" and stated that "...if women come early we shall find that the borderline group is large."

Bloodgood demonstrated the lack of agreement by pathologists in the interpretation of borderline lesions in the following test:

I have submitted over sixty borderline cases to a number of pathologists, and have found that in not a single one has there been uniform agreement as to whether the lesion was benign or malignant.... This is no reflection on the diagnostic abilities of the pathologists; it is simply evidence that at the present time there are certain lesions of the breast about which we apparently do not agree from the microscopic appearance only.

The problems presented by borderline lesions concerned Bloodgood for many years and in 1932 he pointed to the diagnostic and therapeutic uncertainty as "...one of the most important problems in surgery of the breast — the problem of whether the tumor alone should be removed or the complete operation for cancer performed" (1).

The current variability in the interpretation of such lesions was described by Rosai in 1991 (4). Seventeen slides, each with a specific intraepithelial lesion circled, were reviewed by five pathologists. Although none of the slides was interpreted unanimously, all were in agreement that 8 lesions (47 percent) were not carcinoma, differing on whether the process was hyperplasia or atypical hyperplasia. Four lesions were diagnosed as in situ carcinoma by two or three pathologists. One pathologist reported in situ carcinoma in 9 of the 17 while at the other extreme another pathologist concluded that none of the lesions was carcinoma. These were clearly borderline lesions as defined by Bloodgood, leading Dr. Rosai to conclude "...that we are far from having reached uniform diagnostic criteria in this field."

As noted by Rosai, it is widely thought that there is "...a continuum between hyperplasia and carcinoma in situ and that the risk for the development of invasive carcinoma correlates with the degree of proliferation and atypia." Hence, assigning a diagnosis to lesions in this spectrum is also an exercise in estimating the risk for subsequent carcinoma. Some of the limitations which impair the precision of this process are summarized here.

1. *Sampling error*: The excised tissue lacks the most extreme proliferative changes.
2. *Extrapolation inability*: Failure to develop carcinoma after the excision of a proliferative lesion may be attributed to the excision of the lesion in the biopsy. Histologic changes in the biopsy serve as a marker but there is presently no method for determining if similar pathologic changes remain in the breast or if they will develop later. It is not possible to trace a later neoplastic lesion, such as invasive carcinoma, directly to a prior, excised proliferative lesion.
3. *Confounding variables*: These include length of follow-up, family history of breast carcinoma, or parity. Most women with proliferative lesions, even those with the most atypical changes, do not develop carcinoma even after long follow-up. Several investigators have shown that the relative risk for carcinoma following a diagnosis of atypical hyperplasia is greater among women with a history of carcinoma in first degree relatives. Tools are not available to detect morphologic alterations influenced by positive family history or other confounding factors. As a consequence, the classification of proliferative lesions as atypical, precancerous, or borderline on the basis of follow-up results alone, is at best crude.
4. *Lack of Gold Standard*: This has yet to be achieved to distinguish hyperplasia from in situ carcinoma. Rosai has pointed out that "...none of the special techniques that have been employed to date in an attempt to achieve a sharper and more reproducible separation between the various groups has yet fulfilled this goal."

A comparison of photographs of proliferative lesions clearly demonstrates the range of interpretations now assigned to lesions in the broad categories of hyperplasia and in situ carcinoma. These representations are at best informed judgements. There is presently no laboratory test to serve as an objective "gold standard" marker to indicate that a specific lesion is at the level of carcinoma in the breast. If a marker can be identified to distinguish between hyperplasia and in situ carcinoma, it will most likely be found by studying invasive or classic in situ carcinoma rather than among borderline lesions of ambiguous significance. While a standard would resolve many issues relating to diagnostic criteria, sampling and extrapolation would still pose problems in making therapeutic decisions.

In the management of individual patients, pathologists do not differ from their clinical colleagues appreciably with respect to "interobserver variability." Recommendations for the treatment of cancer from surgeons and medical or radiation oncologists may vary substantially. Reaching a therapeutic decision in these circumstances is a judgement based on experience applied specifically to the patient under consideration. A similar process is employed in the pathologic evaluation of borderline proliferative lesions from individual patients.

Interobserver variability in the interpretation of borderline breast lesions has important implications for epidemiologic and clinical studies. The problem is dramatized in the variable interpretation of the cases assembled by Rosai. It is generally agreed that the highest risk of subsequent invasive carcinoma occurs among patients with antecedent in situ lesions, diminishing progressively among those with atypical and simple hyperplastic changes. On the basis of personal criteria, one reviewer in the Rosai study concluded that nine lesions were sufficiently abnormal to be in the highest risk category while another reviewer concluded that four of these

nine warranted an intermediate-risk designation, and five were relatively low-risk lesions. While observer variability can be reduced by standardization of diagnostic criteria, it would not enhance our understanding of how the differing diagnostic interpretations relate to risk (5).

With the foregoing limitations in mind, we describe and illustrate in the following pages our criteria for the diagnosis of a broad range of pathologic conditions including proliferative lesions and in situ carcinoma. The diagnoses offered represent our interpretations for which we take full responsibility. Illustrations included in the volume have been carefully studied and accepted by independent reviewers. They do not differ appreciably from images presented in the prior Fascicle written by McDivitt, Stewart, and Berg. Advances made in coming years should help resolve the diagnostic quandary that now attends lesions variously described as atypical, borderline, precancerous, or in situ carcinoma.

REFERENCES

1. Bloodgood JC. Borderline breast tumors. Encapsulated and non-encapsulated cystic adenomata observed from 1890 to 1931. Am J Cancer 1932;16:103–76.
2. _____. Cancer of the breast. Figures which show that education can increase the number of cures. JAMA 1916;66:552–3.
3. McDivitt RW, Stewart FW, Berg JW. Tumors of the breast. Atlas of Tumor Pathology, 2nd Series, Fascicle 2. Washington D.C.: Armed Forces Institute of Pathology, 1968.
4. Rosai J. Borderline epithelial lesions of the breast. Am J Surg Pathol 1991;15:209–21.
5. Rosen PP. Proliferative breast "disease." An unresolved diagnostic dilemma. Cancer 1993;71:3798–807.
6. Stewart FW. Tumors of the breast. Atlas of Tumor Pathology, Sect. IX–Fascicle 34. Washington D.C.: Armed Forces Institute of Pathology, 1950.

CLASSIFICATION

The classification of mammary neoplasms used in this Fascicle is based on one adopted by the World Health Organization (WHO) in 1981, to provide "histological definitions of cancer types and to facilitate the wide adoption of a uniform nomenclature" (1). We have employed the WHO terminology for almost all tumors. Newly characterized lesions have been added and in some categories subclassification is indicated.

Although the text of the Fascicle employs the diagnostic terms listed in the following classification, the organization differs significantly in some areas. These differences in sequence are readily apparent when the classification is compared with the Table of Contents. Benign tumors of the male breast are grouped together in a single chapter although in the classification gynecomastia appears under Tumor-like Lesions and other benign tumors of the male breast are not separately identified. Carcinomas of the male breast and carcinomas in several unusual clinical situations are listed in a separate category, Unusual Clinical Presentation of Carcinoma. Proliferative lesions that resemble salivary gland adenomas (pleomorphic adenoma or mixed tumor), considered under Other Adenomas in the WHO classification are listed here under Papillary Tumors because they are variants of intraductal papilloma. Adenomyoepithelioma is similarly classified.

HISTOLOGIC CLASSIFICATION OF BREAST TUMORS*

1. Epithelial Tumors
    1.1 Benign
        1.1.1 Papilloma
        1.1.2 Papilloma variants
            1.1.2.1 Adenomyoepithelioma
            1.1.2.2 Mixed tumor (pleomorphic adenoma)
            1.1.2.3 Ductal adenoma
        1.1.3 Florid papillomatosis (adenoma) of nipple
        1.1.4 Syringomatous adenoma of nipple
        1.1.5 Adenoma
            1.1.5.1 Tubular
            1.1.5.2 Lactating
            1.1.5.3 Apocrine
    1.2 Malignant
        1.2.1 Noninvasive
            1.2.1.1 Intraductal carcinoma
                1.2.1.1.1 With Paget disease
            1.2.1.2 Lobular carcinoma in situ
        1.2.2 Invasive
            1.2.2.1 Invasive ductal carcinoma
                1.2.2.1.1 With Paget disease
            1.2.2.2 Invasive ductal carcinoma with a predominant intraductal component

---

*Categories printed in normal type correspond to listings in the WHO Histological Classification of Breast Tumours (1). Other categories, shown in italics, have been added by the authors of this Fascicle.

           4.1.1.7 Lipoma
                  4.1.1.7.1 Adenolipoma
                  4.1.1.7.2 Angiolipoma
           4.1.1.8 Chondroma
           4.1.1.9 Granular cell tumor
        4.1.2 Malignant
           4.1.2.1 Angiosarcoma
           4.1.2.2 Fibrosarcoma
           4.1.2.3 Leiomyosarcoma
           4.1.2.4 Chondrosarcoma
           4.1.2.5 Osteosarcoma
           4.1.2.6 Hemangiopericytoma
           4.1.2.7 Dermatofibrosarcoma protuberans
     4.2 Skin tumors
        4.2.1 Malignant melanoma of nipple
        4.2.2 Squamous cell carcinoma of nipple
        4.2.3 Basal cell carcinoma of nipple
        4.2.4 Neoplasms of mammary skin
     4.3 Lymphoid and hematopoietic tumors
        4.3.1 Non-Hodgkin lymphoma
        4.3.2 Plasmacytoma
        4.3.3 Leukemic infiltration
        4.3.4 Hodgkin disease
5. Mammary Dysplasia/Fibrocystic Changes
     5.1 Ductal hyperplasia
        5.1.1 Atypical ductal hyperplasia
     5.2 Lobular hyperplasia
        5.2.1 Atypical lobular hyperplasia
     5.3 Adenosis
        5.3.1 Sclerosing adenosis
        5.3.2 Adenosis tumor
        5.3.3 Microglandular adenosis
        5.3.4 Tubular adenosis
     5.4 Cysts
     5.5 Fibroadenomatoid hyperplasia
     5.6 Radial sclerosing lesion (radial scar)
6. Tumor-Like Lesions
     6.1 Duct ectasia
     6.2 Inflammatory pseudotumors
        6.2.1 Foreign body reaction
        6.2.2 Fat necrosis
        6.2.3 Infarct
        6.2.4 Infection
     6.3 Hamartoma

REFERENCES

1. World Health Organization. Histological typing of breast tumours. 2nd ed. International Histological Classification of Tumours No. 2. Geneva: World Health Organization, 1981.

ANATOMY

INFANTILE BREAST AND PUBERTY

At birth male and female breasts may have active secretion caused by the transplacental passage of maternal hormones. In some infants this results in bilateral breast enlargement with elaboration of a colostrum-like secretion termed "witch's milk." Microscopically, this is associated with duct dilatation without acinus formation (fig. 1) (3,5).This secretory function can be sustained, in some instances for many months, by squeezing or massaging the breasts. Ordinarily, however, perinatal breast enlargement recedes several months postpartum. Before puberty the breasts in both sexes consist of ducts that manifest variable degrees of branching, lack lobules, and are lined by cuboidal epithelium.

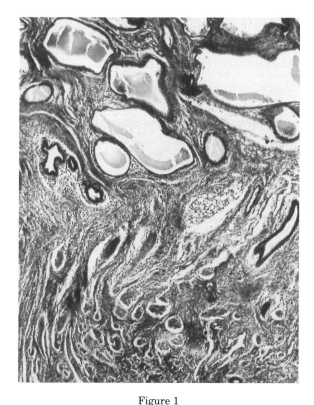

Figure 1
NEONATAL DUCT ECTASIA
Section of breast of newborn infant with dilatation of mammary ducts.

In most female children pubertal breast enlargement begins between 9 and 13 years of age (14). This presents initially as a somewhat rubbery subareolar discoid mass, a result of the proliferation and branching of lactiferous ducts. This development may be asymmetric, and there may not be further growth for months (18). Typically, this breast enlargement coincides with, or antedates, the onset of menses, occasionally by several years. The hallmark of pubertal breast development is the formation of lobules.

Breast development can occur at a much earlier age as a unilateral or bilateral subareolar mass which usually remains stable until the onset of puberty. This enlargement, termed *premature thelarche*, is most likely a manifestation of variable response to endogenous hormone stimulation. Clinical recognition of premature thelarche is essential since excision will result in an amastic adult (11). Histologic examination reveals elongation and branching of mammary ducts with associated intraductal epithelial proliferation as well as the accumulation of fat and connective tissue between the ducts (figs. 2, 3). Lobule formation is not a feature. The ductal epithelial proliferation may be prominent, creating papillary folds that seemingly occlude the duct lumens, intraluminal bridging, and occasional mitoses. The epithelial cells are uniform and there is no necrosis.

MATURE ADULT BREAST

Microanatomy

The normal breast consists of 15 to 25 lactiferous ducts that start in the nipple, branch, and end in the terminal ductal lobular unit. The latter consists of a terminal intralobular duct and multiple lobular ducts, surrounded by intralobular, or perilobular, connective tissue. Whereas extralobular ducts are lined with columnar epithelium, the intralobular and lobular ducts are lined by cuboidal epithelium. Furthermore, extralobular ducts have a prominent coat of elastic fibers while these are absent from intralobular ducts (19).

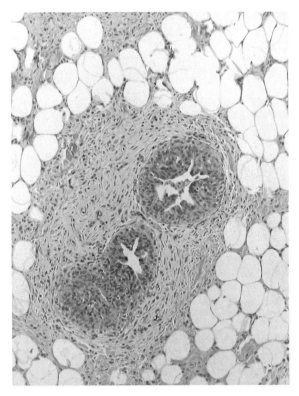

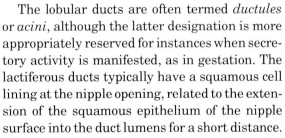

Figure 2
PREMATURE THELARCHE
Proliferation of ducts without associated lobule formation in 9-year-old girl with unilateral breast enlargement. (Figures 2 and 3 are from the same patient.)

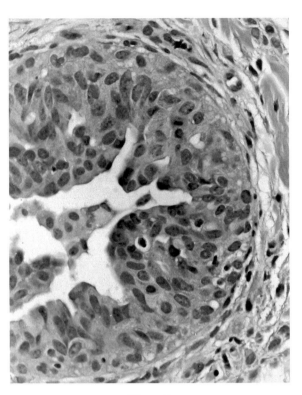

Figure 3
PREMATURE THELARCHE
Higher magnification of a duct revealing intraductal epithelial proliferation. The cells are uniform although they have prominent nuclei.

The lobular ducts are often termed *ductules* or *acini*, although the latter designation is more appropriately reserved for instances when secretory activity is manifested, as in gestation. The lactiferous ducts typically have a squamous cell lining at the nipple opening, related to the extension of the squamous epithelium of the nipple surface into the duct lumens for a short distance.

In addition to lactiferous ducts in the nipple, the small elevations present on the areola, termed *Montgomery tubercles*, are sebaceous glands, each of which is intimately associated with the terminal portion of a lactiferous duct (13). These assume importance in the development of carcinoma in heterotopic autotransplanted nipples, and also in the pathogenesis of persistent subareolar abscesses.

The intralobular connective tissue is a specialized, hormonally responsive tissue that consists of loosely arranged collagen in an acid mucopolysaccharide matrix (12), with fibroblasts, occasional lymphocytes and macrophages, but no fat. The intralobular stroma is quite vascular, in contrast to more densely collagenous, relatively hypocellular, interlobular connective tissue. The interlobular connective tissue becomes progressively fatty after the age of 18 years.

Lymph nodes, usually less than 5 mm in greatest dimension, are present in the interlobular connective tissue in approximately one fourth of breasts (6). They may be situated in any quadrant. In the tail of the breast, it is difficult to distinguish them from low axillary lymph nodes. Intramammary lymph nodes are best appreciated by mammographic examination, and they assume clinical significance by occasionally harboring metastatic carcinoma. The lining of the breast ducts characteristically is composed of two cell types: an inner layer of columnar or cuboidal glandular epithelium and an outer layer of myoepithelium. The number of cell layers of mammary ducts has been a debatable topic among anatomists, related in part to the variable appearance of the lining cells at different times of a woman's reproductive life. The myoepithelium is subtended by a basement membrane, and this, in turn, is surrounded by variable amounts of elastic tissue. While most of the duct system contains a delicate layer of elastic tissue, it is absent around lobular ducts.

Small aggregates of pigment-containing cells occasionally may be seen in the periductal connective tissue. These cells, which have been termed *ochrocytes*, occur in 15 to 20 percent of breasts. They are arranged in variable sized clusters, and possess abundant cytoplasm containing tan to dark brown pigment (4). The pigment does not stain for iron, but it is periodic acid–Schiff positive, resistant to diastase digestion, weakly acid-fast positive, and stainable by lipid dyes. Thus, it has staining properties analogous to ceroid or lipofuscin, and the cells most likely are of histiocytic origin.

After menopause the mammary gland undergoes gradual and progressive involution. This is characterized by lobular atrophy, loss of the intralobular connective tissue, and increased fat in the interlobular connective tissue. Lobular atrophy may contribute to cystic dilatation of ducts, presumably through fusion and unfolding of adjacent lobular ducts. However, in some women occasional normal-appearing lobules may be seen in old age.

Physiologic Anatomy

Menstrual Cycle. The mammary parenchyma undergoes changes during the menstrual cycle parallel to, albeit less pronounced than, comparable changes in the endometrium (7,9,17). These changes are reflected predominantly in lobular ducts and in the intralobular stroma. Thymidine-labeled index values, corresponding to proliferative activity, are proportional to changes in plasma estradiol and progesterone levels (10). Different lobules within the same breast may vary in appearance, necessitating observation of more than one lobule to assess these changes. Lobular ducts become increasingly numerous during the estrogenic phase of the cycle, resulting in an increase in lobular size. They are closely spaced and lumina often appear

to be nearly obliterated by the proliferated epithelial cells. Mitotic figures are characteristically seen in the lobular duct epithelium at this time. The intralobular stroma is compact with cellular collagenous tissue and occasional mononuclear cells.

The progestational phase of the cycle is characterized by increased lobular size, although these changes may vary in different areas of the breast (17). Terminal ducts are lined by luminal columnar cells, with underlying pale eosinophilic basal cells and vacuolated myoepithelial cells. The intralobular stroma becomes less collagenous, and appears less cellular. During the final week of the cycle apocrine-type secretion is evident in the luminal epithelial cells, usually associated with distension of the ductal lumen, and the intralobular stroma appears edematous. Mitoses, rare during the early secretory phase of the cycle, are more numerous premenstrually, and intralobular stromal edema and vascular congestion are prominent (17).

Vacuolation of myoepithelium becomes more conspicuous during the menstrual phase of the cycle. The intralobular stroma becomes compact, and contains numerous mononuclear cells. Sloughing of terminal duct epithelium may be seen, resulting in the appearance of intraluminal debris. In addition, decrease in stromal edema is associated with increasingly prominent metachromatic staining of the intralobular connective tissue, likely corresponding to an increased content of acid mucopolysaccharide.

Pregnancy. Mammary enlargement with increased firmness is one of the earliest signs of pregnancy. This is attributable to proliferation of terminal lobular ducts, resulting in lobular enlargement, progressive effacement of intralobular stroma, and compromise of interlobular stroma (fig. 4).

Secretory vacuoles appear in the lining epithelial cells in the third trimester and secretion is visible in acinar lumens. These changes progress, so that at term the breast has the characteristic lactational appearance, related to secretion in distended acini lined by cells with vacuolated cytoplasm (fig. 5). The latter cells contain cytoplasmic secretory droplets that protrude into acinar lumens resulting in a "hobnail" appearance. During lactation the microscopic appearance of different parts of the breast varies with respect

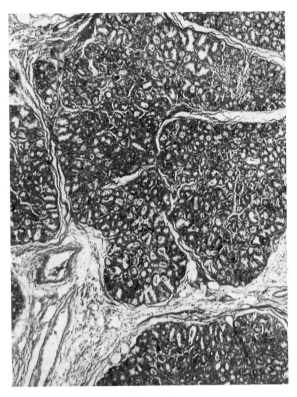

Figure 4
LACTATIONAL HYPERPLASIA
The acinar proliferation results in exclusion of intralobular connective tissue and compromise of interlobular connective tissue. The specimen is from a patient 8 months pregnant.

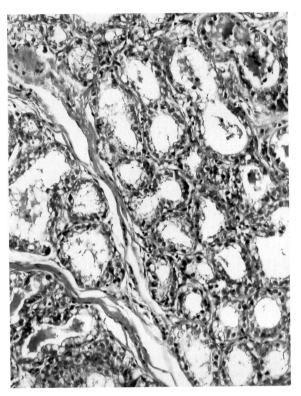

Figure 5
LACTATIONAL HYPERPLASIA
Ectatic acinar lumens are lined by vacuolated epithelium and contain secretion. Such early lactational change may occur late in the third trimester of pregnancy.

to the degree of acinar luminal ectasia, secretion, and lobular size.

With cessation of lactation the breast returns to its so-called resting state, albeit with a variable rate of lobular involution. The involutional changes are characterized by an irregular lobular contour. In contrast to their usual oval to round shape, interspersed small ductules with pyknotic cells and increased numbers of lymphocytes and plasma cells are present (2).

Secretory changes may persist in lobules for years after a pregnancy and must be distinguished from similar alterations that may be present in nonlactating, nonpregnant women (15). Pregnancy-like hyperplasia or so-called "pseudolactational" changes have been associated with hyperprolactinemia as well as phenothiazines, hormonal and antihypertensive agents, and have also been seen in male breasts (8). In most patients, there is no apparent cause.

Pregnancy-like hyperplasia is usually found in isolated lobules surrounded by glands that exhibit no secretory activity (fig. 6). The affected terminal ducts and acinar glands are dilated but contain little or no secretion. The glandular cells have abundant, pale-to-clear, faintly granular or vacuolated cytoplasm, and small darkly-stained nuclei (fig. 7). The luminal cytoplasmic border of the glandular cells tends to be frayed and small cytoplasmic blebs are typically formed. The nucleus may be extruded together with cytoplasm into the glandular lumen (fig. 8). The cells are immunoreactive for alpha-lactalbumin.

Clear cell change is another uncommon benign cytologic alteration of lobules (1). Cells in lobular glands acquire abundant clear or pale finely granular cytoplasm and eccentrically placed small nuclei (fig. 9). They have well-defined cell margins without evidence of luminal secretion or apical cytoplasmic snouts (fig. 10).

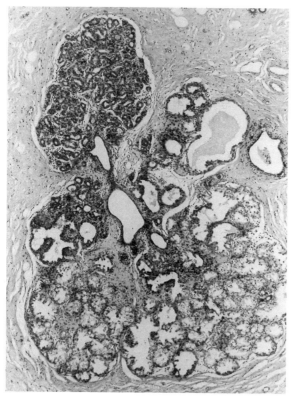

Figure 6
PREGNANCY-LIKE HYPERPLASIA
Part of the lobular complex has expanded acinar glands.
(Figures 6 and 7 are from the same patient.)

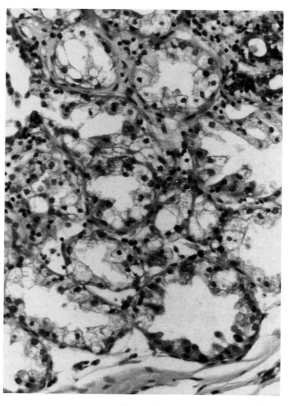

Figure 7
PREGNANCY-LIKE HYPERPLASIA
Cells lining the lobular glands have abundant pale cyto-
plasm and a tendency to form micropapillae.

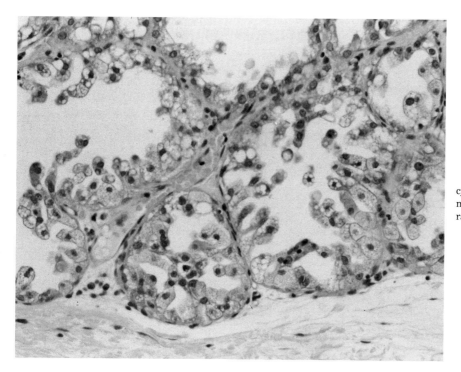

Figure 8
PREGNANCY-LIKE
HYPERPLASIA
Columnar cells with vesicular
cytoplasm and luminal cytoplasmic buds. A micropapillary arrangement of cells is evident.

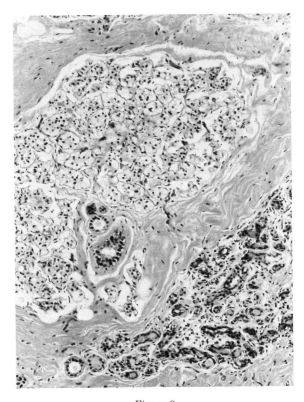

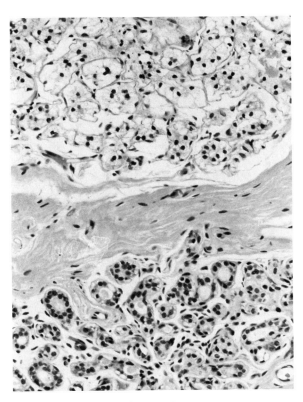

Figure 9
CLEAR CELL CHANGE
The glandular cells in the lobule above have abundant clear cytoplasm. Individual acinar units are obscured.

Figure 10
CLEAR CELL CHANGE
Unaffected lobule below for comparison with clear cell change above.

The clear cytoplasm contains diastase-sensitive PAS-positive glycogen, and the mucicarmine stain is negative. This may represent a form of metaplasia with differentiation towards eccrine sweat gland epithelium (16).

REFERENCES

1. Barwick KW, Kashgarian M, Rosen PP. "Clear-cell" change within duct and lobular epithelium of the human breast. Pathol Annu 1982;17(Pt 1):319–28.
2. Battersby S, Anderson TJ. Histological changes in breast tissue that characterize recent pregnancy. Histopathology 1989;15:415–9.
3. Bluestein DD, Wall GH. Persistent neonatal breast hypertrophy. Am J Dis Child 1963;105:292–4.
4. Davies JD. Pigmented periductal cells (ochrocytes) in mammary dysplasias: their nature and significance. J Pathol 1974;114:205–16.
5. Dossett JA. The nature of breast secretion in infancy. J Pathol Bacteriol 1960;80:93–9.
6. Egan RL, McSweeney MB. Intramammary lymph nodes. Cancer 1983;51:1838–42.
7. Fanger H, Ree HJ. Cyclic changes of human mammary gland epithelium in relation to the menstrual cycle—an ultrastructural study. Cancer 1974;34:574–85.
8. Kiaer HW, Anderson JA. Focal pregnancy-like changes in the breast. Acta Pathol Microbiol Immunol Scand [A] 1977;85:931–41.
9. Longacre TA, Bartow SA. A correlative morphologic study of human breast and endometrium in the menstrual cycle. Am J Surg Pathol 1986;10:382–93.
10. Meyer JS. Cell proliferation in normal human breast ducts, fibroadenomas, and other ductal hyperplasias measured by nuclear labeling with tritiated thymidine. Effects of menstrual phase, age, and oral contraceptive hormones. Hum Pathol 1977;8:67–81.
11. Oberman HA. Breast lesions in the adolescent female. Pathol Annu 1979;14(Pt 1):175–201.

12. Ozzello L, Speer FD. The mucopolysaccharides in the normal and diseased breast. Am J Pathol 1958;34:993–1009.
13. Smith DM, Peters TG, Donegan WL. Montgomery's areolar tubercle. Arch Pathol Lab Med 1982;106:60–3.
14. Steiner MM. Enlargement of breasts during childhood. Pediatr Clin North Am 1955;2:575–93.
15. Tavassoli FA, Yeh IT. Lactational and clear cell changes of the breast in nonlactating, nonpregnant women. Am J Clin Pathol 1987;87:23–9.
16. Vina M, Wells CA. Clear cell metaplasia of the breast: a lesion showing eccrine differentiation. Histopathology 1989;15:85–92.
17. Vogel PM, Georgiade NG, Fetter BF, Vogel FS, McCarty KS Jr. The correlation of histologic changes in the human breast with the menstrual cycle. Am J Pathol 1981;104:23–34.
18. Vorherr H. The breast: morphology, physiology and lactation. New York: Academic Press, 1974:1–19.
19. Wellings SR. Development of human breast cancer. Adv Cancer Res 1980;31:287–314.

DEVELOPMENTAL AND PHYSIOLOGIC ABNORMALITIES

APLASIA AND HYPOPLASIA

While a modest degree of asymmetry of the breasts should be considered normal, unilateral hypoplasia is an uncommon developmental occurrence, often associated with overdevelopment of the contralateral breast. Hypoplasia and aplasia may also be acquired abnormalities, often attributable to irradiation of intrathoracic or chest wall tumors in the prepubertal patient (5).

Hypoplasia should be distinguished from the less common unilateral or bilateral amastia, a congenital abnormality consisting of absence of a nipple, breast ducts, and occasionally the pectoralis major muscle (7,13). Amastia is probably a manifestation of congenital ectodermal dysplasia, based upon sex-linked recessive inheritance, whereas isolated bilateral absence of the breasts represents autosomal recessive transmission. Hypoplasia of the breast and underlying musculature may also be associated with other congenital abnormalities, especially renal malformations.

A developmental abnormality sometimes associated with mammary hypoplasia is unilateral or bilateral nipple dysplasia, resulting in rudimentary, divided, or paired nipples (12). In contrast, inverted nipples are commonplace and result from failure of the central pit of the mammary ridge to proliferate and elevate.

MACROMASTIA

Massive breast enlargement may result from an intrinsic lesion, such as a neglected or rapidly growing malignant neoplasm or, especially in adolescents, from a so-called juvenile fibroadenoma or multiple fibroadenomas. In such instances only one of the breasts is usually involved. In contrast, diffuse enlargement of both breasts, unassociated with any discernable mass, presents most often in adolescence or pregnancy (1). In both of these situations, the enlargement may be considered physiologic, representing an exaggerated response of the breast to hormonal stimulation.

Pubertal (Virginal) Macromastia

Whereas normal breast development occurs over several years until adult dimensions are reached, on occasion the breasts undergo rapid and massive enlargement. The breasts are diffusely enlarged, resulting in flattening of the nipples, and no discrete masses are palpable. Although the enlargement affects both breasts, occasionally they are markedly asymmetric. This is far less common than the occurrence of numerous fibroadenomas as a cause of massive breast enlargement in adolescents. In most instances of pubertal macromastia, the rate of enlargement slows after an initial period of rapid growth, although it usually continues during adolescence. Breast enlargement may assume remarkable dimensions (11). This was most dramatically illustrated by the case described by Durston, who in 1669 recounted a 23-year-old woman whose breasts enlarged "overnight" to a combined weight of 104 pounds (4). Since the breast enlargement will not spontaneously regress, reduction mammoplasty is usually necessary. However, residual breast tissue may continue to enlarge, possibly occasioning the need for additional surgical intervention.

Microscopically, the cardinal feature is the abundance of connective tissue separating mammary ducts (fig. 11) (10). This tissue may be hyalinized or loosely arranged fibrous connective tissue or fat. The duct epithelium may be hyperplastic, although this often is only a focal finding. Lobules usually are poorly developed, and, on occasion, not evident, resulting in microscopic simulation of gynecomastia.

Pregnancy

Massive gestational enlargement of the breast is exceedingly rare. Reviews have noted incidences varying from 1 in 28,000 pregnancies to 1 in 100,000 pregnancies. The breast enlargement commences early in pregnancy, often at the time of, or before, the first missed menstrual period. On occasion the accelerated growth occurs in

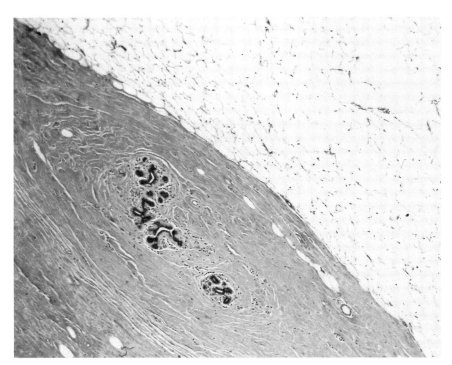

Figure 11
PUBERTAL MACROMASTIA
Massive bilateral enlargement of breasts in a 15-year-old girl. Dense connective tissue surrounds ducts. Note paucity of lobule development.

breasts that previously manifested untoward enlargement prior to the pregnancy. The breasts rapidly grow to extraordinary dimensions, becoming erythematous, edematous, and painful; the overlying skin may ulcerate. To avoid further incapacitating enlargement, lactation is usually suppressed in these patients. Hypercalcemia accompanying this abnormality has been reported, with remission after mastectomy (14).

Postpartum involution is often insufficient to preclude the need for reduction mammoplasty. Patients who have had subsequent pregnancies almost always experience recurrence of this abnormality, even when the pregnancy has terminated in abortion (8). This was exemplified by massive breast growth during pregnancy in a patient who had subcutaneous mastectomy for unrelenting breast enlargement during a previous pregnancy (2).

The microscopic findings in these breasts are far less dramatic than their clinical appearance. Lobular enlargement attributable to the pregnancy is present, as is abundant periductal connective tissue. The latter may be hyalinized or loose and edematous.

ECTOPIC BREAST

Supernumerary Breast

Supernumerary breasts arise from ectopic breast tissue along the milk lines which extend bilaterally from the midaxillae through the normal breasts inferiorly to the medial groin and vulva (3). The embryologic anlage of the milk line is the milk ridge. Supernumerary breasts develop from portions of the milk ridges that fail to atrophy.

Clinically, supernumerary breasts are seen in 1 to 6 percent of adult women and much less often in men (3,6). The majority of patients with clinically evident supernumerary breasts have unilateral axillary breast tissue. In most instances, only the nipple is evident (polythelia), but an areola and underlying mammary ducts may also be present (polymastia).

Supernumerary breast tissue is subject to the changes that occur in the breast with hormonal stimulation, as in pregnancy and lactation. In one report, bilateral vulvar ectopic breast tissue underwent massive enlargement during pregnancy and a postpartum vulvectomy was necessary (9). Another patient had large lactating adenomas excised from the labia majora during the seventh and ninth months of pregnancy (8).

Aberrant Breast

Aberrant breast tissue is defined as mammary glandular parenchyma found beyond the usual anatomic extent of the breast or the milk line.

Aberrant breast tissue does not form a nipple or areola, and is rarely clinically apparent unless it becomes the site of a pathologic process. Ducts and lobules in aberrant breast tissue are structurally normal and histologically indistinguishable from peripheral extensions of the breast.

REFERENCES

1. Beischer NA, Hueston JH, Pepperell RJ. Massive hypertrophy of the breasts in pregnancy: report of 3 cases and review of the literature. Obstet Gynecol Surv 1989; 44:234–43.
2. Boyce SW, Hoffman PG Jr, Mathes SJ. Recurrent macromastia after subcutaneous mastectomy. Ann Plast Surg 1984;13:511–8.
3. De Cholnoky T. Supernumerary breast. Arch Surg 1939;39:926–41.
4. Deaver JB, McFarland J. The breast: its anomalies, its diseases and their treatment. Philadelphia: P. Blaskiston's Son & Co, 1917:111.
5. Furst CJ, Lundell M, Ahlback SO, Holm LE. Breast hypoplasia following irradiation of the female breast in infancy and early childhood. Acta Oncol 1989;28:519–23.
6. Iwai T. A statistical study of the polymastia of the Japanese. Lancet 1907;2:753–9.
7. Kowlessar M, Orti E. Complete breast absence in siblings. Am J Dis Child 1968;115:91–2.
8. Leis SN, Palmer B, Ostberg G. Gravid macromastia. Case report. Scand J Plast Reconstr Surg 1974;8:247–9.
9. Levin N, Diener RL. Bilateral ectopic breast of the vulva. Report of a case. Obstet Gynecol 1968;32:274–6.
10. O'Hara MF, Page DL. Adenomas of the breast and ectopic breast under lactational influences. Hum Pathol 1985;16:707–12.
11. Oberman HA. Breast lesions in the adolescent female. Pathol Annu 1979;14(Pt 1):175–201.
12. Rintala A, Norio R. Familial intra-areolar polythelia with mammary hypoplasia. Scand J Plast Reconstr Surg 1982;16:287–91.
13. Trier WC. Complete breast absence. Case report and review of the literature. Plast Reconstr Surg 1965;36:430–9.
14. Van Heerden JA, Gharib H. Pseudohyperparathyroidism secondary to gigantic mammary hypertrophy. Arch Surg 1988;123:80–2.

INFLAMMATORY AND REACTIVE CONDITIONS

FAT NECROSIS

Fat necrosis of the breast assumes importance because it can simulate carcinoma both clinically and mammographically. While a history of antecedent trauma may be obtained, fat necrosis more commonly results from prior surgical intervention or radiation therapy (2). Following breast-conserving treatment of carcinoma, it may be indistinguishable clinically and mammographically from recurrent carcinoma (1).

The lesion excised early in the course of its evolution contains histiocytes with foamy cytoplasm, as well as larger lipid-filled cysts and occasional multinucleated giant cells. An infiltrate of chronic inflammatory cells, including lymphocytes, plasma cells, and eosinophils is present. As the process evolves, the lesion be-comes surrounded by dense fibrosis with progressive encapsulation of the abnormal area. Foci of calcification at the periphery may be prominent. This end-stage finding can result in a characteristic appearance resembling an egg shell on mammography (fig. 12) (2). However, the earlier lesion causes fibrous retraction of adjacent tissues toward the area of involvement, resulting in an irregular spiculated mass which simulates carcinoma (4).

An unusual variant may present in long-standing posttraumatic fat necrosis with focal or extensive squamous metaplasia (fig. 13) (3). The metaplastic foci involve ducts surrounded by a chronic inflammatory reaction. The compressed or distorted islands of squamous metaplasia may simulate invasive neoplasm; however, there is no evidence of intraductal or invasive ductal carcinoma

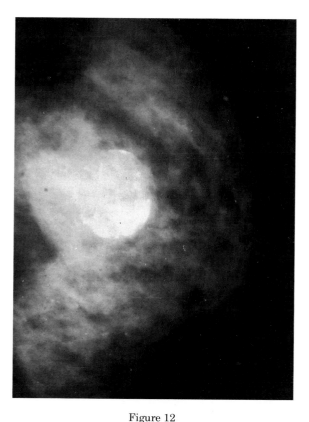

Figure 12
FAT NECROSIS
Peripheral calcification around an area of fat necrosis resulting in mammographic circumscription.

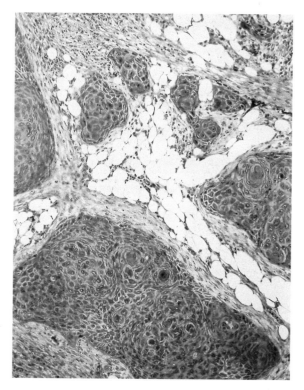

Figure 13
FAT NECROSIS
Nodules of squamous metaplastic epithelium in an area of fat necrosis. The epithelium is well differentiated and keratin whorls are present.

and the squamous cell component, although irregular in configuration, is well differentiated.

HEMORRHAGIC NECROSIS WITH COAGULOPATHY

Extensive hemorrhagic necrosis of the breast may occur shortly after initiation of warfarin treatment. Within a few days after administration of the drug, the patient develops pain and edema of the breast, followed by hemorrhage into the skin and necrosis of underlying tissue. Mastectomy is usually required, and the resulting specimen reveals widespread necrosis of breast tissue associated with multiple thrombi in small blood vessels (5).

This syndrome is attributable to the effect of warfarin in patients with heterozygous protein C deficiency. Warfarin paradoxically initiates thrombosis in capillaries of the skin and subcutaneum, especially in areas of excessive fat, such as the breasts and thighs (6), it reduces the synthesis of the vitamin K–dependent procoagulant factors, and also interferes with the synthesis of vitamin K–dependent inhibitors of coagulation, such as protein C and protein S. Therefore, in contrast to the effect of warfarin in the normal individual, in the patient who already has reduced levels of protein C there is greater reduction in anticoagulant effect than the procoagulant activity, thereby tipping the balance to thrombosis instead of anticoagulation.

LESIONS ASSOCIATED WITH BREAST AUGMENTATION

Women have long sought to augment their breast size through the introduction of foreign materials. Unfortunately, in most instances, these efforts produce only transient improvement and ultimately result in a disfiguring foreign body reaction. The agents utilized in the past have included shellac, glazier's putty, spun glass, epoxy resin, beeswax, and shredded silk (9). Paraffin wax, which enjoyed transient popularity for this purpose, had the unfortunate proclivity to result in oleogranulomas and also to migrate on the chest wall.

One of the first clinical uses of silicones was for injection into the breast for augmentation purposes. Liquid dimethylpolysiloxane, which was widely used in the Orient, is relatively inert;

however, to prevent its migration from the injection site, it was modified by adding fatty acids or vegetable oils to induce fibrosis and limit spread. Unfortunately, this also occasioned granuloma formation, resulting in painful hard lumps in the breast and draining sinus tracts. These complications have discredited the use of injectable silicone for breast augmentation. Microscopically, the injected silicone forms round, doubly refractile sheets in spaces surrounded by histiocytes. Phagocytized refractile, frequently pigmented granules and crystals, representing the supplemental adulterant are often present (figs. 14, 15) (8).

Currently, augmentation mammoplasty involves the placement of an implant consisting of a thin-walled silicone bag containing saline, liquid silicone, or silicone gel usually beneath the pectoral musculature. Formation of a fibrous envelope around the implant, a so-called capsule,

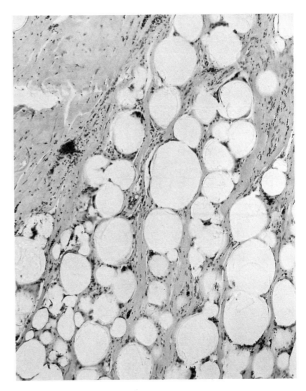

Figure 14
INJECTED SILICONE
This patient received bilateral silicone injections into her breasts 20 years earlier for augmentation purposes. Nodularity has resulted from fibrosis surrounding the silicone and foreign material engulfed by foreign body giant cells. (Figures 14 and 15 are from the same patient.)

with resultant contracture of the prosthesis is an occasional complication, even in the absence of identifiable rupture of the implant (fig. 16) (7). This produces undesirable firmness of the implant and visible distortion of the breast, and may necessitate reoperation. Polyurethane implants have also been utilized. Adjacent tissue may undergo fibrosis; the doubly-refractile crystalline material within foreign body giant cells has a triangular shape, in contrast to the round or ovoid appearance of silicone (fig. 17).

The capsulectomy specimen from such procedures consists of abundant mature scar tissue with mononuclear cells, histiocytes, and foreign body giant cells. Vacuolated spaces containing foreign material, presumably silicone, are present in the dense connective tissue. This may relate to the permeability of the silicone bag to molecules of dimethylpolysiloxane or to shedding of silicone from the surface of the implant (8).

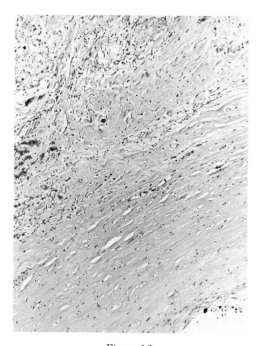

Figure 16
SILICONE IMPLANT
Dense fibrosis with adjacent chronic inflammatory cells produced a capsule surrounding a silicone implant.

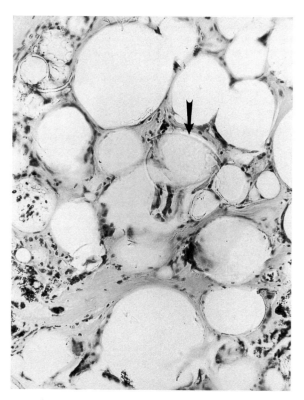

Figure 15
INJECTED SILICONE
Globules of doubly-refractile silicone (arrow) are evident on higher magnification.

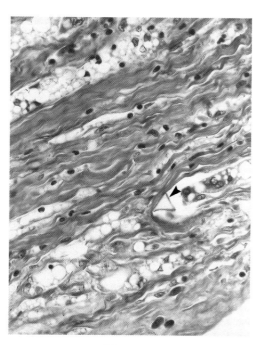

Figure 17
POLYURETHANE IMPLANT
This patient received a polyurethane implant 2 years earlier, following removal of a capsule resulting from a silicone implant. The triangular foreign material (arrow) is related to the polyurethane, while the round globules likely are from the silicone.

On occasion, the axillary lymph nodes contain variably sized vacuoles, either in histiocytes or extracellularly, often surrounded by multinucleated giant cells (10). These vacuoles contain refractile material consistent with silicone. Silicone lymphadenopathy can occur in association with either injection of liquid silicone or silicone implants. This abnormality is usually an incidental finding, lacking clinical significance; however, in some cases, usually associated with injection of silicone or rupture of the prosthesis, it results in lymph node enlargement.

INFLAMMATORY LESIONS IN PREGNANCY AND LACTATION

Puerperal mastitis develops during the early stages of lactation in as many as 5 percent of women (11). It occurs most often in the second and third weeks of lactation, although it may be evident only after the first month. Stasis of milk in distended ducts provides an environment conducive to the growth of bacteria, especially staphylococci.

The usual sequela of mastitis is abscess formation; however, prompt treatment of the mastitis usually prevents this complication. Since management centers on administration of antibiotics, and possibly incision and drainage, the pathologist rarely receives biopsy material from such patients. The fibrosis and associated inflammatory reaction related to a chronic abscess results in distortion of adjacent ducts, and may produce a mass that clinically simulates a neoplasm.

INFARCTS

Although uncommon, infarction of breast lesions may cause clinical and microscopic confusion with carcinoma. Circumscribed areas of coagulation necrosis usually occur in intraductal papillomas or as a complication of pregnancy or lactation. Infarction in fibroadenomas and cystosarcomas is uncommon.

Infarcts of papillomas are usually incidental pathologic findings that rarely result in unique clinical signs. In most instances, only part of the papilloma is involved (12). Infarcted gestational breast tissue produces a painful mass. During pregnancy, the infarct may become quite large because of involvement of confluent hyperplastic lobules or of lactational adenomas (figs. 18, 19).

These adenomas may occur during pregnancy or early in the postpartum period. Infarction is most often an incidental finding since it usually involves only part of the tumor (13), but may occur in more than one fibroadenoma in a given breast.

Infarcts may be confused with carcinoma, especially in intraductal papillomas (15). This is due to inflammation and distortion of ducts at the margin of the infarct, as well as to the occasional presence of squamous metaplasia, more common in infarcted papillomas than in infarction of gestational breast tissue. In addition, enlargement of regional lymph nodes, associated with large lesions, may increase the clinical suspicion of carcinoma.

The pathogenesis of this abnormality is uncertain. Only rarely is thrombotic occlusion of blood vessels evident in these lesions, and it is equally likely that the thrombi are a result of, rather than a cause of, the infarct (14,16).

Figure 18
MAMMARY INFARCT
Infarcted breast tissue (in the lower right corner) is separated by fibrosis from adenomatous tissue with residual lactational change. The mass was removed 2 weeks postpartum. (Figures 18 and 19 are from the same patient.)

NONSPECIFIC INFLAMMATORY LESIONS

Granulomatous Lobular Mastitis

The term *granulomatous mastitis* has come to be associated with a relatively distinct clinicopathologic condition (23,25,28). Going et al. (25) recommended the term *granulomatous lobular mastitis* to separate the lesion from granulomatous forms of periductal mastitis. The alternative diagnosis of postlactational granulomatous mastitis is less satisfactory since the lesion may develop as long as 15 years postpartum (18,22,25).

The etiology of granulomatous lobular mastitis is unknown. The perilobular distribution and granulomatous character of the inflammation suggest a cell-mediated reaction to one or more substances concentrated in the mammary secretion or lobular cells, but no specific antigen has been identified.

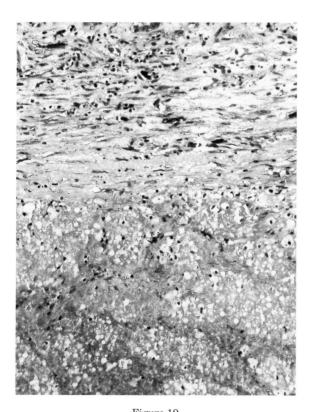

Figure 19
MAMMARY INFARCT
Outlines of ductules are evident in the infarcted tissue.

Clinical Presentation. The lesion usually appears after, rather than during, pregnancy. The mean interval between pregnancy and diagnosis is 2 years. An increased incidence has been reported in women using oral contraceptives (22,30).

The age at diagnosis ranges from 17 to 42 years, with a mean of about 33 years (25). Virtually all patients are parous. They typically present with a distinct, firm to hard mass in any peripheral part of the breast, generally sparing the subareolar region. Bilateral involvement is uncommon (18). The tumors measure up to 8 cm, averaging nearly 6 cm. The clinical findings often suggest carcinoma and mammography has been described as "suspicious" (18,24).

Gross Findings. The specimen typically consists of firm to hard mammary parenchyma containing a distinct mass with a faintly nodular architecture. In some cases, the nodules appear to be small foci of abscess formation. Confluent abscesses are not a characteristic feature.

Microscopic Findings. The primary pathologic change is a granulomatous inflammatory reaction centered on lobules, granulomatous lobulitis (fig. 20). Granulomas composed of epithelioid histiocytes, Langhans giant cells accompanied by lymphocytes, plasma cells, and occasional eosinophils are found within and around lobules. Asteroid bodies are extremely unusual and Schaumann bodies have not been reported in the giant cells. Fat necrosis and abscesses containing polymorphonuclear leucocytes are sometimes present. In the most severe cases, confluent granulomas may obscure or obliterate the lobulocentric distribution of the process, particularly toward the central portion of the tumor. Ducts incorporated in the lesion may become dilated and exhibit periductal or intraductal inflammation, but usually this is relatively inconspicuous. Squamous metaplasia of duct and lobular epithelium is unusual. Stains and cultures for bacteria, acid-fast organisms and fungi are typically negative.

Prognosis and Treatment. In most patients the disease is self-limiting and controlled by a single excisional biopsy. Antibiotics may be helpful, especially if secondary infection occurs. Sarcoidosis and tuberculosis should be considered in the differential diagnosis.

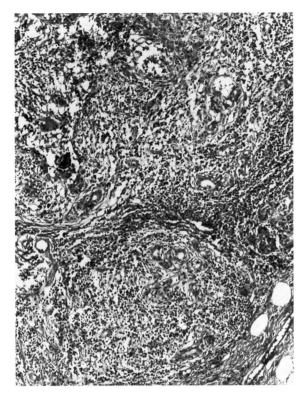

Figure 20
GRANULOMATOUS LOBULAR MASTITIS
Inflammatory reaction in lobules with multinucleated giant cells.

Mammary Duct Ectasia

The term mammary duct ectasia was introduced in 1951 (26). The etiology of this condition is not known. Some authors believe that duct dilatation caused by glandular atrophy and involution in older women is the primary pathologic process, leading to stasis of secretion in ducts followed by leakage of lipid material eliciting periductal inflammation. Others suggest that periductal inflammation resulting from duct obstruction is the underlying abnormality responsible for duct sclerosis, obliteration, and ectasia (20,32).

Duct ectasia, galactorrhea, and lipogranulomatous mastitis have been associated with prolonged phenothiazine treatment (27), a well-documented cause of hyperprolactinemia. However, galactorrhea and lactational hyperplasia do not ordinarily precede the development of duct ectasia.

Clinical Presentation. The earliest symptom is spontaneous, intermittent nipple discharge.

There may be no palpable abnormality. The discharge gives a positive test for blood in about 50 percent of cases. In more advanced cases, subareolar induration progresses to the formation of a mass that may suggest carcinoma clinically. Pain is usually an early symptom in young women while nipple inversion or retraction is often seen at a later age (33). Inversion is generally associated with periductal fibrosis and contracture.

Duct ectasia has been found in women younger than 30 (36) and over 80 years of age but rarely in men (34). The median age in one series of 34 patients was 44 years (36).

Gross Findings. At operation, dilated ducts contain pasty or granular secretion. Calcification is sometimes apparent grossly in the dilated ducts. Abscess-like yellow necrotic areas can be found in the most severe cases.

Microscopic Findings. The ducts contain eosinophilic granular or amorphous proteinaceous material (figs. 21, 22). Usually, there is an admixture of lipid-containing foam cells (so-called colostrum cells) and desquamated duct epithelial cells. Histiocytes in and around the ducts that contain ceroid pigment were termed ochrocytes by Davies (21) (see p. 13). Cholesterol crystals and calcifications may be found in the intraductal debris and in fat necrosis.

Inflammation that features lymphocytes with fewer plasma cells, neutrophils, and histiocytes is present circumferentially throughout the thickness of the duct and in the periductal stroma (fig. 23). Periductal fibrosis and hyperelastosis, often with a lamellar distribution, lead to mural thickening. The duct epithelium is atrophic, flat, and inconspicuous. Epithelial hyperplasia is not a feature of duct ectasia but may be found as a component of coincidental proliferative breast changes. Squamous metaplasia in the lactiferous ducts within the nipple is a factor contributing to duct obstruction and stasis in some cases (figs. 24, 25).

In a later phase, the inflammatory reaction is less conspicuous but the ducts are encased in a thick laminated layer of hyaline fibrous and elastic tissue (20). The duct lumen may be patulous but in some instances the sclerotic process composed of granulation tissue and hyperelastosis narrows or totally occludes the ducts (fig. 26) (19). This has been termed *mastitis obliterans* (32). Remnants of persisting epithelium may

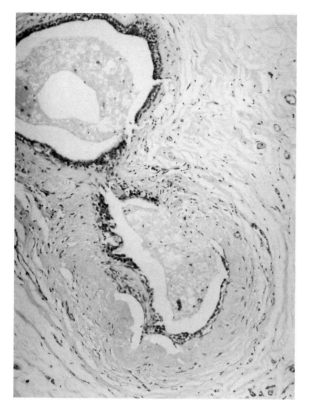

Figure 21
DUCT ECTASIA
Dilated ducts contain sparsely cellular secretion. Lower duct is partially disrupted, releasing stasis material into stroma. This has elicited periductal fibrosis and elastosis.

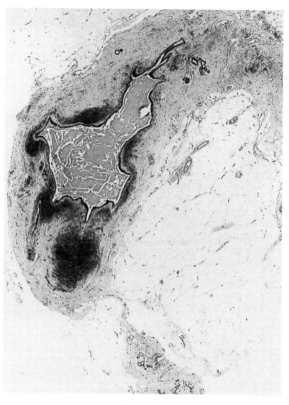

Figure 22
DUCT ECTASIA
Dilated duct containing amorphous stasis material with several lymphoid nodules that tend to form where secondary ducts branch from the main duct. (Figures 22 and 23 are from the same patient.)

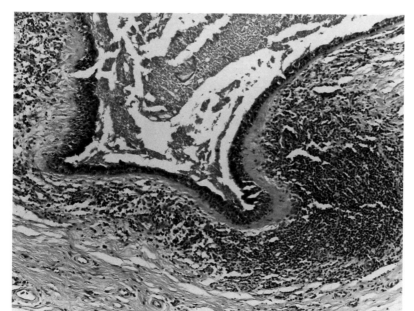

Figure 23
DUCT ECTASIA
In addition to the periductal lymphocytic reaction, noteworthy features are thickened basement membrane and virtual absence of cells in duct contents.

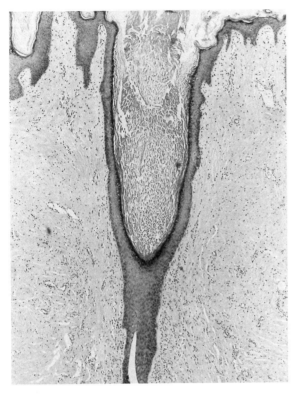

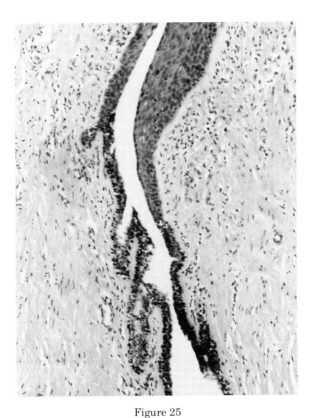

Figure 24

SQUAMOUS METAPLASIA OF LACTIFEROUS DUCT

Plug of keratin debris fills the orifice of a lactiferous duct. Metaplastic squamous epithelium extends into the duct. (Figures 24 and 25 are from the same patient.)

Figure 25

SQUAMOUS METAPLASIA OF LACTIFEROUS DUCT

Proximal extent of squamous metaplasia in duct shown in fig. 24. Note the resultant displacement of the squamo-columnar junction, mild periductal lymphocytic reaction, and beginning of duct dilatation at the lower margin of the photograph.

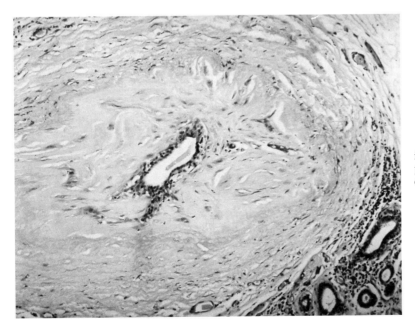

Figure 26

DUCT ECTASIA

The duct lumen is almost obliterated in this late stage lesion characterized by periductal accumulation of collagen and elastic tissue.

proliferate to form secondary glands within the sclerotic duct creating a pattern that resembles a recanalized, healed thrombus in a blood vessel. When the epithelium is totally absent, the duct is reduced to a fibrous scar.

Treatment and Prognosis. The diagnosis of duct ectasia is suggested by symptoms, clinical findings, and mammography, but these are not sufficiently specific to exclude carcinoma in all cases. Consequently, the diagnosis is usually made by excising the affected area. Duct ectasia is not a precancerous condition.

Plasma Cell Mastitis

Ewing is credited with suggesting the term plasma cell mastitis to distinguish a lesion with a very prominent plasma cell component from other forms of mastitis (17). Many authors consider plasma cell mastitis to be a variant of periductal mastitis or mammary duct ectasia (35,37).

Clinical Presentation. Adair (17) described 10 patients with plasma cell mastitis, 29 to 44 years old (average 36 years) all of whom had been pregnant. The average interval between cessation of lactation and the onset of symptoms was 4 years. Patients experienced acute onset of pain, tenderness, redness, and nipple discharge consisting usually of thick secretion.

After the inflammatory symptoms subside, a firm to hard mass of several centimeters remains. Nipple discharge usually persists and nipple retraction is observed in the majority of patients. The mass may be in the periphery of the breast or in a subareolar location. Axillary lymph nodes are often enlarged.

Gross Findings. The indurated affected area has dilated ducts containing thick creamy secretion. Some of the affected ducts appear cystic. Punctate yellow or golden areas of xanthomatous granuloma may be observed.

Microscopic Findings. Two features which distinguish plasma cell mastitis from other forms of mastitis are hyperplasia of ductal epithelium and a marked, diffuse plasma cell infiltrate surrounding ducts and lobules (fig. 27). A histiocytic and sometimes granulomatous reaction to desquamated epithelium and lipid material in the ducts is responsible for areas that appear to be xanthomatous grossly and for the comedo-like character of the duct contents (37).

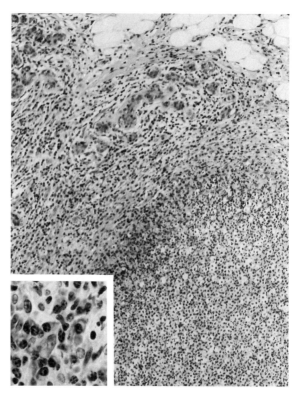

Figure 27
PLASMA CELL MASTITIS
An area of necrosis containing macrophages and plasma cells on the right is surrounded by a lymphoplasmacytic infiltrate. The epithelium and wall of the duct at this site have been obliterated by the inflammatory process. Inset shows plasma cells.

Periductal fibrosis and obliterative proliferation of granulation tissue are not features of plasma cell mastitis.

Prognosis and Treatment. In its acute and mature phases plasma cell mastitis is difficult to distinguish clinically from mammary carcinoma (17,29,31). Fine-needle aspiration biopsy yields a specimen consisting of inflammatory cells in which plasma cells and histiocytes are especially conspicuous. Hyperplastic epithelial cells that may appear typical should not be mistaken for carcinoma.

Excisional biopsy is recommended since cutaneous ulceration and fistulas may develop after the lesion has been incised or only partially removed. Generally, the residual mass is excised after the acute phase has subsided. The acute stage occasionally resolves without a persistent tumor.

SPECIFIC INFECTIONS

Tuberculosis

As tuberculosis has come under better medical control in many parts of the world, infection of the breast is mentioned less frequently as a clinical problem in developed countries (53) but it remains a serious condition in less developed regions. The breast may be unusually resistant to tuberculous infection since mammary lesions were infrequent or absent at autopsy of women who died of tuberculosis (65).

Clinical Presentation. Tuberculous mastitis seems to have a predilection for the lactating breast (38,73), but it may affect the adult female breast at any age and occurs rarely in the male breast as well (64). In younger patients the lesion is more likely to have signs and symptoms of an abscess while in older women tuberculous infection tends to cause a mass that simulates carcinoma. Unilateral tuberculous mastitis is much more common than involvement of both breasts (63).

Infection of the breast may be the primary manifestation of tuberculosis but it is thought that the breasts are infected secondarily in most patients even when the presumed primary focus remains clinically inapparent. The majority of patients also have ipsilateral axillary granulomatous lymphadenitis. Innoculation via the lactiferous ducts, which are particularly dilated during lactation, may account for some pregnancy-associated infections.

The disease has three patterns of clinical presentation (52). The most common form is *nodular mastitis* in which the patient develops a slowly growing, solitary, painless mass with the mammographic appearance of carcinoma (38,51,64, 73). Advanced nodular lesions fixed to the skin may develop draining sinuses. *Diffuse tuberculous mastitis* is characterized by the acute development of multiple painful nodules throughout the breast producing a pattern that can be mistaken for inflammatory carcinoma clinically and mammographically (73). The third or *sclerosing variety* of infection occurs predominantly in elderly women resulting in induration of the breast and in diffuse increased density on mammography (73).

Gross Findings. The specimen consists of nodular, indurated, grey or tan tissue with yellow to white foci of caseous necrosis. Confluent nodular lesions with central necrotic cavitation grossly resemble necrotic carcinoma or a suppurative abscess.

Microscopic Findings. Granulomatous lesions in tuberculous mastitis feature caseous necrosis. In chronic cases fibrosis may be prominent. The granulomas tend to be associated with ducts more than with lobules (figs. 28, 29). Acid-fast bacteria are not detected histologically in most cases (38,52). The diagnosis of granulomatous infection of the breast may be suggested by the findings in a fine-needle aspirate (66,77). Cytologic examination of nipple discharge shows a nonspecific mixture of foamy histiocytes, neutrophils, and necrotic debris.

Treatment and Prognosis. Mastectomy may be necessary for advanced lesions with extensive sinus formation but most patients respond to antibiotic management after excisional biopsy (38,47). Failure to control the lesion has been reported in a few patients who received antibiotic therapy without excision of the lesion (54,66).

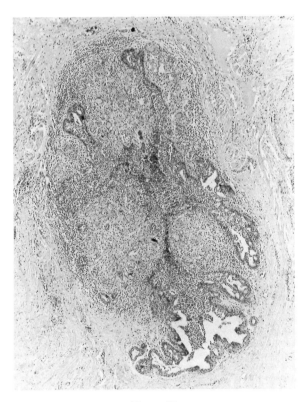

Figure 28
TUBERCULOUS MASTITIS
Granulomatous inflammation of a major lactiferous duct with necrosis of epithelium.

Fungal Infections

Clinically apparent mycotic infections of the breast are uncommon.

Actinomycosis. Infection is usually via the nipple. *Actinomyces bovis* was identified in one case (72). Sinus tracts may develop following incision and drainage or with progression of the untreated lesion. In advanced cases, the infection can extend into the chest wall (69).

The histologic diagnosis is made by demonstrating Gram-positive organisms as filaments or colonies (sulphur granules) in tissue sections or sinus tract drainage. Treatment with penicillin has reportedly been effective (1) but recurrent or advanced infections may require mastectomy.

Histoplasmosis. There have been rare instances of localized mammary *Histoplasma capsulatum* infection (68,70). All were in women 21, 34, and 35 years of age. Each patient presented with a single, unilateral mass. Clinical evaluation in two cases failed to demonstrate

evidence of systemic *H. capsulatum* infection and one patient had an elevated complement fixation test. The excised tumors proved to be multinodular abscesses up to 3 cm in diameter that consisted of confluent necrotizing granulomas in which *H. capsulatum* was demonstrated by a methenamine silver reaction. No organism was isolated in culture from two cases (68).

Blastomycosis. A 4 cm unilateral breast abscess that contained organisms histologically consistent with *Blastomyces dermatitidis* was excised from the para-areolar region of a 30-year-old woman. She had no other evidence of infection and remained well 8 years later (70).

Cryptococcosis. Two instances of cryptococcal mastitis have been described (70,72). One was diagnosed at autopsy. The other patient underwent mastectomy for a mistaken diagnosis of mucinous mammary carcinoma (72).

Parasitic Infections

Filariasis. Mammary filariasis, caused most frequently by *Wuchereria bancrofti,* has been reported from regions where infection with this organism is endemic (45,71). Involvement of the breast occurs in the chronic phase of infection as late as 6 years after last exposure (62). Microfilariae have been found in nipple secretions suggesting that communication may become established between ducts and dilated, ruptured lymphatics (lymphovarix) (58).

The patient usually presents with one or more nontender, painless unilateral masses that may be fixed to the skin and resemble carcinoma. Axillary node enlargement caused by filarial lymphadenitis further complicates the differential diagnosis. Mammary filariasis may occur coincidentally in patients whose primary breast lesion is carcinoma (71).

The majority of the tumors measure 1 to 3 cm and are composed of firm, grey or white tissue that merges with the breast parenchyma. Rarely, thread-like white worms are evident grossly in the lesion (45).

Microscopic examination typically reveals adult filarial worms which may be well preserved or in varying stages of degeneration (fig. 30). The inflammatory reaction is largely granulomatous with the formation of eosinophilic abscesses. Rarely, granulomatous lesions in the

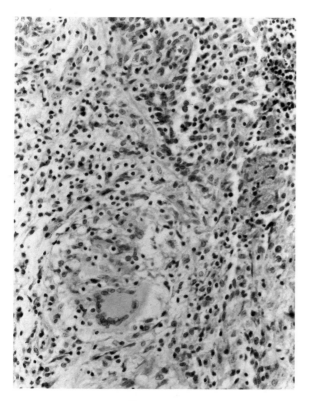

Figure 29
TUBERCULOUS MASTITIS
Langhans-type giant cell and granulomatous inflammation adjacent to necrosis in duct (upper right corner).

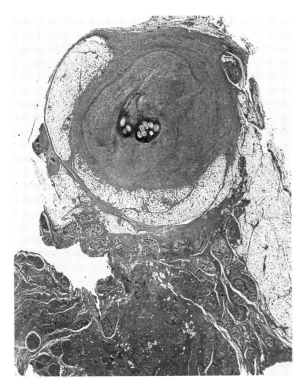

Figure 30
FILARIASIS
Cross sections of the gravid female worm of *W. bancrofti* are evident in exudate that fills the abscess, enclosed in a fibrotic reaction. (Courtesy of Dr. R.C. Neafie and the AFIP.)

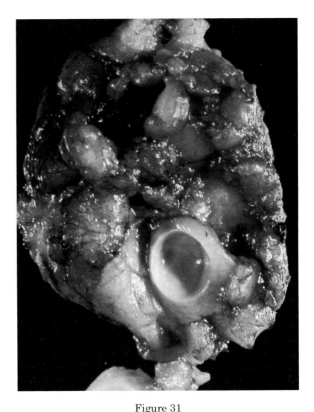

Figure 31
CYSTICERCOSIS
Cyst of *T. solium* in a breast biopsy. (Courtesy of Drs. J.W. Searle and J. Sullivan, Brisbane, Australia.)

breast contain only microfilariae (45,71). Fully degenerated worms are likely to become calcified. Adult worms and microfilariae may also be found in axillary lymph nodes (45).

Zoonotic filarial infections of the breast are much less common than those caused by *W. bancrofti*; most have been reported from North America, Europe, and Asia (39,42,49). Mammary dirofilariasis is usually caused by *Dirofilaria repens* (42), which ordinarily infects cats and dogs, but infestation by *D. tenuis*, which primarily infects raccoons, has been reported (49). The lesions tend to be superficial rather than deeply embedded in the breast parenchyma.

Other Parasites. Infection of the breast by *Schistosoma japonicum* has been reported (76). Mammary coenurosis and cysticercosis, infections caused by the larval stages of tape worms, have been described. Coenurosis results from infestation by tape worms related to the *Taenia* sp. responsible for cysticercosis (41,57); mam-

mary cysticercosis is caused by *T. solium* (fig. 31) (56,60). Mammographically detected calcifications attributed to infection with *Loa loa* were described as having a spiral or vermiform configuration (44,67). Calcifications in the pectoral muscles seen mammographically have been due to infection by *Trichinella* (55).

Miscellaneous Infections

Typhoid Mastitis. Few cases of typhoid mastitis have been reported (40,43). Histologically, the tissue exhibits non-necrotizing granulomatous inflammation with no detectable bacteria.

Cat Scratch Disease. Granulomatous lesions of cat scratch disease were found in intramammary lymph nodes in four women 25 to 56 years of age with 1 to 3 cm tumors in the axillary tail of the breast (59). Microscopic examination of the excised tumors revealed necrotizing granulomas with filamentous and branching Gram-negative Warthin-Starr–positive bacilli in the necrotic centers.

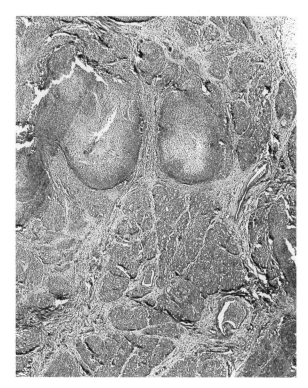

Figure 32
STAPHYLOCOCCAL ABSCESS
Sharply demarcated abscesses contain suppurative inflammation. Clusters of bacteria are present in the central abscess.

Breast Abscess. Lactational mastitis and abscess formation develop as a result of obstruction to flow in one or more major lactiferous ducts. The initial phases of stasis and mastitis are usually sterile. Bacteria isolated from nipple discharge are often skin inhabitants such as streptococci, *Staphylococcus aureus*, and coagulase-negative staphylococci (74). Surgically removed specimens show a mixed acute and chronic inflammatory reaction that may include fat necrosis (fig. 32).

Subareolar Abscess. Nonlactating premenopausal women often experience repeated episodes of subareolar abscess formation. The abscesses evolve slowly, eventually draining through periareolar sinus tracts or mammillary fistulas (48). Subareolar abscesses are usually the result of duct obstruction caused by squamous metaplasia in the terminal portion of one or more lactiferous ducts (50). The nipple discharge that typically occurs when there is duct obstruction due to a papilloma is usually absent

here. Excision of the affected duct, sinus tract, and abscess is successful in most cases (75).

SARCOIDOSIS

Clinical Presentation. Sarcoidosis may present as a primary breast tumor accompanied by lymph node enlargement (80,81), but most mammary lesions are detected after diagnosis of the common clinical manifestations of the disease. Women tend to be in their 20s and 30s. The breast lesion is a firm to hard mass that may be mistaken clinically for carcinoma (83).

Gross Findings. The excised specimen consists of firm to hard, tan tissue. Calcification and necrosis are not features of mammary sarcoidosis. Tumors up to 5 cm in diameter have been reported.

Microscopic Findings. Histologic examination reveals epithelioid granulomas forming nodules among lobules and ducts (fig. 33). Multinucleated giant cells that accompany the granulomas may contain asteroid or Schaumann bodies. Traces of fibrinoid necrosis are found in cellular lesions. A lymphoplasmacytic reaction and fibrosis occur to varying degrees. Small, isolated granulomas with a sparse lymphocytic reaction can be found widely distributed in breast tissue that appears grossly to be unaffected.

The differential diagnosis of granulomatous mastitis includes nonspecific granulomatous mastitis, granulomatous angiopanniculitis of the breast (87), and specific granulomatous infections. Lesions caused by miliary tuberculosis may lack caseous necrosis.

Non-necrotizing sarcoid-like granulomatous inflammation can develop in breast carcinomas and in axillary lymph nodes of patients who have no clinical evidence of sarcoidosis (78,82,86). Bässler and Birke (78) reported sarcoid-like granulomas in axillary lymph nodes from 0.7 percent of patients with breast carcinoma and in the stroma of 0.3 percent of mammary carcinomas. Histologically, it may be difficult to distinguish carcinoma-associated sarcoid-like reactions from coexistent carcinoma in a patient with sarcoidosis (figs. 34, 35) (84,85,86). Little or no fibrosis is seen in carcinoma-associated axillary lymph node granulomas as opposed to long-standing sarcoidosis. Within the breast, the carcinoma-associated granulomatous reaction is restricted to the tumor and immediately surrounding mammary parenchyma.

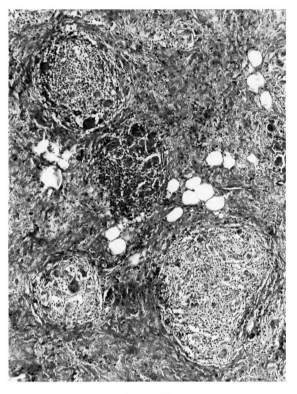

Figure 33
SARCOIDOSIS
Three discrete granulomas with multinucleated giant cells are present in the mammary stroma, largely sparing the lobules.

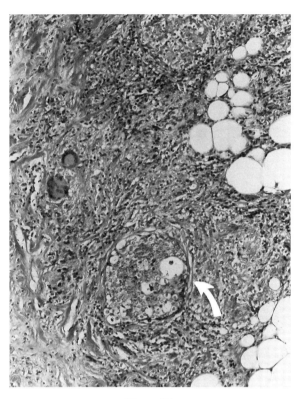

Figure 34
SARCOID-LIKE GRANULOMA AND CARCINOMA
Intraductal carcinoma (arrow) surrounded by granulomatous inflammation. The patient had no clinical manifestations of sarcoidosis.

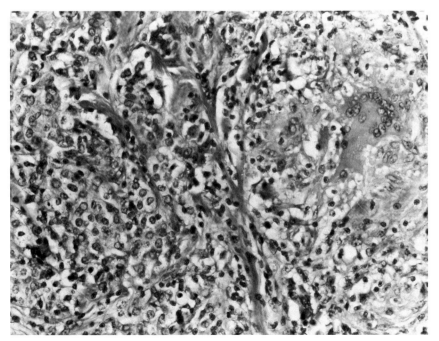

Figure 35
SARCOID-LIKE
GRANULOMA
AND CARCINOMA
Granuloma in invasive lobular carcinoma.

Prognosis and Treatment. The clinical course in women who have generalized sarcoidosis involving the breast depends on the extent of the underlying disease. Mammary lesions are adequately managed by excisional biopsy, which is necessary to rule out carcinoma. Despite significant impairment of cellular immunity and an increased incidence of malignant lymphoma and pulmonary carcinoma (79), there is no evidence that sarcoidosis influences the risk of developing mammary carcinoma or the prognosis if carcinoma develops.

VASCULITIS

Arteritis

The mammary lesions caused by vasculitis often resemble carcinoma clinically. The breasts may be affected as an isolated manifestation or as part of multiorgan involvement. Although there are differences in the histopathologic features of the vasculitis associated with various collagen vascular diseases, the diagnosis of a specific condition is made on the basis of both the clinical and pathologic findings.

Giant Cell Arteritis. Giant cell arteritis limited clinically to the breast has been reported in women 52 to 72 years of age. The lesions were bilateral in three of six cases. The firm to hard, tender or painful tumors measured up to 4 cm and carcinoma was suspected in most cases (100). Most women with giant cell arteritis of the breast have few or no systemic symptoms (90,91).

Microscopically, granulomatous inflammation involves small and medium sized arteries throughout the affected tissue. Veins and arterioles are spared. The reactive process consists of a transmural and perivascular infiltrate composed mainly of lymphocytes, histiocytes, and giant cells (fig. 36). Fibrinoid necrosis is not a consistent feature but fragmentation of the mural elastic fibers is demonstrable with an elastic tissue stain (fig. 37). Calcification develops in

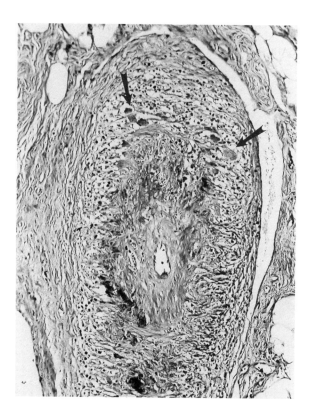

Figure 36
GIANT CELL ARTERITIS
The lumen of this intramammary artery is virtually obliterated by subintimal and mural inflammation, including giant cells (arrows). Note mural calcification in lower part of artery.

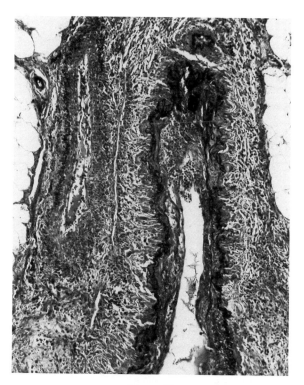

Figure 37
ARTERITIS
Transmural necrotizing inflammation of medium sized arteries in the breast. Elastica is partially destroyed (van Gieson elastic tissue stain).

vessels that are the site of healed arteritis. Edema, fat necrosis, and atrophy of glandular elements occur in the surrounding tissue.

The diagnosis of giant cell arteritis of the breast is made by excisional biopsy. Most patients are treated with adrenal corticosteroids and remain free of systemic symptoms with follow-up of 2 years or less.

Wegener Granulomatosis. The clinical manifestations of Wegener granulomatosis in the breast mimic mammary carcinoma. All patients have been women 40 to 59 years of age (92,93,98). The breast tumor is usually tender. Microscopic examination reveals acute and chronic inflammation of the mammary parenchyma and fat. Portions of the lesion may resemble an abscess. Vessels in necrotic areas and in the surrounding breast exhibit fibrinoid necrosis. Granulomatous foci are present in the affected blood vessels and at the periphery of areas of infarcted breast tissue. Prognosis depends on the severity and extent of systemic involvement.

Polyarteritis. There are several reports of mammary polyarteritis in women 37 to 70 years of age (88). In most cases a unilateral breast lesion was the initial manifestation. Microscopic examination reveals transmural necrotizing vasculitis without giant cell reaction in the breast parenchyma. Eosinophils may be a prominent component of the mixed inflammatory cell infiltrate. The lesion involves arteries of varying size but spares venous channels. Fibrinoid necrosis may be evident as well. Secondary effects in the surrounding breast resulting from ischemic degeneration include acute and chronic inflammation and fat necrosis. After a relatively brief follow-up, all of the patients remain alive, with improvement in systemic symptoms after treatment with corticosteriods.

Scleroderma. Cutaneous involvement of the breast may occur as part of progressive systemic scleroderma. There are several case reports of patients with breast carcinoma who developed scleroderma (94,99,101). The association between mammary carcinoma and scleroderma is probably coincidental, however.

Dermatomyositis. Cutaneous changes and multiple subcutaneous nodules in both breasts and axillae were described in one 49-year-old woman with long-standing dermatomyositis (95). Mammography revealed numerous coarse branching calcifications affecting blood vessels in the skin or subcutaneous tissue.

Phlebitis

Inflammatory lesions of veins within the breast have rarely been encountered. The most common form of phlebitis affecting the mammary region is superficial thrombophlebitis (97). About 25 percent of patients with Mondor disease have been men. Onset is seen after trauma, physical exertion, and surgery performed on the breast or chest wall. Most patients are between 20 and 40 years of age. Physical examination reveals a subcutaneous cord that may be painless or painful and tender. Mondor disease most often involves the upper outer or inframammary portions of the breast and adjacent chest wall.

The diagnosis of Mondor disease is usually established clinically. Mammography confirms the superficial nature of the process (102). Biopsy reveals thrombophlebitis of subcutaneous veins. Subcutaneous thrombophlebitis of the breast and chest wall is a self-limiting condition that resolves over a period of weeks to months after symptomatic treatment. Rare instances of coexistent mammary carcinoma have been reported (89,96)

SECONDARY EFFECTS OF CANCER TREATMENT

Radiation

Long-term clinical effects of therapeutic radiation on the normal breast tissue evolve over a period of months to years (110) and vary greatly among individuals. Most women ultimately exhibit diffuse increased firmness or sclerosis of the breast but in the majority this is mild and the tissue remains elastic. Ptosis, a natural change of aging, is less pronounced in the irradiated breast. Cutaneous atrophy and telangiectasia are likely to be more conspicuous in areas that received a radiation boost.

The major histologic changes in normal breast tissue occur in the terminal duct-lobular units (112). These changes include: collagenization of intralobular stroma; thickening of periacinar and periductal basement membranes; severe atrophy of acinar and ductular epithelium; and cytologic atypia of residual epithelial and

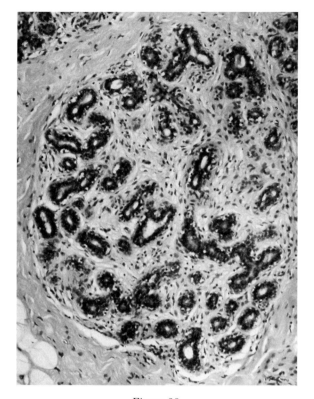

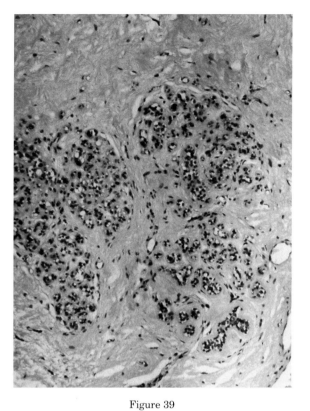

Figure 38
RADIATION
Normal lobule in premenopausal patient prior to radiation. (Figures 38 and 39 are from the same patient.)

Figure 39
RADIATION
Lobule 6 months after radiation showing collagenization of intralobular stroma and glandular atrophy.

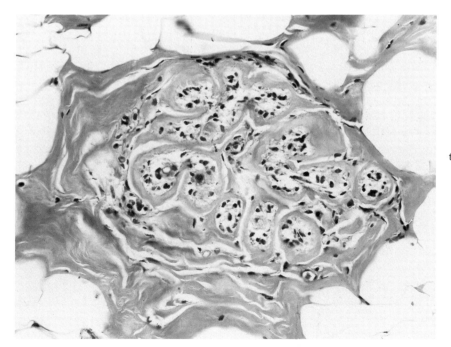

Figure 40
RADIATION
Postradiation lobule showing thickened basement membranes.

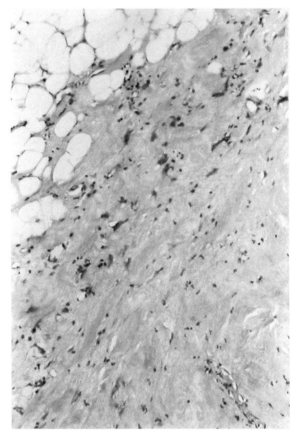

Figure 41
RADIATION
Atypical stromal fibroblasts in radiated breast.

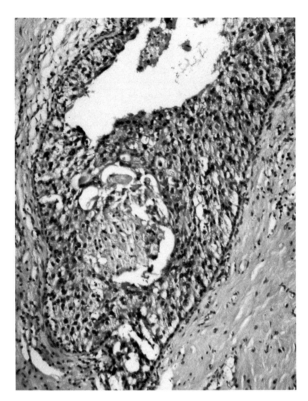

Figure 42
RADIATION
Intraductal carcinoma prior to radiation treatment. (Figures 42 and 43 are from the same patient.)

myoepithelial cells (figs. 38–40). Acinar myoepithelial cells are preserved to a greater extent than the epithelial cells. Atypical fibroblasts are seen in a few cases in the interlobular stroma (fig. 41). The effects of radiation on the larger ducts are much less pronounced.

When a radioactive implant or external boost is used, changes may be more severe than in the surrounding breast. Fat necrosis and atypia of stromal fibroblasts are more common in proximity to such "boosted" or implanted areas. Radiation-induced vascular changes are not ordinarily seen after external beam radiotherapy, but may occur where a boost dose has been delivered. Cytologic and architectural markers of radiation effect in blood vessels include endothelial atypia and myointimal proliferation that leads to vascular sclerosis. In boosted areas, epithelial atypia may occur in the larger ducts. The clinical

and pathologic effects of breast irradiation may be substantially augmented in patients with collagen vascular disease (111).

Cytologic atypia can create diagnostic problems even if one is aware of the typical appearance of radiation-induced atrophy of the breast (103,109,112,113). False-positive needle aspiration cytology diagnoses have been attributed to radiation atypia. In situ lobular and intraductal carcinoma persisting after radiation therapy are largely intact so that the affected lobules and ducts are filled and often expanded with a neoplastic cell population (figs. 42, 43). Frequently, little or no microscopic change is evident when pre- and postradiation samples of in situ carcinoma are compared (figs. 42–45).

Chemotherapy

A chemotherapy effect is most often encountered in the breast when patients with locally advanced or inflammatory carcinoma have been

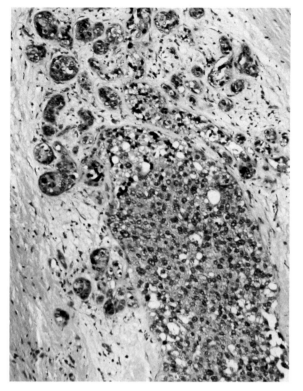

Figure 43
RADIATION
Recurrent intraductal carcinoma after radiation showing no appreciable difference from pretreatment carcinoma in fig. 42.

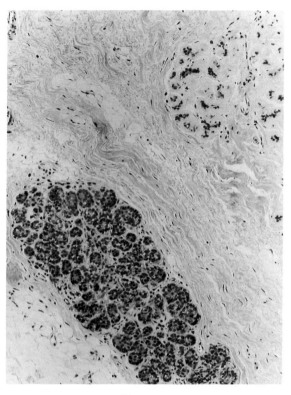

Figure 44
RADIATION
Lobular carcinoma in situ in postradiation breast. Note radiation change in a normal lobule in right corner. (Figures 44 and 45 are from the same patient.)

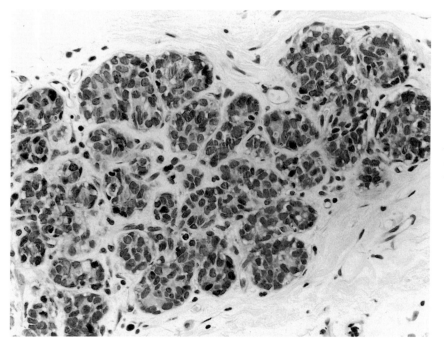

Figure 45
RADIATION
Lobular carcinoma in situ in breast after radiation showing none of the changes observed in radiated non-neoplastic lobules.

given systemic therapy preoperatively. In general, the histopathologic effects of systemic chemotherapy correlate with the extent of clinical response. Chemotherapy-induced changes tend to be similar in the primary tumor and axillary nodal metastases. The most extreme alterations are usually found in patients who appear clinically to have complete resolution of their neoplasm (104,106). On occasion there may be substantial dissociation between the clinical picture after therapy and the histologic findings. When no residual tumor is detectable clinically in the breast, about 60 percent of patients still have persistent carcinoma histologically. Patients who have no residual tumor grossly or histologically have an improved disease-free survival (106).

The most striking manifestation of the treatment effect is a decrease in tumor cellularity (figs. 46, 47). If the breast of a patient who has responded to treatment is examined histologi-

cally, infarcted, necrotic tumor may be found, but in time the degenerated tumor is absorbed, or no residual tumor may be detectable (104). Architectural distortion at sites of prior tumor infiltration is characterized by fibrosis, stromal edema, increased vascularity composed largely of thin-walled vessels, and a chronic inflammatory cell infiltrate (fig. 48).

Residual tumor cells may appear morphologically unaltered but in most cases they exhibit histologic and cytologic changes that reflect treatment effect (104,108). The cells tend to be enlarged and have minute cytoplasmic vacuoles, eosinophilic granules, or both. Some tumor cells have enlarged, pleomorphic and hyperchromatic nuclei (figs. 48–50). Multinucleated cells and abnormal mitotic figures are conspicuous chemotherapy effects. The altered tumor cells may resemble histiocytes especially when present individually, but they retain immunohistochemical reactivity for cytokeratin and epithelial membrane antigen. Aneuploid tumors are more likely than diploid

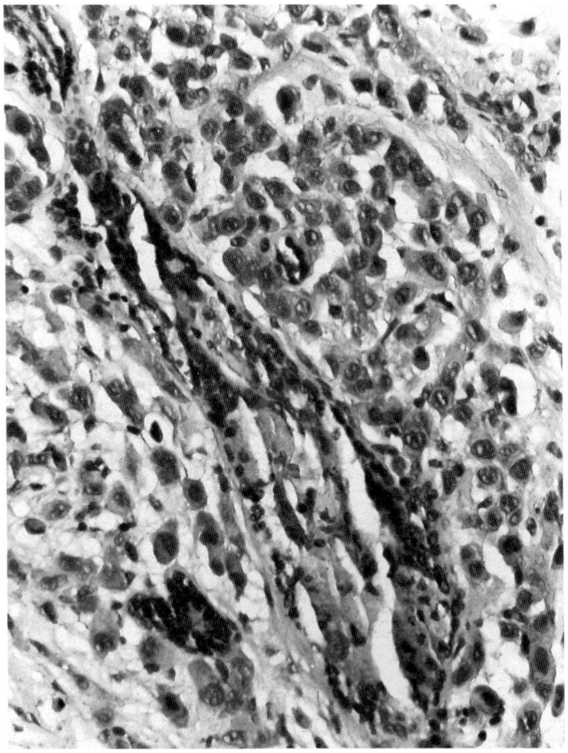

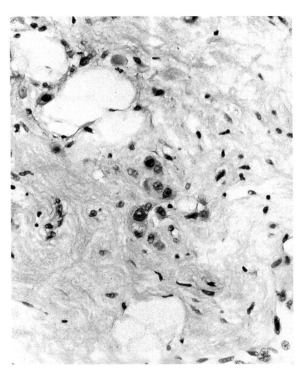

Figure 46
CHEMOTHERAPY EFFECT
Invasive lobular carcinoma prior to chemotherapy in a patient with inflammatory carcinoma and diffuse carcinomatous infiltration of the breast. (Figures 46–48 are from the same patient.)

Figure 47
CHEMOTHERAPY EFFECT
The mastectomy specimen after treatment with cytoxan, adriamycin, and 5-fluorouracil contained only microscopic clusters of carcinoma cells in collagenous stroma.

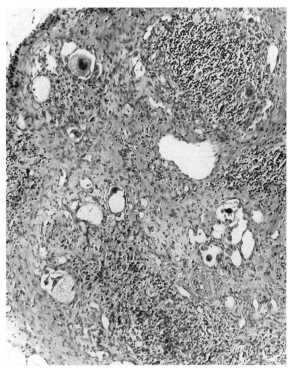

Figure 48
CHEMOTHERAPY EFFECT
Isolated carcinoma cells in lymphatic spaces after chemotherapy surrounded by edematous stroma that contains a lymphoid infiltrate. Tumor cells have enlarged hyperchromatic nuclei.

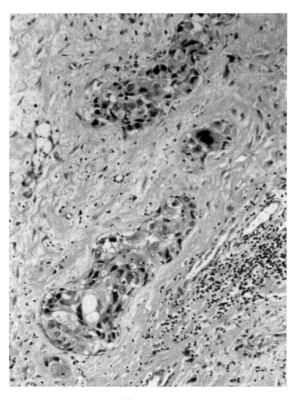

Figure 49
CHEMOTHERAPY EFFECT
In this duct carcinoma after chemotherapy hyperchromatic nuclei and cytoplasmic vacuolization are evident. (Figures 49 and 50 are from the same patient.)

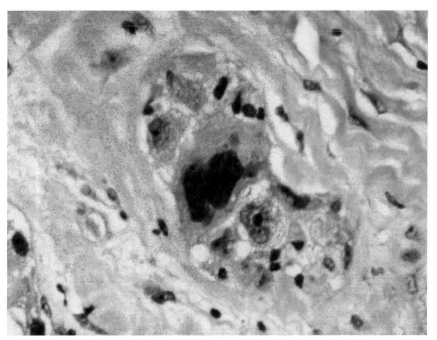

Figure 50
CHEMOTHERAPY EFFECT
Multiple, enlarged hyperchromatic nuclei are present in one cell. Note cytoplasmic vacuolization.

tumors to exhibit histologic and cytologic changes due to chemotherapy (104). Non-neoplastic breast parenchyma is also altered following cytotoxic chemotherapy but the changes are more subtle than those induced in the tumor. The glandular elements undergo diffuse atrophy causing a reduction in the number of lobules and in the size of existing lobules (108). Cytologic atypia may be seen in duct and lobular epithelial cells but in many cases these changes are not attributable specifically to treatment.

Hormone Treatment

Estrogens and androgens have been used to treat mammary carcinoma for approximately 50 years. A detailed examination of the effects of therapeutic doses of estrogen on noncancerous mammary glandular tissue was reported by Huseby and Thomas in 1954 (107). In postmenopausal women normal breast epithelium was stimulated to proliferate, with the elongation of small terminal ducts and the formation of lobules. Epithelial changes were accompanied by the accumulation of interlobular connective tissue. The authors also commented "that the reaction to estrogen administration of certain abnormal, but nonmalignant, epithelial structures was one of proliferation and thus more like that of the normal breast epithelium than like that of the cancerous epithelium."

Further studies of the morphologic changes associated with tumor regression in hormone treated patients were reported by Emerson et al. (105). They noted that low-grade tumors were more likely to respond to treatment and that the duration of regression achieved with such tumors was greater. The extent of hormone-induced changes in normal breast tissue did not correlate with response to treatment.

Antiestrogen treatment with tamoxifen has significantly increased the proportion of immunohistochemically estrogen receptor–positive epithelial cells in normal ducts when compared with untreated normal tissues (114). No concomittant increase in progesterone receptor immunoreactivity was observed.

REFERENCES

Fat Necrosis

1. Bassett LW, Gold RH, Cove HC. Mammographic spectrum of traumatic fat necrosis: the fallibility of "pathognomonic" signs of carcinoma. AJR Am J Roentgenol 1978;130:119–22.
2. Clarke D, Curtis JL, Martinez A, Fajardo L, Goffinet D. Fat necrosis of the breast simulating recurrent carcinoma after primary radiotherapy in the management of early stage breast carcinoma. Cancer 1983;52:442–5.
3. Hurt MA, Dïaz-Arias AA, Rosenholtz MJ, Havey AD, Stephenson HE Jr. Posttraumatic lobular squamous metaplasia of the breast. An unusual pseudocarcinomatous metaplasia resembling squamous (necrotizing) sialometaplasia of the salivary gland. Mod Pathol 1988; 1:385–90.
4 Meyer JE, Silverman P, Gandbhir L. Fat necrosis of the breast. Arch Surg 1978;113:801–5.

Hemorrhagic Necrosis with Coagulopathy

5. Martin BF, Phillips JD. Gangrene of the female breast with anticoagulant therapy: report of two cases. Am J Clin Pathol 1970;53:622–6.
6. Rick ME. Protein C and protein S. JAMA 1990;263:701–3.

Lesions Associated with Breast Augmentation

7. Domanskis EJ, Owsley JQ Jr. Histological investigation of the etiology of capsule contracture following augmentation mammaplasty. Plast Reconstr Surg 1976;58:689–93.
8. Nosanchuk JS. Silicone granuloma in the breast. Arch Surg 1968;97:583–5.
9. Symmers WS. Silicone mastitis in "topless" waitresses and some other varieties of foreign-body mastitis. Br Med J 1968;3:19–22.
10. Truong LD, Cartwright J Jr, Goodman MD, Woznicki D. Silicone lymphadenopathy associated with augmentation mammaplasty. Morphologic features of nine cases. Am J Surg Pathol 1988;12:484–91.

Inflammatory Lesions in Pregnancy and Lactation

11. Eschenbach DA. Acute postpartum infections. Emerg Med Clin North Am 1985;3:87–115.

Infarcts

12. Flint A, Oberman HA. Infarction and squamous metaplasia of intraductal papilloma: a benign breast lesion that may simulate carcinoma. Hum Pathol 1984;15:764–7.

13. Fratamico FC, Eusebi V. Infarct in benign breast diseases. Description of 4 new cases. Pathologica 1988;80: 433–42.
14. Lucey JJ. Spontaneous infarction of the breast. J Clin Pathol 1975;28:937–943.
15. Newman J, Kahn LB. Infarction of fibro-adenoma of the breast. Br J Surg 1973;60:738–40.
16. Wilkinson L, Green WO Jr. Infarction of beast lesions during pregnancy and lactation. Cancer 1964;17: 1567–72.

Nonspecific Inflammatory Lesions

17. Adair FE. Plasma cell mastitis—a lesion simulating mammary carcinoma. A clinical and pathologic study with a report of ten cases. Arch Surg 1933;26:735–49.
18. Brown KL, Tang PH. Postlactational tumoral granulomatous mastitis: a localized immune phenomenon. Am J Surg 1979;138:326–9.
19. Davies JD. Hyperelastosis, obliteration and fibrous plaques in major ducts of the human breast. J Pathol 1973;110:13–26.
20. _____. Inflammatory damage to ducts in mammary dysplasia: a cause of duct obliteration. J Pathol 1975;117:47–54.
21. _____. Pigmented periductal cells (ochrocytes) in mammary dysplasias: their nature and significance. J Pathol 1974;114:205–16.
22. _____, Burton PA. Postpartum lobular granulomatous mastitis [Letter]. J Clin Pathol 1983;36:363.
23. Fletcher A, Magrath IM, Riddell RH, Talbot IC. Granulomatous mastitis: a report of seven cases. J Clin Pathol 1982;35:941–5.
24. Fitzgibbons PL. Granulomatous mastitis. NY State J Med 1990;90:287.
25. Going JJ, Anderson TJ, Wilkinson S, Chetty U. Granulomatous lobular mastitis. J Clin Pathol 1987;40:535–40.
26. Haagenson CD. Mammary-duct ectasia. A disease that may simulate carcinoma. Cancer 1951;4:749–61.
27. Hunter-Craig ID, Tuddenham EG, Earle JH. Lipogranuloma of the breast due to phenothiazine therapy. Br J Surg 1970;57:76–9.
28. Kessler E, Wolloch Y. Granulomatous mastitis: a lesion clinically simulating carcinoma. Am J Clin Pathol 1972;58:642–6.
29. Miller JK. Plasma cell mastitis: a pathologic entity. Am J Surg 1939;43:788–93.
30. Murthy MS. Granulomatous mastitis and lipogranuloma of the breast [Letter]. Am J Clin Pathol 1973;60:432–3.
31. Parsons WH, Henthorne JC, Clark RL Jr. Plasma cell mastitis. Report of five additional cases. Arch Surg 1944;49:86–90.
32. Payne RI, Strauss AF, Glasser RD. Mastitis obliterans. Surgery 1943;14:719–27.
33. Rees BI, Gravelle IH, Hughes LE. Nipple retraction in duct ectasia. Br J Surg 1977;64:577–80.
34. Tedeschi LG, McCarthy PE. Involutional mammary duct ectasia and periductal mastitis in a male. Hum Pathol 1974;5:232–6.
35. Tice GI, Dockerty MB, Harrington SW. Comedomastitis. A clinical and pathologic study of data in 172 cases. Surg Gynecol Obstet 1948;87:525–40.
36. Walker JC, Sandison AT. Mammary-duct ectasia. Br J Surg 1964;51:350–5.
37. Wilhelmus JL, Schrodt GR, Mahaffey LM. Cholesterol granulomas of the breast. A lesion which clinically mimics carcinoma. Am J Clin Pathol 1982;77:592–7.

Specific Infections

38. Alagaratnam TT, Ong GB. Tuberculosis of the breast. Br J Surg 1980;67:125–6.
39. Ashford RW, Dowse JA, Rogers WN, Powell DE. Dirofilariasis of the breast [Letter]. Lancet 1989; 1:1198.
40. Barrett GS, MacDermot J. Breast abscess: a rare presentation of typhoid. Br Med J 1972;2:628–9.
41. Benger A, Rennie RP, Roberts JT, Thornley JH, Scholten T. A human coenurus infection in Canada. Am J Trop Med Hyg 1981;30:638–44.
42. Bennett IC, Furnival CM, Searle J. Dirofilariasis in Australia: unusual cause of a breast lump. Aust NZ J Surg 1989;59:671–3.
43. Campbell FC, Eriksson BL, Angorn IB. Localized granulomatous mastitis—an unusual presentation of typhoid: a case report. S Afr Med J 1980;57:793–5.
44. Carme B, Paraiso D, Gombe-Mbalawa C. Calcifications of the breast probably due to *Loa loa*. Am J Trop Med Hyg 1990;42:65–6.
45. Chen Y, Qun X. Filarial granuloma of the female breast: a histopathological study of 131 cases. Am J Trop Med Hyg 1981;30:1206–10.
46. Davies JA. Primary actinomycosis of the breast. Br J Surg 1951;38:378–81.
47. Dent DM, Webber BL. Tuberculosis of the breast. S Afr Med J 1977;51:611–4.
48. Golinger RC, O'Neal BJ. Mastitis and mammary duct disease. Arch Surg 1982;117:1027–9.
49. Gutierrez Y, Paul GM. Breast nodule produced by dirofilaria tenuis. Am J Surg Pathol 1984;8:463–5.
50. Habif DV, Perzin KH, Lipton R, Lattes R. Subareolar abscess associated with squamous metaplasia of lactiferous ducts. Am J Surg 1970;119:523–6.
51. Hale JA, Peters GN, Cheek JH. Tuberculosis of the breast: rare but still extant. Review of the literature and report of an additional case. Am J Surg 1985;150:620–4.
52. Halstead AC, LeCount ER. Tuberculosis of the mammary gland. Ann Surg 1898;28:685–707.
53. Hamit HF, Ragsdale TH. Mammary tuberculosis [Editorial]. J R Soc Med 1982;75:764–5.
54. Ikard RW, Perkins D. Mammary tuberculosis: a rare modern disease. South Med J 1977;70:208–12.
55. Ikeda DM, Sickles EA. Mammographic demonstration of pectoral muscle microcalcifications. AJR Am J Roentgenol 1988;151:475–6.
56. Kunkel JM, Hawksley CA. Cysticercosis presenting as a solitary dominant breast mass [Letter]. Hum Pathol 1987;18: 1190–1.
57. Kurtycz DF, Alt B, Mack E. Incidental coenurosis: larval cestode presenting as an axillary mass. Am J Clin Pathol 1983;80:735–8.
58. Lahiri VL. Microfilariae in nipple secretion. Acta Cytol 1975;19:154.
59. Lefkowitz M, Wear DJ. Cat-scratch disease masquerading as a solitary tumor of the breast. Arch Pathol Lab Med 1989;113:473–5.

60. Leggett CA. Cystocercosis of the breast. Aust NZ J Surg 1983;53:281.
61. McMeeking AA, Gonzalez R, Hanna B. Mammary tuberculosis. NY State J Med 1989:288–9.
62. Miller MJ, Moore S. Nodular breast lesion caused by Bancroft's filariasis. Can Med Assoc J 1965;93:711–4.
63. Morgen M. Tuberculosis of the breast. Surg Gynecol Obstet 1931;53:593–605.
64. Mukerjee P, Cohen RV, Niden AH. Tuberculosis of the breast. Am Rev Respir Dis 1971;104:661–7.
65. Nagashima Y. Role of tuberculosis of the female breast in presence of tuberculosis of internal organs and especially in miliary tuberculosis. Virchows Arch Pathol Anat 1925;254:185–202.
66. Nayar M, Saxena HM. Tuberculosis of the breast. A cytomorphologic study of needle aspirates and nipple discharges. Acta Cytol 1984;28:325–8.
67. Novak R. Calcifications in the breast in filaria loa infection. Acta Radiol 1989;30:507–8.
68. Osborne BM. Granulomatous mastitis caused by histoplasma and mimicking inflammatory breast carcinoma. Hum Pathol 1989;20:47–52.
69. Pemberton M. A case of primary actinomycosis of the breast. Br J Surg 1942;29:353.
70. Salfelder K, Schwarz J. Mycotic "pseudotumors" of the breast. Report of four cases. Arch Surg 1975;110:751–4.
71. Saxena H, Singh SN, Ajwani KD. Nodular breast lesions caused by filarial worms. Report of three cases. Am J Trop Med Hyg 1975;24:894–6.
72. Symmers WS. Deep-seated fungal infections currently seen in the histopathologic service of a medical school laboratory in Britain. Am J Clin Pathol 1966;46:514–37.
73. Tabár L, Kett K, Németh A. Tuberculosis of the breast. Radiology 1976;118:587–9.
74. Thomsen AC, Espersen T, Maigaard S. Course and treatment of milk stasis, noninfectious inflammation of the breast, and infectious mastitis in nursing women. Am J Obstet Gynecol 1984;149:492–5.
75. Urban JA. Excision of the major ductal system of the breast. Cancer 1963;16:516–20.
76. Varin CR, Eisenberg BL, Ladd WA. Mammographic microcalcifications associated with schistosomiasis. South Med J 1989;82:1060–1.
77. Vassilakos P. Tuberculosis of the breast: cytologic findings with fine-needle aspiration. A case clinically and radiologically mimicking carcinoma. Acta Cytol 1973;17:160–5.

Sarcoidosis

78. Bässler R, Birke F. Histopathology of tumour associated sarcoid-like stromal reaction in breast cancer. An analysis of 5 cases with immunohistochemical investigations. Virchows Arch [A] 1988;412:231–9.
79. Brincker H, Wilbek E. The incidence of malignant tumours in patients with respiratory sarcoidosis. Br J Cancer 1974;29:247–51.
80. Fitzgibbons PL, Smiley DF, Kern WH. Sarcoidosis presenting initially as breast mass: report of two cases. Hum Pathol 1985;16:851–2.
81. _____. Granulomatous mastitis. NY State J Med 1990;90:287.
82. Gorton G, Linell F. Malignant tumors and sarcoid reactions in regional lymph nodes. Acta Radiol 1957; 47:381–92.
83. Milward TM, Gough MH. Granulomatous lesions in the breast presenting as carcinoma. Surg Gynecol Obstet 1970;130:478–82.
84. Prior JT. Boeck's sarcoid with coexisting carcinoma. Am J Surg 1952;83:201–4.
85. Shah AK, Solomon L, Gumbs MA. Sarcoidosis of the breast coexisting with mammary carcinoma. NY State J Med 1990;90:331–3.
86. Symmers WS. Localized tuberculoid granulomas associated with carcinoma. Their relationship to sarcoidosis. Am J Pathol 1951;27:493–521.
87. Wargotz ES, Lefkowitz M. Granulomatous angiopanniculitis of the breast. Hum Pathol 1989;20:1084–8.

Vasculitis

88. Chaitin B, Kohout ND, Goldman RL. Focal arteritis of the breast. Angiology 1981;32:334–7.
89. Chiedozi LC, Aghahowa JA. Mondor's disease associated with breast cancer. Surgery 1988;103:438–9.
90. Clement PB, Senges H, How AR. Giant cell arteritis of the breast: case report and literature review. Hum Pathol 1987;18:1186–9.
91. Cook DJ, Bensen WG, Carroll JJ, Joshi S. Giant cell arteritis of the breast. Can Med Assoc J 1988;139:513–5.
92. Deininger HK. Wegener granulomatosis of the breast. Radiology 1985;154:59–60.
93. Elsner B, Harper FB. Disseminated Wegener's granulomatosis with breast involvement. Report of a case. Arch Pathol 1969;87:544–7.
94. Forbes AM, Woodrow JC, Verbov JL, Graham RM. Carcinoma of the breast and scleroderma: four further cases and a literature review. Br J Rheumatol 1989;28:65–9.
95. Gyves-Ray KM, Adler DD. Dermatomyositis: an unusual cause of breast calcifications. Breast Dis 1989; 2:195–201.
96. Miller DR, Cesario TC, Slater LM. Mondor's disease associated with metastatic axillary nodes. Cancer 1985;56:903–4.
97. Mondor H. Tronculite sous-cutanee subaigne de la paroi thoracique antero-laterale. Mem Acad Chir 1939; 65:1271–8.
98. Pambakian H, Tighe JR. Breast involvement in Wegener's granulomatosis. J Clin Pathol 1971;24:343–7.
99. Papasavvas G, Goodwill CJ. Scleroderma and breast carcinoma. Br J Rheumatol 1989;28:366–7.
100. Potter BT, Housley E, Thomson D. Giant-cell arteritis mimicking carcinoma of the breast. Br Med J (Clin Res Ed) 1981;282:1665–6.
101. Roumm AD, Medsger TA Jr. Cancer and systemic sclerosis. An epidemiologic study. Arthritis Rheum 1985;28:1336–40.
102. Tabár L, Dean PB. Mondor's disease: clinical, mammographic and pathologic features. Breast 1981;7:18–20.

Secondary Effects of Cancer Treatment

103. Bondeson L. Aspiration cytology of radiation-induced changes of normal breast epithelium. Acta Cytol 1987;31:309–10.

104. Briffod M, Spyratos F, Tubiana-Hulin M, et al. Sequential cytopunctures during preoperative chemotherapy for primary breast carcinoma. Cytomorphologic changes, initial tumor ploidy, and tumor regression. Cancer 1989;63:631–7.

105. Emerson WJ, Kennedy BJ, Taft EB. Correlation of histological alterations in breast cancer with response to hormone therapy. Cancer 1960;13:1047–52.

106. Feldman LD, Hortobagyi GN, Buzdar AU, Ames FC, Blumenschein GR. Pathological assessment of response to induction chemotherapy in breast cancer. Cancer Res 1986; 46:2578–81.

107. Huseby RA, Thomas LB. Histological and histochemical alterations in the normal breast tissues of patients with advanced breast cancer being treated with estrogenic hormones. Cancer 1954;7:54–74.

108. Kennedy S, Merino MJ, Swain SM, Lippman ME. The effects of hormonal and chemotherapy on tumoral and non-neoplastic breast tissue. Hum Pathol 1990;21:192–8.

109. Peterse JL, Thunnissen FB, Van Heerde P. Fine needle aspiration cytology or radiation-induced changes in nonneoplastic breast lesions. Possible pitfalls in cytodiagnosis. Acta Cytol 1989;33:176–80.

110. Pierquin B, Grimard L, Marinello G. Normal-tissue tolerance in the irradiation of female breast. Front Radiat Ther Oncol 1989;23:341–8.

111. Robertson JM, Clarke DH, Pevzner MM, Matter RC. Breast conservation therapy. Severe breast fibrosis after radiation therapy in patients with collagen vascular disease. Cancer 1991;68:502–8.

112. Schnitt SJ, Connolly JL, Harris JR, Cohen RB. Radiation-induced changes in the breast. Hum Pathol 1984;15:545–50.

113. Vilcoq JR, Calle R, Stacey P, Ghossein NA. Outcome of treatment by tumorectomy and radiotherapy of patients with operable breast cancer. Int J Radiat Oncol Biol Phys 1981;7:1327–32.

114. Walker KJ, Price-Thomas JM, Candlish W, Nicholson RI. Influence of the antiestrogen tamoxifen on normal breast tissue. Br J Cancer 1991;64:764–8.

BENIGN PROLIFERATIVE LESIONS

Many terms have been used to collectively characterize a pathologic spectrum of seemingly related clinically benign breast abnormalities. These include palpably irregular and painful breasts, often with discrete lumps or multiple nodules with some fluctuation of symptoms in relation to the menstrual cycle. Microscopic changes include cystically dilated ducts, apocrine metaplasia of the ductal epithelium, interlobular and intralobular fibrosis, adenosis, and intraductal epithelial proliferation. Because of a diagnostic kinship with intraductal carcinoma, the latter abnormality will be considered in the Intraepithelial Carcinoma chapter.

Diagnostic terms such as *chronic cystic mastitis*, *periductal mastitis*, *mammary dysplasia*, *cystic mastalgia,* and *fibrocystic disease* have achieved variable popularity in encompassing these pathologic findings. Until recently, fibrocystic disease was the term most widely used. However, the lack of specificity of this term resulted in inappropriate inference as to its malignant potential; furthermore, these abnormalities do not represent a specific disease, but rather a variable end-organ response to hormonal stimuli (5).

There is now general agreement that the term fibrocystic disease should be discarded, that *fibrocystic changes* or *fibrocystic condition* are preferred diagnostic terms, and that the microscopically detected component elements should be specified in a pathologic diagnosis (2). An alternative is to consider a number of benign breast disorders as "aberrations of normal development and involution." Accordingly, the acronym ANDI is used as a broad generic designation encompassing the aforementioned fibrocystic changes as well as mastalgia, fibroadenoma, intraductal papilloma, nipple inversion, pregnancy-related duct hyperplasia, and mammary duct ectasia (4).

Fibrocystic changes are extremely common. In a 1951 autopsy study, Frantz et al. (3) found microscopic evidence of these alterations in 58 percent of cases (3). A more recent autopsy study indicated that fibrosis was the most common breast abnormality, and that epithelial hyperplasia and cystic ducts were seen in only 39 and 61 percent, respectively, of grossly abnormal breasts (1). This study also showed that the patterns of breast density, occasionally utilized by radiologists as prognostic indicators for risk of subsequent carcinoma, correlate with the extent of fibrosis.

CYSTS AND APOCRINE METAPLASIA

Mammary cysts arise in the terminal ductal lobular unit of the duct system, probably by the unfolding of adjacent ductules. The cysts can be single or multiple, unilocular or multilocular, and of microscopic or gross dimension. Leakage of secretions from cystic ducts may result in periductal chronic inflammation and fibrosis. The cysts are lined by flattened epithelium or by cuboidal or columnar cells which frequently manifest apocrine metaplasia. The apocrine epithelium may project into the cyst lumen as small papillary projections (fig. 51). Some have suggested that most breast cysts commence in apocrine metaplasia of lobular duct epithelium or are derived from intraductal epithelial hyperplasia (7,10,11).

The significance of apocrine metaplastic epithelium is open to debate. Apocrine metaplasia is an extremely common finding in breast biopsies and an increased incidence of subsequent carcinoma in patients with apocrine metaplastic cysts has been noted, especially grossly evident cysts lined by apocrine epithelium (6,9). Further support for such an association is the observation that a protein isolated from cyst fluid (GCDFP-15) can be localized immunohistochemically in the cytoplasm of apocrine metaplastic epithelium and in intraductal and invasive carcinomas, especially neoplasms with apocrine features (8).

FOCAL FIBROSIS

This is a poorly defined condition referring to a breast mass resulting from abundant parvicellular connective tissue engulfing atrophic ducts and lobules. Haagensen (13) first suggested this as a distinct clinical entity in

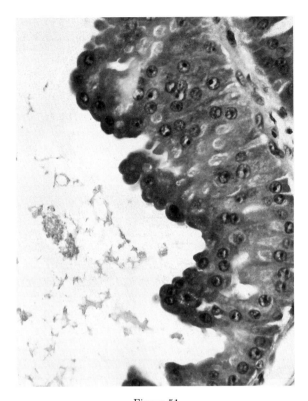

Figure 51
CYSTIC DUCT LINED BY
MULTILAYERED APOCRINE EPITHELIUM
The metaplastic apocrine epithelium is thickened as a result of cellular crowding.

1956, and proposed the term *fibrous disease*. Other names for this condition include fibrous mastopathy (14), fibrosis of the breast (17), fibrous tumor (15), and focal fibrous disease (16).

While there is no question that this is a clinical entity, there is considerable doubt whether it is a pathologic condition (12). It most likely represents a variation of the normal involution of the breast rather than a specific lesion.

Clinical Presentation. Most of these tumors occur in premenopausal women, with the peak incidence in the fourth and fifth decades of life. However, the majority of patients reported by Rivera-Pomar et al. (16) were in their thirties.

The lesion forms a firm mass, most often in the upper outer quadrant of the breast. It rarely attains large size. There is no associated skin retraction. Multiple nodules may be present.

Microscopic Findings. Microscopically, the lesion consists of broad areas of parvicellular fibrous connective tissue separating atrophic

ducts and lobules, replacing the intralobular connective tissue. Both Rivera-Pomar et al. (16) and Minkowitz et al. (14) subdivided these masses into three types, depending on the relative amounts of periductal stroma and the degree of ductal atrophy. A periductal lymphocytic infiltrate is common.

Differential Diagnosis. This condition should be distinguished from mammary hamartoma, especially if the hamartoma is composed predominantly of dense connective tissue. The distinctive feature of hamartomas is sharp circumscription, evident grossly and mammographically. Fibromatosis must be considered in the differential diagnosis since this lesion also has an infiltrating contour. Fibromatosis is characterized by greater stromal cellularity.

Treatment. Treatment is by local excision. Because there is poor gross circumscription, the surgeon may have difficulty in ascertaining the margins of the lesion. This is not of great concern, since focal fibrosis is perfectly innocuous with little tendency for recurrence.

ADENOSIS AND VARIANT LESIONS

Adenosis

Adenosis implies an elongation of the terminal ductules of the mammary lobule resulting in a caricature of the lobule. It is significant because of the possible confusion by the pathologist with invasive carcinoma. The abnormality presents in various growth patterns. In the prototype lesion, lobulocentric ductular proliferation is circumscribed, consisting of epithelial and myoepithelial cells associated with variable amounts of fibrosis. When the fibrosis is minimal, the lesion may be termed *florid adenosis* while the designation *sclerosing adenosis*, indicates prominent interductular fibrosis. The florid pattern is probably the earliest manifestation of the lesion that evolves, with progressive stromal proliferation and ductular attenuation, into the sclerosing pattern.

Confluence of adjacent lobulocentric areas of adenosis may result in a clinically evident mass termed *adenosis tumor* or *tumoral adenosis*. *Apocrine adenosis* refers to lesions with prominent metaplasia of the ductular epithelium. Other variants, including *tubular adenosis*, *adenomyoepithelial adenosis*, and *microglandular adenosis* will be described below.

Clinical Presentation. Adenosis most commonly occurs in women in their third and fourth decades of life. It is usually a nonpalpable lesion, not grossly visible, solely of microscopic significance. It presents as an incidental finding in biopsy material or is recognized in mammograms because clustered microcalcifications commonly develop in adenosis.

In contrast to carcinoma, no clinical retraction signs are produced. Confluent adenosis that forms an adenosis tumor also lacks retraction signs, but may result in a firm, mobile, rubbery mass which usually is less than 2 cm in diameter.

Microscopic Findings. The circumscribed area of apparent ductular proliferation constituting adenosis results from a numerical increase in ductules as well as from elongation of lobular ductules with associated myoepithelial and stromal proliferation. These foci commonly are multiple in the breast and their circumscription is best appreciated on low-power examination. The affected ducts have an oval to elongated contour and consistently contain well-defined epithelial and myoepithelial layers. This contrasts with the angulated shape and absence of myoepithelium and basal lamina in tubular carcinoma (25).

In most instances the caliber of the affected ductules is greater at the periphery than at the center of the lesion, contrasting with the relatively uniform dimensions of neoplastic ducts in tubular carcinoma (fig. 52). The ductules at the periphery of adenosis nodules may be dilated and even cystic. Small ducts proliferating adjacent to the adenosis may invaginate into the cysts, ultimately producing small papillomas (figs. 53–55). Most intraductal papillomas with adenosis that comprise one type of radial scar probably arise in this manner (29).

Microcalcifications are common in areas of adenosis within the ductule lumens. This most likely represents calcification of luminal content rather than dystrophic calcification. The epithelial lining of the ductules lacks atypism, although occasional mitoses may be present.

Central attenuation of ductules may progress to virtual absence of the epithelial layer, resulting solely in spindled myoepithelial cells surrounded by dense connective tissue. The entire abnormality may consist of this pattern, with minimal, if any, evidence of tubule formation.

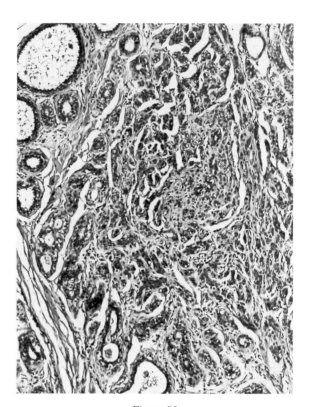

Figure 52
SCLEROSING ADENOSIS
The calibre of the ducts at the periphery of the lesion is greater than that of the central ducts.

Such foci may create diagnostic confusion with invasive lobular carcinoma. Nonetheless, the nodular lobulocentric character of the lesion usually is retained (figs. 56–58).

Occasional invasion of nerves by the ductular elements of the lesion results in additional confusion with carcinoma (fig. 59) (35). The nerves can be surrounded by the ducts or small ducts may be present within the substance of the nerve. The ductules retain their banal appearance and two-cell composition. Invasion of the blood vessel walls may also be seen (20).

Variant Patterns

Adenosis Tumor. This is a clinically and grossly recognizable breast mass formed by contiguous foci of adenosis (28). There may be dense fibrosis at the confluence of the adenosis nodules, and the entrapped ducts at this site may simulate invasive growth.

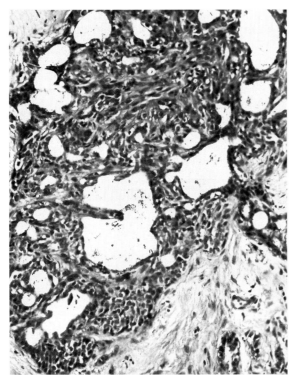

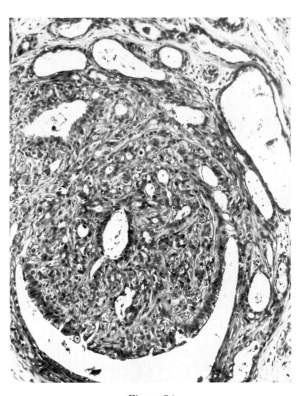

Figure 53
SCLEROSING ADENOSIS
The origin of a small intraductal papilloma in an area of adenosis is illustrated in a single lesion. Ectatic ducts contrast with attenuated ducts in this circumscribed area of adenosis. (Figures 53–55 are from the same patient.)

Figure 54
SCLEROSING ADENOSIS
Invagination of adenosis into peripheral cystic duct.

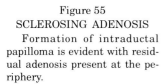

Figure 55
SCLEROSING ADENOSIS
Formation of intraductal papilloma is evident with residual adenosis present at the periphery.

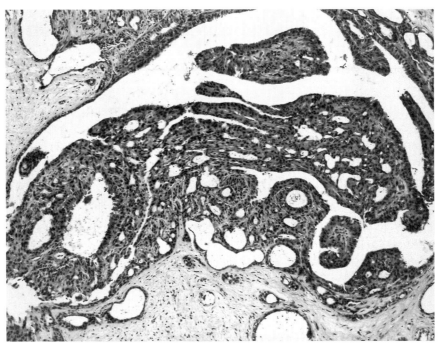

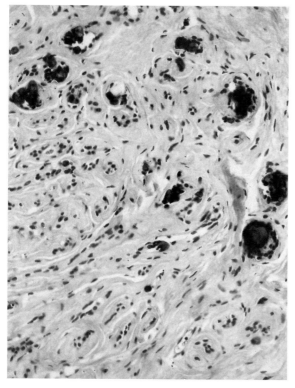

Figure 56
SCLEROSING ADENOSIS
Markedly attenuated ducts that contain microcalcifications are present at the periphery of the lesion. (Figures 56–58 are from the same patient.)

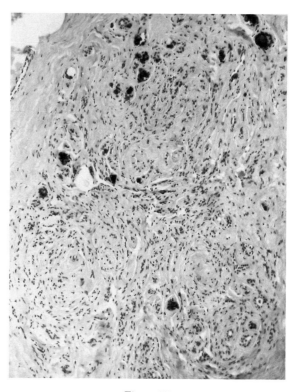

Figure 57
SCLEROSING ADENOSIS
A circumscribed area of adenosis probably involving three adjacent lobules is depicted.

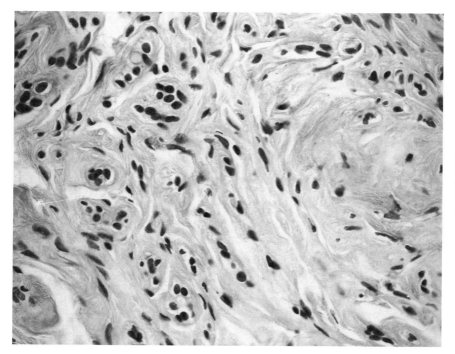

Figure 58
SCLEROSING ADENOSIS
Higher magnification demonstrates absence of ductal epithelium. In contrast to invasive lobular carcinoma, the myoepithelial cells have uniform spindled nuclei.

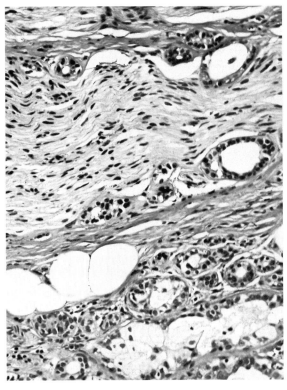

Figure 59
SCLEROSING ADENOSIS
Small bland ducts are present immediately adjacent to a branch of a peripheral nerve.

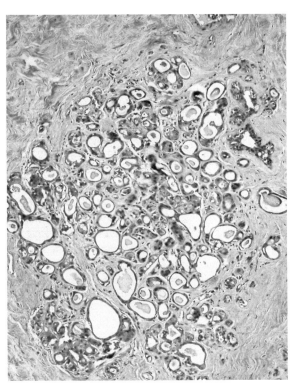

Figure 60
APOCRINE ADENOSIS
The circumscription of sclerosing adenosis is present with ectatic ducts most numerous at the periphery. (Figures 60 and 61 are from the same patient.)

Blunt Duct Adenosis. This term was coined by Foote and Stewart (24) to refer to an aggregate of ducts that apparently end abruptly without forming lobules. The blunt end ducts may have dilated lumens, resulting in an aggregate of microcysts or may manifest multilayering of epithelium. The lining epithelium is often composed of tall columnar cells with luminal snouts surrounded by myoepithelial cells that also appear hyperplastic. In the latter, intraductal hyperplasia or atypical lobular hyperplasia may occur, often with associated apocrine metaplasia. Small intraductal papillomas may be seen. It is probable that the cystic pattern is an end-stage of the abnormality.

Adenosis in Fibroadenomas. Sclerosing adenosis may occur focally, or as the predominant pattern in fibroadenomas. Fibrocystic changes in these tumors are common; moreover, since both lesions arise from the mammary lobule, their concurrence should not be surprising (30). As is true elsewhere in the breast, the area of adenosis must be distinguished from the unusual occurrence of invasive carcinoma in this setting.

Apocrine Adenosis. Apocrine metaplasia is a common finding in adenosis (fig. 60). Especially when associated with nuclear hypertrophy and prominent nucleoli, this metaplastic change may result in a microscopic picture that simulates carcinoma (figs. 61–63) (18). The cytoplasm is often focally clear as well as eosinophilic and granular. The nodular lobulocentric configuration of the area of adenosis is retained, and duct lumens are preserved. Moreover, other areas of adenosis in the adjacent breast lack apocrine epithelium or possess it only in small foci.

Tubular Adenosis. This pattern is characterized by numerous elongated and seemingly interdigitated ductules of relatively uniform size (29). These lack the circumscribed whorled arrangement of more typical examples of adenosis (figs. 64, 65). Microcalcifications are common, and a two-cell layer is uniformly evident (fig. 66).

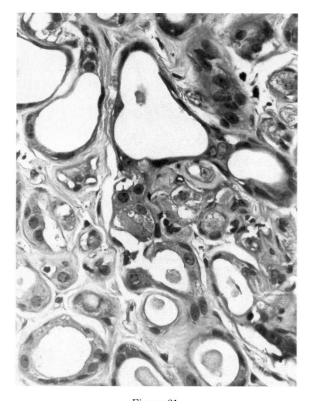

Figure 61
APOCRINE ADENOSIS
These ductules are lined by apocrine epithelium with large nuclei and prominent nucleoli.

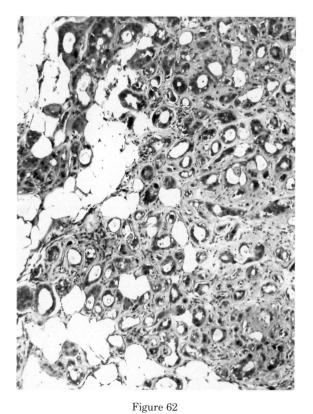

Figure 62
APOCRINE ADENOSIS
This area of adenosis is less circumscribed than is usual, increasing the potential for confusion with carcinoma.

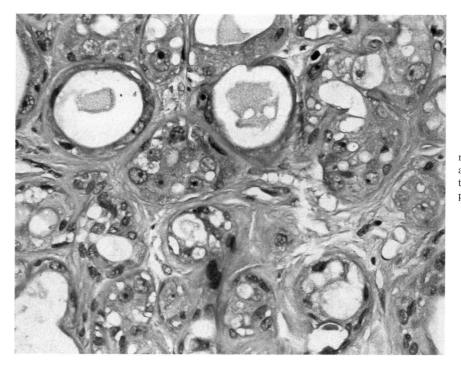

Figure 63
APOCRINE ADENOSIS
Large nuclei with prominent nucleoli are present in an area of apocrine metaplasia. The epithelium has vacuolated cytoplasm.

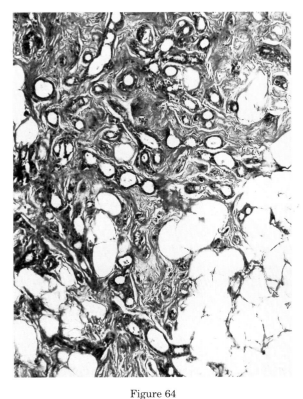

Figure 64
TUBULAR ADENOSIS
Irregular tubules lacking a lobulocentric distribution branch through mammary stroma.

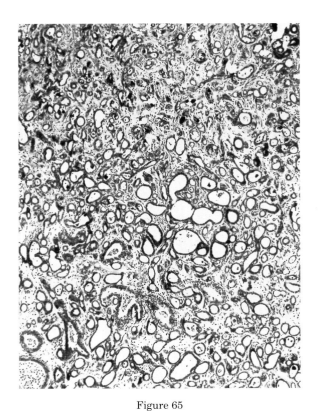

Figure 65
TUBULAR ADENOSIS
Poorly circumscribed aggregate of ducts that are elongated and appear to branch in three dimensions. (Figures 65 and 66 are from the same patient.)

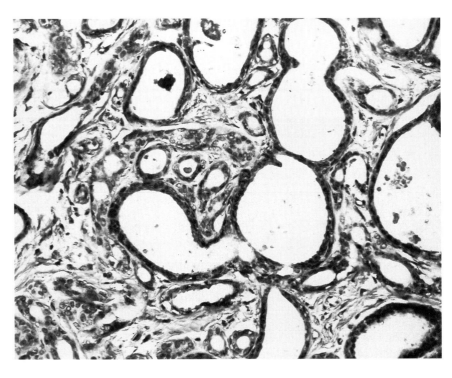

Figure 66
TUBULAR ADENOSIS
Ductal branching is evident as is lining of the ducts by epithelium and myoepithelium.

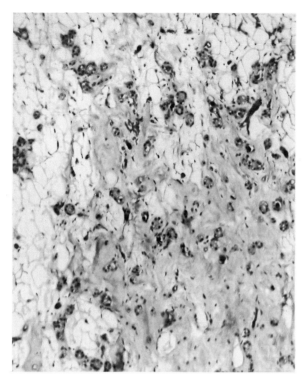

Figure 67
MICROGLANDULAR ADENOSIS
Haphazard distribution of ducts of uniform size. Extension into fat may cause confusion with invasive carcinoma.

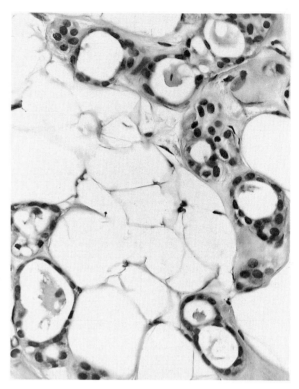

Figure 68
MICROGLANDULAR ADENOSIS
Lining epithelium has uniform nuclei and focally vacuolated cytoplasm. Myoepithelium is absent. The luminal secretion stains positively with the periodic acid–Schiff reagent.

Microglandular Adenosis. Microglandular adenosis differs from other forms of adenosis since the glandular units are haphazardly scattered rather than lobulocentric, lacking the characteristic whorled appearance (fig. 67). Some authors have reported that the myoepithelial layer is absent (32,34) while others claim to have found such cells with immunohistochemical studies (19). Although usually an incidental microscopic finding, these lesions occasionally result in a clinically and grossly identifiable mass. Small round glands are distributed haphazardly in fibrofatty mammary stroma resulting in an infiltrative growth pattern. The intervening stroma may consist of fat or hypocellular collagenous tissue much less cellular than the desmoplastic stroma of a carcinoma (34). The glands or ductules are round to oval and the epithelial lining usually is cuboidal, with discrete, bland nuclei and abundant, frequently clear cytoplasm (figs. 68, 69). Apocrine snouts are inconspicuous. The lumen characteristically contains eosinophilic, PAS-positive secretion that may calcify.

Adenomyoepithelial Adenosis. This rare lesion has a pattern resembling microglandular adenosis but the glands contain a prominent myoepithelial layer (27). The lesion consists of multiple foci of haphazardly arranged ductules with luminal secretion and lining epithelium similar to microglandular adenosis. However, in contrast to the latter lesion, there is greater variation in shape and size of the ducts and the lining epithelium may be tall columnar. Most significant is the presence of a peripheral layer of myoepithelial cells that may manifest hyperplasia. Squamous metaplasia may be present. Apocrine metaplasia has been described in this setting; however, application of the term apocrine adenosis for the abnormality results in confusion with the more common appearance of apocrine adenosis described above (21).

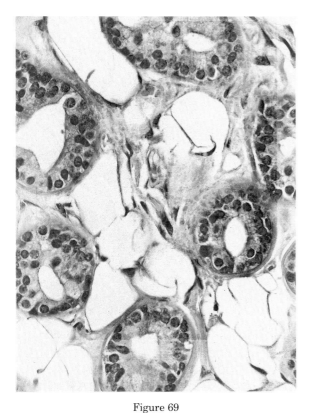

Figure 69
MICROGLANDULAR ADENOSIS
Multilayering of epithelial cells associated with granular cytoplasm.

Differential Diagnosis. Florid, tubular, and microglandular patterns of adenosis are likely to be confused with tubular carcinoma, and sclerotic areas of adenosis with severe attenuation of ducts may resemble invasive lobular carcinoma.

Microglandular adenosis may present a problem in differential diagnosis due to the apparent absence of a myoepithelial layer and the disorderly arrangement of glands. The round profile of the glands, the bland character of the cuboidal epithelial cells with frequent cytoplasmic vacuolation, and luminal secretion help distinguish it from tubular carcinoma.

Sclerosing adenosis with marked ductular attenuation is distinguished from small foci of invasive lobular carcinoma by the retention of a nodular lobulocentric configuration and the absence of cytologic pleomorphism. In this form of adenosis, which lacks evident ductules, the persisting cellular elements usually are spindled myoepithelial cells. Classic invasive lobular carcinoma is composed of rounded cells arranged in rather rigid

linear arrays. Invasive lobular carcinoma may be present in multiple isolated microscopic foci but a lobulocentric distribution is absent.

Prognosis and Treatment. Accurate diagnosis of adenosis is important to avoid confusion with invasive carcinoma rather than for its prognostic implications for the patient. Emphasis on this differential diagnostic problem in educational programs over the past half century has led to increasingly accurate recognition of the lesion by pathologists. The less common variant forms, noted above, cause the greatest degree of diagnostic difficulty.

Adenosis is a manifestation of fibrocystic change that is generally considered to lack significance as a risk factor for subsequent carcinoma. However, a recent study questions this (26). In addition, microglandular adenosis is subject to changes leading to invasive carcinoma in which the cells have granular or clear cytoplasm (33). Neoplastic transition has been associated with the appearance of pleomorphic glands in the lesion. Such atypical microglandular adenosis should be completely excised.

Carcinoma in Adenosis

The finding of noninvasive carcinoma arising in an area of adenosis is unusual (31), although it is not uncommon for adenosis to be invaded by carcinoma from another part of the breast. Since sclerosing adenosis and fibroadenomas are derived from the mammary lobule, it is not surprising that lobular carcinoma in situ arises in these lesions more often than intraductal carcinoma (figs. 70, 71). Although the number of cases reported is small, noninvasive carcinoma may arise in adenosis tumor more often than in other forms of adenosis (28).

While carcinoma localized to an area of adenosis implies a favorable prognosis, the majority of reported patients with noninvasive carcinoma arising in adenosis also had foci of noninvasive carcinoma elsewhere in the breast. However, none had axillary lymph node metastases (23).

Appropriate therapy depends on distinguishing this uncommon presentation of noninvasive carcinoma from invasive carcinoma. This distinction is more difficult when adenosis is involved by in situ lobular rather than intraductal carcinoma. Identification of a myoepithelial layer surrounding the neoplastic ducts is useful in resolving difficult cases (22).

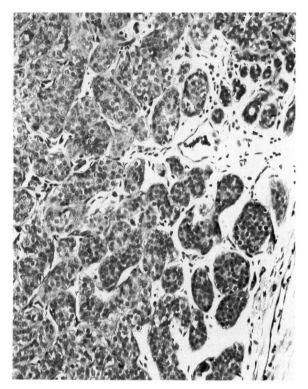

Figure 70
CARCINOMA IN ADENOSIS
Lobular carcinoma in situ arising in sclerosing adenosis. Note uninvolved glands in the upper right corner.

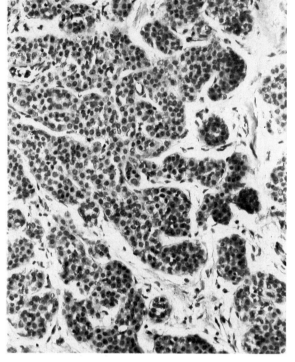

Figure 71
CARCINOMA IN ADENOSIS
The tubular pattern of adenosis is evident in this area at the periphery of the lesion.

RADIAL SCLEROSING LESION

This is a localized, nonencapsulated stellate lesion consisting of a fibroelastotic core and radiating bands of fibrous connective tissue containing lobules manifesting adenosis and ducts with papillary or diffuse intraductal hyperplasia (fig. 72). The lesion has been given various names, including sclerosing papillomatosis, sclerosing papillary proliferation (39), nonencapsulated sclerosing lesion (40), infiltrating epitheliosis (37), indurative mastopathy (47), radial scar (43), obliterative mastopathy (41), and scleroelastotic lesion (38). All of these refer to the radial character of the lesion, as well to its central hyalinizing fibrosis and elastosis with entrapped ducts and lobules (46). However, none of these terms is entirely satisfactory. Since the lesion may contain adenosis or papilloma alone or in combination, a name referring only to one component is suboptimal (infiltrating epitheliosis, sclerosing papillomatosis, sclerosing papillary prolifera-

tion). On the other hand, terms that refer only to the stromal component are nonspecific (scleroelastic lesion) as are names that refer to palpatory findings (indurative mastopathy), since the majority of these lesions are not palpable. Radial scar suggests histogenesis in a scarring process, but a postinflammatory pathogenesis is entirely hypothetical. As a consequence, we prefer the term radial sclerosing lesion; it describes the configuration of the process histologically and mammographically, but is sufficiently nonspecific to encompass the broad range of microscopic components encountered in these lesions.

Clinical Presentation. These lesions are most often of microscopic dimension and therefore not palpable. Their frequency in reported series depends on the thoroughness with which the breast is examined by the pathologist. When large, the stellate appearance can be confused with carcinoma, both grossly and radiologically. The mammogram shows delicate linear densities radiating from a dense central nidus resulting

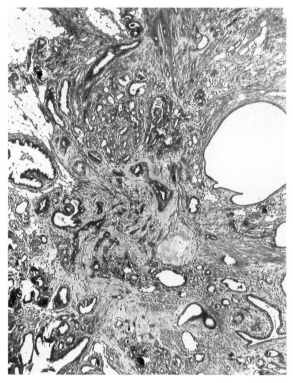

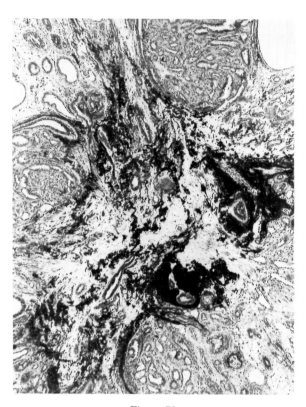

Figure 72
RADIAL SCLEROSING LESION
This epithelial proliferation is composed largely of adenosis surrounding the central area of fibrosis and elastosis with entrapped ducts. Cysts are commonly present at the periphery of a radial sclerosing lesion.

Figure 73
RADIAL SCLEROSING LESION
Central elastosis in the lesion is emphasized here with the elastica stain.

from the alternating interdigitation of fat and cysts with bands of connective tissue. Failure to visualize many of the lesions by X ray is due to the absence of this mixture of fat and collagen at the periphery. Microcalcifications are most often seen in the mammogram when the lesion contains areas of adenosis since this component is more likely to develop calcifications than is isolated duct hyperplasia.

The frequency of these lesions in pathologic studies is variable. Wellings and Alpers (49), using serial subgross examination, found radial sclerosing lesions in 14 percent of breasts. Nielsen et al. (45) examined multiple tissue blocks from breasts obtained at autopsy and noted radial sclerosing lesions in 28 percent of adult women. Fisher et al. (40) studying biopsy specimens, detected them in 4 percent of breasts (40). In the majority of patients these lesions are multicentric and bilateral.

Gross Findings. While most of these lesions are visualized solely on microscopic examination, many identified by the radiologist may be seen on gross examination. The central area is characteristically white and retracted from surrounding tissue, resembling a scar. It often contains chalky streaks, thereby simulating the appearance of a carcinoma (pl. I). Narrow bands of connective tissue extend into the adjacent fat from this central nidus. Other lesions form a less discrete area of fibrosis, lacking the more characteristic stellate appearance.

Microscopic Findings. The central nidus of characteristic lesions consists of fibrosis and elastosis engulfing attenuated ducts. These ducts are haphazardly arranged and distorted, but they are consistently lined by epithelium and myoepithelium. The fibrosis forms dense bundles of collagen, which contrast with the somewhat basophilic, amorphous areas of elastosis (fig. 73). Areas of elastosis can be highlighted with elastica stains that emphasize periductal condensation.

PLATE I

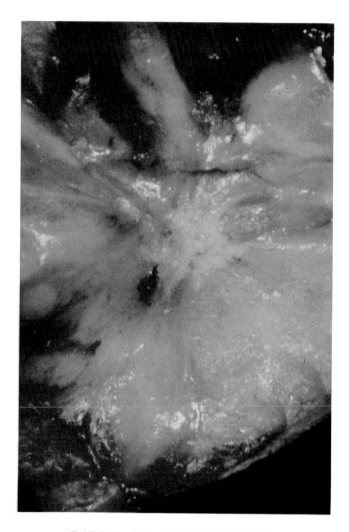

RADIAL SCLEROSING LESION

The irregular scar at the center of the lesion, representative of the area of dense fibrosis and elastosis, resembles a carcinoma.

Central elastosis and associated ductal distortion may be less evident in very small lesions. In such instances the radiating growth pattern related to adenosis is present, and periductal elastosis may not be appreciated in routinely stained sections.

Foci of sclerosing adenosis and intraductal hyperplasia, often papillary in configuration, with associated fibrosis, comprise the periphery of the lesion. The nodular areas of adenosis and intraductal epithelial proliferation may be retracted toward the nidus. Ducts in this location may be cystic and have apocrine epithelium; the cysts sometimes dominate the microscopic picture. In addition, squamous metaplasia may be present in ducts (fig. 74) and, rarely, small areas of central necrosis are present in proliferative ducts. This finding should not be regarded as evidence of carcinoma arising in the radial sclerosing lesion when the proliferative epithelium resembles the epithelium of hyperplastic ducts that lack necrosis.

Although periductal elastosis may be seen in the periphery, irregular "clouds" of elastosis are restricted to the center of the lesion. As noted above, microcalcifications may occur in the areas of adenosis. Entrapped nerves may be present in this area. Most important is the failure of any of the ducts to extend into adjacent fat.

These lesions are most common in breasts with multiple foci of adenosis, suggesting that this process contributes to the formation of radial sclerosing lesions (48). The presence of both adenosis and papillary intraductal hyperplasia is in keeping with the occasional detection of transitional growth patterns suggesting an occasional kinship between the two proliferative abnormalities (46).

Differential Diagnosis. The distinction of this lesion from invasive carcinoma, especially the tubular variety, is important. Tubular carcinoma often has a stellate configuration but the neoplastic ducts consistently lack a myoepithelial investment and they may invade adjacent fat. It may prove helpful to demonstrate the myoepithelial layer with immunohistochemical methods (42). In addition, the connective tissue surrounding ducts of invasive tubular carcinoma typically is loosely arranged, in contrast to the dense fibroelastotic stroma in the center of these lesions. Many radial sclerosing lesions have a cystic apocrine component that is not a regular feature of tubular carcinoma.

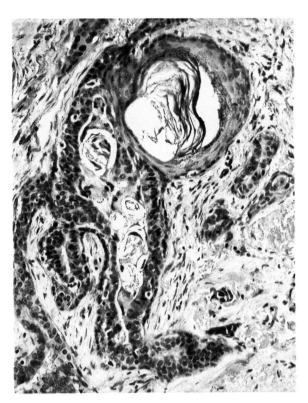

Figure 74
RADIAL SCLEROSING LESION
Squamous metaplasia of small duct in the center of a lesion.

Prognosis and Treatment. There is debate as to whether these lesions are precursors to tubular carcinoma, a speculation first proposed by Linell et al. (43) and furthered by Fisher et al. (40). Wellings and Alpers (45) could neither confirm nor deny the premalignant character of radial sclerosing lesions, yet concluded that they represent a marker of increased risk of subsequent carcinoma. However, most authors have concluded that they are benign abnormalities with little increased risk of subsequent carcinoma. Nielsen et al. (44,45) found no difference in the frequency of these lesions among women with and without breast carcinoma at autopsy. Andersen and Gram (36) in a follow-up study of 32 women with these lesions found only 1 patient who subsequently developed carcinoma over a mean interval of 19.5 years. In common with the majority of authors, Rickert et al. (47) concluded that these were benign variants of adenosis which progressed to sclerosis rather than carcinoma.

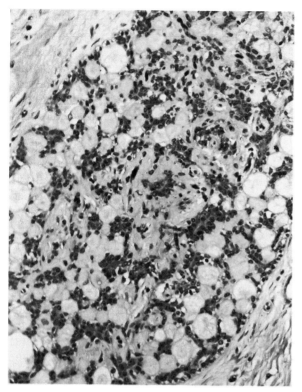

Figure 75
COLLAGENOUS SPHERULOSIS
Circumcribed lesion with acellular spherules surrounded by narrow cords of epithelium. Mucin-containing glands characteristic of adenoid cystic carcinoma are absent. (Figures 75 and 76 are from the same patient.)

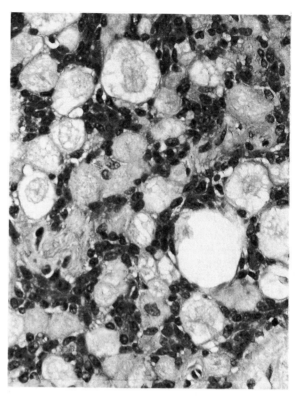

Figure 76
COLLAGENOUS SPHERULOSIS
Higher magnification indicates the uniformity and lack of atypism of the epithelial cells.

While carcinomas may arise in radial sclerosing lesions, this occurs infrequently and there is insufficient evidence to consider them premalignant. In this respect, radial sclerosing lesions are similar to other benign lobular duct–derived lesions such as sclerosing adenosis and fibroadenoma. Therefore, local excision is adequate treatment, and there is little reason for particularly vigorous follow-up of these patients.

COLLAGENOUS SPHERULOSIS

This is a peculiar form of intraductal epithelial proliferation detected as an incidental microscopic finding during examination of a breast biopsy (50). Most characteristic of the lesion is the presence of well-circumscribed, acellular, 20 to 100 micron spherules surrounded by narrow cords of bland, ovoid to round cells that stain positively for actin, suggesting myoepithelial differentiation (figs. 75, 76). The epithelial proliferation is associated with duct ectasia, and, aside from the presence of the spherules, is comparable to that seen in intraductal hyperplasia. These foci most commonly are solitary, although they can be multiple.

The spherules are eosinophilic and fibrillar, and appear to consist of basement membrane material. Some spherules coalesce, others seem hollow, and they are rarely calcified. The condition may be seen in approximately 1 to 2 percent of biopsies, and is commonly associated with other conditions, such as sclerosing adenosis, intraductal papillomas, or radial sclerosing lesions. There is no evidence to suggest that this lesion results in an increased risk of carcinoma. The resemblance of the lesion to adenoid cystic carcinoma has led to the suggested designation of adenoid cystic hyperplasia (51).

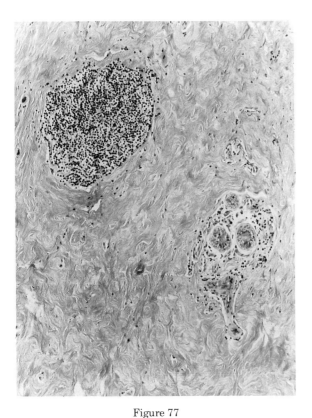

Figure 77
DIABETIC MASTOPATHY
Lymphocytic infiltrate localized around small blood vessels that largely spares the lobule.

DIABETIC MASTOPATHY

The occurrence of fibrous tumor-forming stromal proliferation in patients with diabetes mellitus was first noted in 1984 (56) and subsequently described as mastopathy in insulin-dependent diabetics (52), fibrous disease in juvenile diabetes (53), and diabetic mastopathy (57). Alterations in collagen metabolism that occur in diabetics may contribute to this lesion.

Clinical Presentation. All reported examples of diabetic mastopathy have been in females. Most were 20 years or less in age when type I insulin-dependent diabetes mellitus was diagnosed. Two patients with type II diabetes have been described (57). The mean ages at onset of diabetes in two studies were 12 and 13 years, respectively (53,56). Age at biopsy ranged from 19 to 63 years with a mean of 34 to 40 years in four studies. The interval between onset of diabetes and detection of the breast lesion has averaged about 20 years. Bilateral lesions have been diagnosed in

about 50 percent of reported cases. The majority of the patients had complications of juvenile onset diabetes such as retinopathy and renal impairment.

The initial clinical symptom is a firm to hard nontender tumor. The mammogram reveals localized increased density but no changes specifically associated with this condition.

Gross Findings. The tumors measured 2 to 6 cm in one study. Most specimens do not contain a visible tumor, but a distinct firm or hard mass is palpable and the area of involvement has a firm edge when bisected. The palpable lesion consists of homogeneous white to pale grey tissue that may be trabeculated but is often indistinguishable from the surrounding fibrous breast parenchyma. Cysts and other gross alterations of proliferative breast disease are not an integral part of diabetic mastopathy.

Microscopic Findings. The tissue consists of collagenous stroma with a slightly increased density of fibroblasts when compared to the surrounding breast tissue. Polygonal epithelioid fibroblasts are found dispersed in the collagen among more characteristic spindly fibroblasts. The stromal cells exhibit no cytologic abnormalities. Multinucleated stromal cells and mitotic activity are not part of this proliferative process. Mature lymphocytes are clustered circumferentially around and in the walls of small blood vessels throughout the lesion but they tend to spare lobules and ducts (fig. 77). Germinal centers are rarely formed. Stromal collagen fibers may appear prominent but they do not have a keloidal appearance. Histochemical studies have failed to demonstrate any unusual or specific features in the collagen (54). The lymphocytic infiltrate is composed predominantly of B cells, a feature suggested to be associated with diabetic mastitis since nondiabetic mastitis has a higher proportion of T cells (57). However, Schwartz and Strauchen (55) studied eight patients with a lesion they characterized as lymphocytic mastopathy and reported that only one had diabetes mellitus but in all cases the lymphocytic infiltrate had a B-cell phenotype.

Prognosis and Treatment. Diabetic mastopathy appears to be a self-limiting stromal abnormality of premenopausal women. Tumors have recurred in the ipsilateral breast in a minority of cases. These patients are prone to asynchronous, as well as synchronous bilateral involvement. Excisional biopsy is adequate treatment.

REFERENCES

1. Bartow SA, Black WC, Waeckerlin RW, Mettler FA. Fibrocystic disease: a continuing enigma. Pathol Annu 1982;17(Pt 2):93–111.
2. Cancer Committee of the College of American Pathologists. Is "fibrocystic disease" of the breast precancerous? Arch Pathol Lab Med 1986;110:171–3.
3. Frantz VK, Pickren JW, Melcher GW, Auchincloss H Jr. Incidence of chronic cystic disease in so-called "normal breasts." Cancer 1951;4:762–83.
4. Hughes LE, Mansel RE, Webster DJ. Aberrations of normal development and involution (ANDI): a new perspective on pathogenesis and nomenclature of benign breast disorders. Lancet 1987;2:1316–9.
5. Love SM, Gelman RS, Silen W. Fibrocystic "disease" of the breast—a nondisease? N Engl J Med 1982;307:1010–4.

Cysts and Apocrine Metaplasia

6. Haagensen CD. Diseases of the breast. Philadelphia: WB Saunders Co, 1986:259–65.
7. Martin JE, Gallager HS. Reflections on benign disease: a radiographic-histologic correlation. In: Gallager HS, ed. Early breast cancer detection and treatment. New York: John Wiley and Sons, 1975:177–81.
8. Mazoujian G, Pinkus GS, Davis S, Haagensen DE Jr. Immunohistochemistry of a gross cystic disease fluid protein (GCDFP-15) of the breast. A marker of apocrine epithelium and breast carcinomas with apocrine features. Am J Pathol 1983;110:105–12.
9. Page DL, Vander Zwaag R, Rogers LW, Williams LT, Walker WE, Hartmann WH. Relation between component parts of fibrocystic disease complex and breast cancer. JNCI 1978;61:1055–63.
10. Vilanova JR, Simon R, Alvarez J, Rivera-Pomar JM. Early apocrine change in hyperplastic cystic disease. Histopathology 1983;7:693–8.
11. Wellings SR, Alpers CE. Apocrine cystic metaplasia: subgross pathology and prevalence in cancer-associated versus random autopsy breasts. Hum Pathol 1987;18:381–6.

Focal Fibrosis

12. Azzopardi JG. Problems in breast pathology. Philadelphia: WB Saunders Co, 1979:89–90.
13. Haagensen CD. Diseases of the breast. Philadelphia: WB Saunders Co, 1956:191.
14. Minkowitz S, Hedayati H, Hiller S, Gardner B. Fibrous mastopathy. Cancer 1973;32:913–6.
15. Puente JL, Potel J. Fibrous tumor of the breast. Arch Surg 1974;109:391–4.
16. Rivera-Pomar JM, Vilanova JR, Burgos-Bretones JJ, Arocena G. Focal fibrous disease of breast. A common entity in young women. Virchows Arch [A] 1980;386:59–64.
17. Vassar PS, Culling CF. Fibrosis of the breast. Arch Pathol 1959;67:128–33.

Adenosis and Variant Lesions

18. Carter DJ, Rosen PP. Atypical apocrine metaplasia in sclerosing lesions of the breast: a study of 51 patients. Mod Pathol 1991;4:1–5.
19. Diaz NM, Wick MR, McDivitt RW. Microglandular adenosis of the breast: an immunohistochemical comparison with tubular carcinoma [Abstract]. Mod Pathol 1991;4:10A.
20. Eusebi V, Azzopardi JG. Vascular infiltration in benign breast disease. J Pathol 1976;118:9–16.
21. _____, Casadei GP, Bussolati G, Azzopardi JG. Adenomyoepithelioma of the breast with a distinctive type of apocrine adenosis. Histopathology 1987;11:305–15.
22. _____, Collina G, Bussolati G. Carcinoma in situ in sclerosing adenosis of the breast: an immunocytochemical study. Semin Diagn Pathol 1989;6:146–52.
23. Fechner RE. Lobular carcinoma in situ in sclerosing adenosis. A potential source of confusion with invasive carcinoma. Am J Surg Pathol 1981;5:233–9.
24. Foote FW, Stewart FW. Comparative studies of cancerous versus noncancerous breasts. Ann Surg 1945;121:6–53.
25. Jao W, Recant W, Swerdlow MA. Comparative ultrastructure of tubular carcinoma and sclerosing adenosis of the breast. Cancer 1976;38:180–6.
26. Jensen RA, Page DL, DuPont WD, Rogers LW. Invasive breast cancer risk in women with sclerosing adenosis. Cancer 1989;64:1977–83.
27. Kiaer H, Nielsen B, Paulsen S, Sörensen IM, Dyreborg U, Blichert-Toft M. Adenomyoepithelial adenosis and low-grade malignant adenomyoepithelioma of the breast. Virchows Arch [A] 1984;405:55–67.
28. Nielsen BB. Adenosis tumour of the breast—a clinicopathological investigation of 27 cases. Histopathology 1987;11:1259–75.
29. Oberman HA. Benign breast lesions confused with carcinoma. In: McDivitt RW, Oberman HA, Ozzello L, Kaufman N, eds. The breast. Baltimore: Williams & Wilkins, 1984:1–33.
30. _____, French AJ. Chronic fibrocystic disease of the breast. Surg Gynecol Obstet 1961;112:647–52.
31. _____, Markey BA. Noninvasive carcinoma of the breast presenting in adenosis. Mod Pathol 1991;4:31–5.

32. Rosen PP. Microglandular adenosis. A benign lesion simulating invasive mammary carcinoma. Am J Surg Pathol 1983;7:137–44.

33. Rosenblum MK, Purrazzella R, Rosen PP. Is microglandular adenosis a precancerous disease? A study of carcinoma arising therein. Am J Surg Pathol 1986;10:237–45.

34. Tavassoli FA, Norris HJ. Microglandular adenosis of the breast. A clinicopathologic study of 11 cases with ultrastructural observations. Am J Surg Pathol 1983; 7:731–7.

35. Taylor HB, Norris HJ. Epithelial invasion of nerves in benign diseases of the breast. Cancer 1967;20:2245–9.

Radial Sclerosing Lesion

36. Andersen JA, Gram JB. Radial scar in the female breast. A long-term follow-up study of 32 cases. Cancer 1984;53:2557–60.

37. Azzopardi JG. Problems in breast pathology. Philadelphia: WB Saunders Co, 1979:174–88.

38. Eusebi V, Grassigli A, Grosso F. Lesioni focali sclero-elastotiche mammarie simulanti il carcinoma infiltrante. Pathologica 1976; 68:507–18.

39. Fenoglio C, Lattes R. Sclerosing papillary proliferations in the female breast. A benign lesion often mistaken for carcinoma. Cancer 1974;33:691–700.

40. Fisher ER, Palekar AS, Kotwal N, Lipana N. A nonencapsulated sclerosing lesion of the breast. Am J Clin Pathol 1979;71:240–6.

41. Hamperl H. Strahlige narben und obliterierende mastopathie. Virchows Arch [A] 1975;369:55–68.

42. Hijazi YM, Lessard JL, Weiss MA. Use of anti-actin and S-100 protein antibodies in differentiating benign and malignant sclerosing breast lesions. Surg Pathol 1989; 2:125–35.

43. Linell F, Ljungberg O, Andersson I. Breast carcinoma. Aspects of early stages, progression and related problems. Acta Pathol Microbiol Immunol Scand [A] 1980;Suppl 272:1–233.

44. Nielsen M, Christensen L, Andersen J. Radial scars in women with breast cancer. Cancer 1987;59:1019–25.

45. _____, Jensen J, Andersen JA. An autopsy study of radial scar in the female breast. Histopathology 1985;9:287–95.

46. Oberman HA. Benign breast lesions confused with carcinoma. In: McDivitt RW, Oberman HA, Ozzello L, Kaufman N, eds. The breast. Baltimore: Williams & Wilkins, 1984:1–33.

47. Rickert RR, Kalisher L, Hutter RV. Indurative mastopathy: a benign sclerosing lesion of breast with elastosis which may simulate carcinoma. Cancer 1981;47:561–71.

48. Rosen PP, Oberman HA. Tumors of the breast. Proceedings of the 53rd Annual Anatomic Pathology Slide Seminar of the American Society of Clinical Pathologists. Chicago: ASCP Press, 1987:69–73.

49. Wellings SR, Alpers CE. Subgross pathologic features and incidence of radial scars in the breast. Hum Pathol 1984;15:475–9.

Collagenous Spherulosis

50. Clement PB, Young RH, Azzopardi JG: Collagenous spherulosis of the breast. Am J Surg Pathol 1987; 11:411–7.

51. Rosen PP. Adenoid cystic carcinoma of the breast. A morphologically heterogeneous neoplasm. Pathol Annu 1989; 24(Pt 2):237–54.

Diabetic Mastopathy

52. Byrd BF Jr, Hartmann WH, Graham LS, Hogle HH. Mastopathy in insulin-dependent diabetics. Ann Surg 1987;205:529–32.

53. Gump FE, McDermott J. Fibrous disease of the breast in juvenile diabetes. NY State J Med 1990;90:356–7.

54. Minkowitz S, Hedayati H, Hiller S, Gardner B. Fibrous mastopathy: a clinical histopathologic study. Cancer 1973;32:913–6.

55. Schwartz IS, Strauchen JA. Lymphocytic mastopathy. An autoimmune disease of the breast? Am J Clin Pathol 1990;93:725–30.

56. Soler NG, Khardori R. Fibrous disease of the breast, thyroiditis, and cheiroarthropathy in Type I diabetes mellitus. Lancet 1984;1:193–5.

57. Tomaszewski JE, Brooks JS, Hicks D, LiVolsi VA. Diabetic mastopathy: an autoimmune mastitis? Hum Pathol 1992;23:780–6.

BENIGN EPITHELIAL LESIONS

ADENOMAS

Many breast lesions have been categorized as adenomas, including tubular, lactating, apocrine, and ductal adenomas. The designation has also been applied to pleomorphic adenomas, which closely simulate salivary gland tumors of the same name. All have in common a predominance of benign epithelial elements, a variable stromal component, and circumscription.

Tubular Adenoma

These are circumscribed benign tumors consisting of uniform sized ducts lined by a single layer of epithelium and myoepithelium. They have also been termed "pure" adenomas (15). Most are less than 4 cm in diameter and sharply demarcated from adjacent breast tissue. They are far less common than fibroadenomas.

They present clinically as discrete, freely movable masses, unassociated with nipple discharge or retraction signs, and are most common in young women. In this regard they are indistinguishable from fibroadenomas. There is no association between the occurrence of these tumors and oral contraceptive use or pregnancy (7).

Grossly, these are circumscribed, soft to somewhat rubbery, tan masses. The ducts comprising the lesion are round to oval, in close proximity to one another, and, in contrast to those in fibroadenomas, they are not elongated or compressed (fig. 78). The tubules are lined by a single layer of epithelium subtended by a layer of myoepithelium. While a connective tissue stromal component envelops each duct, it is much less conspicuous, and more uniformly arranged than in fibroadenomas. Cytoplasmic vacuolation of the epithelial cells is not a prominent feature, although eosinophilic secretion may be present in occasional duct lumens. The latter is unassociated with pregnancy or hormonal treatment (14).

These findings may be present focally in a mass that is typical of fibroadenoma, indicating a relationship between the two lesions (fig. 79). In such tumors, the two growth patterns are usually distinct but lack an intervening fibrous separation (7). Ultrastructurally, the ducts of tubular adenomas, and especially their associated epithelial-stromal junctions, are similar to

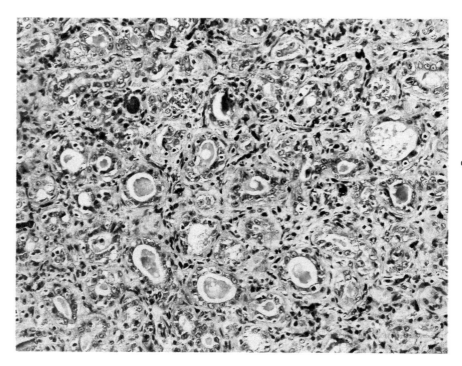

Figure 78
TUBULAR ADENOMA
The tumor is comprised of ducts of uniform size.

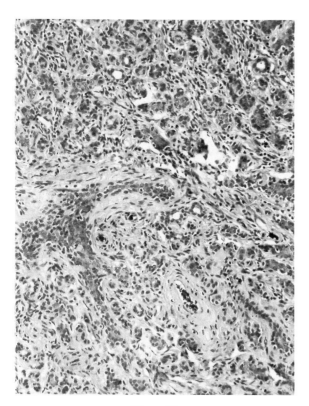

Figure 79
TUBULAR ADENOMA
A tubular adenoma pattern of growth is present above with compressed and elongated ducts, typical of a fibroadenoma, below.

normal breast, differing from the partly disrupted epithelial-stromal junctions seen in fibroadenomas (12). There may be a histogenetic relationship between tubular adenoma and a lactating adenoma.

Tubular adenomas do not recur after local excision. In the only patient reported to have malignant change in one of these tumors (8), metastatic carcinoma in the liver prompted reexamination of an adenoma removed from the breast a month earlier, and a minute area of invasive carcinoma was discovered. Nevertheless, it seems reasonable to conclude that these tumors do not impart an increased risk of carcinoma.

Lactating Adenoma

Lactating adenomas characteristically present as enlarging masses during lactation, although the patient is often first aware of the abnormality during pregnancy. These adenomas are circumscribed benign tumors composed predominantly of glandular structures with scanty stroma with prominent secretory change in the ducts. The histologic findings relate to the stage of pregnancy, and approximate the changes in the adjacent breast. If removed during pregnancy, the secretory changes are less prominent than if the tumor is removed postpartum. This raises the question of whether these are unique tumors or whether they are focally hyperplastic lobules.

Lactating adenomas seem to arise most often in preexisting fibroadenomas or, on occasion, in tubular adenomas (15). As a rule, changes of pregnancy are only focally evident in fibroadenomas, often seeming to spare the tumor, and may be out of sequence with those in the rest of the breast. Origin in tubular adenomas is a more likely possibility, prompting the view that the two lesions represent the same process examined during different physiologic states (7). This opinion has been challenged by finding lactating adenomas with lactational changes somewhat out of phase with the adjacent breast, leading to the opinion that the adenomas were unique lesions (9). The occurrence of tubular adenomas in postpartum patients who first noted the mass during pregnancy, suggests that tubular adenomas may result from involution of a preexisting lactational adenoma (14).

These tumors are usually less than 5 cm in diameter, although occasionally they may be much larger. Typically, they are soft, sharply circumscribed, and consist of ducts with a paucity of surrounding stroma. The ducts contain luminal secretion and are lined by secretory epithelium with cytoplasm distended by lipid-filled vacuoles containing intraluminal secretion. There is no cytologic atypia. Papillary clusters of epithelial cells with an increased nuclear to cytoplasmic ratio may be seen. This feature may cause a false diagnosis of carcinoma in a fine-needle aspiration cytologic specimen (14). Infarction of these lesions may result in a painful mass. Infarcted lactating adenomas may assume considerable size. In this situation, the patient usually becomes aware of a mass earlier in pregnancy, and pain and sudden enlargement occasions its removal.

Apocrine Adenoma

While apocrine metaplasia of ductal epithelium is an extremely common finding in a variety of breast abnormalities, the formation of a clinically and pathologically discrete lesion composed solely of benign ducts lined by apocrine epithelium is extremely unusual (3,19). All of the reported cases have occurred in young women and the tumors have been less than 2 cm in diameter.

Cystic ducts lined by papillary projections of benign apocrine epithelium differentiate these lesions from tubular adenomas. There is no increased incidence of subsequent carcinoma and no tendency for recurrence after tumor removal.

Adenolipoma

Circumscribed masses of mature adipose tissue engulfing mammary ducts may present as palpable or mammographically distinct lesions. These are uncommon, and when their consistency is compared to adjacent breast masses they may be clinically undetectable. Although these lesions were originally termed *adenolipomas* (18), they are best considered variants of mammary hamartoma, as suggested by Arrigoni et al. (1).

Ductal Adenoma

Azzopardi and Salm (2) described this as a solid benign lesion of breast ducts in 1984. Ductal adenomas present as discrete sclerotic nodules, solitary or multiple, although instances of multicentricity appear to involve the same duct system. They rarely exceed 2 cm in greatest dimension. The mean age of the patients in Azzopardi and Salm's series was 51 years.

Most characteristic microscopically is the circumscription of the lesion with intermixture of hyalinizing fibrosis and partly attenuated ductal elements in a nodular pattern surrounded by fibrosis. The lesional ducts are uniformly lined by epithelial and myoepithelial cells, and have a clearly defined basement membrane that can be emphasized with stains for type IV collagen.

In most tumors the lesion appears to be present, at least in part, within a duct lumen associated with a thickened duct wall, suggesting derivation from an intraductal papilloma. Less often, origin from a papilloma is obliterated and the nodules distort adjacent breast tissue; there may be radiating arrangement of the nodular epithelial component with scar-like central fibrosis (fig. 80). Ducts at the periphery of the

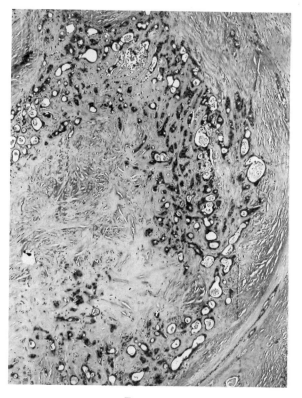

Figure 80
DUCTAL ADENOMA
Circumscribed lesion consisting of dense central fibrosis and peripherally arranged bland ducts.

lesion may have greater luminal calibre than those approaching the center and often contain small sclerotic papillomas.

As in sclerosing adenosis where there is extreme attenuation of ducts, only the spindled myoepithelium may be seen and there may be foci of apparent myoepithelial overgrowth (figs. 81–83). Apocrine metaplasia of the ductal epithelium is present in over half of cases and occasional cells with foamy cytoplasm may be seen. Epithelial cells infrequently manifest nuclear pleomorphism and large nucleoli, possibly attributable to apocrine metaplasia (fig. 84) (6). Microcalcifications are occasionally present and may coalesce to form large densities.

Although ductal adenomas resemble sclerotic intraductal papillomas, Azzopardi and Salm (2) noted that they do not arise particularly in the subareolar region, that they involve small to mid-sized ducts, and that they only rarely are associated with a history of a nipple discharge.

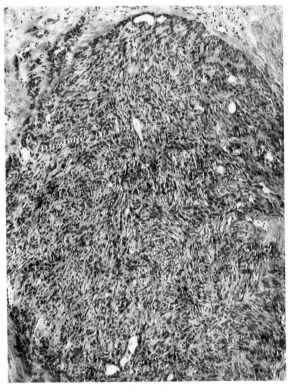

Figure 81
DUCTAL ADENOMA
Nodular lesion composed predominately of spindle cells.
(Figures 81–83 are from the same patient.)

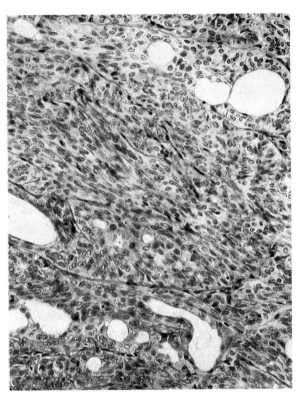

Figure 82
DUCTAL ADENOMA
Spindle cells mingled with residual ducts.

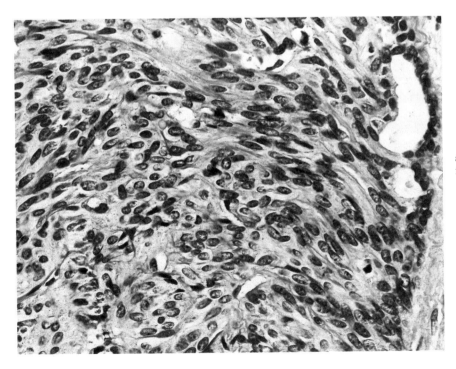

Figure 83
DUCTAL ADENOMA
Spindled myoepithelial cells surround a small duct at the periphery of the tumor.

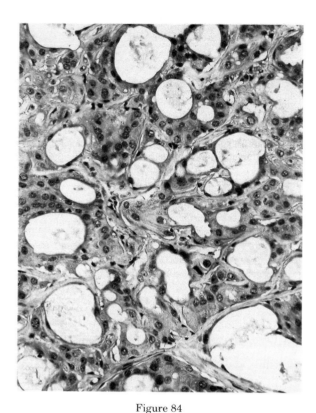

Figure 84
DUCTAL ADENOMA
Ducts lined by apocrine cells may cause confusion with carcinoma.

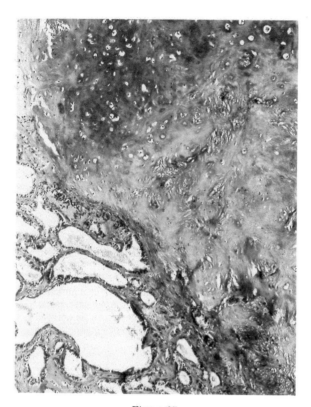

Figure 85
PLEOMORPHIC ADENOMA
Fibrosis with chondroid metaplasia is associated with ectatic mammary ducts.

Lammie and Millis (10) recently reported, however, that ductal adenomas in 8 of their 14 patients were located adjacent to the nipple. Several of the lesions arose in major ducts and 2 patients had blood-stained nipple discharge. Moreover the epithelial component of ductal adenomas and nipple adenomas resembled sclerosing adenosis. Therefore, they hypothesized that sclerosing adenosis may contribute to the pathogenesis of both lesions, although these tumors may evolve from sclerotic intraductal papillomas.

Ductal adenomas are benign. There is no tendency for recurrence after complete excision and no evidence of an increased risk of subsequent carcinoma. It is important to recognize these lesions to avoid possible misinterpretation as a carcinoma.

Pleomorphic "Adenoma" ("Mixed Tumor")

These uncommon breast tumors have histologic features that resemble pleomorphic adenomas (benign mixed tumors) of the salivary glands. They form discrete, firm masses in the breast. All but one of the reported cases have occurred in females (11). The tumors characteristically are solitary, although occasionally multiple, and closely approximated (20). Most are less than 2 cm in greatest dimension; however, a remarkable case of a 17-cm-diameter tumor has been reported (21). Prominent chondroid and osseous metaplasia is a consistent feature. Calcification is common and may be prominent on mammogram (fig. 85).

These tumors are extremely common in dogs, where they comprise almost half of all breast tumors (13). Neutered dogs have a much lower incidence than nonneutered animals, suggesting a hormonal influence. Although only a few cases have been analyzed, elevated estrogen receptor values have been found in human tumors.

The so-called pleomorphic "adenoma" of the breast is an intraductal papilloma with stromal metaplasia, resulting principally from myoepithelial cell proliferation (4). The mesenchymal component is considered to be a result of the multipotential differentiation of myoepithelial cells to form myoid, chondroid, and osseous tissues (16). Evidence for derivation from intraductal papillomas is found in the association with papillomas in most of these tumors, as well as their frequent juxta-areolar location (5). The prominent myoepithelial component suggests an association with ductal adenomas and adenomyoepitheliomas since these tumors are also derived from intraductal papillomas.

The most important differential diagnostic consideration is metaplastic carcinoma. Pseudosarcomatous examples of metaplastic carcinoma, although often circumscribed, manifest at least focal areas of cellular pleomorphism in the metaplastic stroma and usually have recognizable foci of intraductal or invasive carcinoma. Primary sarcomas of the breast with osseous and chondroid components have microscopic features of sarcoma and also lack the epithelial component of metaplastic carcinoma.

Pleomorphic adenomas are benign. Flow cytometric studies indicate a diploid cell population. Treatment consists of adequate local excision. Since local recurrence has been reported, clinical follow-up is recommended (17). If a tumor initially diagnosed as a pleomorphic adenoma of the breast recurs, the lesion should be carefully reevaluated to rule out metaplastic carcinoma.

INTRADUCTAL PAPILLOMA

These discrete benign papillary epithelial tumors arise in the mammary ducts. Although most common in subareolar lactiferous ducts, they may occur elsewhere in the breast, occasionally in cystically dilated ducts where the appellation, *intracystic papilloma*, is appropriate. Dilated ducts containing solitary large intraductal or intracystic papillomas have been termed *papillary cystadenomas*. Multiple intraductal papillomas are far less common and typically involve an aggregate of adjacent ducts in the periphery of the breast, likely representing involvement of several foci in one or two duct systems. Bilateral involvement is rare.

Intraductal papilloma should be distinguished from papillomatosis, a term synonymous with intraductal epithelial hyperplasia. Papillomatosis is a nonspecific term since a variety of microscopic patterns have been associated with it. Microscopic foci of duct hyperplasia may be found in conjunction with intraductal papillomas.

Clinical Presentation. Solitary intraductal papillomas commonly arise in lactiferous ducts and at least 70 percent of patients present with a serous or bloody nipple discharge (27). Less commonly, the patient notices a subareolar mass, although this is more often detected by the examining physician. The perceived mass is the dilated duct, often with surrounding reaction, rather than the papilloma. Solitary intracystic papillomas present as mass lesions in the periphery of the breast or as densities on mammography. The cystic component is better appreciated on ultrasonography or by injection of air into the cystic duct.

Multiple papillomas, in contrast to subareolar solitary papillomas, present as masses in the periphery of the breast. Patients with solitary intraductal papillomas tend to be paramenopausal or postmenopausal, with a peak age incidence in the sixth decade of life, while those with multiple papillomas are usually ten years younger.

Intraductal papillomas also occur in males. In a recently reported case, a papilloma in a male was associated with chronic phenothiazine administration (38), although the majority of male lesions lack a causal association.

Gross Findings. An intraductal papilloma is characteristically found in a dilated duct that may result in a palpable mass. They may be grossly or only microscopically evident. Subareolar intraductal papillomas can attain a diameter of 3 to 4 cm but often much of the lesion is the dilated duct rather than the papilloma. Evidence of recent or past hemorrhage may be seen around the associated duct. Intracystic papillomas, however, often result in palpable masses of considerable size. A 15-cm lesion resulted from the presence of approximately 440 g of blood under pressure in a cystic duct containing a papilloma 4 cm in diameter (37).

Microscopic Findings. The prototype of a benign intraductal papilloma consists of an orderly proliferation of ductal epithelium on well-defined fibrovascular stalks. The epithelium, distributed in a single layer, has little cellular pleomorphism or nuclear hyperchromasia with minimal mitotic activity. The stalk-like projections arise from a single base or from several foci in a dilated duct. A myoepithelial layer is present between the fibrovascular stalk and the epithelial cells. The remainder of the epithelium lining the cystically dilated duct lacks abnormal proliferative activity. Fusion of adjacent papillary processes in portions of a papilloma may result in the formation of duct-like spaces in the lesion lined by myoepithelium and epithelium (fig. 86) (29).

Benign papillomas commonly possess areas of apocrine metaplasia. These are usually focal (figs. 87, 88) (30). Areas of adenosis may be present, often near the base of the lesion (28). This configuration should be distinguished from small foci of intraductal papillary proliferation surrounded by adenosis, often seen as a benign proliferative change in mammary lobules. These areas of papillary intraductal hyperplasia, indistinguishable from small intraductal papillomas, are derived from ectatic ducts at the periphery of an area of adenosis in contrast to larger solitary lesions (31).

Hyalinizing fibrosis is characteristically seen in papillomas, usually commencing at the axis and extending outward to involve the entire lesion (figs. 89, 90). Entrapment of epithelial elements

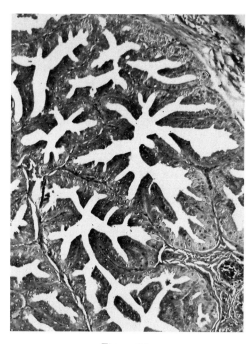

Figure 87
APOCRINE INTRADUCTAL PAPILLOMA
The epithelium lining the papillary fibrovascular fronds was entirely apocrine in this lesion. (Figures 87 and 88 are from the same patient.)

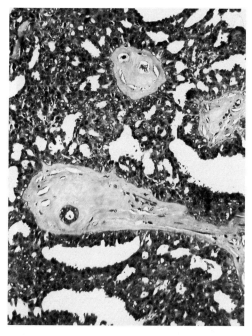

Figure 86
INTRADUCTAL PAPILLOMA
Fusion of adjacent papillary processes composed of epithelial and myoepithelial cells results in the formation of gland-like spaces.

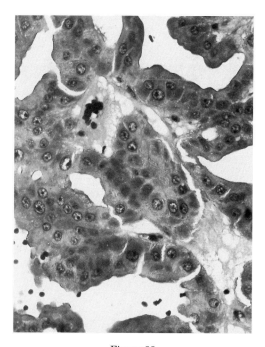

Figure 88
APOCRINE INTRADUCTAL PAPILLOMA
The apocrine epithelium contains large nuclei and prominent nucleoli.

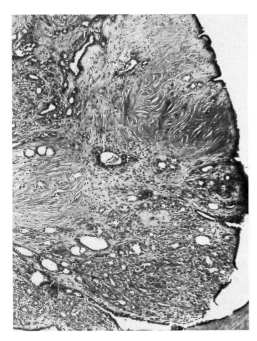

Figure 89
INTRADUCTAL PAPILLOMA
Fibrosis separating ducts at the base of a papilloma results in a pattern that simulates sclerosing adenosis. (Figures 89 and 90 are from the same patient.)

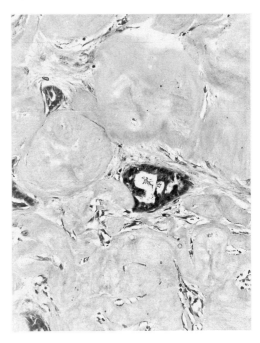

Figure 91
INTRADUCTAL PAPILLOMA
Small ducts surrounded by hyalinized connective tissue in papilloma.

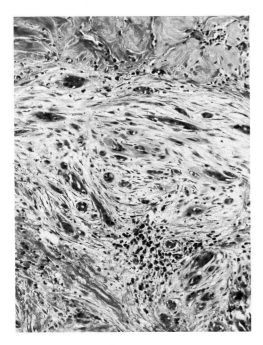

Figure 90
INTRADUCTAL PAPILLOMA
Fibroblastic proliferation, chronic inflammation, and hyalinizing fibrosis are evident here at the base of a papilloma.

by fibrosis may create concern that carcinoma is present (fig. 91). In some lesions the fibrosis may be extensive, virtually obliterating the papilloma, and resembling a nodular scar containing occasional benign epithelial elements. This is the basis for the previously noted association with ductal adenoma.

The papilloma may extend into other levels or branches of the affected duct, resulting in additional areas of involvement or stromal invasion. Although fibrosis may distort the duct, the consistent presence of surrounding myoepithelium permits these foci to be recognized as part of the intraductal lesion and not as evidence of invasion.

Multiple intraductal papillomas produce a mass lesion resulting from involvement of more than one duct system or multiple foci of a single duct system. Three-dimensional microscopic reconstruction studies have shown that these lesions, also termed peripheral papillomas, arise in the terminal duct lobular unit (TDLU) of the duct system whereas solitary papillomas, or central papillomas, usually develop in large segmental ducts, occasionally extending into adjacent smaller ducts but not into the TDLU (33,34). Progression

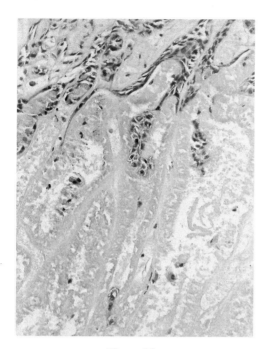

Figure 92
INFARCTED INTRADUCTAL PAPILLOMA
Infarcted papillary fronds below are associated with viable epithelium above.

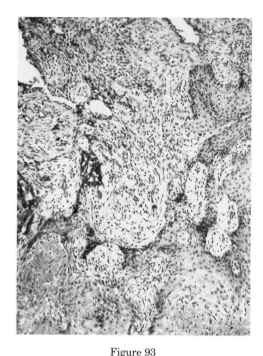

Figure 93
INFARCTED INTRADUCTAL PAPILLOMA
Squamous metaplasia and fibrosis in the wall of a duct containing an infarcted papilloma. (Figures 93–96 are from the same patient.)

from benign papilloma to atypism or carcinoma in adjacent small papillomas in the involved duct system can be demonstrated. Wellings et al. (41) concluded that seemingly large ducts containing papillomas in the periphery of the breast may actually be involved TDLUs with associated unfolding of adjacent lobular ducts (41).

Multiple papillomas, which have a propensity for recurrence as well as for an increased risk of carcinoma, may manifest prominent hyperplasia of the epithelium and myoepithelium (26,32,42). These lesions may be accompanied by intraductal hyperplasia, with or without atypism, in adjacent ducts. This difference distinguishes multiple papillomas from an exaggeration of duct hyperplasia in fibrocystic change, a more diffuse process often affecting much of the breast.

Infarction of intraductal papillomas is relatively uncommon. In most instances no associated cause is evident although hyperprolactinemia was described in a 19-year-old patient (40). Necrosis may involve the entire papilloma or, more often, only a portion. The general outline of the papilloma is preserved in the area of infarction, and foci of dystrophic calcification may be

present (fig. 92). The surrounding tissue usually contains fibroblastic proliferation and collagenization, which may entrap persisting intact duct-like elements of the papilloma. These small ducts may be distorted and their haphazard arrangement can even suggest carcinoma. Squamous metaplasia of viable ductal epithelium may occur adjacent to the infarcted area (fig. 93) (24).

Squamous metaplasia of intraductal papillomas most often occurs as small areas in association with foci of infarction; however, in some instances it is florid, and the pseudoinfiltrative pattern of growth may simulate carcinoma (figs. 94–96). Whether such cases constitute a separate lesion or whether there is obliteration of evidence of a preexisting infarct is difficult to ascertain (39). It has been suggested that the myoepithelial cells, rather than the epithelial cells, undergo squamous metaplasia in these situations (35).

Intraductal papillomas possess a layer of myoepithelial cells but this component is not equally evident in all portions of the lesion. In some areas the distribution of these cells is discontinuous or absent. Alternatively, they may be

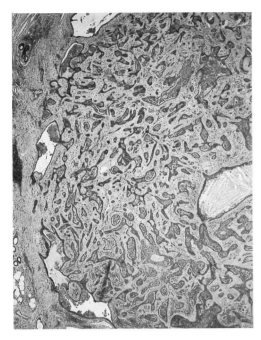

Figure 94
INTRADUCTAL PAPILLOMA
WITH SQUAMOUS METAPLASIA
This low-power view shows an intraductal papilloma with prominent squamous metaplasia. The lumen of the duct containing the papilloma is visible on the left.

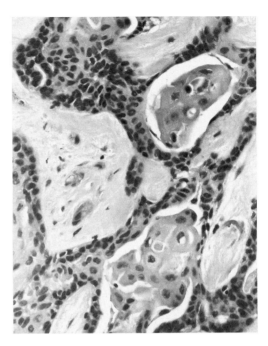

Figure 96
INTRADUCTAL PAPILLOMA
WITH SQUAMOUS METAPLASIA
These elongated ducts centrally located in the papilloma contain keratinized squamous cells.

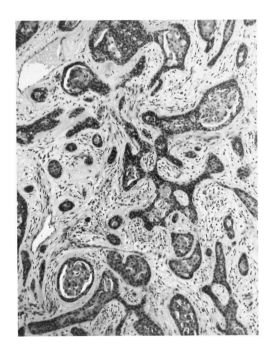

Figure 95
INTRADUCTAL PAPILLOMA
WITH SQUAMOUS METAPLASIA
This view shows the haphazard arrangement of ductal components in the papilloma.

hyperplastic and in rare tumors may dominate the microscopic picture, filling the involved duct to efface the underlying papilloma (fig. 97). An unusual variant of this process occurs when the myoepithelial cells assume a myoid, spindle cell configuration (figs. 98–100).

Differential Diagnosis. The most important consideration in the histologic diagnosis of papillomas is to determine if carcinoma has developed in the lesion. Carcinoma that has arisen in the epithelium of a papilloma exhibits one of the conventional growth patterns of intraductal carcinoma.

Frozen Section. While most intraductal papillomas can readily be diagnosed on frozen section, at times it can be very difficult to recognize carcinoma in a papilloma by this procedure. Frozen section examination of these small papillary tumors may interfere with the quality of subsequent paraffin sections. Since the pathologist cannot anticipate the microscopic findings and since there is little need for rapid diagnosis of this lesion for the management of the patient, it is advisable to defer the diagnosis to paraffin sections when a papillary lesion is suspected.

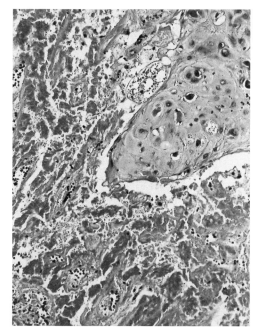

Figure 97
INFARCTED INTRADUCTAL PAPILLOMA
Higher magnification reveals metaplastic epithelium surrounded by necrotic tissue.

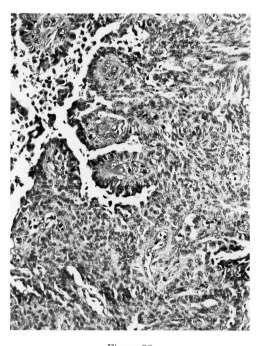

Figure 98
INTRADUCTAL PAPILLOMA WITH SPINDLE CELLS
Papilloma with a predominant spindle cell pattern. The spindle cells are covered by cuboidal to columnar epithelium located on the surface of the papilloma. (Figures 98 and 99 are from the same patient.)

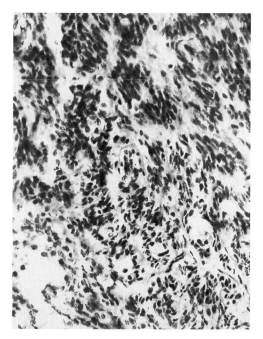

Figure 99
INTRADUCTAL PAPILLOMA WITH SPINDLE CELLS
Packets of spindle cells comprise solid portions of the lesion. The ductal epithelium is markedly attenuated in this area.

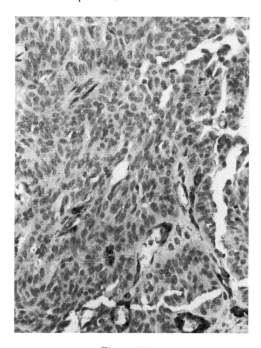

Figure 100
INTRADUCTAL PAPILLOMA WITH SPINDLE CELLS
The spindle cells are not reactive with anti-actin. Actin reactivity is present in vascular elements which are darkly stained below.

Cytology. Fine-needle aspiration cytologic examination of papillary lesions is increasingly performed, especially for intracystic lesions in the periphery of the breast. The procedure holds little value for subareolar papillomas which should be surgically excised and assessed by conventional histopathologic techniques. Cytologic examination of material from a nipple discharge may be diagnostic if carcinoma cells are identified, but cannot be relied upon to rule out carcinoma if the cellular composition is benign.

Aspirated cell clusters from intracystic papillomas are papillary in configuration and a fibrovascular core may occasionally be evident (23). The cells are diploid while cells from intracystic papillary carcinomas may manifest low-grade aneuploidy. Although cellular monomorphism is seen in malignant papillary lesions, a low degree of nuclear atypism is present. The cells aspirated from a papillary carcinoma may have a poorly defined cribriform arrangement. Papillary carcinomas characteristically lack discernible myoepithelial cells.

Prognosis and Treatment. Solitary subareolar or intracystic intraductal papillomas are benign; however, for many years there has been debate as to whether they may be precursors of papillary carcinoma, or whether they may predispose the breast to an increased risk of carcinoma. Most follow-up studies have failed to demonstrate an increased carcinoma risk associated with these lesions. Discrepancies in reported series may be related to the presence of intraductal hyperplasia with atypism elsewhere in the breast of patients with intraductal papillomas who subsequently develop carcinoma.

Foci of carcinomatous change are occasionally present in an otherwise benign solitary papilloma. Often there are foci of intraductal carcinoma in ducts adjacent to such a papilloma. The clinical significance of such areas is poorly understood. It is possible that they represent an uncommon progression from a benign intraductal papilloma to an intraductal papillary carcinoma. These foci of malignant change in an otherwise benign solitary lesion do not warrant overly aggressive treatment and may be controlled by wide excision possibly supplemented with radiation. Solitary papillomas lack implication for an increased risk of subsequent carcinoma in the remainder of the breast and may be

safely treated by local excision (36). On the other hand, multiple intraductal papillomas, which produce a mass in the periphery of the breast, are more often associated with concurrent or subsequent carcinoma. Two of the six patients reported by Carter (22) developed carcinoma, and a similar incidence of associated carcinoma has been noted by others (25).

FLORID PAPILLOMATOSIS OF THE NIPPLE

This lesion is defined in the WHO classification of breast tumors (56) as "a benign epithelial tumor arising in the nipple ducts and showing an intraductal proliferation, often combined in the more advanced stages of its evolution, with a tubular component.... The lesion should be distinguished from discrete papillomas occurring in the subareolar area."

The literature is replete with alternative names for this disease. Before the lesion was well characterized, the terms adenoma or papillomatosis were used. Handley and Thackray (48) preferred adenoma of the nipple, pointing to the absence of papillary components in some lesions. Perzin and Lattes (52) urged the name papillary adenoma since the main feature of the lesion is a papillary proliferation.

None of these terms is an improvement on florid papillomatosis proposed in 1955 by Jones (49), which recognizes that duct hyperplasia is the dominant feature in most cases (fig. 101). Except for location in the nipple, the proliferative patterns of florid papillomatosis are identical to those encountered in radial sclerosing lesions throughout the breast.

Clinical Presentation. The majority of the patients are 40 to 50 years of age (48,49,52,56) with diagnosis ranging from birth (54) to 89 years (45,53). Bilateral involvement is extremely uncommon (43,48).

Fewer than 5 percent of the reported cases of florid papillomatosis of the nipple were in men (50,53–55). The age at diagnosis in men ranged from 43 to 83 years with all but one patient older than 65 years. Three of the 10 male patients had concurrent ipsilateral breast carcinoma (46,54).

Most of these tumors are present for no more than a few months before the patient seeks medical attention. However, there are instances on

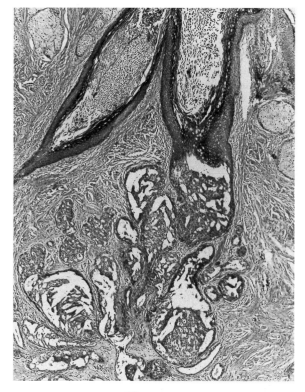

Figure 101
FLORID PAPILLOMATOSIS
Clinically inapparent stage in the formation of the lesion arising in the terminal lactiferous duct at the squamocolumnar junction. (Fig. 9B from Rosen PP, Caicco JA. Florid nipple papillomatosis. Am J Surg Pathol 1986;10:87–101.)

record in which the lesion was reportedly present for 10 (45,53), 11 (48), 14 (55), 15 (54), and 20 (52) years. Flow cytometry in two cases revealed diploid cells with relatively high S-phase fractions of 10.9 and 34.4 percent (51). The most frequent presenting symptom is discharge that is often bloody. Pain, itching, or burning sensations are not unusual. Small lesions may not cause nipple enlargement but in most cases the nipple is enlarged and a mass can be palpated. The surface of the nipple may appear granular or ulcerated and can be mistaken for Paget disease clinically.

Gross and Microscopic Findings. The lesions may be grouped by growth pattern into four categories. In three subtypes one particular structural feature dominates while the fourth group is comprised of tumors that exhibit mixed patterns.

Thus far, no prognostic significance has been attached to these subtypes nor is there evidence that they differ in pathogenesis. However, some clinicopathologic correlations have been noted.

Sclerosing papillomatosis (radial sclerosing) pattern. This lesion typically presents as a discrete tumor. Scaling of the nipple skin may occur but redness, ulceration, and inflammation are rare. About 50 percent of the patients have nipple discharge which is serous rather than bloody.

Histologically, the lesion is indistinguishable from radial sclerosing lesions encountered elsewhere in the breast. Exuberant ductal hyperplasia is arranged in papillary, solid, tubular, and glandular structures that are distorted by stromal proliferation (figs. 102, 103). Foci of myoepithelial cell hyperplasia can usually be identified (fig. 104) (51). Myoepithelial cells may be inconspicuous or absent.

The overlying cutaneous squamous epithelium is usually intact and hyperplastic. Squamous cysts are commonly formed in the terminal portions of lactiferous ducts. Focal comedo-type necrosis may be found in the hyperplastic duct epithelium sometimes associated with scattered mitoses in epithelial cells. Apocrine metaplasia and extension of glandular epithelium to the nipple surface are uncommon and not prominent when present.

Papillomatosis pattern. These patients usually complain of bleeding from the nipple. The nipple often appears ulcerated or inflamed and the clinical diagnosis is likely to be Paget disease or carcinoma. Microscopic examination reveals florid papillary hyperplasia of ductal epithelium causing expansion and crowding of the affected ducts (figs. 105–107). Focal epithelial necrosis and scattered mitotic figures may be found. These tumors lack the sclerosing stromal proliferation that characterizes the radial sclerosing lesion. Hyperplastic glandular tissue may replace the overlying squamous epithelium over part or all of the nipple surface. Squamous-lined cysts and apocrine metaplasia are not prominent in these lesions.

Adenosis pattern. The lesion produces a discrete nodule within the nipple which may have a bloody or serous discharge. The nipple may appear ulcerated, inflamed, and swollen, but the epidermis is usually hyperplastic and intact. Microscopic examination reveals glandular

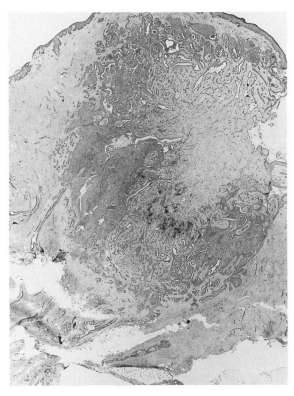

Figure 102
FLORID PAPILLOMATOSIS
Sclerosing variant with a central area of fibrosis and a small area of superficial erosion. (Fig. 1A from Rosen PP, Caicco JA. Florid nipple papillomatosis. Am J Surg Pathol 1986;10:87–101.) (Figures 102–104 are from the same patient.)

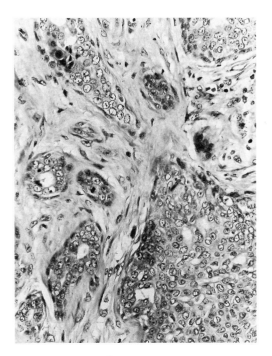

Figure 103
FLORID PAPILLOMATOSIS
Nests of hyperplastic duct epithelium appear detached in the sclerotic stroma. (Fig. 1B from Rosen PP, Caicco JA. Florid nipple papillomatosis. Am J Surg Pathol 1986;10:87–101.)

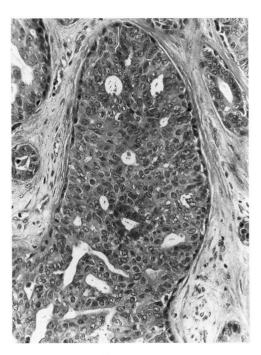

Figure 104
FLORID PAPILLOMATOSIS
Myoepithelial cell hyperplasia at the periphery of a duct.

structures arranged in the pattern of sclerosing adenosis (figs. 108, 109). Myoepithelial hyperplasia accompanies the epithelial proliferation.

Mixed proliferative pattern. Patients with this type of florid papillomatosis report various symptoms including scaling, bleeding, pain, or burning and ulceration. Examination usually reveals a mass or nodule in the nipple and the surface typically appears eroded. As a consequence, the clinical diagnosis is often carcinoma or Paget disease or both.

Microscopic examination reveals varying combinations of the other three patterns. Prominent features include superficial squamous metaplasia of ducts with cysts, apocrine metaplasia, and acanthosis of the overlying epithelium (fig. 110). Focal necrosis may be found in duct epithelium. Mitotic activity is minimal (fig. 111). Adenosis occurs in about one third of these lesions (figs. 112, 113).

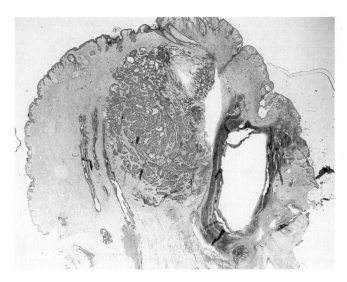

Figure 105
FLORID PAPILLOMATOSIS
Papillomatosis variant characterized by a complex pattern of duct hyperplasia with minimal sclerosis. Defect in the tissue is the site of a recent biopsy. (Figures 105 and 106 are from the same patient.)

Figure 106
FLORID PAPILLOMATOSIS
Branching fronds of hyperplastic epithelium in dilated duct. Note relatively orderly distribution of cells with predominantly basal nuclear orientation along fibrovascular stroma. Epidermis of the nipple is seen above.

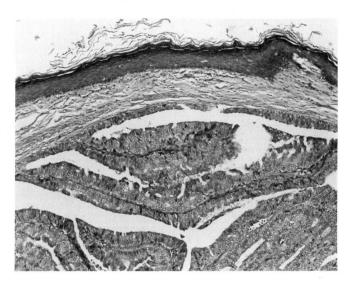

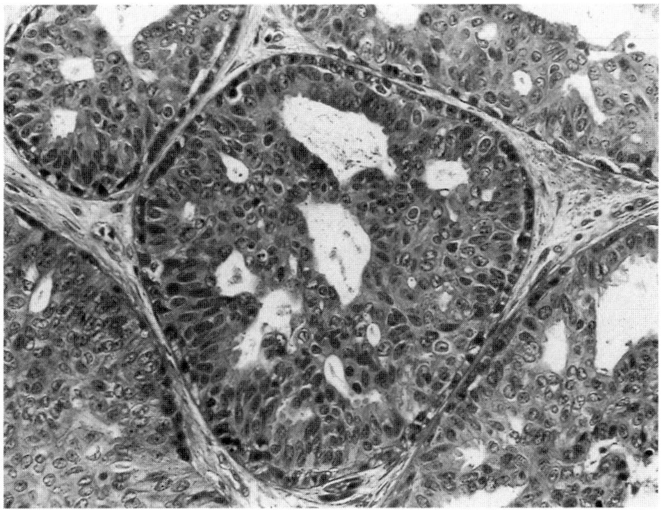

Figure 107
FLORID PAPILLOMATOSIS
WITH ATYPICAL HYPERPLASIA
Although basal nuclear orientation is focally preserved, much of the epithelium has a disorderly growth pattern and lacks stroma. Hyperplastic myoepithelial cells are focally present at the periphery of the ducts.

Figure 108
FLORID PAPILLOMATOSIS
Adenosis variant that is a compact nodular proliferation similar to florid adenosis elsewhere in the breast. (Fig. 3A from Rosen PP, Caicco JA. Florid nipple papillomatosis. Am J Surg Pathol 1986; 10:87–101.) (Figures 108 and 109 are from the same patient.)

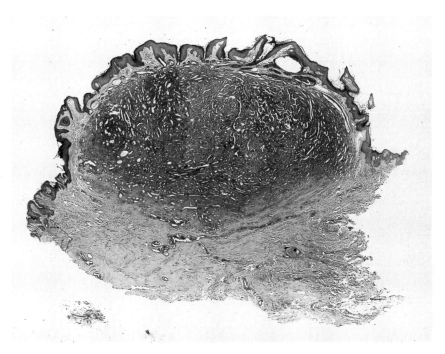

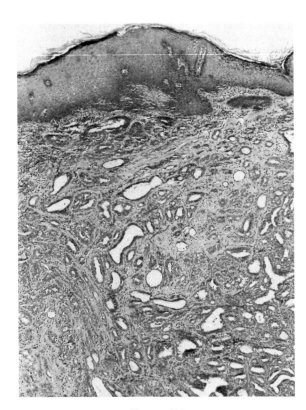

Figure 109
FLORID PAPILLOMATOSIS
Compact arrays of ductules in adenosis lesion beneath the intact nipple epidermis.

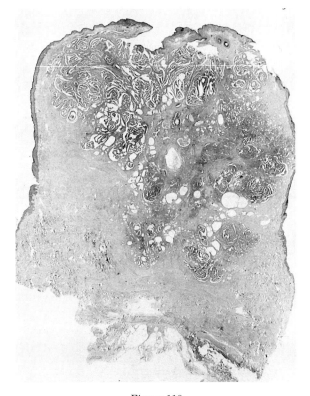

Figure 110
FLORID PAPILLOMATOSIS
Mixed type of lesion with papilloma in upper region, sclerosis in the center, and prominent adenosis on the right. Note cysts throughout the tumor. (Figures 110–112 are from the same patient.)

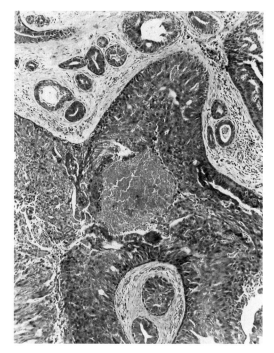

Figure 111
FLORID PAPILLOMATOSIS
Focal necrosis in a hyperplastic duct in an area of sclerosis.

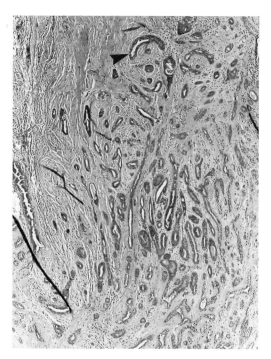

Figure 113
FLORID PAPILLOMATOSIS
Ductular proliferation in this part of the lesion has a syringomatous pattern. Note comma-shaped ductules (arrow). (Fig. 7A from Rosen PP, Caicco JA. Florid nipple papillomatosis. Am J Surg Pathol 1986;10:87–101.)

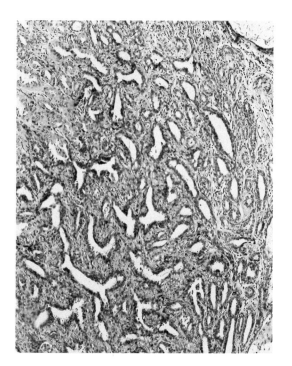

Figure 112
FLORID PAPILLOMATOSIS
Adenosis in an example of mixed florid papillomatosis. Hyperplastic myoepithelial cells fill space between the glands.

Florid Papillomatosis and Mammary Carcinoma. A review of the literature reveals that 37 of 224 (16.5 percent) patients with florid papillomatosis also had mammary carcinoma Nineteen had carcinoma that arose coincidentally, but separately in the same breast. Coincidental carcinomas are usually of the ductal variety. One patient had a separate invasive lobular carcinoma (44) while three patients developed carcinoma in a breast from which florid papillomatosis had been previously excised (52,54).

Carcinoma arose directly from florid papillomatosis in eight patients (three men (46, 54) and five women (44,47,54)). Two of the men and three of the women had intraductal carcinoma; the others had invasive carcinomas.

Carcinoma of the contralateral breast was reported in seven women. Three had bilateral breast carcinoma with florid papillomatosis as a separate coincidental lesion in one breast. The other four patients had florid papillomatosis in the nipple of one breast and carcinoma only in the contralateral breast.

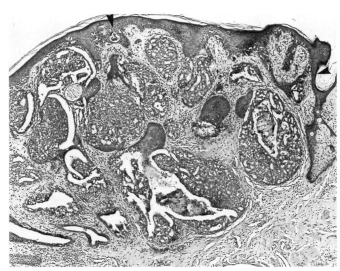

Figure 114
INTRADUCTAL CARCINOMA
IN FLORID PAPILLOMATOSIS
Lesion in the nipple of an adult man. Ducts are very atypical and interpreted as intraductal carcinoma focally because of association with Paget disease. Arrows indicate Paget disease in epidermis. (Figures 114 and 115 are from the same patient.)

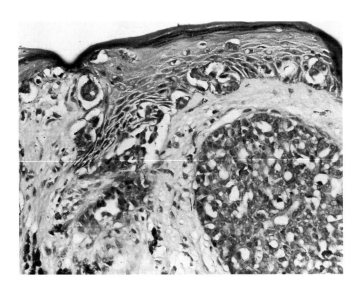

Figure 115
INTRADUCTAL CARCINOMA
IN FLORID PAPILLOMATOSIS
Paget disease in epidermis.

Carcinoma and florid papillomatosis of the nipple are each uncommon lesions of the male breast. Their coexistence in nearly 50 percent of male patients reported to have florid papillomatosis suggests this may be a precancerous lesion in men, especially since all of the carcinomas seem to have arisen in the nipple lesion. The evidence indicating that florid papillomatosis is precancerous in women is less substantial. Nonetheless, a woman with florid papillomatosis should have both breasts carefully examined clinically and radiologically to exclude an independent coincidental carcinoma. If the florid papillomatosis lesion is completely excised and found not to harbor carcinoma, the risk for sub-

sequently developing carcinoma in the same breast seems to be relatively low.

It may be difficult to detect carcinoma arising in florid papillomatosis of the nipple. Hyperplastic areas often exhibit atypical features that may include comedo-type necrosis as well as cribriform and micropapillary growth patterns, mitoses, and cytologic atypia. In the absence of definitive evidence of invasion, Paget disease of the nipple epidermis is the most reliable evidence for a diagnosis of carcinoma arising in florid papillomatosis (figs. 114, 115). A diagnosis of carcinoma is extremely difficult to substantiate when Paget disease or invasive carcinoma are absent (figs. 116–121).

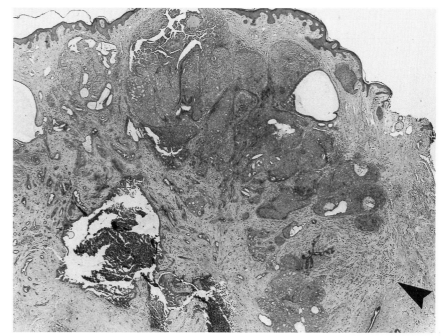

Figure 116
INVASIVE CARCINOMA IN
FLORID PAPILLOMATOSIS
Overview of nipple excised after biopsy in region of hemorrhagic defect (lower left) showed florid papillomatosis. Arrow indicates invasive carcinoma. There is no Paget disease in epidermis. (Fig. 5B from Rosen PP, Caicco JA. Florid nipple papillomatosis. Am J Surg Pathol 1986;10:87–101.) (Figures 116–118 are from the same patient.)

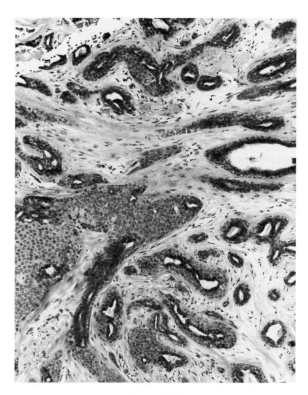

Figure 117
INVASIVE CARCINOMA
IN FLORID PAPILLOMATOSIS
Area of sclerosis with focal solid epithelial proliferation accompanied by myoepithelial hyperplasia. By itself, in the absence of Paget disease or an invasive component, this is interpreted as atypical hyperplasia.

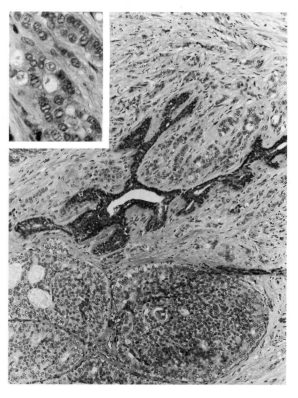

Figure 118
INVASIVE CARCINOMA
IN FLORID PAPILLOMATOSIS
Invasive duct carcinoma surrounds a lactiferous duct in the center. Inset shows a magnified view of the invasive component. (Fig. 5C from Rosen PP, Caicco JA. Florid nipple papillomatosis. Am J Surg Pathol 1986;10:87–101.)

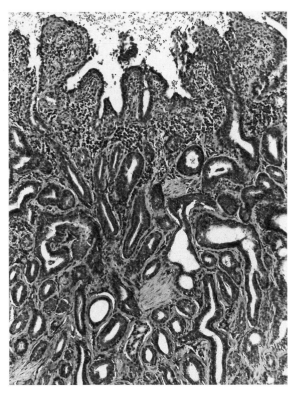

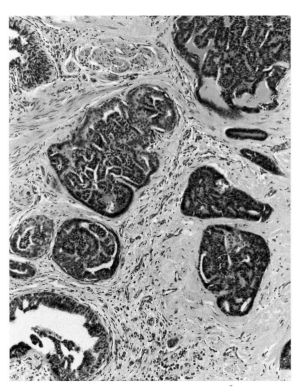

Figure 119
FLORID PAPILLOMATOSIS
AND AXILLARY NODE METASTASES

Superficial portion of the lesion showing erosion and adenosis pattern. (Fig. 7A from Rosen PP, Caicco JA. Florid nipple papillomatosis. Am J Surg Pathol 1986;10:87–101.) (Figures 119–121 are from the same patient.)

Figure 120
FLORID PAPILLOMATOSIS
AND AXILLARY NODE METASTASES

The most atypical proliferation seen in the lesion. No Paget disease or invasive carcinoma was identified in the nipple lesion or in the breast at mastectomy.

Figure 121
FLORID PAPILLOMATOSIS
AND AXILLARY
NODE METASTASES

One axillary lymph node contained metastatic carcinoma with this glandular pattern. (Fig. 7C from Rosen PP, Caicco JA. Florid nipple papillomatosis. Am J Surg Pathol 1986;10:87–101.)

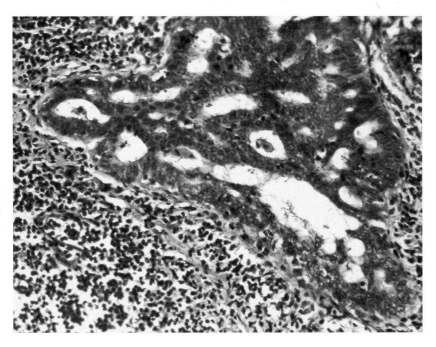

Prognosis and Treatment. Complete excision is recommended treatment for florid papillomatosis. This often requires removal of the nipple. Incisional biopsy or needle biopsy are not satisfactory to exclude the possibility of carcinoma arising in the lesion. Local recurrence may follow subtotal excision (52,54,55), but a substantial number of patients have reportedly remained asymptomatic after incomplete excision. Mastectomy is not indicated as primary treatment of florid papillomatosis unassociated with carcinoma.

SYRINGOMATOUS ADENOMA

This benign locally infiltrating neoplasm of the nipple has a close histopathologic resemblance to microcystic adnexal carcinoma (59) and sclerosing sweat gland duct (syringomatous) carcinoma (57).

Clinical Presentation. The 18 female patients with this lesion reported since 1983 (58,60,62,63) ranged from 11 to 67 years of age at diagnosis (median age, 36 years). One man was 76 years old (62). Syringomatous adenomas are unilateral lesions affecting either breast with approximately equal frequency. The initial symptom is a mass in the nipple or subareolar region. Ulceration and erosion are not seen.

Gross Findings. The excised tumors have measured 1 to 3.5 cm, with a mean of 1.7 cm. Most consist of ill-defined, firm to hard, grey, tan, or white tissue. Discrete nodules and microcystic areas have been noted infrequently.

Microscopic Findings. The lesion consists of tubules, ductules, and strands composed of small, uniform generally basophilic cells infiltrating the dermis of the skin and the stroma of the nipple (fig. 122). Hyperplasia of the epidermis is slight in most cases but occasionally pseudoepitheliomatous hyperplasia may be seen. Neoplastic glands sometimes appear to be connected with the basal layer of the epidermis.

The ducts lined by one or more layers of cells have teardrop, comma-like, and branching shapes with lumens that are usually open and round in cross section (figs. 123, 124). A layer of myoepithelial cells is not apparent (fig. 125). Mitoses are virtually absent and nuclei lack prominent nucleoli or pleomorphism. The lumens are empty or they contain deeply eosinophilic, retracted secretion. Squamous differentiation sometimes results in keratotic cysts (fig. 126).

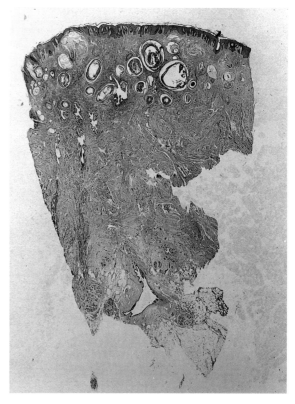

Figure 122
SYRINGOMATOUS ADENOMA
Syringomatous glands are most prominent in nipple just beneath the epidermis where keratotic cysts have been formed. Glandular proliferation extends around lactiferous ducts. (Fig. 1A from Rosen PP. Syringomatous adenoma of the nipple. Am J Surg Pathol 1983;7:739–45.) (Figures 122–125 are from the same patient.)

The syringomatous tubules diffusely infiltrate the periductal stroma of the nipple and in larger lesions may extend into the subareolar breast parenchyma. Invasion into the smooth muscle bundles of the nipple is common and occasionally perineural invasion is observed.

Lesions to be considered in the differential diagnosis of syringomatous adenoma include florid papillomatosis and tubular carcinoma which rarely occurs near the nipple. Despite some structural similarities between the two lesions, syringomatous adenoma and low-grade adenosquamous carcinoma (61) are not, as has been suggested (60), variants of the same neoplastic process. Syringomatous adenoma arises in the nipple and secondarily involves the breast parenchyma underlying the nipple. Low-grade

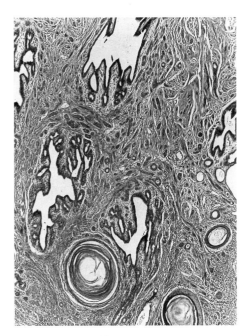

Figure 123
SYRINGOMATOUS ADENOMA
Transverse section of the nipple showing syringomatous glands around lactiferous ducts. (Fig. 1B from Rosen PP. Syringomatous adenoma of the nipple. Am J Surg Pathol 1983;7:739–45.)

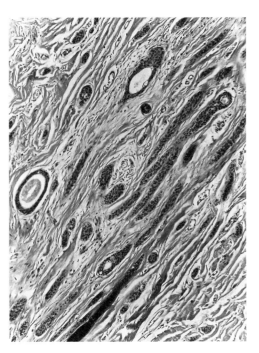

Figure 124
SYRINGOMATOUS ADENOMA
Longitudinal section revealing characteristic syringomatous comma-shaped ducts. (Fig. 1C from Rosen PP. Syringomatous adenoma of the nipple. Am J Surg Pathol 1983;7:739–45.)

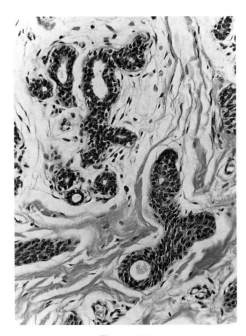

Figure 125
SYRINGOMATOUS ADENOMA
Syringomatous ducts next to a normal terminal duct lobular unit. Note the absence of myoepithelial cells in the neoplastic ducts. (Fig. 1D from Rosen PP. Syringomatous adenoma of the nipple. Am J Surg Pathol 1983;7:739–45.)

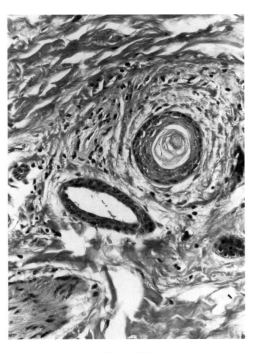

Figure 126
SYRINGOMATOUS ADENOMA
Keratinization in one of two syringomatous ducts.

adenosquamous carcinoma develops peripherally, but may involve the nipple secondarily. It is accompanied by intraductal carcinoma and cartilaginous metaplasia has been found.

Prognosis and Treatment. Most patients have been treated by local excision, which in some instances has required removing the entire nipple. Reexcision is indicated if the margins appear involved (60). There is a 30 percent recurrence rate after incomplete excision (60,62). The time to recurrence has varied from less than 1 year to 4 years. No patients developed metastases in regional lymph nodes or at distant sites and there is no evidence of an association with mammary adenocarcinoma.

SUBAREOLAR SCLEROSING
DUCT HYPERPLASIA

Sclerosing papillary hyperplasia of ducts refers to radial sclerosing lesions arising from the subareolar lactiferous ducts. The term subareolar sclerosing duct hyperplasia (64) should be used when a radial sclerosing lesion occurs in the subareolar region without involving the nipple to distinguish this tumor from florid papillomatosis of the nipple (65) because the clinical presentations of the conditions differ, and to facilitate future studies in etiologic and prognostic differences.

Clinical Presentation. The age at diagnosis ranges from 26 to 73 years, averaging about 50 years. The presenting symptom is a mass located beneath the nipple or the areola; no lesions have been found within the nipple. Erosion or ulceration of the nipple surface are absent. Nipple retraction may occur and some patients have bloody discharge. The mammographic findings may suggest carcinoma.

Gross Findings. The specimen contains a firm to hard, round or oval tumor with indistinct borders measuring up to 2 cm (average 1.2 cm). Excision generally spares the nipple since the lesion is located in the underlying mammary parenchyma (fig. 127).

Microscopic Findings. The histologic structure is similar to that of other radial sclerosing lesions. Sclerosis and elastosis are most marked toward the center of the tumor while duct hyperplasia is especially prominent at the periphery (figs. 128, 129). Most of the tumor has a rounded margin created by the nodular expansion of a few

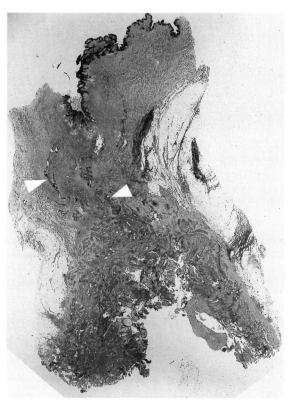

Figure 127
SUBAREOLAR SCLEROSING DUCT HYPERPLASIA
Low magnification view of a vertical section of the lesion beneath and at the margin of the nipple. Lactiferous ducts (arrows) indicate direction of nipple which was not resected. (Fig. 1A from Rosen PP. Subareolar sclerosing duct hyperplasia of the breast. Cancer 1987;59:1927–30.) (Figures 127–129 are from the same patient.)

large ducts (figs. 130, 131). Scattered mitotic figures may be seen in the epithelium or in hyperplastic myoepithelial cells found throughout much of the lesion. Focal comedonecrosis is infrequently found in the hyperplastic duct epithelium. In contrast to radial sclerosing lesions that develop elsewhere in the breast, subareolar sclerosing duct hyperplasia generally lacks cysts, apocrine changes, and squamous metaplasia. Carcinoma may arise in subareolar sclerosing duct hyperplasia just as it infrequently occurs in radial sclerosing lesions.

Prognosis and Treatment. Treatment is by excisional biopsy, usually performed through a circumareolar incision, sparing the nipple. The tumor may recur after incomplete excision but in most cases the patients have remained well

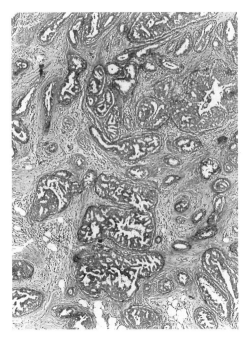

Figure 128
SUBAREOLAR SCLEROSING DUCT HYPERPLASIA
Complex papillary duct proliferation with laciform and microgland-forming patterns.

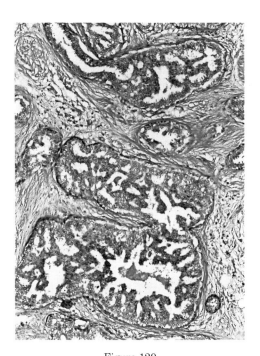

Figure 129
SUBAREOLAR SCLEROSING DUCT HYPERPLASIA
Hyperplastic myoepithelial cells outline epithelial hyperplasia in these ducts. (Fig. 1D from Rosen PP. Subareolar sclerosing duct hyperplasia of the breast. Cancer 1987;59:1927–30.)

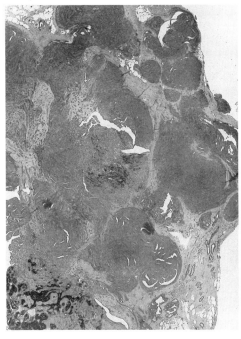

Figure 130
SUBAREOLAR SCLEROSING DUCT HYPERPLASIA
Transverse section of the tumor formed by relatively solid hyperplasia in ducts surrounding foci of sclerosis and papilloma. (Figures 130 and 131 are from the same patient.)

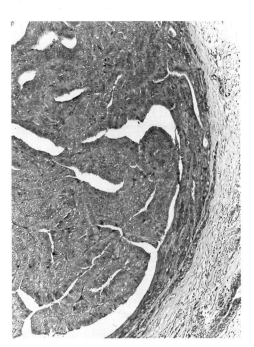

Figure 131
SUBAREOLAR SCLEROSING DUCT HYPERPLASIA
Compact papillary duct hyperplasia with circumscribed border.

for up to 4 years after initial treatment. At present, there is no evidence that this condition is a precancerous one, but longer follow-up is necessary for further evaluation.

MYOEPITHELIAL NEOPLASMS

Mammary neoplasms composed entirely or in part of myoepithelial cells are uncommon. Cameron et al. (68) commented that "purely myoepithelial benign tumours are called 'myoepitheliomas' or even myomas; if epithelial cells participate in their structure the term 'adenomyoepithelioma' seems appropriate... [and] if we are left with a purely myothelial malignant tumour, the term 'myothelial sarcoma' or even leiomyosarcoma seems suitable." Morphologic similarities between certain tumors of the breast, salivary glands, and skin appendage glands reflect the contribution of myoepithelial cells to these lesions.

Adenomyoepithelioma

The first full description of adenomyoepithelioma of the breast was published in 1970 by Hamperl (77). With the exception of two studies consisting of 13 and 18 cases (72,81) descriptions of these lesions are limited to case reports (76,78,83,87,88).

Clinical Presentation. All cases of adenomyoepithelioma have been in women aged 27 to 80 years (average 60 years). Most patients present with a solitary unilateral painless mass located in a peripheral portion of the breast. Occasionally, the lesions have been central or near the areola (77). The mammographic findings were suspicious in some patients (76,81). Estrogen receptors have usually been positive while progesterone receptors have been negative.

Gross Findings. The grossly measured size of adenomyoepitheliomas has varied from 0.5 to more than 5.0 cm, with a median size of 1.5 cm. With rare exceptions, the tumors have been described as well circumscribed, firm or hard; lobulation is often noted (fig. 132). Small cysts were observed in a few cases (76,81).

Microscopic Findings. Microscopically, most adenomyoepitheliomas are circumscribed and composed of aggregated nodules (fig. 133). Some consist largely or entirely of intraductal papillary elements. The papillary intraductal component can extend into ducts outside the grossly recognizable lesion and this may be re-

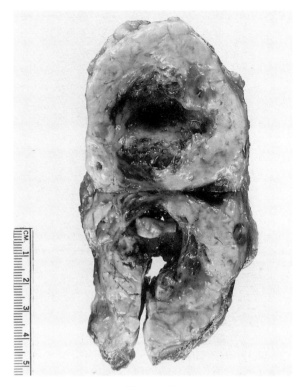

Figure 132
ADENOMYOEPITHELIOMA
Gross appearance of an unusually large, bisected tumor with a central cavity in which there are papillomatous nodules. Note the bosselated contour.

sponsible for recurrence after seemingly adequate excision. Some of these lesions have been termed *ductal adenomas*, an inappropriate designation (see p. 69) (66,76).

The most distinctive microscopic pattern features a balanced proliferation of round, oval, or tubular glandular elements with intervening islands and bands of polygonal myoepithelial cells that have clear cytoplasm (figs. 134, 135). In some tumors the clear myoepithelial cells are numerous resulting in extensive zones virtually devoid of glands (figs. 136–138). Other lesions feature the glandular component that may proliferate in broad bands and trabeculae separated by strands of delicate fibrovascular stroma (figs. 139, 140). In papillary regions, distinct polygonal myoepithelial cells accompany the epithelium in its various branches and ramifications.

The epithelial cells tend to have sparse, darkly staining cytoplasm and hyperchromatic nuclei. Squamous, apocrine, and sebaceous metaplasia

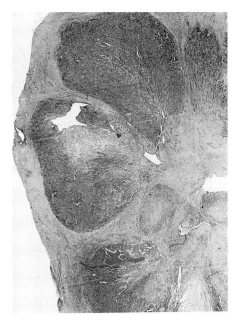

Figure 133
ADENOMYOEPITHELIOMA
Multinodular configuration, intraductal papillary proliferation, and central sclerosis are shown here at low magnification. (Fig. 1A from Rosen PP. Adenomyoepithelioma of the
breast. Hum Pathol 1987;18:1232–7.)

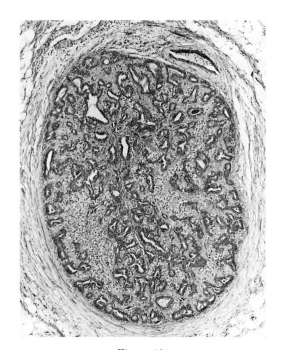

Figure 134
ADENOMYOEPITHELIOMA
Intraductal component in which pale bands of
myoepithelial cells separate adenomatous proliferation of
ductal epithelium.

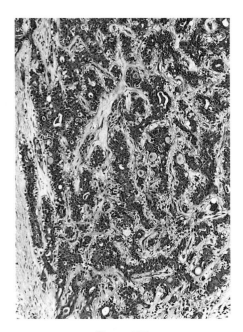

Figure 135
ADENOMYOEPITHELIOMA
Glandular units outlined by myoepithelial cells are sepa-
rated by delicate fibrovascular stroma. (Fig. 1B from Rosen
PP. Adenomyoepithelioma of the breast. Hum Pathol 1987;18:
1232–7.) (Figures 135 and 136 are from the same patient.)

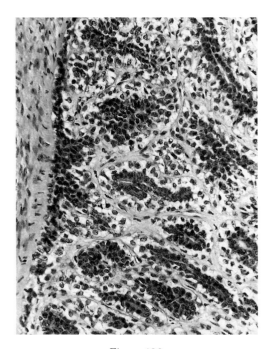

Figure 136
ADENOMYOEPITHELIOMA
Myoepithelial cells with clear cytoplasm are sufficiently
numerous to crowd the epithelium and expand into the stroma.

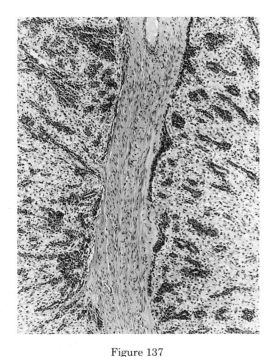

Figure 137
ADENOMYOEPITHELIOMA
Marked overgrowth of myoepithelial cells in two adjacent nodules separated by a stromal band.

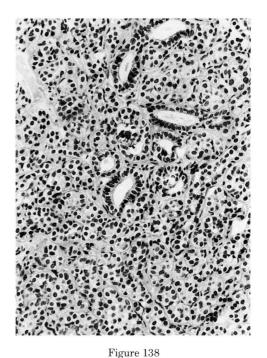

Figure 138
ADENOMYOEPITHELIOMA
Myoepithelial cells have virtually replaced glandular elements. Note tendency of the myoepithelial cells to form small alveolar clusters.

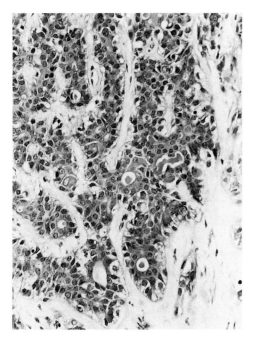

Figure 139
ADENOMYOEPITHELIOMA
Where glandular elements are numerous, lumens with secretion are formed. Glandular elements enmeshed in fibrosis at the margin on the right simulate invasion. (Figures 139 and 140 are from the same patient.)

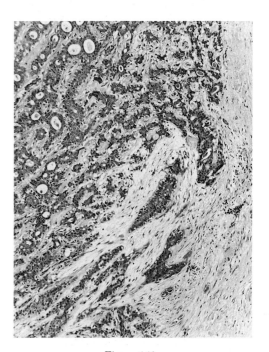

Figure 140
ADENOMYOEPITHELIOMA
Isolated myoepithelial cells with clear vacuolated cytoplasm are present.

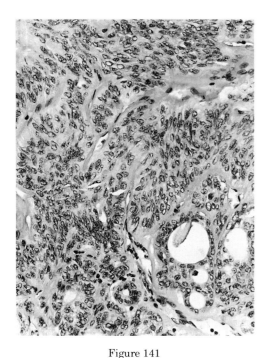

Figure 141
ADENOMYOEPITHELIOMA
View to show transition from adenomatous to myomatous growth.

may be present focally. Cytologic atypia and mitotic activity are infrequent or absent in most cases. However, in very rare instances, the epithelial component exhibits exaggerated proliferation accompanied by cytologic atypia and mitoses that may constitute carcinoma arising in an adenomyoepithelioma (84). The carcinomatous component may metastasize to axillary lymph nodes (84).

The extent to which myoepithelial cells assume a spindly, myoid shape varies greatly. Tumors composed entirely of these cells with no identifiable epithelial cells are classified as myoepitheliomas, an extreme variant of the group of myoepithelial neoplasms. Many adenomyoepitheliomas have foci of spindle cell myoid growth. Palisading of spindle cells and alveolar clustering of polygonal cells are common myoid patterns (fig. 141). Cytologic atypia of myoepithelial cell nuclei may be encountered in lesions in which there is a tendency to form spindle cells (fig. 142, 143). Atypical features include scattered mitotic figures, nuclear pleomorphism, nuclear hyperchromasia,

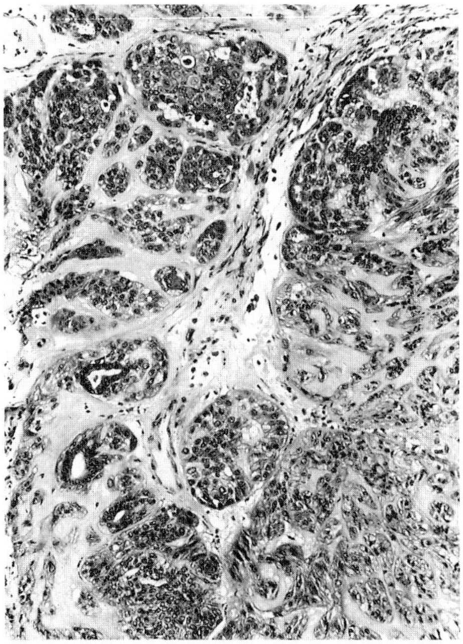

Figure 142
ADENOMYOEPITHELIOMA
Myoepithelial proliferation in which atypical myoepithelial cells have hyperchromatic nuclei and retain epithelioid characteristics. (Fig. 2A from Rosen PP. Adenomyoepithelioma of the breast. Hum Pathol 1987;18:1232–7.)

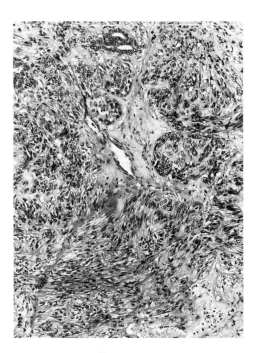

Figure 143
ADENOMYOEPITHELIOMA
Atypical myomatous proliferation with residual glandular elements above. Note palisading of spindle cells that have hyperchromatic nuclei. (Fig. 2B from Rosen PP. Adenomyoepithelioma of the breast. Hum Pathol 1987;18:1232–7.)

and occasional multinucleated cells. Myoid hyperplasia may give rise to areas with leiomyomatous features (75); this process infrequently produces leiomyosarcoma.

Histochemistry, Immunohistochemistry, and Electron Microscopy. Generally, the diverse cellular components exhibit expected histochemical properties. Glands may contain PAS- or mucicarmine-positive secretion but intracytoplasmic secretion is minimal or absent. The cytoplasm of glandular cells tends to be strongly reactive with antibodies to cytokeratin and the luminal surfaces of these cells are positive for CEA and epithelial membrane antigen (fig. 144). While most of the epithelial cells are S-100 negative, small groups may be strongly reactive for this antigen.

Polygonal and spindle myoepithelial cells are not reactive for epithelial membrane antigen or CEA. Anti-actin staining tends to be more conspicuous in spindle than clear polygonal cells and no reactivity is seen in epithelial cells (figs. 145, 146). Some myoepithelial cells are S-100 positive in virtually all tumors but the intensity

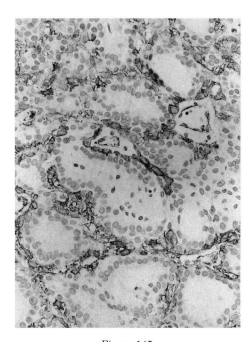

Figure 145
ADENOMYOEPITHELIOMA
Immunoperoxidase stain for actin highlights some myoepithelial cells (CGA7, muscle actin, avidin-biotin).

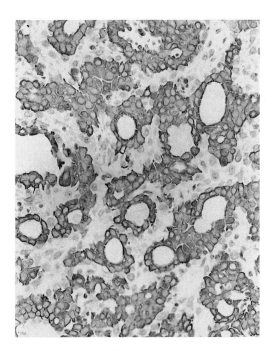

Figure 144
ADENOMYOEPITHELIOMA
Immunohistochemical stain for low molecular weight cytokeratin accentuates glandular cells leaving myoepithelial cells unstained (anti-AE1, avidin-biotin).

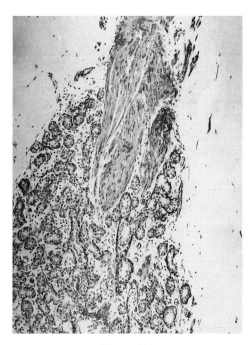

Figure 146
MYOID METAPLASIA OF LOBULE
Bundles of smooth muscle cells merging with this lobule are derived from myoepithelial cells normally present in lobular glands. Both cell types are immunoreactive for muscle common antigen in this section (HHF-35, avidin-biotin).

and uniformity of reactivity vary considerably. There does not appear to be a consistent relationship between staining with anti-actin and anti-S-100 antibodies.

Several papers have described the ultrastructural features of individual lesions classified as adenomyoepitheliomas (72,74,88). These case reports have consistently documented the presence of epithelial and myoepithelial components in the lesions. Polygonal and spindle myoepithelial cells have desmosomes that may be well or poorly formed and interdigitating cell processes. The cytoplasm contains tonofilaments and subplasmalemmal pinocytotic vesicles. Bundles of cytofilaments are prominent in the cytoplasm of myoepithelial cells, sometimes arranged in perinuclear bundles or peripheral arrays along which fusiform densities or condensation zones are commonly found. Distinct basal lamina material is seen around and among the myoepithelial cells.

Prognosis and Treatment. Adenomyoepithelioma is a benign tumor that can be treated by local excision (76). Local recurrence is rare, usually more than 2 years after the initial excision (79,81,84,87). Recurrence may be attributed to incomplete excision. The multinodular character of the lesion and peripheral intraductal extension are contributory factors. Reexcision may be performed, especially for multinodular lesions with peripheral intraductal extension. Adenomyoepithelioma is not particularly related to the development of mammary adenocarcinoma. Carcinoma may be detected coincidentally as a separate lesion (66), or rarely it may arise within the tumor.

Myoepithelioma

Myoepithelial neoplasms of the breast are extremely uncommon and reports are limited to individual case studies. Hamperl's review of the subject in 1970 (77) described lesions composed of epithelioid and spindle myoepithelial cells. Toth (86) described a myoepithelioma that presented as a painful, hard breast tumor. The specimen was grossly nodular and consisted microscopically of dilated ducts "filled with cellular adenomatous intraductal papillomas" in which "the proliferating myoepithelial elements almost filled the ducts . . . with leiomyoma-like tumors the spindle cells of which formed either bundles

or whorl-like patterns." The myoepithelial nature of the spindle cells was confirmed by electron microscopy.

Tumors referred to as muscular (71) and myoid (70) hamartomas probably arise from hyperplastic myoepithelial cells. Davies and Riddell (71) noted "the intimate relationship of the smooth muscle to the lobular epithelium" in one of their cases and suggested that "the smooth muscle is of myoepithelial origin." Three patients, 38 to 61 years of age, with myoid hamartomas studied by electron microscopy were described by Daroca (70). A 54-year-old patient with a similar lesion was reported by Eusebi et al. (74).

Cameron et al. (68) described a 40-year-old woman with a 5 x 7 cm adenomyoepitheliomatous tumor in which a portion of the lesion was a highly cellular spindle cell neoplasm. One year after treatment by mastectomy the patient developed a local recurrence involving fat and skeletal muscle consisting entirely of spindle cells with no epithelial structures. The authors stated that "if confronted exclusively with this picture, one would come to the diagnosis 'leiomyosarcoma'."

Several spindle cell neoplasms composed entirely of myoepithelial cells have been described (67,73,80,82,84,85). The histogenesis of these lesions was confirmed by electron microscopy and in most instances by immunohistochemistry (67,80, 82,84,85). Light microscopy revealed interlacing bundles of spindle cells sometimes arranged in a storiform pattern (figs. 147–150). Cytoplasm of the cells tended to be eosinophilic or clear. Three tumors had few or no mitotic figures and a benign clinical course with a relatively short follow-up (73,80,82). Numerous mitoses were present in two other tumors. Metastatic tumor was found in an axillary lymph node of one of these patients (84) and the other died of pulmonary metastases 6 months after diagnosis. Estrogen and progesterone receptor analyses were negative in both malignant myoepithelial neoplasms.

The differential diagnosis of spindle cell myoepithelial tumors includes metaplastic carcinoma, primary spindle cell sarcoma such as leiomyosarcoma or fibrous histiocytoma, myofibroblastoma, and metastatic tumor. The issue can usually be resolved by considering the clinical history, as well as careful histologic and immunohistochemical analysis, but electron microscopy may sometimes be required.

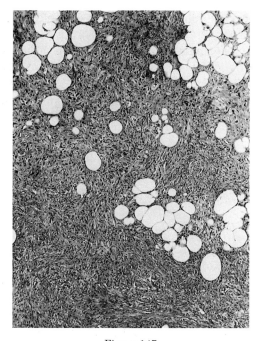

Figure 147
MYOEPITHELIOMA
Invasive densely cellular spindle cell lesion. (Figures 147–150 are from the same patient.)

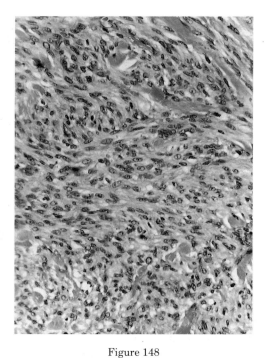

Figure 148
MYOEPITHELIOMA
Magnified view of lesion showing plump interlacing spindle cells with oval nuclei.

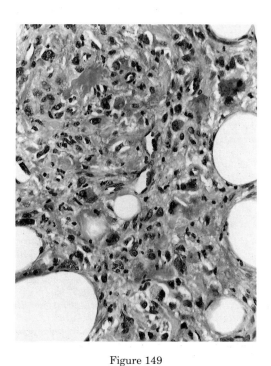

Figure 149
MYOEPITHELIOMA
Polygonal cells with hyperchromatic nuclei may be present in these tumors.

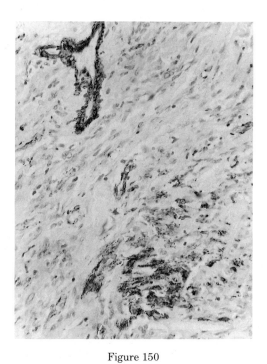

Figure 150
MYOEPITHELIOMA
Immunohistochemical stain for actin reveals focal reactivity among spindle cells and strong staining of myoepithelial cells in a duct above (CGA7, muscle common actin, avidin-biotin).

Myoepithelial neoplasms composed of polygonal cells with clear cytoplasm have received less attention than spindle cell myoepithelial tumors. The histogenesis of these tumors is usually not recognized and most are probably misclassified as clear cell, apocrine, secretory, or signet-ring cell carcinoma. An invasive clear cell myoepithelial neoplasm in a 77-year-old woman was documented by electron microscopy and immunohistochemistry (69). The 3.5 cm tumor was treated only by excisional biopsy and no follow-up information was provided. Remarkably high levels of estrogen receptor (470 fmol/mg protein) were detected in the lesion.

REFERENCES

Adenomas

1. Arrigoni MG, Dockerty MB, Judd ES. The identification and treatment of mammary hamartoma. Surg Gynecol Obstet 1971;133:577–82.
2. Azzopardi JG, Salm R. Ductal adenoma of the breast: a lesion which can mimic carcinoma. J Pathol 1984; 144:15–23.
3. Baddoura FK, Judd RL. Apocrine adenoma of the breast: a report of a case with investigation of lectin binding patterns in apocrine breast lesions. Mod Pathol 1990;3:373–6.
4. Ballance WA, Ro JY, El-Naggar AK, Grignon DJ, Ayala AG, Romsdahl MG. Pleomorphic adenoma (benign mixed tumor) of the breast: an immunohistochemical, flow cytometric, and ultrastructural study and review of the literature. Am J Clin Pathol 1990;93:795–801.
5. Chen KT. Pleomorphic adenoma of the breast. Am J Clin Pathol 1990;93:792–4.
6. Gusterson BA, Sloane JP, Middwood C, et al. Ductal adenoma of the breast—a lesion exhibiting a myoepithelial/epithelial phenotype. Histopathology 1987;11:103–10.
7. Hertel BF, Zaloudek C, Kempson RL. Breast adenomas. Cancer 1976;37:2891–905.
8. Hill RP, Miller FN. Adenomas of the breast. With case report of carcinomatous transformation in an adenoma. Cancer 1954;7:318–24.
9. James K, Bridger J, Anthony PP. Breast tumour of pregnancy ("lactating adenoma"). J Pathol 1988;156:37–44.
10. Lammie GA, Millis RR. Ductal adenoma of the breast— a review of fifteen cases. Hum Pathol 1989;20:903–8.
11. Makek M, von Hochstetter AR. Pleomorphic adenoma of the human breast. J Surg Oncol 1980;14:281–6.
12. Moross T, Lang AP, Mahoney L. Tubular adenoma of breast. Arch Pathol Lab Med 1983;107:84–6.
13. Moulton JE, Taylor DO, Dorn CR, Andersen AC. Canine mammary tumors. Pathol Vet 1970;7:289–320.
14. O'Hara MF, Page DL. Adenomas of the breast and ectopic breast under lactational influences. Hum Pathol 1985;16:707–12.
15. Persaud V, Talerman A, Jordan R. Pure adenoma of the breast. Arch Pathol 1968;86:481–83.
16. Smith BH, Taylor HB. The occurrence of bone and cartilage in mammary tumors. Am J Clin Pathol 1969;51:610–8.
17. Söreide JA, Anda 0, Eriksen L, Holter J, Kjellevold KH. Pleomorphic adenoma of the human breast with local recurrence. Cancer 1988;61:997–1001.
18. Tedeschi CG. Mammary lipoma. Arch Pathol 1948;46:386–97.
19. Tesluk H, Amott T, Goodnight JE Jr. Apocrine adenoma of the breast. Arch Pathol Lab Med 1986;110:351–2.
20. Willën R, Uvelius B, Cameron R. Pleomorphic adenoma in the breast of a human female. Aspiration biopsy findings and receptor determinations. Acta Chir Scand 1986;152:709–13.
21. Williams RW, Leach WB. Mixed tumor of female breast of unusual duration and size. South Med J 1975;68:97–100.

Intraductal Papilloma

22. Carter D. Intraductal papillary tumors of the breast. A study of 78 cases. Cancer 1977;39:1689–92.
23. Corkill ME, Sneige N, Fanning T, El-Naggar A. Fine-needle aspiration cytology and flow cytometry of intracystic papillary carcinoma of breast. Am J Clin Pathol 1990; 94:673–80.
24. Flint A, Oberman HA. Infarction and squamous metaplasia of intraductal papilloma: a benign lesion that may simulate carcinoma. Hum Pathol 1984;15:764–7.
25. Haagensen CD, Bodian C, Haagensen DE. Breast carcinoma: risk and detection. Philadelphia: WB Saunders Co, 1981:146–237.
26. _____, Stout AP, Phillips JS. The papillary neoplasms of the breast. I. Benign intraductal papilloma. Ann Surg 1951;133:18–36.
27. Moross T, Lang AP, Mahoney L. Tubular adenoma of breast. Arch Pathol Lab Med 1983;107:84–6.
28. Murad TM, Contesso G, Mouriesse H. Papillary tumors of large lactiferous ducts. Cancer 1981;48:122–33.
29. _____, Swaid S, Pritchett P. Malignant and benign papillary lesions of the breast. Hum Pathol 1977;8:379–90.
30. Nielsen BB. Oncocytic breast papilloma. Virchows Arch [A] 1981;393:345–51.

31. Oberman HA. Benign breast lesions confused with carcinoma. In: McDivitt RW, Oberman HA, Ozzello L, Kaufman N, eds. The breast. Baltimore: Williams & Wilkins, 1984:1–33.

32. O'Hara MF, Page DL. Adenomas of the breast and ectopic breast under lactational influences. Hum Pathol 1985;16:707–12.

33. Ohuchi N, Abe R, Kasai M. Possible cancerous change of intraductal papillomas of the breast. A 3-D reconstruction study of 25 cases. Cancer 1984;54:605–11.

34. _____, Abe R, Takahashi T, Tezuka F. Origin and extension of intraductal papillomas of the breast: a three-dimensional reconstruction study. Breast Cancer Res Treat 1984;4:117–28.

35. Reddick RL, Jennette JC, Askin FB. Squamous metaplasia of the breast. An ultrastructural and immunologic evaluation. Am J Clin Pathol 1985;84:530–3.

36. Rosen PP. Arthur Purdy Stout and papilloma of the breast. Am J Surg Pathol 1986;10(Suppl 1):100–7.

37. Roy I, Meakins JL, Tremblay G. Giant intraductal papilloma of the breast: a case report. J Surg Oncol 1985;28:281–3.

38. Sara AS, Gottfried MR. Benign papilloma of the male breast following chronic phenothiazine therapy. Am J Clin Pathol 1987;87:649–50.

39. Söderstrom KO, Toikkanen S. Extensive squamous metaplasia simulating squamous cell carcinoma in benign breast papillomatosis. Hum Pathol 1983;14:1081–2.

40. Walker AN, Betsill WL. Infarction of intraductal papilloma associated with hyperprolactinemia. Arch Pathol Lab Med 1980;104:280.

41. Wellings SR, Jensen HM, Marcum RG. An atlas of subgross pathology of human breast with special reference to possible precancerous lesions. JNCI 1975;55:231–73.

42. Willén R, Uvelius B, Cameron R. Pleomorphic adenoma in the breast of a human female. Aspiration biopsy findings and receptor determinations. Acta Chir Scand 1986;152:709–13.

Florid Papillomatosis of the Nipple

43. Bergdahl L, Bergman F, Rais O, Westling P. Bilateral adenoma of nipple. Report of a case. Acta Chir Scand 1971;137:583–6.

44. Bhagavan BS, Patchefsky A, Koss LG. Florid subareolar duct papillomatosis (nipple adenoma) and mammary carcinoma: report of three cases. Hum Pathol 1973;4:289–95.

45. Brownstein MH, Phelps RG, Magnin PH. Papillary adenoma of the nipple: analysis of fifteen new cases. J Am Acad Dermatol 1985;12:707–15.

46. Burdick C, Rinhart RM, Matsumoto T, O'Connell TJ, Heisterkamp CW. Nipple adenoma and Paget's disease in a man. Arch Surg 1965;91:835–8.

47. Gudjónsdóttir Å, Hägerstrand I, Östberg G. Adenoma of the nipple with carcinomatous development. Acta Pathol Microbiol Immunol Scand [A] 1971;79:676–80.

48. Handley RS, Thackray AC. Adenoma of nipple. Br J Cancer 1962;16:187–94.

49. Jones DB. Florid papillomatosis of the nipple ducts. Cancer 1955;8:315–9.

50. Miller G, Bernier L. Adenomatose erosive du mamelon. Can J Surg 1965;8:261–6.

51. Myers JL, Mazur MT, Urist MM, Peiper SC. Florid papillomatosis of the nipple: immunohistochemical and flow cytometric analysis of two cases. Mod Pathol 1990;3:288–93.

52. Perzin KH, Lattes R. Papillary adenoma of the nipple (florid papillomatosis, adenoma, adenomatosis). A clinicopathologic study. Cancer 1972;29:996–1009.

53. Richards AT, Jaffe A, Hunt JA. Adenoma of the nipple in a male. S Afr Med J 1973;47:581–3.

54. Rosen PP, Caicco JA. Florid papillomatosis of the nipple. A study of 51 patients including nine with mammary carcinoma. Am J Surg Pathol 1986;10:87–101.

55. Taylor HB, Robertson AG. Adenomas of the nipple. Cancer 1965;18:995–1002.

56. World Health Organization. Histological typing of breast tumours. 2nd ed. International Histological Classification of Tumours No. 2. Geneva: World Health Organization, 1981:19.

Syringomatous Adenoma

57. Cooper PH, Mills SE, Leonard DD, et al. Sclerosing sweat duct (syringomatous) carcinoma. Am J Surg Pathol 1985;9:422–33.

58. Ferrari A, Roncalli M. Adenoma siringomatoso della mammella. Istocitopatologia 1984;6:231–4.

59. Goldstein DJ, Barr RJ, Santa Cruz DJ. Microcystic adnexal carcinoma: a distinct clinicopathologic entity. Cancer 1982;50:566–72.

60. Jones MW, Norris HJ, Snyder RC. Infiltrating syringomatous adenoma of the nipple. Am J Surg Pathol 1989;13:197–201.

61. Rosen PP, Ernsberger D. Low grade adenosquamous carcinoma. A variant of metaplastic mammary carcinoma. Am J Surg Pathol 1987;11:351–8.

62. _____. Syringomatous adenoma of the nipple. Am J Surg Pathol 1983;7:739–45.

63. Ward BE, Cooper PH, Subramony C. Syringomatous tumor of the nipple. Am J Clin Pathol 1989;92:692–6.

Subareolar Sclerosing Duct Hyperplasia

64. Rosen PP. Subareolar sclerosing duct hyperplasia of the breast. Cancer 1987;59:1927–30.

65. _____, Caicco JA. Florid papillomatosis of the nipple. A study of 51 patients, including nine having mammary carcinoma. Am J Surg Pathol 1986;10:87–101.

Myoepithelial Neoplasms

66. Azzopardi JG, Salm R. Ductal adenoma of the breast: a lesion which can mimic carcinoma. J Pathol 1984; 144:15–23.

67. Bigotti G, Di Giorgio CG. Myoepithelioma of the breast: histologic, immunologic and electromicroscopic appearance. J Surg Oncol 1986;32:58–64.

68. Cameron HM, Hamperl H, Warambo W. Leiomyosarcoma of the breast originating from myoepithelium (myoepithelioma). J Pathol 1974;114:89–92.

69. Cartagena N Jr, Cabello-Inchausti B, Willis I, Poppiti R Jr. Clear cell myoepithelial neoplasm of the breast. Hum Pathol 1988;19:1239–43.

70. Daroca PJ Jr, Reed RJ, Love GL, Kraus SD. Myoid hamartomas of the breast. Hum Pathol 1985;16:212–9.

71. Davies JD, Riddell RH. Muscular hamartomas of the breast. J Pathol 1973;111:209–11.

72. Decorsiere JB, Thibaut I, Bouissou H. Les proliférations àdeno-myoepithéliales du sein. Ann Pathol 1988;8:311–6.

73. Erlandson RA, Rosen PP. Infiltrating myoepithelioma of the breast. Am J Surg Pathol 1982;6:785–93.

74. Eusebi V, Casadei GP, Bussolati G, Azzopardi JG. Adenomyoepithelioma of the breast with a distinctive type of apocrine adenosis. Histopathology 1987;11:305–15.

75. _____, Cunsolo A, Fedeli F, Severi B, Scarani P. Benign smooth muscle metaplasia in breast. Tumori 1980;66:643–53.

76. Gusterson BA, Sloane JP, Middwood C, et al. Ductal adenoma of the breast—a lesion exhibiting a myoepithelial/epithelial phenotype. Histopathology 1987;11:103–10.

77. Hamperl H. The myoepithelia (myoepithelial cells): normal state; regressive changes; hyperplasia; tumors. Curr Top Pathol 1970;53:161–220.

78. Jabi M, Dardick I, Cardigos N. Adenomyoepithelioma of the breast. Arch Pathol Lab Med 1988;112:73–6.

79. Kiaer H, Nielsen B, Paulsen S, Sörensen IM, Dyreborg V, Blichert-Toft M. Adenomyoepithelial adenosis and low grade adenomyoepithelioma of the breast. Virchows Arch [A] 1984;405:55–67.

80. Rode L, Nesland JM, Johannessen JV. A spindle cell breast lesion in a 54-year-old woman. Ultrastruct Pathol 1986;10:421–5.

81. Rosen PP. Adenomyoepithelioma of the breast. Hum Pathol 1987;18:1232–7.

82. Schürch W, Potvin C, Seemayer TA. Malignant myoepitheliomas (myoepithelial carcinoma) of the breast: an ultrastructural and immunocytochemical study. Ultrastruct Pathol 1985;8:1–11.

83. Tamura S, Enjoji M, Toyoshima S, Terasaka R. Adenomyoepithelioma of the breast. A case report with an immunohistochemical study. Acta Pathol Jpn 1988; 38:659–65.

84. Tavassoli FA. Myoepithelial lesions of the breast. Myoepitheliosis, adenomyoepithelioma, and myoepithelial carcinoma. Am J Surg Pathol 1991;15:554–68.

85. Thorner PS, Kahn HJ, Baumal R, Lee K, Moffat W. Malignant myoepithelioma of the breast: an immunohistochemical study by light and electron microscopy. Cancer 1986;57:745–50.

86. Töth J. Benign human mammary myoepithelioma. Virchows Arch [A] 1977;374:263–9.

87. Young RH, Clement PB. Adenomyoepithelioma of the breast. A report of three cases and review of the literature. Am J Clin Pathol 1988;89:308–14.

88. Zarbo RJ, Oberman HA. Cellular adenomyoepithelioma of the breast. Am J Surg Pathol 1983;7:863–70.

FIBROEPITHELIAL NEOPLASMS

FIBROADENOMATOUS TUMORS

Fibroadenoma

These are clinically and pathologically discrete tumors that manifest proliferation of epithelial and stromal elements. The predominant abnormality is the stromal proliferation and, as a consequence, semantic purists have preferred the designation adenofibroma. However, in common parlance, as well as in such influential documents as the International Histological Classification of Tumors, the popularity of the term fibroadenoma has prevailed. The tumor arises from the ducts and stroma of the terminal part of the mammary duct system and can be characterized as a giant lobule formed by exaggerated and uncoordinated epithelial and stromal growth (3,9).

Clinical Presentation. Fibroadenomas are the most common breast tumor in adolescent and young adult women, with a peak age incidence in the third decade. They account for the majority of all lesions which occasion breast biopsy in this age group, presenting as well-circumscribed, freely movable, nonpainful masses. The tumors are most often solitary; however, as many as 25 percent of patients have multiple fibroadenomas in one or both breasts or they develop subsequent tumors (15). There is a higher incidence in black patients (4).

Although common in young women, they are much less prevalent in postmenopausal patients. This suggests that some fibroadenomas regress with age if left untreated, an observation supported by the relatively small size and marked sclerotic character of fibroadenomas in the postmenopausal breast.

Gross Findings. Fibroadenomas are round to oval, rubbery, firm masses whose circumscription allows them to be "shelled out" by the surgeon. They appear encapsulated and have a bulging, uniform, gray-white, fleshy cut surface. Slit-like spaces or small cysts often are evident.

Microscopic Findings. The stroma consists of fibroblastic proliferation with interspersed collagen. It has been suggested that myoepithelial cells and myofibroblasts are stromal components, but the fibroblast is the predominant stromal cell (21). There may be variable stromal cellularity, ranging from hypercellularity to a hypocellular, avascular, even hyalinized, stroma usually accompanied by atrophic ducts, a retrogressive change seen in aged patients (9). Stromal calcification may be present in longstanding tumors. The gross appearance of encapsulation is a result of compression of adjacent tissue.

The ducts may be distorted into elongated and compressed slit-like structures, resulting in the so-called intracanalicular pattern. In other tumors, ducts not compressed by the proliferating connective tissue produce a pericanalicular growth pattern. This subclassification is of little practical value, because a mixture of these growth patterns is often present in a single lesion, and the patterns have no relevance to treatment. However, a fibroadenoma with an extreme intracanalicular pattern may be mistaken for a cystosarcoma.

Fibrocystic changes are evident in approximately 50 percent of fibroadenomas (17). These may consist of apocrine metaplasia of the ductal epithelium, adenosis, or intraductal hyperplasia, with more than one of these findings usually present. Sclerosing adenosis may result in a pattern that simulates invasive carcinoma, especially on frozen section (figs. 151, 152). In most instances the adenosis is focal within the tumor, and the areas of extreme ductal attenuation contain myoepithelial cells. Intraductal hyperplasia in a fibroadenoma does not appear to be associated with an increased risk for subsequent carcinoma (figs. 153, 154) (11). In addition, there is no association between the extent of intraductal hyperplasia and use of oral contraceptives (5,16).

Rarely, otherwise characteristic fibroadenomas may contain bundles of smooth muscle cells (fig. 155) (8). In reported cases, proximity of the tumor to the areola suggests that the muscle may be related to muscle from the nipple. Squamous metaplasia of the ductal epithelium can occasionally result in a confusing microscopic growth pattern (fig. 156) (22), and may result in keratin cysts. Squamous metaplasia of the epithelium, as well as osteochondroid or lipocytic stromal metaplasia, are more common in cystosarcomas.

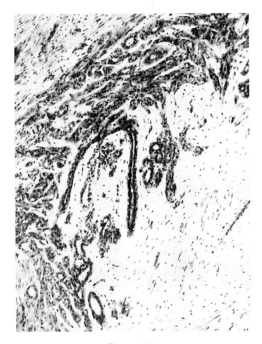

Figure 151
ADENOSIS IN FIBROADENOMA
In this area of adenosis at the edge of a fibroadenoma ductules lack cellular pleomorphism. They are lined by epithelium and myoepithelium.

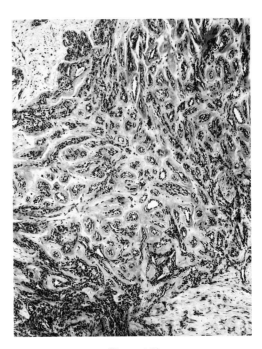

Figure 152
ADENOSIS IN FIBROADENOMA
Focal aggregate of small ducts associated with periductal fibrosis in a fibroadenoma. In other areas the microscopic pattern was typical of a fibroadenoma.

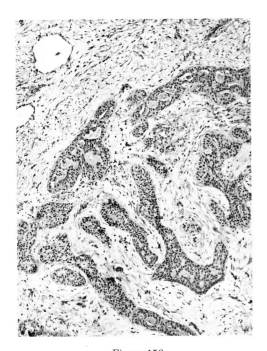

Figure 153
DUCTAL HYPERPLASIA IN FIBROADENOMA
Focal intraductal proliferation in a fibroadenoma. (Figures 153 and 154 are from the same patient.)

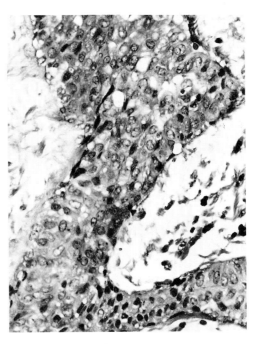

Figure 154
DUCTAL HYPERPLASIA IN FIBROADENOMA
The ducts are filled with a polymorphous cell population.

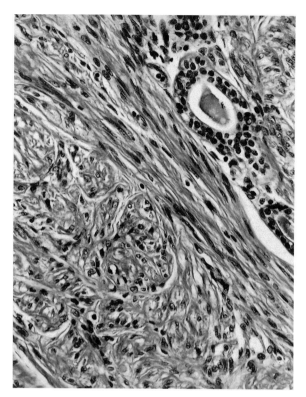

Figure 155
SMOOTH MUSCLE IN FIBROADENOMA
Smooth muscle was present in a small area of the lesion.

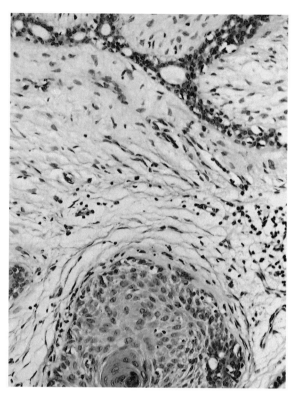

Figure 156
SQUAMOUS METAPLASIA IN FIBROADENOMA
Focal squamous metaplasia with keratinization.

Infarction in the absence of pregnancy is rare (14). However, recognition of such foci is important to prevent confusion with necrotic carcinoma. When circumscribed nodules are infarcted in pregnant patients it is difficult to determine whether the preexisting lesion was a fibroadenoma, a tubular adenoma, or a lactational adenoma, especially when typical fibroadenomatous tissue is not evident.

Benign multinucleated giant cells may be seen in the stroma of fibroadenomas, just as they may occur in mammary stroma in otherwise unremarkable biopsies (1). These cells are of mesenchymal origin and should not be mistaken for malignant cells.

Differential Diagnosis. The microscopic appearance of fibroadenomas is among the most distinctive of any tumor. Diagnostic problems result from an incorrect frozen section diagnosis of a fibroadenoma that contains sclerosing adenosis. The presence of spindled myoepithelial cells in adenosis is a helpful diagnostic finding.

Distinguishing fibroadenomas from tubular adenomas is not of critical importance, since both are benign lesions unassociated with any increased risk for subsequent carcinoma. Moreover, as noted in the discussion of tubular adenomas, there is a morphologic kinship between the two lesions. Although some fibroadenomas with an otherwise characteristic microscopic appearance may become unusually large, these tumors should not be classified as juvenile fibroadenomas or as cystosarcoma phyllodes; the latter tumors are characterized by prominent stromal cellularity.

Frozen Section. Since fibroadenomas are easily recognized grossly, there is no reason to perform a frozen section examination. Although the uncommon occurrence of carcinoma presenting in a fibroadenoma may be overlooked by this approach, it is highly unlikely today that definitive treatment would be based on the frozen section diagnosis. Far greater harm would result from the misdiagnosis of an area of adenosis in a fibroadenoma as invasive carcinoma.

Cytology. A fine-needle aspiration specimen from a fibroadenoma shows a distinctive cytologic pattern consisting of tightly arranged clusters of cells that often appear to branch. These cells are uniform, contain scant cytoplasm, and represent the ductal component of the tumor. Spindled cells or isolated oval nuclei also are seen, singly or in clusters, corresponding to the stroma. This diagnostic pattern is not evident in all fibroadenomas since very little cellular material is obtained from those with hyalinized stroma and atrophic ducts.

Prognosis and Treatment. These tumors may be excised with narrow margins of normal tissue. There is no evidence of an increased risk of malignant change to cystosarcoma after the excision in this fashion. Recurrent fibroadenomas in other terminal duct lobular units may represent a field effect rather than recurrence of the previously excised lesion or can result from incomplete removal of fibroadenomas that appear to be encapsulated grossly but are not encapsulated microscopically. If the tumor is shelled out, a remnant may be left behind but this rarely results in clinical recurrence.

Sclerosing Lobular Hyperplasia

This palpable tumor is characterized by prominent hyperplasia of lobules and an associated proliferation of stroma (10) which may be cellular, especially at the periphery, but sclerotic centrally (fig. 157). This abnormality most likely represents a form of local parenchymal overgrowth. It is most common in young women, with approximately one third the incidence of fibroadenomas.

Grossly, the masses consist of soft to rubbery, circumscribed, mobile nodules. In contrast to fibroadenomas, where the lobular architecture is lost, these lesions consist of enlarged, easily recognizable lobules. Nevertheless, the kinship of this lesion to fibroadenomas is seen in incipient fibroadenomatous areas, so-called fibroadenomatoid mastopathy, as well as the frequent coexistence of sclerosing lobular hyperplasia with fibroadenomas. These lesions are benign and not associated with an increased risk for carcinoma in the affected breast.

Juvenile Fibroadenoma

In contrast to the usual fibroadenoma, these tumors occur most often in young girls. They are characterized by stromal hypercellularity and by hyperplasia of ductal epithelium with occasional atypical features (20). This tumor has been called fetal fibroadenoma, cellular fibroadenoma, and benign cystosarcoma phyllodes. None of these terms is completely satisfactory; these tumors lack the overall microscopic appearance of cystosarcomas, and the occasional occurrence of the tumor in patients older than 30 years belies the specificity of the term, juvenile fibroadenoma. Cellular fibroadenoma has also been applied to benign cystosarcomas. Therefore, despite its imprecision, juvenile fibroadenoma is preferred, as it connotes a distinctive tumor that occurs most often in adolescent girls.

Clinical Presentation. These tumors form discrete masses that often manifest rapid growth and attain large size. They most commonly occur in paramenarchal children or in adolescents and occasionally in older patients. The majority are solitary, painless, firm, movable masses. Most of

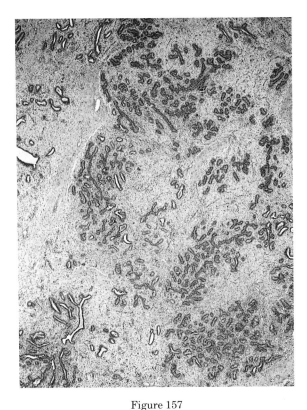

Figure 157
SCLEROSING LOBULAR HYPERPLASIA
Nodular lesion consisting of apparent enlargement of lobule with associated central fibrosis.

the patients note rapid growth of the tumor. Breast asymmetry is present if the tumor attains large size.

Multiple tumors are uncommon and occur most often in blacks (6). It is not possible to determine whether the metachronous tumors are new lesions or recurrences. These may present in one breast, but more often both breasts are asymmetrically involved. Multiple tumors may result in breast enlargement. In addition, these patients have a propensity to develop recurrent tumors after operative removal of the masses, although this phenomenon tends to decrease after 20 years of age. Recurrent tumors may have the microscopic pattern of adult-type fibroadenoma while others may have a cellular stroma comparable to that of juvenile fibroadenomas.

Gross Findings. These masses are soft to rubbery and circumscribed. Slit-like spaces may be evident on the cut surface. Size varies from microscopic to tumors large enough to distort the breast.

Microscopic Findings. The overriding characteristic of these circumscribed tumors is engulfment of ducts by a cellular stroma (fig. 158). A pericanalicular arrangement of the ducts is most common, although a mixture of intracanalicular and pericanalicular patterns may be present. In most tumors the ducts are widely separated by the stromal component; however, in some tumors lobules are recognizable. Broad areas of collagenization may be present.

The stromal cells lack cellular atypism and mitoses are sparse, usually no more than 1 to 3 per 10 high-power fields. The spindled cells appear to be fibroblastic in origin, a conclusion supported by ultrastructural studies as well as the lack of staining of the cells for S-100 protein (21). Multinucleated stromal cells may be present. There is no stromal overgrowth to the extent that a low-power (X40) microscopic field is occupied solely by stroma unaccompanied by ducts.

In contrast to the usual fibroadenoma, conspicuous intraductal hyperplasia may occur (fig. 159). This can result in expansion of duct lumens by hyperplastic epithelium with solid, cribriform and micropapillary patterns. The epithelial proliferation may have severely atypical features that border histologically on intraductal carcinoma (13). However, there is also usually conspicuous proliferation of myoepithelial cells.

The microscopic pattern of multiply-presenting fibroadenomas is similar to that of solitary juvenile tumors, but variability of patterns may be seen among the lesions. Some of the synchronous and recurrent tumors may be typical adult-type fibroadenomas with pericanalicular or intracanalicular growth, and others may be tubular adenomas.

Differential Diagnosis. It is important to recognize these lesions as benign. The absence of atypism of stromal cells and of stromal overgrowth, the paucity of abnormal mitotic activity, and the sharp circumscription of the tumor attest to its indolent character. Distinguishing a juvenile fibroadenoma from a benign cystosarcoma phyllodes is usually not difficult since the latter tumor most often has an exaggerated intracanalicular growth pattern with the formation of leaf-like projections of tumoral tissue into the elongated ducts. The stroma in cystosarcomas

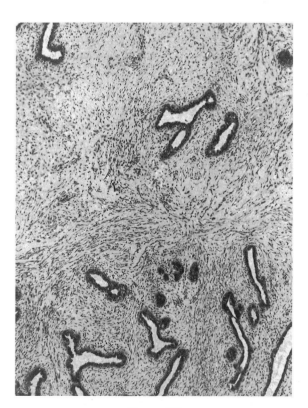

Figure 158
JUVENILE FIBROADENOMA
This tumor, found in a 24-year-old woman, had prominent stromal cellularity separating ducts. The tumor lacked an intracanalicular pattern and the stroma was more cellular than in a typical adult fibroadenoma.

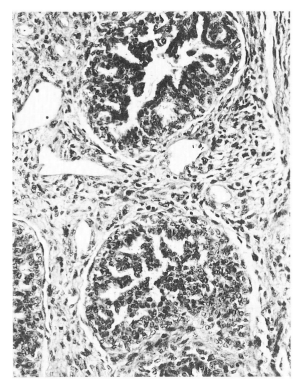

Figure 159
JUVENILE FIBROADENOMA
Intraductal hyperplasia in a rapidly enlarging 5-cm tumor from a 13-year-old girl.

usually is more cellular adjacent to ducts, whereas in juvenile fibroadenomas the stromal proliferation tends to be more uniform. A significant reason for distinguishing the two tumors is that an adolescent patient with a juvenile fibroadenoma should have an excision which spares as much of the adjacent breast as possible, while greater concern for local recurrence of the phyllodes tumor should result in assurance of its total removal by wider excision.

Prognosis and Treatment. The solitary tumors are benign and have little tendency for recurrence. Emphasis should be on preservation of breast tissue in these young patients so that normal breast development can occur. Even when the tumor occupies most of the breast in a paramenarchal patient, preservation of seemingly minimal amounts of normal tissue can result in normal development. When there is severe atypism of the ductal epithelium, long-term follow-up should be conducted, although thus far no predisposition to develop carcinoma has been demonstrated in these patients.

Patients with multiple, successive tumors are more difficult to manage. Even after removal of all grossly evident masses, recurrent lesions may develop within months and necessitate repeat excision. Because of frustration with apparent failure of excision of the lesions, some of these patients ultimately may elect to have a mastectomy. However, there appears to be a reduced tendency for clinically evident recurrences among patients over 20 years of age.

Carcinoma in Fibroadenoma

Invasive carcinoma may secondarily involve fibroadenomas or, less often, may arise in the tumor itself. Origin in a fibroadenoma can be established with confidence if the invasive lesion is confined to the fibroadenoma or if an in situ element is present.

The mean age of patients with carcinoma occurring in a fibroadenoma is 43 years, approximately two decades older than the average age of patients with fibroadenomas (19,23). In most instances there are no clinical or gross findings that would suggest carcinomatous change in a fibroadenoma. The extent of the carcinoma may vary from a small focus of involvement to almost complete replacement of the epithelial component of the tumor.

Lobular carcinoma in situ is much more common than intraductal carcinoma in this setting (figs. 160, 161) (2). This may relate to the derivation of fibroadenomas from the terminal duct lobular unit (3). Noninvasive carcinoma is a rare finding in more than one fibroadenoma in a breast (2,12); all reported examples of this occurrence have been lobular carcinoma in situ. Intraductal carcinoma arising in a fibroadenoma has the same histologic features as intraductal carcinoma in nonfibroadenomatous tissue, and usually grows with a comedo or cribriform pattern.

Foci of invasive carcinoma may occur in association with a noninvasive component, most often with the pattern of invasive lobular carcinoma. It is essential to distinguish this from sclerosing adenosis involving a fibroadenoma. Immunohistochemical stains demonstrate myoepithelial cells, indicative of adenosis rather than lobular carcinoma.

Treatment of fibroadenomas containing carcinoma requires ascertaining the extent of malignant change in the breast. Even when the fibroadenoma only harbors noninvasive carcinoma, clinically inapparent areas of invasive carcinoma are present elsewhere in the breast in about half of the patients (18). A potential for recurrence as invasive carcinoma exists for lesions treated solely by local excision if other foci of carcinoma are overlooked (12). Lobular carcinoma in situ arising in a fibroadenoma has the same implication for bilateral involvement as when it arises elsewhere in the mammary parenchyma. Consequently, treatment depends upon the type and extent of carcinoma and should be the same as for patients with comparable lesions not affecting a fibroadenoma (7).

CYSTOSARCOMA PHYLLODES

Cellular periductal stromal tumors of the breast have been known by a variety of names since their initial description as neoplasms by Johannes Muller over 150 years ago. His original designation, cystosarcoma phyllodes, implied a fleshy tumor having a leaf-like pattern and cysts on gross examination of its cut surface. Muller did not attribute malignant potential to the tumor; in fact, he considered them to be perfectly innocent lesions.

Since that time, over 50 names have been suggested for this lesion. The World Health Organization monograph on the Histological Classification of Breast Tumors (43) classifies these tumors under the generic term phyllodes tumors, with the following definition:

> ...a more or less circumscribed neoplasm having a foliated structure and composed of connective tissue and epithelial elements analogous to a fibroadenoma but characterized by a greater connective tissue cellularity.

This definition implies a close relation to fibroadenoma, and leaves open the histogenetic question of the possible origin of the tumor from a preexisting fibroadenoma. It also correctly emphasizes the importance of the stromal component in assessing malignant potential.

It has been suggested that the microscopically benign tumors be termed cellular fibroadenomas or periductal fibromas, and that the malignant tumors can be termed periductal sarcomas, possibly adding

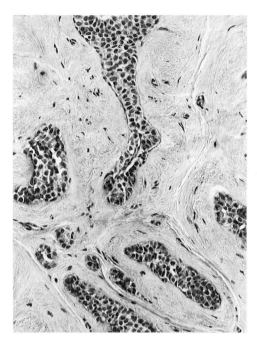

Figure 160
LOBULAR CARCINOMA IN FIBROADENOMA
Increased cellularity of ducts in fibroadenoma due to lobular carcinoma in situ. (Figures 160 and 161 are from the same patient.)

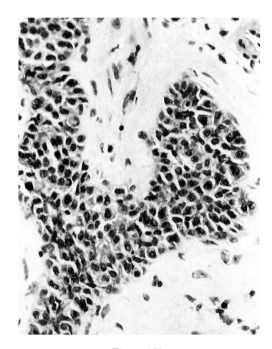

Figure 161
LOBULAR CARCINOMA IN FIBROADENOMA
Magnified view showing cells typical of lobular carcinoma in situ. Note loss of cohesion among the neoplastic cells.

the degree of differentiation. Microscopically borderline neoplasms should be considered low-grade sarcomas. The term cystosarcoma phyllodes continues to be widely used. Therefore, it is necessary to append the prefatory terms "benign" or "malignant" to this designation. The latter group should be subdivided into low-grade and high-grade tumors. Most tumors previously characterized as "borderline" fall in the low-grade group.

Clinical Presentation. These tumors account for less than 1 percent of breast tumors and represent approximately 2 to 3 percent of fibroepithelial neoplasms. Patients present with a discrete, palpable breast mass. Circumscription is evident on mammography. There usually is a history of rapid enlargement of the tumor, although some patients note sudden rapid growth of a preexisting lesion that had been of constant size over several years.

Although rare in children, there are well-documented examples of malignant cystosarcoma phyllodes that recurred and metastasized in this age group. Most tumors diagnosed as benign cystosarcomas in adolescents represent juvenile fibroadenomas (36), and reports of carcinosarcomas in juveniles most likely represent examples of malignant cystosarcoma phyllodes.

These tumors also occur in men, who present with breast enlargement, occasioning the diagnosis of gynecomastia. All male patients have been middle-aged to elderly (34).

Gross Findings. The masses are discrete and may have a variegated cut surface. Some tumors are tan to grey with a firm consistency. Others are soft and even gelatinous. The tumors tend to have a lobulated, bulging cut surface with clefts and polypoid areas. Foci of necrosis and hemorrhage suggest malignant change. The size of the tumor varies from 1 cm to more than 15 cm and is an unreliable indicator of whether the tumor is benign or malignant (32).

Microscopic Findings. The overall microscopic pattern is an exaggeration of that of an intracanalicular fibroadenoma (fig. 162). The ductal component is elongated and lines polypoid structures that appear to invaginate into epithelial-lined cysts. These structures account for the leaf-like gross appearance that gives the tumor its name. The microscopic hallmark of these tumors is their stromal cellularity which exceeds that seen

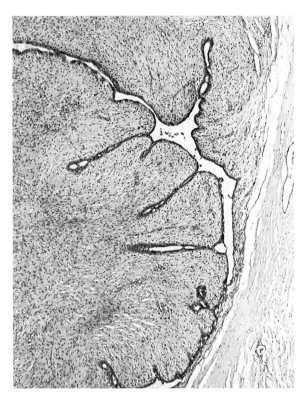

Figure 162
BENIGN CYSTOSARCOMA PHYLLODES
Tumor with a sharply defined margin. The epithelial component is elongated and appears to form a leaf-like structure.

in fibroadenomas (fig. 163). This cellularity is most pronounced adjacent to intratumoral ducts. Mitotic activity is relatively more prominent in the periductal stroma (fig. 164).

Some investigators have advocated subdividing cystosarcoma phyllodes into benign, malignant, and borderline groups on the basis of histologic features (39). However, the usefulness of the latter category has been challenged (30), and it seems preferable to regard such tumors as malignant, albeit of low histopathologic grade. These have a greater tendency for local recurrence than benign cystosarcomas, although there is little of the risk of metastatic spread associated with malignant cystosarcomas.

No single microscopic feature is wholly reliable in predicting the clinical behavior of cystosarcoma phyllodes (35). Assessment of the malignant potential of these tumors rests on the microscopic features of the stromal cells. The microscopic patterns

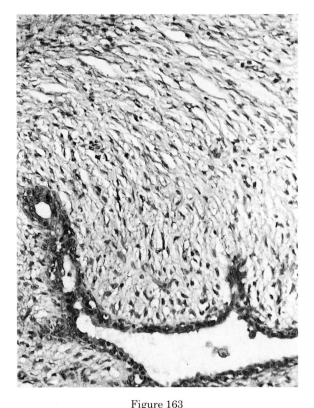

Figure 163
BENIGN CYSTOSARCOMA PHYLLODES
The degree of stromal cellularity exceeds that of a fibroadenoma, although this may vary within an individual tumor.

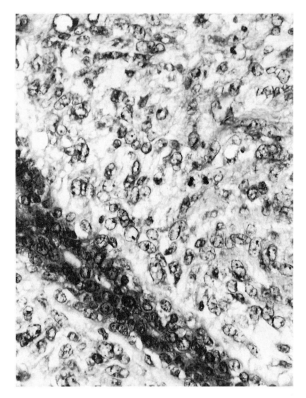

Figure 164
BENIGN CYSTOSARCOMA PHYLLODES
Nuclear pleomorphism and increased mitotic activity adjacent to a duct.

are often heterogeneous, necessitating thorough sampling. This is especially important at the periphery of the tumor. Reported instances of metastases from microscopically benign tumors may represent failure to detect sarcomatous foci through inadequate sampling.

Benign cystosarcomas lack cellular atypism or increased mitotic activity and have a microscopically clearly defined margin. Malignant change is characterized by stromal hypercellularity with associated cellular atypism and prominent mitotic activity (fig. 165), generally exceeding 5 mitoses per 10 high-power fields. In addition, stromal overgrowth at the expense of the ductal component, especially at the periphery of the tumor, is an indication of a heightened potential for local recurrence (30,42). This is denoted by the absence of ductal elements in a X40 low-power field. Other factors that have an adverse prognostic influence are tumor necrosis and the presence of heterologous stromal elements (26). Multinu-

cleated giant cells may be associated with the stromal proliferation, creating a resemblance to malignant fibrous histiocytoma (fig. 166).

The margin of the tumor may infiltrate adjacent breast tissue, even though the tumor grossly appears circumscribed. Tumors with a microscopically invasive border have an increased risk of local recurrence and comprise the majority of low-grade malignant cystosarcomas.

The stromal cells stain positively with antibodies to vimentin, and may also be immunoreactive for desmin and S-100 protein. Both immunohistochemically and ultrastructurally, the majority of tumor cells are fibroblasts, although occasional cells have properties of myofibroblasts (24). Flow cytometric studies of malignant tumors indicate a high proliferative index and aneuploidy; however, low-grade malignant tumors lack either characteristic (33). The latter studies correlate with the clinical course, suggesting that ploidy analysis may have prognostic usefulness (27).

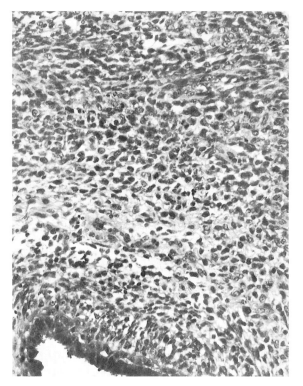

Figure 165
MALIGNANT CYSTOSARCOMA PHYLLODES
The neoplastic stromal cells that separate the ductal component of this tumor manifest increased mitotic activity and have sarcomatous characteristics.

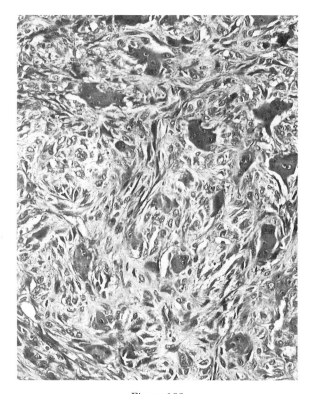

Figure 166
MALIGNANT CYSTOSARCOMA PHYLLODES
Multinucleated giant cells amidst the stromal proliferation in this malignant tumor.

Metaplastic change may involve ductal and stromal components. Squamous metaplasia of the ductal epithelium does not influence the clinical course of the tumor. In some instances keratin cysts are prominent, resulting in grossly recognizable white or pearly nodules (fig. 167). Although squamous cell carcinoma has been reported as arising in cystosarcomas, the documentation is not fully convincing (25).

The stromal component of benign cystosarcomas may undergo metaplastic change into bone, cartilage, adipose tissue, or smooth and striated muscle (fig. 168). Comparable sarcomatous elements have been observed in malignant cystosarcoma phyllodes. Malignant tumors with lipocytic transformation of the stroma usually have the appearance of well-differentiated liposarcomas, and are most often seen in young women (figs. 169, 170) (37). The cells in the immediate vicinity of the ducts lack cytoplasmic vacuolation. These well-differentiated tumors have an indolent clinical course if completely excised.

Occasionally, multifocal cystosarcomas occur, a situation much less frequent than breasts harboring multiple fibroadenomas (40). In addition, lobules adjacent to the neoplasm may have hypercellular intralobular connective tissue, comparable to that in cystosarcomas.

The epithelial component of these tumors may manifest epithelial hyperplasia, sometimes with extreme atypia, but malignant change is uncommon (fig. 171). Myoepithelial hyperplasia invariably accompanies the epithelial proliferation in these lesions. Only a few cases of in situ or invasive carcinoma arising in cystosarcomas have been reported, including examples of intraductal carcinoma and lobular carcinoma in situ (fig. 172) (28,31).

Differential Diagnosis. As noted above, juvenile fibroadenomas may have cellular stroma; however, the spindle cells lack atypism or increased mitotic activity. Moreover, they are sharply circumscribed tumors and often manifest hyperplasia of the ductal epithelium.

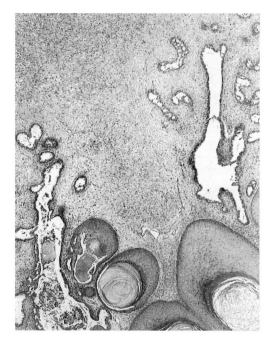

Figure 167
MALIGNANT CYSTOSARCOMA PHYLLODES
This circumscribed tumor had grossly evident keratin
cysts due to squamous metaplasia of the ductal epithelium.

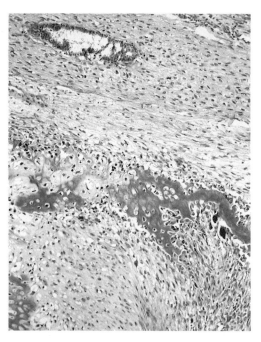

Figure 168
MALIGNANT CYSTOSARCOMA PHYLLODES
Osteochondroid metaplasia. A duct is evident above.

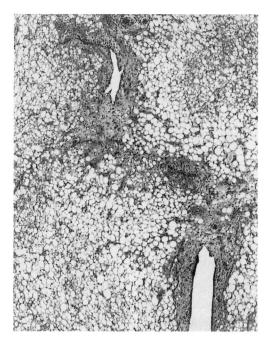

Figure 169
MALIGNANT CYSTOSARCOMA PHYLLODES
Stromal lipocytic metaplasia resulting in a pattern of
well-differentiated liposarcoma in a fibroepithelial tumor.
(Figures 169 and 170 are from the same patient.)

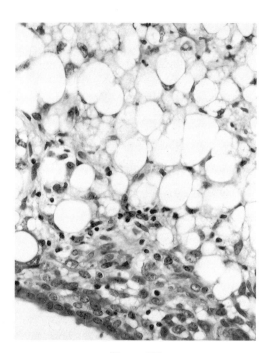

Figure 170
MALIGNANT CYSTOSARCOMA PHYLLODES
Vacuolation is not pronounced adjacent to ductal epithelium.

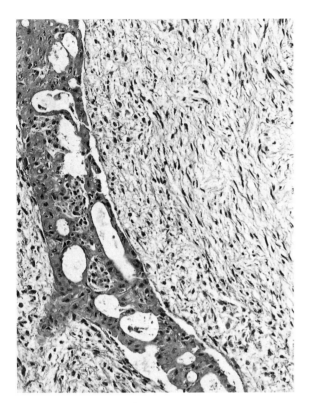

Figure 171
BENIGN CYSTOSARCOMA PHYLLODES
Intraductal hyperplasia with apocrine characteristics.

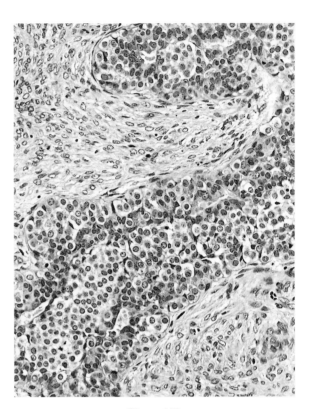

Figure 172
BENIGN CYSTOSARCOMA PHYLLODES
WITH LOBULAR CARCINOMA
Lobular carcinoma in the epithelium of a tumor that had histologically benign stroma.

Carcinosarcoma of the breast is characterized by independent malignant stromal and epithelial components. Each of these elements is discrete and of separate origin. Such tumors are exceedingly rare, and are either instances of carcinoma arising in a malignant cystosarcoma or collision tumors formed by the merging of separate carcinomatous and sarcomatous lesions.

Metaplastic carcinoma, especially with a predominant spindle cell growth pattern, may be confused with cystosarcoma phyllodes. Although an exaggerated intracanalicular growth pattern is not seen in metaplastic carcinoma, the spindle cell variant often has cysts lined by neoplastic ductal, or more often squamous, epithelium. Recognition that the epithelial component of such tumors has malignant characteristics permits differentiation from cystosarcoma. Transition is typically seen between the epithelial and spindle cells in metaplastic carcinoma while these components remain discrete in cystosarcomas.

In some malignant tumors, extensive stromal overgrowth may obliterate the epithelial component, resulting in a specimen that is indistinguishable from a sarcoma especially in a small biopsy. Diagnosis of cystosarcoma phyllodes requires demonstration of the ductal component, which can be identified when the entire tumor is generously sampled.

Prognosis and Treatment. Local recurrence is more frequent than metastasis. Initial recurrences may mirror the microscopic pattern of the original tumor. Consequently, the recurrence of a microscopically benign tumor typically contains well-differentiated ductal and stromal components. In other tumors dedifferentiation of the stromal component and progressive exclusion of ducts is evident. This is especially true of multiple recurrences, where the tumor may evolve to consist entirely of malignant mesenchymal elements.

Metastases are hematogenous and most often involve the lungs. They usually contain only the mesenchymal elements. Axillary lymph node metastases are extremely rare and occur in less than 1 percent of malignant cystosarcomas.

Treatment of cystosarcomas is influenced by the relative size of the tumor and the breast, and histologic features of the tumor. Total excision is of paramount importance to achieve clear surgical margins. There is a substantial risk of local recurrence if the tumor is simply enucleated. Gross circumscription perceived by the surgeon may be deceptive, as the microscopic margin of the neoplasm may be infiltrative. When the tumor is small and the breast is large, wide local excision is feasible; however, when the reverse is true, mastectomy may prove necessary. In general, stromal overgrowth and the presence of an infiltrating tumor border are most closely associated with local recurrence.

Even tumors that microscopically appear benign have the potential for recurrence (29). In most cases, local recurrence of benign tumors does not adversely affect survival. However, these tumors must be thoroughly sampled for malignant foci. Recurrence of malignant tumors after local excision requires mastectomy (41). Progressive dediffer entiation may be seen with subsequent recurrences, culminating in additional chest wall recurrences and metastases. Nonetheless, only a small proportion of adequately treated cystosarcomas recur locally or metastasize.

Since these tumors spread hematogenously, axillary lymph node dissection is unnecessary except when the breast also harbors carcinoma or there is clinical evidence of nodal involvement. Hormonal receptor determinations have not proven useful in the management, or in assessing prognosis of cystosarcomas. Flow cytometric data suggest that patients with tumors having an S-phase fraction greater than 5 percent have a shorter disease-free survival than those with tumors of lower proliferative fraction. DNA ploidy has not been shown to correlate with survival or local recurrence (38).

REFERENCES

Fibroadenomatous Tumors

1. Berean K, Tron VA, Churg A, Clement PB. Mammary fibroadenoma with multinucleated stromal giant cells. Am J Surg Pathol 1986;10:823–7.
2. Buzanowski-Konakry K, Harrison EG Jr, Payne WS. Lobular carcinoma arising in fibroadenoma of the breast. Cancer 1975;35:450–6.
3. Demetrakopoulos NJ. Three-dimensional reconstruction of a human mammary fibroadenoma. Q Bull Northwest Univ Med Sch 1958;32:221–8.
4. Farrow JH, Ashikari H. Breast lesions in young girls. Surg Clin North Am 1969;49:261–9.
5. Fechner RE. Fibroadenomas in patients receiving oral contraceptives: a clinical and pathologic study. Am J Clin Pathol 1970;53:857–64.
6. Fekete P, Petrek J, Majmudar B, Someren A, Sandberg W. Fibroadenomas with stromal cellularity. A clinicopathologic study of 21 patients. Arch Pathol Lab Med 1987;111:427–32.
7. Fondo EY, Rosen PP, Fracchia AA, Urban JA. The problem of carcinoma developing in a fibroadenoma: recent experience at Memorial Hospital. Cancer 1979;43:563–7.
8. Goodman ZD, Taxy JB. Fibroadenomas of the breast with prominent smooth muscle. Am J Surg Pathol 1981;5:99–101.
9. Kern WH, Clark RW. Retrogression of fibroadenomas of the breast. Am J Surg 1973;126:59–62.
10. Kovi J, Chu HB, Leffall LD Jr. Sclerosing lobular hyperplasia manifesting as a palpable mass of the breast in young black women. Hum Pathol 1984;15:336–40.
11. LiVolsi VA, Stadel BV, Kelsey JL, Holford TR. Fibroadenoma in oral contraceptive users. A histopathologic evaluation of epithelial atypia. Cancer 1979;44:1778–81.
12. McDivitt RW, Stewart FW, Farrow JH. Breast carcinoma arising in solitary fibroadenomas. Surg Gynecol Obstet 1967;125:572–6.
13. Mies C, Rosen PP. Juvenile fibroadenoma with atypical epithelial hyperplasia. Am J Surg Pathol 1987;11:184–90.
14. Newman J, Kahn LB. Infarction of fibroadenoma of the breast. Br J Surg 1973;60:738–40.
15. Oberman HA. Breast lesions in the adolescent female. Pathol Annu 1979;14(Pt 1):175–201.
16. _____. Hormonal contraceptives and fibroadenomas of the breast. N Engl J Med 1971;284:984.
17. _____, French AJ. Chronic fibrocystic disease of the breast. Surg Gynecol Obstet 1961;112:647–52.
18. Ozzello L, Gump FE. The management of patients with carcinomas in fibroadenomatous tumors of the breast. Surg Gynecol Obstet 1985;160:99–104.

19. Pick PW, Iossifides IA. Occurrence of breast carcinoma within a fibroadenoma. A review. Arch Pathol Lab Med 1984;108:590–4.

20. Pike AM, Oberman HA. Juvenile (cellular) adenofibromas. A clinicopathologic study. Am J Surg Pathol 1985;10:730–6.

21. Reddick RL, Shin TK, Sawhney D, Siegal GP. Stromal proliferations of the breast: an ultrastructural and immunohistochemical evaluation of cystosarcoma phyllodes, juvenile fibroadenoma, and fibroadenoma. Hum Pathol 1987;18:45–9.

22. Salm R. Epidermoid metaplasia in mammary fibroadenoma with formation of keratin cysts. J Pathol Bacteriol 1957;74:221–2.

23. Yoshida Y, Takaoka M, Fukumoto M. Carcinoma arising in fibroadenoma: case report and review of the world literature. J Surg Oncol 1985;29:132–40.

Cystosarcoma Phyllodes

24. Auger M, Hanna W, Kahn HJ. Cystosarcoma phyllodes of the breast and its mimics. An immunohistochemical and ultrastructural study. Arch Pathol Lab Med 1989;113:1231–5.

25. Austin WE, Fidler HK. Carcinoma developing in fibroadenoma of the breast. Am J Clin Pathol 1953;23:688–90.

26. Cohn-Cedermark G, Rutqvist LE, Rosendahl I, Silverswärd C. Prognostic factors in cystosarcoma phyllodes. A clinicopathologic study of 77 patients. Cancer 1991;68:2017–22.

27. El-Naggar AK, Ro JY, McLemore D, Garnsy L. DNA content and proliferative activity of cystosarcoma phyllodes of the breast. Potential prognostic significance. Am J Clin Pathol 1990;93:480–5.

28. Grove A, Deibjerg Kristensen L. Intraductal carcinoma within a phyllodes tumor of the breast: a case report. Tumori 1986;72:187–90.

29. Hajdu SI, Espinosa MH, Robbins GF. Recurrent cystosarcoma phyllodes. A clinicopathologic study of 32 cases. Cancer 1976;38:1402–6.

30. Hart WR, Bauer RC, Oberman HA. Cystosarcoma phyllodes. A clinicopathologic study of twenty-six hypercellular periductal stromal tumors of the breast. Am J Clin Pathol 1978;70:211–6.

31. Knudsen PJ, Ostergaard J. Cystosarcoma phyllodes with lobular and ductal carcinoma in situ. Arch Pathol Lab Med 1987;111:873–5.

32. McDivitt RW, Urban JA, Farrow JH. Cystosarcoma phyllodes. Johns Hopkins Med J 1967;120:33–45.

33. Murad TM, Hines JR, Bauer K. Histopathological and clinical correlations of cystosarcoma phyllodes. Arch Pathol Lab Med 1988;112:752–6.

34. Nielsen VT, Andreasen C. Phyllodes tumour of the male breast. Histopathology 1987;11:761–2.

35. Norris HJ, Taylor HB. Relationship of histologic features to behavior of cystosarcoma phyllodes: analysis of ninety-four cases. Cancer 1967;20:2090–9.

36. Oberman HA. Breast lesions in the adolescent female. Pathol Annu 1979;14(Pt 1):175–201.

37. _____, Nosanchuk JS, Finger JE. Periductal stromal tumors of breast with adipose metaplasia. Arch Surg 1969;98:384–7.

38. Palko MJ, Wang SE, Shackney SE, Cottington EM, Levitt SB, Hartsock RJ. Flow cytometric S fraction as a predictor of clinical outcome in cystosarcoma phyllodes. Arch Pathol Lab Med 1990;114:949–52.

39. Pietruszka M, Barnes L. Cystosarcoma phyllodes. A clinicopathologic analysis of 42 cases. Cancer 1978;41:1974–83.

40. Salm R. Multifocal histogenesis of a cystosarcoma phyllodes. J Clin Pathol 1978;31:897–903.

41. Salvadori B, Cusumano F, Del Bo R, et al. Surgical treatment of phyllodes tumors of the breast. Cancer 1989;63:2532–6.

42. Ward RM, Evans HL. Cystosarcoma phyllodes. A clinicopathologic study of 26 cases. Cancer 1986;58:2282–9.

43. World Health Organization. Histological typing of breast tumors. 2nd ed. International Histological Classification of Tumours No. 2. Geneva: World Health Organization, 1981:19.

◇◇◇

TNM STAGING OF BREAST CARCINOMA

The currently recommended staging system for breast carcinoma was adopted in 1989 by the American Joint Committee on Cancer (AJCC) (1) and the International Union Against Cancer (UICC) (4). Staging is based on characteristics of the primary tumor (T), extent of regional axillary node metastases (N), and distant metastases (M). The designation TNM has been chosen for clinical classification and pTNM refers to pathologic staging.

This classification applies only to carcinoma that has been histologically confirmed. The anatomic subsite in the breast of the primary tumor should be recorded but is not an element in classification. The seven sites identified in the female breast are the nipple, the central subareolar region, the four quadrants, and the axillary tail. The male breast is considered to be a single site. All other staging categories apply equally to carcinoma of the male breast.

When multiple carcinomas are present simultaneously in one breast, "the tumor with the highest T category should be used for classification. Simultaneous *bilateral* breast cancers should be classified independently."

Clinical staging may be employed in some circumstances but is less accurate than pathologic staging since there is a tendency to overestimate the size of the primary tumor and inaccurately assess the axillary lymph nodes for the presence of metastatic carcinoma. The false-positive and false-negative rates for clinical axillary lymph node staging are 30 to 40 percent (2). Rosen et al. (3) compared clinical and pathologic staging of the axillary lymph nodes of 203 patients treated by modified or radical mastectomy. Overall error rates were 33 and 38 percent for patients with T1 and T2 tumors, respectively. After surgery, 48 percent of patients classified clinically as T2N0 proved to be pathologically T2N1 (false negative) and 41 percent of women staged clinically as T1N1 were pathologically staged as T1N0 (false positive).

The following pages duplicate the text of the TNM staging classification as published by the AJCC and the UICC. Diagrams included in the UICC Atlas have been omitted.

A. REGIONAL LYMPH NODES

1. **Axillary (ipsilateral) and interpectoral (Rotter nodes)**: lymph nodes along the axillary vein and its tributaries, which may be divided into the following levels:

   a. Level I (low-axilla): lymph nodes lateral to the lateral border of pectoralis minor muscle.

   b. Level II (mid-axilla): lymph nodes between the medial and lateral borders of the pectoralis minor muscle and the interpectoral (Rotter) lymph nodes.

   c. Level III (apical axilla): lymph nodes medial to the medial margin of the pectoralis minor muscle including those designated as the subclavicular, infraclavicular, or apical.

Note: Intramammary lymph nodes are coded as axillary lymph nodes.

2. **Internal mammary (ipsilateral)**: lymph nodes in the intercostal spaces along the edge of the sternum in the endothoracic fascia.

Any other lymph node metastasis is coded as a distant metastasis (M1), including supraclavicular, cervical, or contralateral internal mammary lymph nodes.

B. TNM CLINICAL CLASSIFICATION

T - Primary Tumor

TX Primary tumor cannot be assessed

T0 No evidence of primary tumor

Tis Carcinoma in situ: intraductal carcinoma, or lobular carcinoma in situ, or Paget disease of the nipple with no tumor

Note: Paget disease associated with a tumor is classified according to the size of the tumor.

T1 Tumor 2 cm or less in greatest dimension

   T1a 0.5 cm or less in greatest dimension

   T1b More than 0.5 cm but not more than 1 cm in greatest dimension

T1c More than 1 cm but not more than 2 cm in greatest dimension

T2 Tumor more than 2 cm but not more than 5 cm in greatest dimension

T3 Tumor more than 5 cm in greatest dimension

T4 Tumor of any size with direct extension to chest wall or skin

Note: Chest wall includes ribs, intercostal muscles, and serratus anterior muscle but not pectoral muscle.

T4a Extension to chest wall

T4b Edema (including peau d'orange), or ulceration of the skin of the breast, or satellite skin nodules confined to the same breast

T4c Both 4a and 4b, above

T4d Inflammatory carcinoma

Notes: Inflammatory carcinoma of the breast is characterized by diffuse, brawny induration of the skin with an erysipeloid edge, usually with no underlying palpable mass. If the skin biopsy is negative and there is no localized, measurable primary cancer, the T category is pTX when pathologically staging a clinical inflammatory carcinoma (T4d).

Dimpling of the skin, nipple retraction or other skin changes, except those in T4, may occur in T1, T2, or T3 without affecting the classification.

N - Regional Lymph Nodes

NX Regional lymph nodes cannot be assessed (e.g. previously removed)

N0 No regional lymph node metastasis

N1 Metastasis to movable ipsilateral axillary node(s)

N2 Metastasis to ipsilateral axillary node(s) fixed to one another or to other structures

N3 Metastasis to ipsilateral internal mammary lymph node(s)

M - Distant Metastasis

MX Presence of distant metastasis cannot be assessed

M0 No distant metastasis

M1 Distant metastasis (includes metastasis to supraclavicular lymph nodes)

The category M1 may be further specified according to the following notation:

Pulmonary	PUL	Bone marrow	MAR
Osseous	OSS	Pleura	PLE
Hepatic	HEP	Peritoneum	PER
Brain	BRA	Skin	SKI
Lymph nodes	LYM	Other	OTH

C. pTNM PATHOLOGICAL CLASSIFICATION

pT - Primary Tumor

The pathological classification requires the examination of the primary carcinoma with no gross tumor at the margins of resection. A case can be classified pT if there is only microscopic tumor in a margin.

The pT categories correspond to the T categories.

pN - Regional Lymph Nodes

The pathological classification requires the resection and examination of at least the low axillary lymph nodes (level II). Such a resection will ordinarily include 6 or more lymph nodes.

pNX Regional lymph nodes cannot be assessed (not removed for study or previously removed)

pN0 No regional lymph node metastasis

pN1 Metastasis to movable ipsilateral axillary node(s)

pN1a Only micrometastasis (none larger than 0.2 cm)

pN1b Metastasis to lymph node(s), any larger than 0.2 cm

pN1bi Metastasis in 1 to 3 lymph nodes, any more than 0.2 cm and all less than 2.0 cm in greatest dimension

pN1bii Metastasis to 4 or more lymph nodes, any more than 0.2 cm and all less than 2.0 cm in greatest dimension

pN1biii Extension of tumor beyond the capsule of a lymph node, metastasis less than 2.0 cm in greatest dimension

pN1biv Metastasis to a lymph node 2.0 cm or more in greatest dimension pN2 Metastasis to ipsilateral axillary lymph nodes that are fixed to one another or to other structures

pN3 Metastasis to ipsilateral internal mammary lymph node(s)

pM - Distant Metastasis

The pM categories correspond to the M categories.

D. G HISTOPATHOLOGICAL GRADING

GX Grade of differentiation cannot be assessed

G1 Well differentiated

G2 Moderately differentiated

G3 Poorly differentiated

G4 Undifferentiated

E. R CLASSIFICATION

The absence or presence of residual tumor after treatment may be described by the symbol R.

RX Presence of residual tumor cannot be assessed

R0 No residual tumor

R1 Microscopic residual tumor

R2 Macroscopic residual tumor

F. STAGE GROUPING

Stage	T	N	M
Stage 0	Tis	N0	M0
Stage I	T1	N0	M0
Stage IIA	T0	N1	M0
	T1	N1	M0
	T2	N0	M0
Stage IIB	T2	N1	M0
	T3	N0	M0
Stage IIIA	T0	N2	M0
	T1	N2	M0
	T2	N2	M0
	T3	N1, N2	M0
Stage IIIB	T4	Any N	M0
	Any T	N3	M0
Stage IV	Any T	Any N	M1

REFERENCES

1. American Joint Committee on Cancer. Manual for staging of cancer. 3rd ed. Philadelphia: JB Lippincott Co, 1989:93–9.
2. Kinne DW. Staging and follow-up of breast cancer patients. Cancer 1991;67:1196–8.
3. Rosen PP, Fracchia AA, Urban JA, Schottenfeld D, Robbins GF. "Residual" mammary carcinoma following simulated partial mastectomy. Cancer 1975;35:739–47.
4. Spiessl B, ed. International Union Against Cancer. TNM-Atlas: illustrated guide to the TNM/pTNM-classification of malignant tumours. 3rd ed. Berlin: Springer-Verlag, 1989:174–83.

INTRAEPITHELIAL (PREINVASIVE OR IN SITU) CARCINOMA

LOBULAR CARCINOMA IN SITU AND ATYPICAL HYPERPLASIA

Foote and Stewart (13) introduced the term lobular carcinoma in situ (LCIS) to describe "a disease of small lobular ducts and lobules." They described almost all the important clinical and pathologic features of the disease including the inconspicuous character of LCIS which cannot be detected by clinical or gross pathologic examination, its multicentricity, the pagetoid extension in ducts and the rarity of true Paget disease, signet ring cells as a feature of LCIS, the association with infiltrating lobular carcinoma, and the coexistence of LCIS with other patterns of carcinoma, including ordinary duct carcinoma and tubular carcinoma.

Since lobular carcinoma in situ is a microscopic lesion that does not form a palpable tumor, the incidence is unknown. When it occurs alone, LCIS constitutes 1 to 6 percent of mammary carcinomas and 30 to 50 percent of noninvasive carcinomas (31,35). In retrospective reviews, each involving several thousand breast specimens, the frequency of LCIS was 3.9 percent (18), 1.5 percent (5), 1.4 percent (34), and 0.6 percent (45). One study reported that previously unrecognized LCIS was found in 64 of 8,609 (0.7 percent) biopsies originally diagnosed as benign (34). Nielsen et al. (26) examined breasts from young women, many of whom died unexpectedly, including only one with previously diagnosed breast carcinoma and found LCIS in 4 of 110 (3.6 percent) cases. Three autopsy studies of more than 300 women failed to detect any LCIS (1,14,21).

Clinical Presentation. LCIS is typically discovered by coincidence in breast tissue removed for proliferative lesions that cause a mass or in apparently normal tissue surrounding a benign tumor such as a fibroadenoma. Associated benign processes may cause mammographic abnormalities that lead to a biopsy in which LCIS is detected. Calcifications are rare but occur commonly in coexisting lesions such as sclerosing adenosis (19) or in nearby normal lobules and ducts (29). Mammography is not an effective method for detecting LCIS (23) and cannot be depended upon to assess multicentricity or bilaterality of the disease.

The age distribution of LCIS is similar to that of most other forms of mammary carcinoma. However, it occurs infrequently in the absence of other forms of carcinoma in women younger than 35 or older than 75 years of age. The average age at diagnosis ranges from 44 to 54 years (37). In a consecutive series of more than 1,000 patients treated for breast carcinoma the mean age of women with LCIS (53 years) was not significantly different from that of patients with infiltrating duct carcinoma (57 years) (32).

Documentation of bilaterality is uncertain because few surgeons routinely biopsy the contralateral breast or perform bilateral mastectomy for this disease. Newman (25) found bilateral LCIS in 33 percent of 18 women who had a contralateral biopsy. Lewison and Finney (22) found bilateral disease in 7 of 15 (46 percent) women who had tissue from both breasts examined, and Haagensen (16) found bilateral LCIS in 25 of 84 (30 percent) patients. Urban (43) systematically performed contralateral biopsies for all types of breast carcinoma and reported finding concurrent contralateral LCIS in 9 of 22 (40 percent) patients. Sunshine et al. (41) reported that 21 of 36 (67 percent) women with LCIS treated by bilateral mastectomy had LCIS in their opposite breast.

These data on the bilaterality of LCIS provide compelling evidence that both breasts are frequently affected by the disease, often at the same time. When the ipsilateral breast contains only LCIS, contralateral LCIS will be found in approximately one of every three breasts biopsied. When contralateral mastectomy is performed, bilaterality can be demonstrated in two thirds of patients. Conceivably, the proportion of bilaterality could be increased further by whole organ serial sectioning, but there are women with LCIS who do not have simultaneous bilaterality and may never have both breasts affected by LCIS or any other form of mammary carcinoma.

Multicentricity and bilaterality are interrelated characteristics of mammary carcinomas. Carcinomas associated with a high frequency of

Table 1

FINDINGS AT MASTECTOMY AFTER BIOPSY DIAGNOSIS OF LOBULAR CARCINOMA IN SITU

Researchers		Mastectomy Findings		
	Biopsy Diagnosis (No. patients)	Carcinoma		No Carcinoma
		Intraepithelial No. patients (%)	Invasive No. patients (%)	No. patients (%)
Rosen et al. (33)	LCIS (50)	30 (60)	2 (4)	18 (36)
Carter and Smith (9)	LCIS (49)	31 (63)	3 (6)	15 (31)
Shah et al. (39)	LCIS (40)	26 (65)	2 (5)	12 (30)

bilaterality are also likely to occur in multicentric foci in the affected breast. Multicentric foci of carcinoma have been found in 60 to 85 percent of patients undergoing mastectomy for LCIS (3,10, 22,33,44); of these, 90 percent have been LCIS. Invasive carcinoma has been unexpectedly found in 4 to 6 percent of mastectomies performed after a biopsy diagnosis of LCIS (Table 1) (9,33,39).

Gross Findings. LCIS does not, by itself, result in a grossly apparent pathologic alteration in breast tissue but the tissue which harbors LCIS often appears abnormal as a result of co-existing benign proliferative lesions. In patients with very florid and extensive LCIS, the cut surface of the breast tissue may have a faintly granular appearance when viewed at an angle because the affected lobules are sufficiently enlarged to be visible.

Microscopic Findings. LCIS arises from the terminal ducts in the postmenopausal atrophic breast but from the terminal duct lobular complex in premenopausal women. The microscopic anatomic distribution of LCIS in lobules and terminal ducts influences the histopathologic findings in a given case.

In the typical lobular form of LCIS, neoplastic cells replace the normal epithelium of acini and intralobular ductules (fig. 173). The abnormal cells are usually sufficiently numerous to cause expansion of these structures as well as enlargement of the entire lobule in comparison with uninvolved lobules in the adjacent breast. However, unwarranted emphasis has been given to lobular distension as a diagnostic feature. According to Foote and Stewart (13) this is not a requirement for diagnosis and no yardstick permits accurate evaluation of what constitutes lobular distension. Comparison of adjacent involved and uninvolved lobules is not reliable because lobular diameters vary considerably within a section and from case to case (figs. 174, 175). In one study there was a slight but statistically insignificant trend for a greater risk of subsequent carcinoma when distension was minimal than when it was marked (34). Others found a slight but insignificant increase in the risk of subsequent intraductal or invasive carcinoma with maximum distention (16). If the diagnosis of LCIS is to be meaningful because it identifies a lesion associated with a substantial risk of later carcinoma, then lobular distension cannot be regarded as an important diagnostic criterion in lesions that have reached an acceptable qualitative level of cytologic abnormality.

Quantitative factors have been included among the diagnostic criteria for LCIS. The question of how much lobular involvement is necessary for the diagnosis remains unanswered. While some authors require at least two lobules exhibiting diagnostic features (20), others feel that one fully affected lobule is sufficient evidence for the diagnosis (18,34). The latter position is based on the observation that the risk of subsequent intraductal or invasive carcinoma did not prove to be related to the number of affected lobules in biopsy specimens of patients not treated by mastectomy (34). There was no significant difference in risk between patients

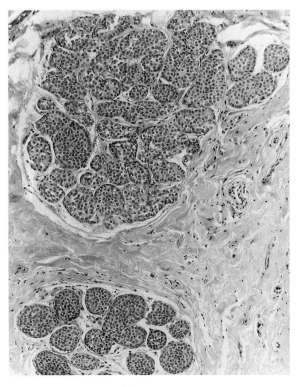

Figure 173
LOBULAR CARCINOMA IN SITU
Normal epithelium in two lobules has been entirely replaced by uniform population of neoplastic cells that fill acinar glands. Individual glands are rounded and discrete. (Figures 173 and 182 are from the same patient.)

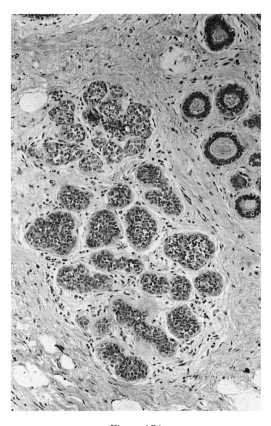

Figure 174
LOBULAR CARCINOMA IN SITU
Neoplastic acini are not appreciably larger than those of the adjacent uninvolved lobule with microcystic change.

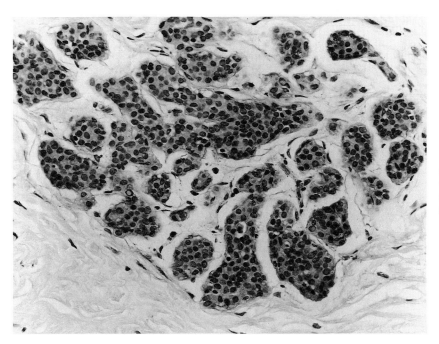

Figure 175
LOBULAR CARCINOMA
IN SITU
Magnified view of lobule similar to the one in figure 174. Discrete acini with haphazardly arranged monomorphic cells that have uniform dark nuclei and scant cytoplasm.

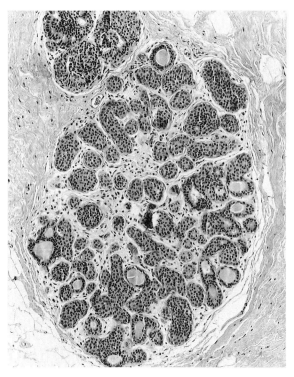

Figure 176
LOBULAR CARCINOMA IN SITU
Partially affected lobule in which approximately 80 percent of acini have been filled by neoplastic cells. (Figures 176 and 177 are from the same patient.)

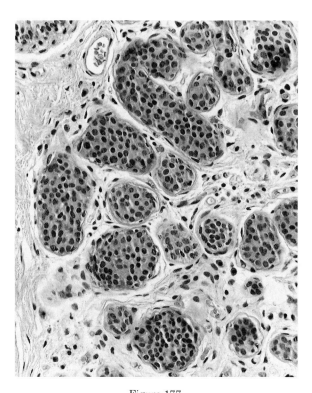

Figure 177
LOBULAR CARCINOMA IN SITU
Magnified view of figure 176 showing discrete acinar units filled with monomorphic cells in a disorderly distribution not oriented to the basement membrane.

with one or with two affected lobules and thus there is no logical reason for drawing a distinction between one and two involved lobules as a basis for the diagnosis of LCIS.

Partial involvement of one or more lobules is not an uncommon finding in a patient whose biopsy also contains many completely affected lobules (figs. 176, 177). In some cases the only evidence of a neoplastic lobular proliferation is one lobule in which some, but not all, of the acini are involved (figs. 178, 179). The complete absence of glandular lumens throughout the lobule is not necessary for the diagnosis of LCIS. It has been suggested arbitrarily that at least 50 percent (28) or 75 percent (31) of one lobule be involved to establish a diagnosis of LCIS and that specimens with smaller lesions be included in the category of atypical lobular hyperplasia (figs. 180, 181).

Loss of cohesion is a characteristic of neoplastic cells in LCIS although this may not be readily apparent in acini filled and expanded by the process. When loss of cohesion is prominent and

the neoplastic cells have a dissociated distribution, spaces may be created between them that can be mistaken for glandular lumens. However, the neoplastic cells here are not arranged in the orderly evenly spaced fashion that characterizes non-neoplastic cells persisting around true glandular lumens.

Typically, the neoplastic cells are described as having scant cytoplasm and small, round, cytologically bland nuclei that lack nucleoli (fig. 182). This is the cytologic pattern referred to as type A by Haagensen and associates (18). However, considerable cytologic pleomorphism may be encountered and the more varied cells are classified as type B. Type A cells tend to have a diploid DNA content whereas type B cells are largely hyperdiploid (fig. 183) (46), have more abundant cytoplasm, and larger more pleomorphic nuclei that sometimes have nucleoli. The cytologic features of type B cells sometimes resemble those of intraductal carcinoma. When the lesion is composed entirely of type B cells, the distinction between LCIS and

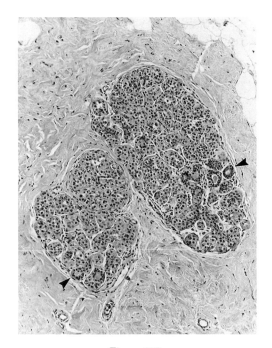

Figure 178
LOBULAR CARCINOMA IN SITU
Neoplastic cells fill most acini in two adjacent lobules. Arrows indicate unaffected glands. (Figures 178 and 179 are from the same patient.)

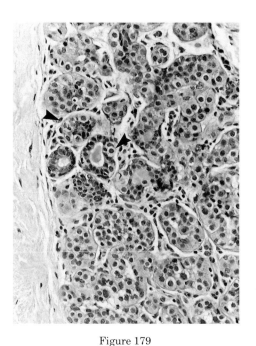

Figure 179
LOBULAR CARCINOMA IN SITU
Magnified view of part of lobule in figure 178 showing pagetoid spread of neoplastic cells into normal acinar epithelium (arrows).

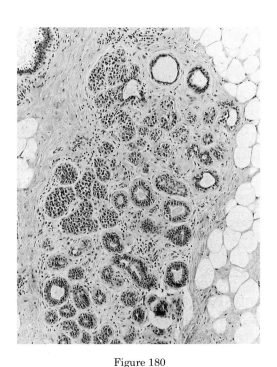

Figure 180
ATYPICAL LOBULAR HYPERPLASIA
Neoplastic cells occupy less than 50 percent of acinar units in this lobule. (Figures 180 and 181 are from the same patient.)

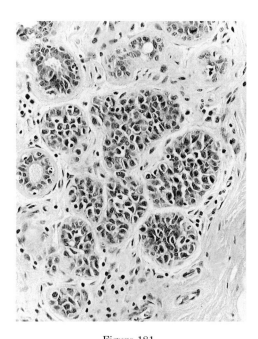

Figure 181
ATYPICAL LOBULAR HYPERPLASIA
Magnified view of part of lobule in figure 180. Note loss of cohesion among neoplastic cells and pagetoid spread in acinar epithelium. Replacement of acinar epithelium by the neoplastic cells shown here with loss of cohesion and disorderly arrangement would be diagnostic of lobular carcinoma in situ if present more widely in the lobule.

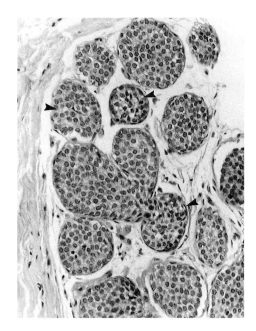

Figure 182
LOBULAR CARCINOMA IN SITU
Characteristic cytologic appearance of neoplastic cells with uniform round nuclei. Many of the cells have minute cytoplasmic vacuoles that are barely perceptible at this magnification (arrows). Mucicarmine stain was positive in many cells.

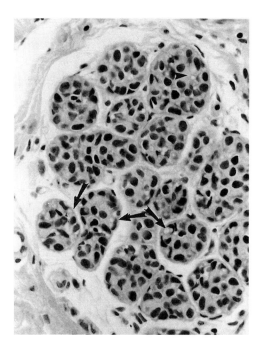

Figure 184
LOBULAR CARCINOMA IN SITU
Magnified view of lobule similar to figure 182. Many tumor cells contain small, indistinct cytoplasmic mucin vacuoles (arrows).

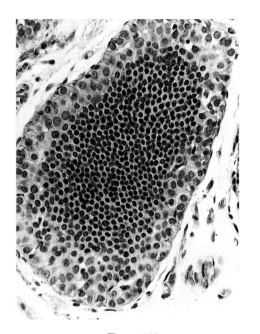

Figure 183
LOBULAR CARCINOMA IN SITU
Magnified view of acinar gland showing the typical distribution of type A cells crowded in the center and type B cells at the periphery.

intralobular extension of intraductal carcinoma may be difficult to establish. Type B LCIS is predominantly a lobular lesion in which duct involvement is typically a minor component that has a pagetoid distribution. The ductal component lacks comedo, cribriform, or papillary growth patterns typical of duct carcinoma.

Intracytoplasmic vacuoles that contain mucinous secretion are almost always present in at least some LCIS cells (fig. 184) (4,15). These can be highlighted with a stain for intracellular mucin such as mucicarmine or Alcian blue–PAS (15). An extreme manifestation of this phenomenon is the formation of signet ring cells that have a cytoplasmic vacuole due to mucin accumulation (fig. 185) (7). Because intracytoplasmic mucin vacuoles are uncommon in the cells of ductal carcinoma and are virtually absent in hyperplastic lesions of duct or lobular epithelium, their presence is an important but not a necessary criterion for the diagnosis of LCIS (4,7,15).

LCIS typically involves intralobular and extralobular or terminal ductules as well as acinar units within the lobule (figs. 186, 187). Extralobular LCIS occurs in 65 to 75 percent of patients

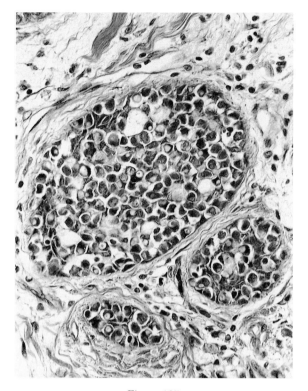

Figure 185
LOBULAR CARCINOMA IN SITU
Pronounced signet ring cell formation in lobular carcinoma in situ.

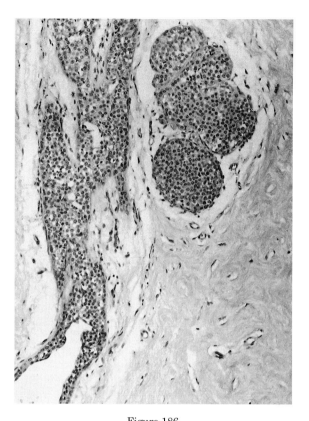

Figure 186
LOBULAR CARCINOMA IN SITU
Neoplastic cells fill acinar units of a lobule and much of a terminal duct. Pagetoid extension of neoplastic cells beneath duct epithelium is seen in lower left corner.

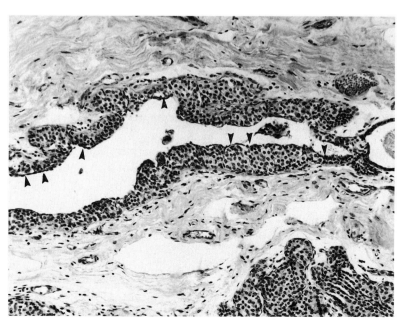

Figure 187
LOBULAR CARCINOMA IN SITU
Duct involvement by lobular carcinoma in situ. Solid layer of neoplastic cells extends beneath duct epithelium persisting as a thin layer at the luminal surface (small arrows). Duct epithelium is lifted where it is undermined by the "advancing" neoplastic proliferation. (Fig. 9 from Rosen PP, Kosloff C, Lieberman PH, Adair F, Braun DW Jr. Lobular carcinoma in situ of the breast. Detailed analysis of 99 patients with an average follow-up of 24 years. Am J Surg Pathol 1978;2:225–51.)

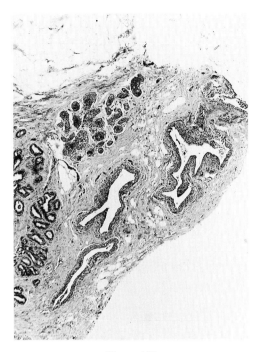

Figure 188
LOBULAR CARCINOMA IN SITU
Lesion involving a lobule (left center) and ducts. (Figures 188–190 are from the same patient.)

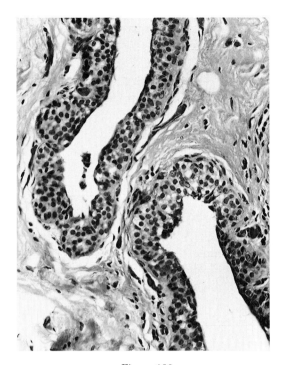

Figure 190
LOBULAR CARCINOMA IN SITU
Layer of neoplastic cells beneath attenuated duct epithelial cells which form a dark line at the luminal surface.

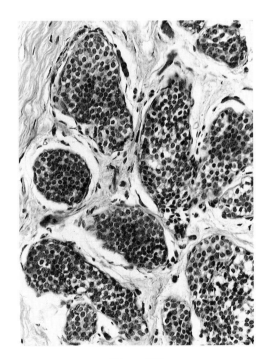

Figure 189
LOBULAR CARCINOMA IN SITU
Acinar glands in the lobule shown in figure 188 filled by uniform neoplastic cells.

(2,11,16). In postmenopausal patients with atrophic lobular breast tissue, duct involvement may be the only manifestation of LCIS (figs. 188–190) (16,17). The irregular configuration of these ductules has been described as saw-toothed or resembling a clover leaf (figs. 191–193). The neoplastic cells may be distributed continuously along the ductal system, undermining and ultimately displacing the normal ductal epithelium. Clusters of LCIS cells arising beneath the non-neoplastic ductal epithelium form buds projecting into the surrounding stroma around the periphery of the duct. When this occurs, the normal glandular epithelium often persists, having been elevated and pushed toward the lumen. The myoepithelial layer, only preserved to a variable extent, is often absent. LCIS cells may also be found singly or in small groups within the epithelium in a pattern that resembles Paget disease of the nipple, so-called pagetoid spread. Usually this process is limited to secondary and tertiary or terminal ductules. It is unusual to detect pagetoid spread in the epithelium of large, lactiferous ducts but this

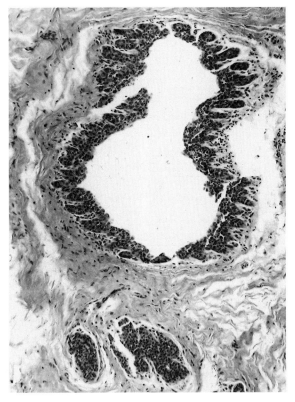

Figure 191
LOBULAR CARCINOMA IN SITU
Fully developed "saw-tooth" or serrated pattern. In this postmenopausal patient, the neoplastic process was limited to ducts, many of which had this pattern. Ductules also involved by LCIS are present below.

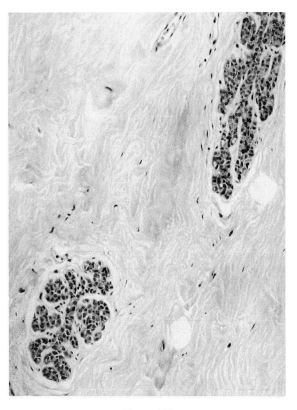

Figure 192
LOBULAR CARCINOMA IN SITU
Clover leaf configuration in atrophic terminal duct lobular units in a postmenopausal woman. (Figures 192 and 193 are from the same patient.)

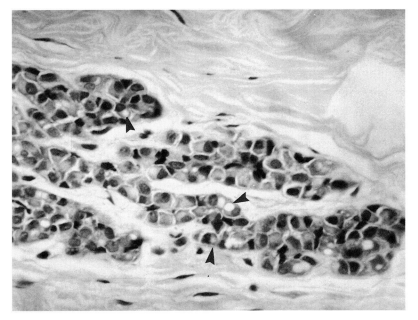

Figure 193
LOBULAR CARCINOMA IN SITU
Neoplastic cells in the clover leaf pattern of postmenopausal lobular carcinoma in situ. Atrophic glandular structures here lack the round contour seen in the premenopausal breast. Cytologic features typically seen in this setting are cytoplasmic vacuoles (arrows) that contain mucin (signet ring cells), darkly stained irregular nuclei, relatively dense eosinophilic cytoplasm, and loss of cohesion. This cytologic appearance has been described as "myoid" because of a superficial resemblance to myoblasts.

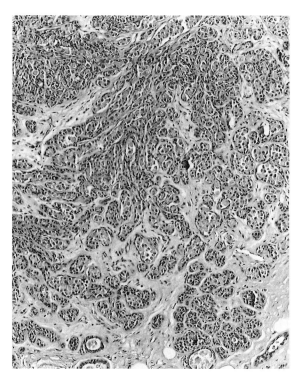

Figure 194
LOBULAR CARCINOMA IN SITU
IN SCLEROSING ADENOSIS
Complex pattern formed by proliferation of neoplastic epithelial cells and myoepithelial cells. (Figures 194–196 are from the same patient.)

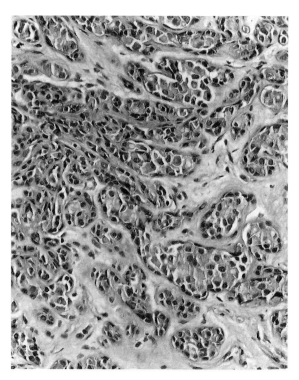

Figure 195
LOBULAR CARCINOMA IN SITU
IN SCLEROSING ADENOSIS
Neoplastic cells filling tubules some of which are outlined by myoepithelial cells. Indistinct tubular or glandular borders, disruption of basement membranes, or cells seemingly isolated in the stroma should not be regarded as evidence of invasion within sclerosing adenosis involved by lobular carcinoma in situ.

may occur when lobules in or near the nipple are affected by LCIS (36). Paget disease of the surface of the nipple is not a feature of LCIS.

LCIS has been encountered in fibroadenomas, in sclerosing adenosis in intraductal papillomas, and in radial sclerosing lesions. The diagnosis of LCIS under these circumstances rests largely on the identification of the appropriate cytologic features. The demonstration of intracytoplasmic mucin droplets is especially helpful for distinguishing between florid adenosis and LCIS in adenosis since this finding is virtually never seen in benign lobular proliferations (figs. 194, 195). The lobular configuration is radically distorted in sclerosing lesions and as a result it is difficult to exclude invasion in such foci (12). However, careful inspection usually reveals the underlying lobular pattern of sclerosing adenosis (figs. 196, 197). This architectural pattern can be accentuated with the reticulin stain and by the immunohistochemical demonstration of laminin or type IV collagen. At-

tenuated spindle-shaped myoepithelial cells that proliferate in sclerosing adenosis usually persist even when the lesion is colonized by LCIS (figs. 198, 199). Invasion should not be diagnosed as long as the neoplastic cells remain confined to the configuration of sclerosing adenosis.

LCIS usually involves the epithelium of a papilloma by pagetoid spread (figs. 200–202). The preexisting ductal epithelium is elevated and persists over the neoplastic cell layer. This process must be distinguished from the uncommon situation of LCIS merging with intraductal carcinoma (figs. 203–205).

Electron microscopic studies have documented the origin of LCIS from lobular epithelial cells (24,27,42). Intracytoplasmic lumina lined by microvilli are seen ultrastructurally in the typical case. Myoepithelial cells have been demonstrated

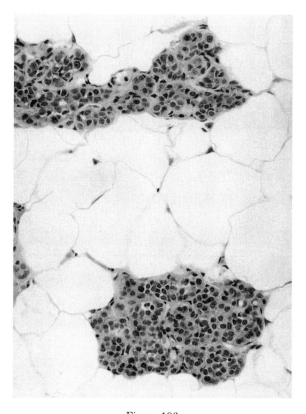

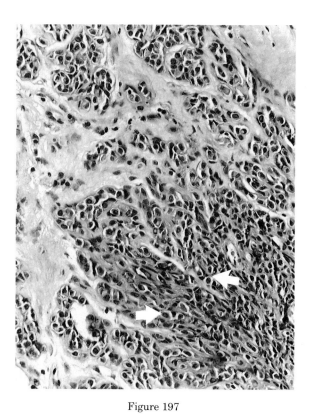

Figure 196
LOBULAR CARCINOMA IN SITU
Although this simulates invasive carcinoma, the internal alveolar configuration of lobular carcinoma in situ is retained.

Figure 197
LOBULAR CARCINOMA IN SITU
IN SCLEROSING ADENOSIS
Pagetoid spread of neoplastic cells into glandular units distorted by myoepithelial cell proliferation (arrows).

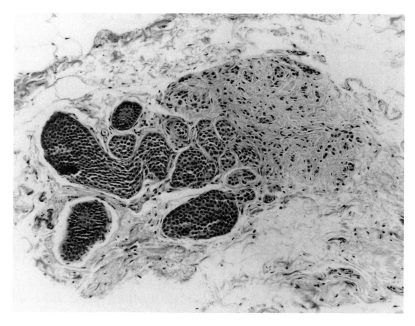

Figure 198
LOBULAR CARCINOMA IN SITU
WITH MICROINVASION
Invasive carcinoma cells form a small nodule in contiguity with in situ lobular carcinoma. Note loss of lobular pattern in invasive component where tumor cells are present individually or in linear strands.

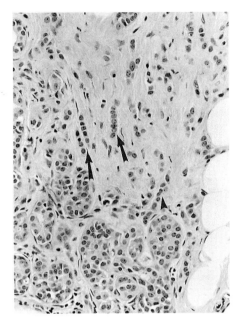

Figure 199
LOBULAR CARCINOMA IN SITU IN SCLEROSING
ADENOSIS WITH MICROINVASION

Invasive lobular carcinoma cells form linear strands (arrows) in fibrous stroma, unaccompanied by myofibroblastic proliferation. The adjacent in situ component is part of a large focus of sclerosing adenosis diffusely involved by lobular carcinoma in situ.

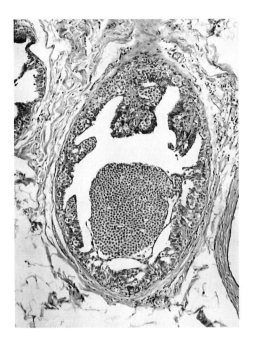

Figure 200
LOBULAR CARCINOMA IN SITU IN PAPILLOMA

Neoplastic cells spreading in a pagetoid fashion beneath papillary duct epithelium and forming a polypoid mass in the duct lumen. (Figures 200 and 201 are from the same patient.)

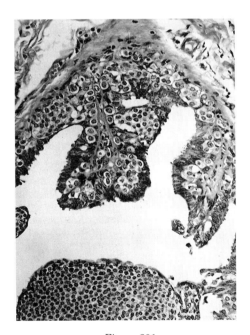

Figure 201
LOBULAR CARCINOMA IN SITU IN PAPILLOMA

Magnified view of papillary hyperplasia showing pagetoid lobular carcinoma in situ beneath persisting duct epithelium.

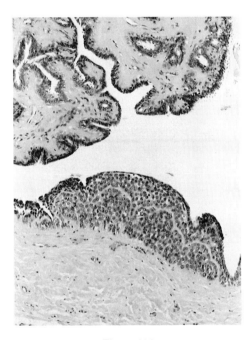

Figure 202
LOBULAR CARCINOMA
IN SITU IN PAPILLOMA

Plaque-like pattern of pagetoid lobular carcinoma in situ beneath duct epithelium in the wall of a duct that contained an intraductal papilloma.

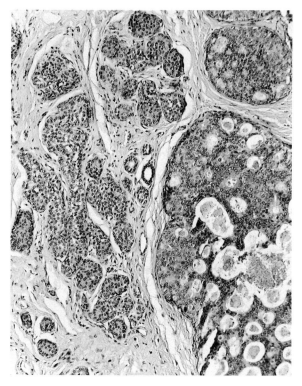

Figure 203
LOBULAR CARCINOMA IN SITU MERGING
WITH INTRADUCTAL CARCINOMA

Separate adjacent foci of cribriform intraductal carcinoma and lobular carcinoma in situ. (Fig. 2A from Rosen PP. Coexistent lobular carcinoma in situ and intraductal carcinoma in a single lobular-duct unit. Am J Surg Pathol 1980;4:241–6.) (Figures 203–205 are from the same patient.)

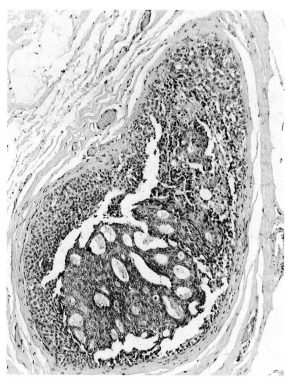

Figure 204
LOBULAR CARCINOMA IN SITU MERGING
WITH INTRADUCTAL CARCINOMA

Cribriform intraductal carcinoma fills the center of the duct and lobular carcinoma in situ is distributed around the periphery. (Fig. 2B from Rosen PP. Coexistent lobular carcinoma in situ and intraductal carcinoma in a single lobular-duct unit. Am J Surg Pathol 1980;4:241–6.)

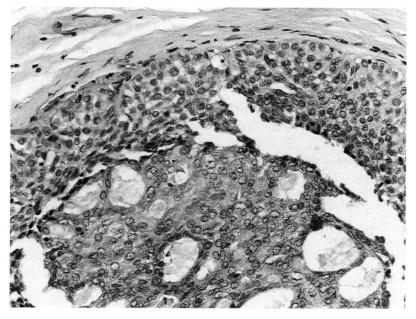

Figure 205
LOBULAR CARCINOMA IN SITU
MERGING WITH
INTRADUCTAL CARCINOMA

Magnified view of figure 204 showing different growth patterns and cytology in the two components.

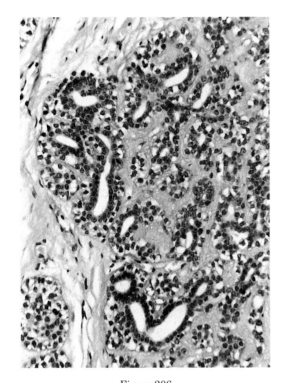

Figure 206
MYOEPITHELIAL HYPERPLASIA
Glandular epithelial cells are displaced by the proliferation of clear round myoepithelial cells.

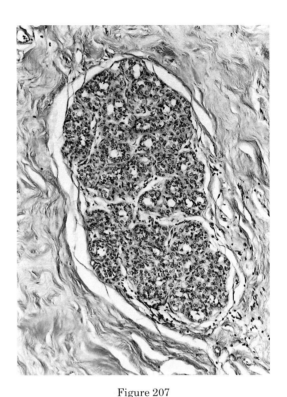

Figure 207
ATYPICAL LOBULAR HYPERPLASIA
At low magnification many acinar lumens appear to be preserved and individual acinar glands are poorly defined.

by electron microscopy and by immunohistochemistry (8). The distribution of these cells tends to be disordered and they are less numerous or absent when LCIS is associated with invasive lobular carcinoma (8).

Differential Diagnosis. A number of proliferative and cytologic alterations that should be distinguished from LCIS affect the terminal duct lobular units. These include pregnancy-like "pseudolactational" hyperplasia, myoepithelial hyperplasia, clear cell change, and atypical lobular hyperplasia. Pseudolactational hyperplasia occurs in premenopausal women who are not pregnant and in postmenopausal women while clear cell change is found mainly in premenopausal women. Usually, only a few isolated lobules are affected. Pregnancy-like hyperplasia and clear cell change will be described later.

Hyperplasia of myoepithelial cells in lobules results in expansion of the myoepithelial component displacing the epithelial cells (fig. 206). However, lobular acini usually retain some identifiable glandular cells. Hyperplastic myoepithelial cells

are characterized by clear cytoplasm and small, round, hyperchromatic nuclei.

In atypical lobular hyperplasia (ALH) the glandular proliferation has some features of LCIS but the changes are not sufficient to establish the diagnosis. There are no universally accepted criteria for the precise distinction between atypical lobular hyperplasia and LCIS; the diagnosis depends upon qualitative and quantitative factors.

From the qualitative point of view, ALH is characterized by the presence within a lobule of abnormal cells resembling the cells seen in LCIS. In the most inconspicuous and least well-developed configuration, the neoplastic proliferation replaces the normal glandular cells and disrupts the lobular structure by effacing the lumens while not expanding the acinar units (figs. 207, 208). As the process evolves, the accumulation of a greater number of neoplastic cells causes some acinar expansion but the borders of acinar units and intralobular ductules remain indistinct (figs. 209, 210). Clear delineation of intralobular acinar units is an important feature that distinguishes

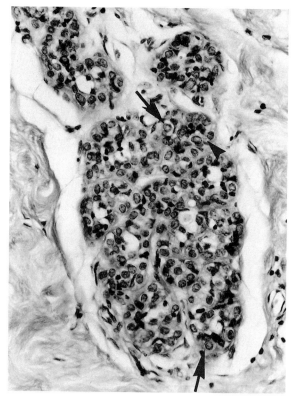

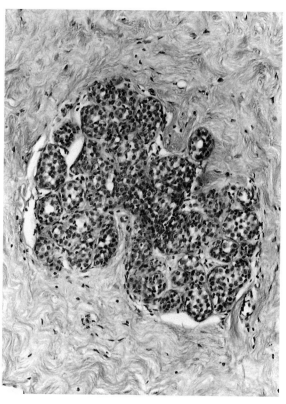

Figure 208
ATYPICAL LOBULAR HYPERPLASIA

An early stage in which haphazardly dispersed atypical cells (arrows) have partially replaced the normal cellular constituents of the lobule. The "busy" appearance of the lobule is in part due to the pyknotic nuclei of degenerating cells. Individual acinar glands are poorly defined.

Figure 209
ATYPICAL LOBULAR HYPERPLASIA

An advanced lesion in which a number of acinar units have been expanded and stand out at the left margin of the lobule. (Figures 209 and 210 are from the same patient.)

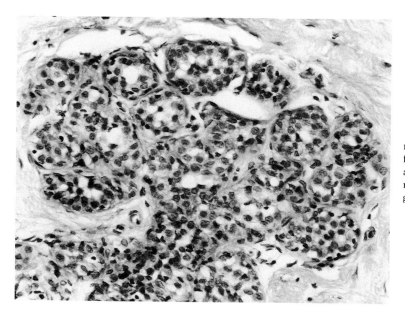

Figure 210
ATYPICAL LOBULAR HYPERPLASIA

There is some loss of cohesion among neoplastic cells that have almost entirely filled and have caused slight expansion of acinar units. Note marginal orientation of nuclei within individual acini and heterogeneous population of cells.

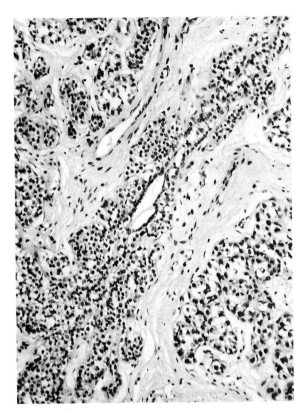

Figure 211
ATYPICAL LOBULAR HYPERPLASIA
OF TERMINAL DUCT
Clover leaf pattern of proliferation around a terminal duct. Non-neoplastic duct epithelium is preserved around the duct in the center. (Figures 211 and 212 are from the same patient.)

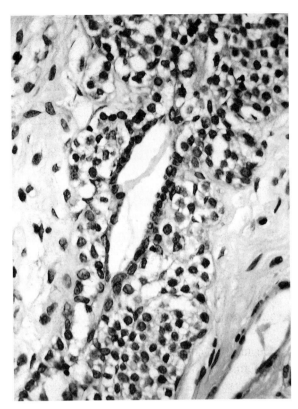

Figure 212
ATYPICAL LOBULAR HYPERPLASIA
OF TERMINAL DUCT
Magnified view of figure 211 showing ill-defined glandular proliferation surrounding the terminal duct.

LCIS from ALH, especially in the premenopausal breast (figs. 211, 212). This phenomenon reflects the accumulation in the acinar unit of a sufficient number of neoplastic cells to expand the gland to a round or oval configuration.

Prognosis. In virtually all cases mastectomy will "cure" a patient whose breast biopsy shows LCIS because at this stage the lesion has not become invasive and does not have access to the blood stream or lymphatics. Cure must be interpreted in this setting as largely preventive. Mastectomy has been recommended because of the 4 to 6 percent risk of unsuspected concurrent invasion in the biopsied breast and the risk that invasive carcinoma might develop later in the affected breast.

The majority of patients with LCIS not treated by mastectomy remain well. Studies of more than

25 women followed for at least 15 years have demonstrated subsequent ipsilateral carcinoma in 17.4 to 22 percent of the patients (5,16,34), and subsequent contralateral carcinoma in 9.7 to 23 percent of patients. The risk of carcinoma increases with longer follow-up. When compared with age-matched normal women, the observed frequency of carcinoma exceeds the expected rate by 5.9 (16) to 9 (34) times. The risk for women with a positive family history of breast carcinoma is especially high (13.8 times expected rate) (32).

The risk of subsequent carcinoma is not related to the number of lobules with LCIS in the original biopsy. Cases in which LCIS cells were small (so-called "type A") have essentially the same frequency of later carcinoma as cases with large (so-called "type B") cells. Carcinoma is most frequent, with an earlier onset, in cases that have both types of cells (large and small) (32,34).

Approximately 25 percent of carcinomas that arise in patients with LCIS are infiltrating lobular carcinomas; histologically favorable types of carcinoma account for less than 15 percent. The majority of patients develop invasive duct carcinomas.

Treatment. The three treatment choices generally considered are: 1) no surgery after the diagnostic biopsy, relying on clinical follow-up to detect subsequent carcinoma; 2) bilateral mastectomy; and 3) ipsilateral mastectomy. The opposite breast may be biopsied and contralateral mastectomy performed if carcinoma is found. It is advisable that these alternatives for treatment be discussed with the patient.

The nonsurgical clinical follow-up approach is a lifetime undertaking in view of the relatively high frequency of late-occurring carcinomas. While clinical follow-up is increasingly recommended for, or selected by, LCIS patients there is no consensus regarding the optimal follow-up program. Mortality due to breast cancer among untreated patients in one retrospective study of LCIS patients was nearly 11 times greater than expected (34). It remains to be seen whether mortality can be reduced by detecting subsequent carcinomas through close clinical surveillance. Data from the SEER Program (40) and others (38) indicate that when detected, subsequent invasive carcinomas of 1 cm or less have axillary metastases in 13 to 16 percent of cases. In one series with no systematic follow-up of LCIS patients, about 50 percent had nodal metastases when carcinoma was later detected (34). A study of more carefully followed patients showed axillary metastases in 26 percent and nearly 25 percent later developed systemic metastases (32).

Subcutaneous mastectomy, whether unilateral or bilateral, may leave an appreciable amount of breast tissue, especially if the nipple is preserved. Lobular tissue has been described in the nipple (36). If surgical treatment is elected, it should remove all breast parenchyma because of the known multicentric nature of the disease and the possibility of a coexistent occult invasive lesion. Total mastectomy with low axillary dissection is the preferred operation. This procedure preserves the pectoral musculature and fold, thereby providing the best setting for reconstruction.

Conclusions regarding bilateral risk have been based largely on studies in which only the breast that harbored LCIS had been biopsied. The status of the opposite breast in these cases was unknown. Bilaterality of LCIS occurs frequently, but it is unproven whether it occurs in every patient. While the overall risk of subsequent ipsilateral and contralateral carcinoma may have been equal in retrospective studies, the risk is not necessarily equal for both breasts in each patient. Biopsy of the opposite breast may identify patients with the greatest risk of subsequent contralateral carcinoma. The biopsy should be substantial to provide adequate material for histologic examination. When there is no clinical abnormality that warrants biopsy, the specimen should be taken from the upper outer quadrant. There seems little justification for routinely carrying out a contralateral mastectomy without a prior biopsy, although some patients may choose this approach.

There is little experience other than surgical with treatment of LCIS. No systematic study of radiation therapy has been undertaken and this is not a recommended therapeutic approach. LCIS that appears histologically unaffected by radiation has been observed in mastectomies from patients with recurrent carcinoma following lumpectomy and irradiation. Atrophy of radiated non-neoplastic lobules is invariably seen in the same specimens.

Patients receiving tamoxifen as adjuvant therapy following invasive carcinoma had a lower than expected frequency of contralateral carcinoma (6). The possibility that an antiestrogen might inhibit the evolution of LCIS was suggested in 1978 (34). Recently initiated trials have employed tamoxifen in patients with LCIS or other markers of high breast cancer risk (30), but at present this must be regarded as experimental treatment.

INTRADUCTAL CARCINOMA AND ATYPICAL HYPERPLASIA

Carcinoma of the breast arises within the duct system, frequently in the terminal duct lobular unit. Intraductal carcinoma, also termed *noninvasive carcinoma* or *ductal carcinoma in situ*, is the culmination of a continuum starting with focal or circumferential multilayering of the normal single cell epithelial lining of the duct resulting in bland hyperplasia, and evolving through progressively increasing atypism. It must be inferred that the ductal epithelium, at some point, undergoes a change to a preneoplastic character and subsequently to a neoplastic one (94).

While there is general agreement with this progression, some dispute the concept of an unbroken spectrum linking hyperplasia to carcinoma (47). The time required for these transitions undoubtedly is extremely variable, and it is likely that the process may be halted and possibly reversed in some stages. The microscopic criteria for recognizing progression of ductal hyperplasia remain, at best, inexact and subjective. There is no specific morphologic marker or constellation of markers to distinguish between intraductal epithelial cells committed to neoplastic proliferation and those that are not (83). Not only the epithelium, but also the periductal stroma, participate in this process. Periductal and stromal elastosis progressively increase in prominence when one compares breasts containing bland intraductal hyperplasia to those with atypical hyperplasia and intraductal carcinoma (79).

Although this abnormality usually initially affects the terminal duct lobular unit, the calibre of involved ducts at the time of diagnosis suggests that extralobular ducts are most often involved. This is acknowledged by the use of the prefix "intraductal." However, this level of ductal involvement is often more apparent than real, and results from the unfolding and coalescence of ductules within the lobule to form larger structures (95). However, there are clearly instances of intraductal carcinoma limited to the major ductal system or the terminal lactiferous ducts indicating origin at this level rather than in the terminal duct lobular unit. The continued use of "intraductal" relates more to the pattern of involvement than to the level of the duct system involved.

Intraductal epithelial proliferation usually is included in the category of proliferative or fibrocystic changes. However, the importance of the diagnostic distinction of bland intraductal hyperplasia from intraductal hyperplasia with atypism, and the difficulty in distinguishing the latter lesion from intraductal carcinoma, as well as the association with an increased risk of subsequent carcinoma, warrants separate consideration of the topic.

The microscopic distinction between the various manifestations of intraductal epithelial proliferation is, to some extent, subjective and arbitrary. Nevertheless, recognition of these proliferative abnormalities is important for the clinical management of the patient, since studies have shown that intraductal hyperplasia is associated with an increased risk for the development of carcinoma (50,55). This risk is greater when there is epithelial atypism, and the risk is further increased when there is a history of breast carcinoma in a first degree relative (77).

Intraductal Hyperplasia

Intraductal hyperplasia is a very common microscopic finding, frequently coexisting with other fibrocystic changes. *Epitheliosis* and *papillomatosis* are synonymous terms. The latter implies that the proliferation has a papillary appearance and results in confusion with multiple intraductal papillomas. Since hyperplastic duct lesions do not always have a papillary configuration, papillomatosis is not a useful term in this setting.

Duct hyperplasia must be distinguished from adenosis, a caricature of the lobule resulting from proliferation and elongation of lobular ducts lined by myoepithelium and epithelium without associated intraductal epithelial proliferation. Duct hyperplasia ordinarily does not produce a grossly identifiable lesion and, unless it is associated with microcalcification or with extensive fibrosis, it does not produce a mammographic abnormality.

Microscopically, intraductal hyperplasia results in a varied growth pattern. Only a few ducts in a high-power field may be involved, or the process can occupy most of the ducts in a section. The epithelial proliferation may range from a sparse, often focal, increase in the number of cells lining the duct, to occlusion and distension of the duct by proliferating cells (fig. 213).

Myoepithelial and epithelial cells participate in the cellular proliferation (fig. 214, 215). In some instances the hyperplasia is papillary, varying from the formation of multiple micropapillae within a duct to small intraductal papillomas with delicate fibrovascular cores. Ribbons or bridges of proliferating epithelium often grow into the lumen of the involved duct and these may merge with one another to form secondary lumens. The cells in these areas tend to be arrayed parallel to the long axis of the ribbon or of the fenestration, resulting in apparent streaming of the cells (fig. 216). The ribbons may have a rigid or wavy appearance. The proliferating cells can form small tufts which protrude into the duct lumen, or virtually solid intraductal nodules.

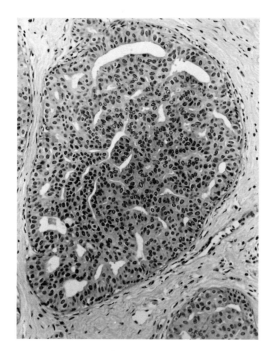

Figure 213
INTRADUCTAL HYPERPLASIA
Distension of a duct by a cellular proliferation in which the spaces formed by anastomosis of cellular columns are irregular and slit-like.

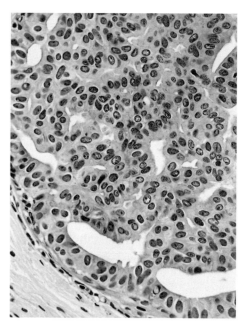

Figure 214
INTRADUCTAL HYPERPLASIA
The cell population consists of a mixture of oval to spindled epithelial cells and elongated myoepithelial cells with denser nuclear chromatin. (Figures 214 and 215 are from the same patient.)

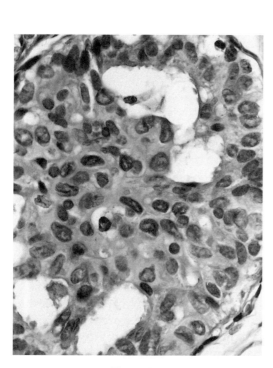

Figure 215
INTRADUCTAL HYPERPLASIA
The heterogeneity of the cellular proliferation is more apparent at higher magnification.

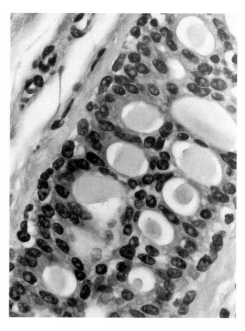

Figure 216
INTRADUCTAL HYPERPLASIA
Spindled epithelial cells appear to be arranged parallel to the long axis of intraductal cellular bridges. The cell bridges merge in the center of the duct to form secondary round lumens. Myoepithelial cells are evident along the borders of the duct.

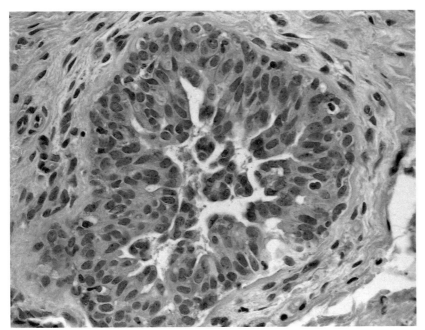

Figure 216A
MICROPAPILLARY
INTRADUCTAL
HYPERPLASIA
Multilayering of epithelial cells resulting in papillary fronds. Note the parallel alignment of most of the proliferating cells and the uniformity of nuclei.

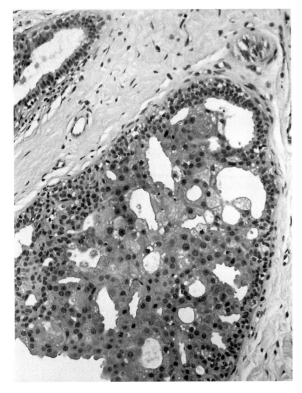

Figure 217
INTRADUCTAL HYPERPLASIA
Apocrine metaplasia forming secondary lumens that contain foam cells.

While the epithelial cells adjacent to the ductal basement membrane have a columnar or cuboidal appearance, in bland intraductal hyperplasia the cells tend to be smaller and often are flattened toward the lumen. A heterogeneous cellular composition characteristically is present throughout, resulting from the multiplication of epithelium and myoepithelium as well as from nuclear pleomorphism and variation in the shape and arrangement of the epithelial cells.

Cellular proliferation sometimes results in micropapillae that may simulate micropapillary intraductal carcinoma. This pattern, referred to as *micropapillary hyperplasia*, resembles epithelial hyperplasia occasionally seen in gynecomastia (fig. 216A). It is not associated with an increased risk of subsequent carcinoma. The columnar epithelium lining the ducts is uniform, lacks atypism, and the hyperchromatic cells in the micropapillae do not extend to the basement membrane (92).

The presence of foamy cells and occasional apocrine metaplastic cells in the proliferative epithelium connotes a benign process (fig. 217). Infrequent mitoses may be present in the epithelial cells, but abnormal mitotic figures are not a feature of hyperplasia. Intraductal lumens formed by cellular proliferation tend to be variable in size and shape, usually having an oval or slit-like configuration with greater calibre at the periphery of the involved duct than at the center (figs. 213, 217, 218). Rather than having a smooth surface, the lumen usually has a scalloped or uneven contour. Most often it is free of secretion, although occasionally, especially when the lumens are ectatic, eosinophilic fluid may be present. Coagulation necrosis is not found in intraductal hyperplasia except in the context of a radial sclerosing lesion.

Intraductal Hyperplasia with Atypism

Defining the borderline between intraductal hyperplasia and intraductal hyperplasia with atypism is important because of the increased risk for subsequent carcinoma associated with the latter proliferative lesion (52). Observer variation is a considerable problem in distinguishing between proliferative lesions that seemingly constitute a continuum. Nonetheless, by defining certain criteria for atypism, authors have demonstrated an association between these microscopic patterns and an increased incidence of subsequent carcinoma in carefully studied populations. The designation of atypism therefore has the potential for identifying patients who are at greater than average risk for the future development of breast cancer. Most of these studies indicate that the presence of intraductal hyperplasia is associated with a moderately increased risk of subsequent invasive carcinoma and that there is an approximate doubling of this risk in the setting of atypical intraductal hyperplasia. The risk of carcinoma is increased in either breast, even if atypia has been demonstrated histologically in only one breast.

Significant obstacles to the clinical use of this information include the subjectivity of the diagnosis, resulting in variability of interobserver interpretation, inconsistency of diagnosis by the same observer, the thoroughness of the pathologic examination of the specimen, and the problem of obtaining a biopsy that is representative of proliferative changes in the breast. Frequently the diagnosis of atypism is used indiscriminately when a pathologist has difficulty in distinguishing between hyperplasia and carcinoma. Subsequent review of such cases may, in some instances, result in the diagnosis of florid, albeit ordinary, intraductal hyperplasia, while in others it may result in the diagnosis of intraductal carcinoma.

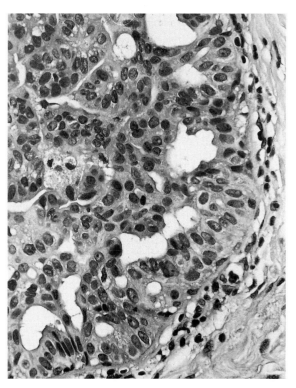

Figure 218
INTRADUCTAL HYPERPLASIA
The secondary lumens at the periphery of the duct have irregular shapes. Columnar epithelium persists around much of the border of the duct. (Figures 218 and 219 are from the same patient.)

While there is no disagreement that progressive atypism of the intraductal epithelial proliferation is associated with an increased risk of carcinoma, there is some difficulty in applying this information to the clinical care of individual patients. In addition to the issues already raised regarding the definition of atypism, it must be emphasized that the risk for developing carcinoma is influenced by many other factors. The relative importance of proliferative breast changes among other known risk factors for individual patients remains uncertain.

Distinguishing between intraductal hyperplasia with atypism and intraductal carcinoma can be difficult, especially when dealing with well-differentiated, noncomedo intraductal carcinomas. Assessment of proliferative rate and various immunohistochemical markers have been utilized, with variable success, to make the distinction. Aneuploidy is more common in intraductal carcinomas than in atypical hyperplasias and this feature correlates with lack of cytologic and architectural differentiation. However, ploidy does not allow a distinct separation between the two lesions in the individual case (53). Strong immunoreactivity for high molecular weight keratins is prominent in atypical hyperplasias while most, but not all, examples of intraductal carcinoma are nonreactive. Myoepithelial cell participation, which may be confirmed immunohistochemically, is most prominent in hyperplasia but generally is confined to the periphery of the involved duct in atypical hyperplasia and carcinoma (80).

More than two decades ago, Black and Chabon (51) developed a five-step numerical grading system to evaluate the progression of atypical changes and intraductal proliferation, culminating in carcinoma. They defined atypism as a multilayering of cells with progressive loss of nuclear polarity. Cytologic features associated with atypism were enlargement of nuclei and nucleoli (50). The authors demonstrated that patients with intraductal atypia defined by their criteria had an increased risk of developing cancer.

In the most extensive investigation to date, DuPont and Page (57) studied more than 10,000 breast biopsies from over 3,000 women who had a median follow-up of 17 years. The microscopic criteria for atypical hyperplasia were comparable to those used by Black et al., but the authors referred specifically to lesions that had some, but not all, of the features of intraductal carcinoma (78). Even when duct involvement was fully consistent with intraductal carcinoma, unless more than one duct was involved the lesion was termed *atypical hyperplasia* (77a). DuPont and Page demonstrated that patients with atypical hyperplasia had a relative risk of subsequent invasive cancer 5.3 times that of women in the general population who lacked proliferative disease. This risk was almost doubled if the woman had a history of breast cancer in a first degree relative with the effect maximal in the first ten years after the breast biopsy (56).

While this study is extremely useful in defining a pattern of intraductal epithelial proliferation of intermediate risk between bland hyperplasia and carcinoma, the microscopic classification of lesions in the study was, of necessity, retrospective. Even in such a controlled study, which contrasts with the interpretation of a biopsy in the usual diagnostic setting, disagreement between pathologists on initial review occurred in 10 percent of cases. Furthermore, it could be anticipated that the highly selective definition of atypical hyperplasia would result in a cohort of patients with a prognosis intermediate between that of hyperplasia and intraductal carcinoma.

The prognosis associated with some but not all of the features of atypical hyperplasia was not clear since these cases were included in a group that also had a large number of women with bland hyperplasia. In addition, the validity of regarding a single duct with characteristic intraductal carcinoma as atypical hyperplasia merely because it is the sole area of involvement in a biopsy is questionable, especially when it is appreciated that less than half of all patients with intraductal carcinoma treated solely by local excision eventually develop invasive carcinoma, even when more than one duct is affected.

An increased risk of developing invasive carcinoma associated with atypical intraductal hyperplasia was also demonstrated by Tavassoli and Norris (91) in a study of almost 200 women. They found that 2.6 percent of patients with ordinary intraductal hyperplasia and 9.8 percent of women with atypical intraductal hyperplasia subsequently developed invasive carcinoma. A family history of carcinoma at least doubled the risk of subsequent invasive carcinoma among patients with either bland or atypical intraductal hyperplasia.

The criteria for atypical intraductal hyperplasia utilized by Tavassoli and Norris were in part similar to those of Page et al., but they insisted that the diagnosis of intraductal carcinoma be limited to lesions with an aggregate diameter of at least 2 mm, regardless of the number of ducts involved. Smaller foci, even with histologic characteristics of intraductal carcinoma, were classified as atypical intraductal hyperplasia. These criteria increased the number of atypical hyperplastic lesions by including cases regarded as carcinoma in other series and thereby worsened the apparent prognosis of hyperplastic lesions.

The subjectivity involved in diagnosing a borderline intraductal epithelial proliferation was pointed out by Rosai who described the variation in assessment of a small group of such lesions by pathologists with expertise in this area (82). To emphasize the continuum of hyperplasia, atypical hyperplasia, and intraductal carcinoma, he suggested that consideration be given to a system

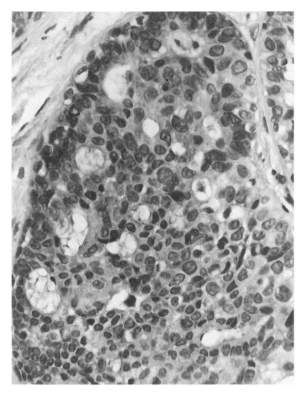

Figure 219
INTRADUCTAL HYPERPLASIA
The secondary lumens adjacent to the basement membrane are more rounded than the smaller central lumens and the cell population is heterogeneous.

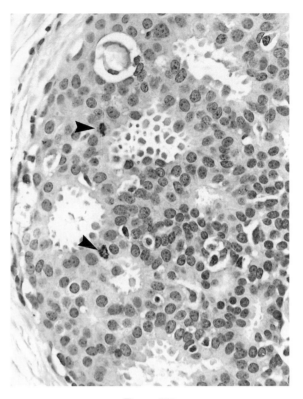

Figure 220
INTRADUCTAL HYPERPLASIA WITH ATYPISM
Intraductal proliferation wherein cells lack "streaming" and are arranged haphazardly in cellular bridges with mitotic activity (arrows). However, the secondary lumens have irregular shapes.

comparable to that utilized for intraepithelial proliferations of the uterine cervix, i.e., mammary intraepithelial neoplasia or MIN, with an associated grading system to indicate the level of severity. While of conceptual interest, this suggestion does not eliminate the necessity for distinguishing between proliferative categories, regardless of the terminology employed, and definitions for grades of mammary intraepithelial neoplasia are yet to be established.

The diagnosis of atypical hyperplasia is employed to indicate that a patient has an increased risk of developing invasive carcinoma. This information must be utilized in combination with other factors to determine appropriate treatment. Other considerations include a family history of breast carcinoma, age, ease of subsequent breast examination clinically and mammographically, extent of the microscopic abnormality, and the willingness of the patient to adhere to a rigorous follow-up program. The patient with atypical intraductal hyperplasia and a history of breast cancer in a first degree relative has a risk of subsequent invasive carcinoma comparable to that of the patient with intraductal carcinoma.

In this presentation, an intraductal epithelial proliferative lesion that has some, but not all, of the features of intraductal carcinoma is referred to as atypical hyperplasia. Emphasis is placed on well-characterized cytologic and architectural features that identify intraductal carcinoma. The photomicrographs accompanying this chapter are classified based on this rather simplistic and arbitrary definition (figs. 219–225). The extent of involvement, as discussed above, is of uncertain importance in determining appropriate treatment, especially since it may vary with the size of the specimen and the completeness of sampling.

Basing the diagnosis of intraductal carcinoma on the number of ducts involved (77) or on the size of the area of involvement (91), may lack

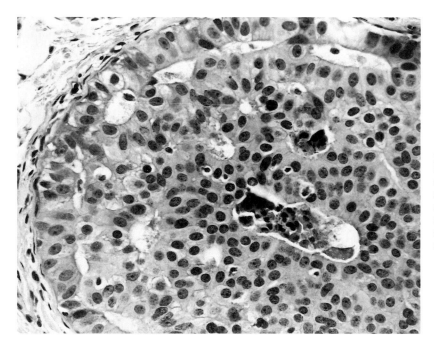

Figure 221
INTRADUCTAL HYPERPLASIA
WITH ATYPISM
Cells comprising the hyperplastic process are uniform in shape and size. Small foci of necrosis with dystrophic calcification are present. The secondary lumens are irregular and most numerous at the periphery of the duct. A distinct single layer of duct epithelial cells is applied to the basement membrane.

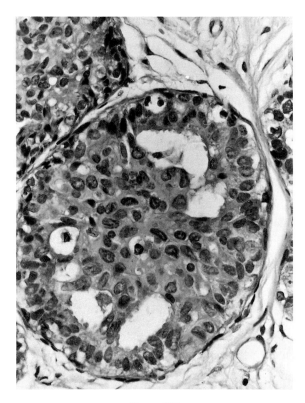

Figure 222
INTRADUCTAL HYPERPLASIA WITH ATYPISM
Secondary lumens are rounded and the cell population appears to be heterogeneous.

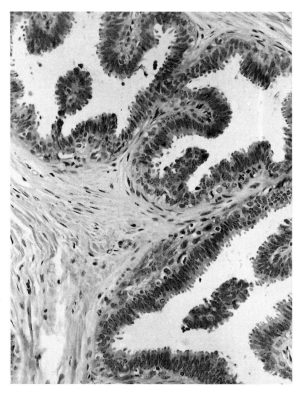

Figure 223
INTRADUCTAL HYPERPLASIA
WITH ATYPISM
Ducts are lined by crowded, hyperplastic, tall columnar cells forming small papillae. Although secondary lumens are not formed, this pattern is of prognostic concern.

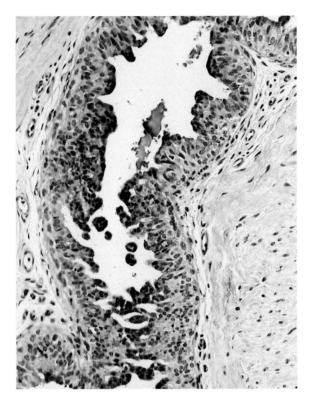

Figure 224
INTRADUCTAL HYPERPLASIA WITH ATYPISM
Papillary proliferation of multilayered ductal epithelium. Only a portion of the duct circumference was involved. (Figures 224 and 225 are from the same patient.)

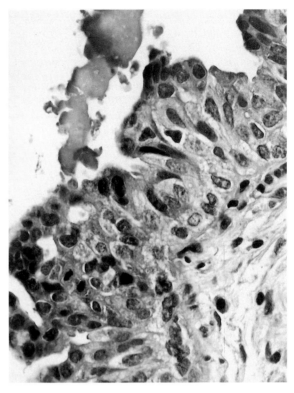

Figure 225
INTRADUCTAL HYPERPLASIA WITH ATYPISM
Epithelial and myoepithelial cells participate in the proliferative process.

relevance in management of the individual patient. It provides a basis for understanding the significance of the microscopic findings and for relating them to other factors in assigning definitive treatment. Therefore, these quantitative factors are not included here among the fundamental criteria for the diagnosis and classification of proliferative ductal lesions.

Intraductal Carcinoma

In simplest terms, this diagnosis applies to carcinoma with cytologic features and a growth pattern attributed to duct carcinoma confined to the mammary ducts at any level, including the lobular ducts. The pathologic definition of intraductal carcinoma specifically excludes invasion of the mammary stroma. Clinical definitions that include carcinomas where a proportion of the neoplasm is invasive (65) are inaccurate and misleading, resulting in inappropriate rates of recurrence

and death due to disease as well as an excessive frequency of axillary lymph node metastases.

Intraductal carcinoma may have a variety of growth patterns including micropapillary (clinging) (48), papillary, solid, comedo, or cribriform in pure form or in combination. It must be appreciated that invasive carcinoma may commingle with foci of intraductal carcinoma, and in some instances the noninvasive carcinoma may comprise a large portion of the tumor.

Clinical Presentation. Intraductal carcinoma is usually a nonpalpable lesion recognized by abnormalities seen mammographically, or discovered as an incidental finding in a biopsy performed for another lesion that produced a clinically detectable mass or mammographic abnormality. Intraductal carcinoma with comedonecrosis usually has dystrophic calcifications recognized as irregularly shaped microcalcifications on a mammogram, often resembling casts of the involved duct. The increased frequency of diagnosis of intraductal carcinoma in recent years may be attributed to the growing popularity of mammography.

Less often, involvement of multiple adjacent ducts by intraductal carcinoma, especially if associated with prominent periductal fibrosis, produces a palpable mass. Nipple discharge is the least common manner of presentation.

The incidence of intraductal carcinoma has been based most often on clinical studies. In a detailed study of hundreds of step sections through both breasts examined in autopsies of 77 adult women without previous breast cancer, 1 invasive carcinoma and 14 intraductal carcinomas were discovered, resulting in an incidence of occult carcinoma exceeding 25 percent (74).

Many intraductal carcinomas go unrecognized and are diagnosed in retrospect when the patient presents with an invasive carcinoma. Even when we are certain that a lesion microscopically is intraductal carcinoma, it cannot be determined with confidence whether it would progress to invasion if not excised. Until the assessment of the risk of such lesions improves, it is appropriate to consider them all as potentially committed to invasion and to treat the patient accordingly, thereby affording the best chance for long-term survival.

Gross Findings. While most intraductal carcinomas are not visible grossly, an exception must be made for tumors with comedonecrosis. As is implied by the prefix, comedo, the necrotic cores may be expressed from the sectioned surface of the biopsy specimen as soft, thin cylinders. In addition, if periductal fibrosis is pronounced, firmness of the area of involvement may be evident.

Microscopic Findings. The cellular composition of intraductal carcinoma may be well differentiated, consisting of a monotonous proliferation of rather uniform epithelial cells with an increased nuclear to cytoplasmic ratio and rounded, central nuclei (fig. 226). This is particularly true of carcinomas with orderly micropapillary and cribriform growth patterns. In other instances, especially in comedocarcinomas, cytologic and nuclear pleomorphism and hyperchromasia, as well as abnormal mitoses, are evident. Mitoses are not a useful differential diagnostic criterion as they are uncommon in intraductal hyperplasia and intraductal carcinoma, although they are somewhat more frequent in the latter lesion. Some comedo intraductal carcinomas

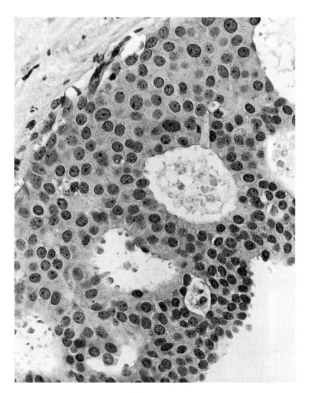

Figure 226
INTRADUCTAL CARCINOMA
Periphery of a duct containing cribriform intraductal carcinoma. Note the uniform cells arranged haphazardly or at right angles to the long axis of the intraductal column.

have numerous mitoses but they rarely present a diagnostic problem. In some instances intraductal carcinoma may be composed of apocrine cells, often with cytoplasmic vacuolation or clear cytoplasm.

Myoepithelial proliferation is not part of intraductal carcinoma. Although the neoplastic intraluminal component uniformly lacks myoepithelial cells, the marginal myoepithelial layer is sometimes maintained. The myoepithelial layer may be hyperplastic but most often it is inconspicuous and discontinuous, having been replaced in part by proliferating carcinoma cells. The carcinoma cells along the basement membrane exhibit loss of basal polarity and cellular crowding may be manifested by overlapping nuclei, a rather characteristic feature of all forms of intraductal carcinoma.

Intraductal carcinomas possess variable hormonal receptor expression. Studies using immunohistochemical methods have shown that approximately 50 percent of micropapillary, solid,

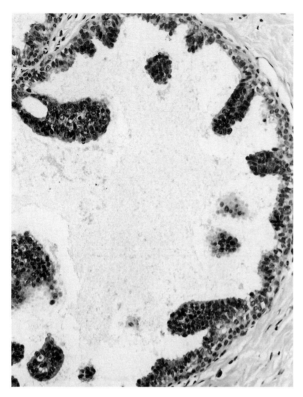

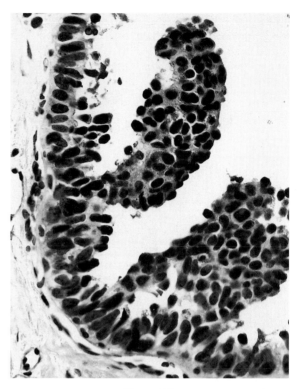

Figure 227
INTRADUCTAL CARCINOMA
Micropapillary growth pattern in which discontinuous cellular fragments are related to the plane of sectioning. (Figures 227 and 228 are from the same patient.)

Figure 228
INTRADUCTAL CARCINOMA
The micropapillae lack fibrovascular cores. The cells adjacent to the basement membrane manifest crowding and are cytologically identical to cells in the micropapillae.

and cribriform intraductal carcinomas show nuclear staining for estrogen receptors in contrast to only about 20 percent of comedocarcinomas, suggesting an inverse relationship between nuclear hormonal receptor activity, cytologic differentiation, and histologic subtypes (62).

One or more growth patterns may be seen in a given case. These have more than diagnostic importance since they differ with respect to DNA content, proliferative activity, and the potential for stromal invasion.

Intraductal carcinoma that is low grade cytologically usually has a micropapillary or cribriform appearance. The micropapillary pattern consists of bulbous, seemingly fragile, neoplastic epithelial projections protruding into the lumen of the duct (fig. 227). These projections are composed of relatively uniform cells with small nuclei, arranged haphazardly or at right angles to the long axis of the papillae. Fibrovascular cores are inapparent. Separated cell nests, appearing to float in the

lumen, are portions of micropapillae not entirely in the plane of section. Thickened micropapillae represent coalescence of adjacent fronds. The tumor cells have an increased nuclear-cytoplasmic ratio and mitoses are rare. Micropapillary intraductal carcinoma should be distinguished from intraductal hyperplasia with atypism that has a micropapillary pattern (figs. 228–230).

When the intraductal carcinoma does not form micropapillae, the neoplastic cells may extend into the duct lumen as ribbons or bridges. Fusion or anastomosis of the bridges may produce cellular arcades or a cribriform pattern with multiple fenestrations (figs. 231, 232). The epithelial bridges sometimes form arches around the periphery of the duct, resulting in a "Roman bridge" pattern of growth (fig. 233). The fenestrations are rounded, "punched out" spaces which tend to be uniform in size and arrangement throughout the duct, in contrast to intraductal hyperplasia in which the lumens are more prominent peripherally (fig. 234).

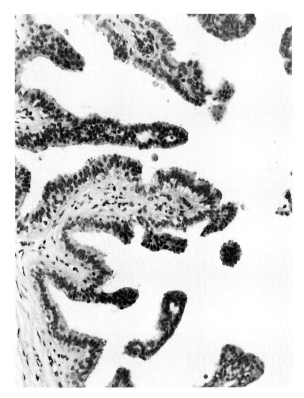

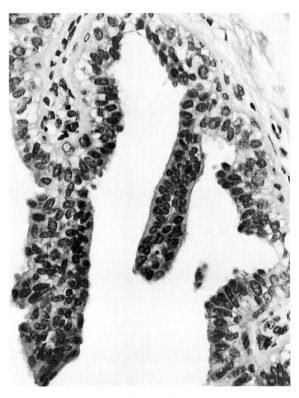

Figure 229
PAPILLARY INTRADUCTAL HYPERPLASIA
WITH ATYPISM
An isolated focus of intraductal proliferation resembling micropapillary carcinoma. (Figures 229 and 230 are from the same patient.)

Figure 230
PAPILLARY INTRADUCTAL HYPERPLASIA
WITH ATYPISM
The cell population is more uniform than in the malignant lesion shown in figures 227 and 228.

Figure 231
INTRADUCTAL CARCINOMA
The cribriform growth pattern results from the merging of intraductal bridges of epithelial cells. (Figures 231 and 232 are from the same patient.)

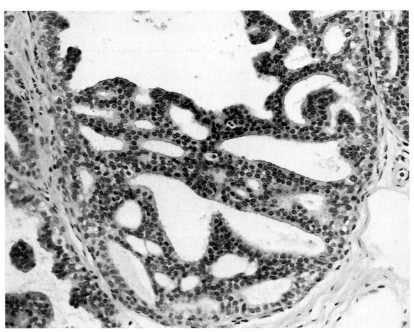

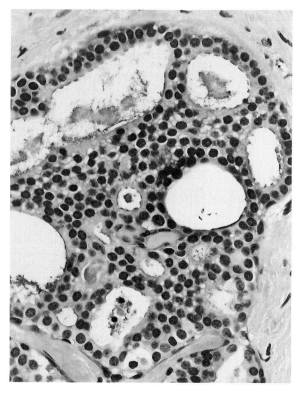

Figure 232
INTRADUCTAL CARCINOMA
This histologic pattern features a uniform cell population.

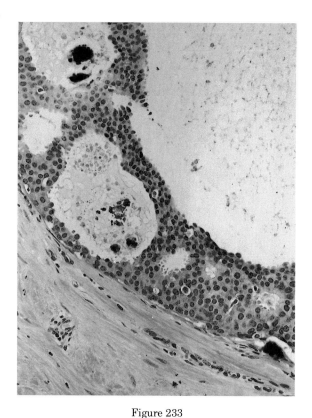

Figure 233
INTRADUCTAL CARCINOMA
An ectatic duct lined by relatively uniform neoplastic cells with prominent secondary lumen formation, resulting in a "Roman bridge" appearance.

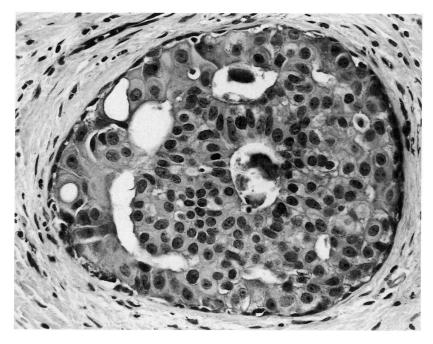

Figure 234
INTRADUCTAL HYPERPLASIA
WITH ATYPISM
An isolated focus of intraductal epithelial proliferation detected on mammography because of focal micro-calcifications. Although the cytologic findings are suggestive of intraductal carcinoma, the irregular shapes and variable sizes of the secondary lumens are indicative of a hyperplastic lesion.

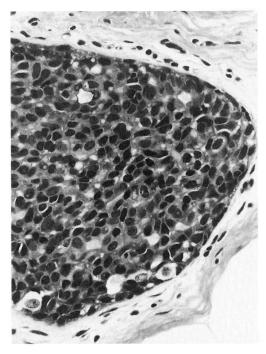

Figure 235
INTRADUCTAL CARCINOMA
Solid growth pattern with occlusion and distension of ducts by proliferation of cells possessing prominent nuclear pleomorphism.

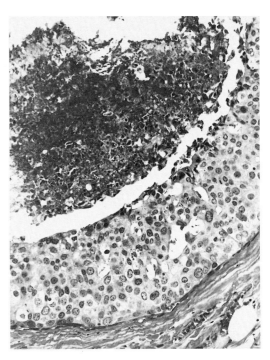

Figure 237
INTRADUCTAL CARCINOMA
Central necrosis with dystrophic calcification, resulting in the pattern of comedonecrosis. (Figures 237 and 238 are from the same patient.)

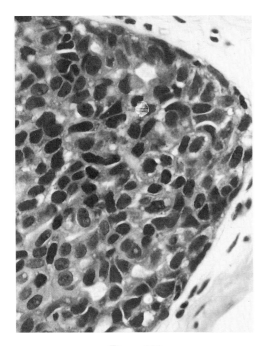

Figure 236
INTRADUCTAL CARCINOMA
Cellular pleomorphism is more pronounced than in the micropapillary or cribriform patterns.

Another distinction is the relative uniformity of size of the lumens, characteristic of intraductal carcinoma to a greater degree than the rounded contour of the lumen. The cells comprising the bridges are arranged haphazardly or transversely to the long axis and do not manifest the streaming pattern seen in hyperplasia.

The involved duct may largely be filled with neoplastic cells of a single type, resulting in a solid growth pattern (figs. 235, 236). In contrast to a solid form of hyperplasia, the epithelial proliferation lacks a myoepithelial component. The cells are of a single type and have well-defined margins. Moreover, there may be considerable cellular pleomorphism and abnormal mitotic activity. Spindling of the cells is usually absent. Nuclei tend to be hyperchromatic and to have conspicuous nucleoli.

Coagulation necrosis is particularly common in solid intraductal carcinoma, resulting in a central necrotic core and the pattern of so-called comedonecrosis (fig. 237). Cell outlines may be visible in the area of necrosis and histiocytes are relatively infrequent. Dystrophic calcification of the necrotic

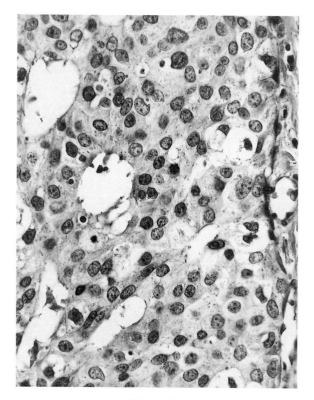

Figure 238
INTRADUCTAL CARCINOMA
The duct is lined by neoplastic cells with greater pleomorphism than in the micropapillary or cribriform types of carcinoma.

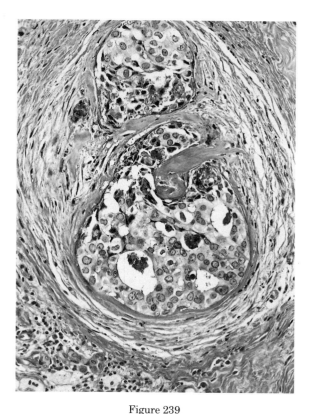

Figure 239
INTRADUCTAL CARCINOMA
Prominent periductal fibrosis and elastosis surround foci of intraductal carcinoma.

core is visible on mammography. Necrosis and calcification occur less often in cribriform and micropapillary intraductal carcinoma.

Comedonecrosis is associated with considerable cellular pleomorphism, nuclear atypism, and increased mitotic activity of the viable cellular component (fig. 238). These findings parallel the increased proliferative activity of this form of intraductal carcinoma in comparison to other growth patterns, and may account for its apparently more rapid progression to invasive carcinoma (73). This pattern also is more likely to be associated with oncogene expression than are other patterns. Strong staining for c-*erb*B-2(HER2/*neu*) oncogene was noted not only in most comedocarcinomas but also in association with comedonecrosis in intraductal carcinomas of mixed microscopic types (72). This staining is very uncommon in atypical intraductal hyperplasia.

Periductal fibrosis, elastosis, and lymphocytic reaction may obscure duct outlines and make it

difficult to evaluate the lesion for invasion (fig. 239). Microinvasion can be diagnosed with confidence when carcinoma cells individually or in small groups are found detached in the periductal stroma in a fashion that does not represent tangential sectioning of the intraductal lesion. To make this distinction is sometimes difficult.

The so-called clinging growth pattern implies that a single layer, or a few layers, of neoplastic cells line the lumen of a duct that is otherwise patent (fig. 240). The epithelium usually has a micropapillary or bridging configuration. Rarely, it is arranged in a relatively flat band of cells. Nuclei are typically hyperchromatic. There is considerable cytologic variability among nuclei from case to case, ranging from low to high nuclear grade.

Intraductal cystic hypersecretory lesions include cystic hypersecretory hyperplasia and cystic hypersecretory carcinoma (63,85), where the intraductal component is a variant of clinging intraductal carcinoma with a prominent

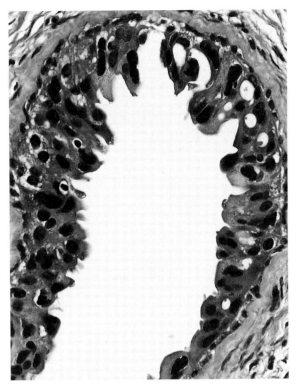

Figure 240
INTRADUCTAL CARCINOMA
Multilayered, pleomorphic neoplastic cells line a patent duct resulting in "clinging" growth pattern in this example of apocrine intraductal carcinoma.

micropapillary pattern. However, the overall appearance of the lesion warrants consideration as a separate entity.

Signet ring growth is an unusual pattern of intraductal carcinoma (59). Cells with eccentric and compressed nuclei and clear to ground-glass cytoplasm fill the involved ducts. The cytoplasm stains positively with the periodic acid–Schiff or Alcian blue methods. Involved ducts may also contain epithelial cell–lined lumens. Although most examples of invasive carcinoma with a signet ring cell growth pattern appear to represent invasive lobular carcinoma, at least some may arise from an intraductal lesion.

An endocrine pattern of intraductal carcinoma was recently described (54). The lesion has an organoid appearance and manifests prominent argyrophilia, thereby resembling a carcinoid tumor. Neoplastic cells either solidly fill the duct or are papillary and arranged in a variety of patterns, forming tubules, pseudorosettes, pali-

sades, or ribbons. The significance of this growth pattern is related to the possible elaboration of hormones, such as corticotropins.

Intraductal carcinoma may initially present in areas of adenosis or in fibroadenomas. The significance of this occurrence and related diagnostic problems have been discussed.

Microinvasion. Of critical importance to the diagnosis of intraductal carcinoma is the integrity of the basement membrane. Ultrastructural studies have revealed protrusion of carcinoma cells through gaps in the basal lamina of the duct before evidence of invasion can be seen with light microscopy (75). This phenomenon, as well as incomplete sampling, undoubtedly accounts for very rare instances of axillary node metastases in women with intraductal carcinoma. Nevertheless, light microscopy, and not electron microscopy, is utilized clinically to assess the presence of invasion.

The recognition of invasion may be difficult. Sections of lobular cancerization where intraductal carcinoma extends into lobular ducts, can simulate invasion; the same effect may result from sections through small ducts (figs. 241, 242). In both situations the plane of section results in seemingly detached cell aggregates mimicking invasion. The presence of a myoepithelial layer around the involved small ducts is a helpful indication that these cells are not invasive. Although invasion is diagnosed by disruption and penetration through the intact basement membrane, this may be extremely difficult to assess in some lesions. The reticulin stain has been more useful for defining an intact basement membrane than the periodic acid–Schiff technique or the immunohistochemical stain for laminin (60), but the results of any of these studies are inconsistent because staining of the basement membrane may be discontinuous even when there is no invasion. Periductal fibrosis, elastosis, and a periductal lymphocytic infiltrate may obscure the basement membrane, further complicating assessment of stromal invasion.

The importance of determining the presence or absence of invasion outweighs biochemical hormonal receptor studies. Small tissue specimens should not be partially sacrificed for hormone receptor analysis. Immunocytochemical determination of hormonal receptors is possible in paraffin sections of intraductal carcinoma.

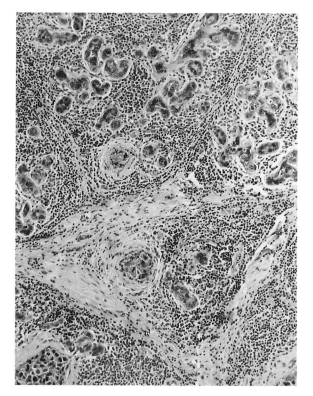

Figure 241
INTRADUCTAL CARCINOMA
Extension of intraductal carcinoma into lobular ducts. The prominent lymphocytic infiltrate is not a specific feature of intraductal carcinoma extending into lobules. (Figures 241 and 242 are from the same patient.)

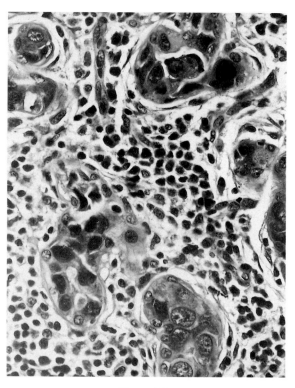

Figure 242
INTRADUCTAL CARCINOMA
The degree of cellular pleomorphism exceeds that of lobular carcinoma in situ in this example of duct carcinoma in lobular glands.

Frozen Section. Of obvious critical importance in the management of the patient is the distinction between intraductal carcinoma and intraductal hyperplasia. Similarly, the recognition of stromal invasion is of both prognostic and therapeutic significance. Therefore, the availability of an optimally prepared section is necessary. It is best to avoid frozen section assessment, especially of nonpalpable lesions.

In addition, the surgeon should be cautioned not to remove the lesion with cautery. This creates thermal artefact at the excised margin which may obliterate critical findings. If cautery is required for hemostasis, it is best employed after the biopsy specimen has been removed,

Prognosis and Treatment. The importance of intraductal carcinoma relates to its potential to eventuate into invasive ductal carcinoma. This has been assessed in several studies, usually related to lesions that mistakenly were diagnosed originally as benign. It is evident that only a fraction of incompletely treated intraductal carcinomas progress to invasive carcinoma. Unfortunately, we are unable to predict with accuracy those neoplasms that are capable of progression.

An early example of such a study was reported from Memorial Hospital in New York (49). Six of 10 women with originally undiagnosed micropapillary noninvasive carcinoma developed invasive carcinoma, and a seventh had recurrent intraductal carcinoma in the same breast after a mean interval of 9.7 years. In a later review of these patients, as well as 5 additional patients, Rosen et al. (84) found that 8 of 15 women subsequently developed invasive carcinoma, and 2 others developed clinically manifest intraductal carcinoma in the same breast.

Page et al. (76) found that 7 of 28 women with intraductal carcinoma treated solely by biopsy developed invasive carcinoma in the same breast after an average interval of 6.1 years. The patients had micropapillary and cribriform forms of intraductal carcinoma. Although small foci of necrosis were present in the latter lesions, none had fully developed comedonecrosis.

More recently, Eusebi et al. (58) assessed the progress of 28 women with originally "benign" breast biopsies subsequently diagnosed as intraductal carcinoma. The clinging carcinoma pattern was found in 21 patients. Only 1 of the 7 women with intraductal carcinoma, other than that of the clinging type, developed recurrent invasive carcinoma. This was the sole patient having a neoplasm with the pattern of comedonecrosis. Two of the 21 women with unrecognized lesions subsequently diagnosed as intraductal carcinoma with the growth pattern of clinging carcinoma developed invasive carcinoma, and 2 others developed recurrent intraductal carcinoma.

Lagios et al. (69) studied 79 patients diagnosed as having intraductal carcinoma who were treated by wide local excision without either postoperative irradiation or lymph node dissection. All of these patients had microscopic confirmation of seemingly complete excision of the neoplasm. These lesions were studied by a serial subgross method, correlated with specimen radiography, and all were less than 2.5 cm in greatest diameter. Ten percent of the patients developed recurrent carcinoma in the vicinity of the biopsy site after a median follow-up of 4 years. Half of the recurrences were invasive carcinoma. Following re-excision in one patient and mastectomy in the remainder, all of the patients were free of carcinoma at the time of the report. The carcinomas that recurred had a high nuclear grade and comedonecrosis, whereas none of the micropapillary or cribriform carcinomas of low nuclear grade recurred.

Treatment of intraductal carcinoma is variable, with mastectomy favored by some and wide local excision, usually followed by irradiation, recommended by others. Although mastectomy has a cure rate of nearly 100 percent, and circumvents the issues of multicentricity, recurrence, and occult invasive growth, there is an increasing trend toward breast conservation treatment. This requires rigorous long-term monitoring of the patient, with regular physical examination as frequently as every 4 months, and mammography as often as every 6 months for the first 2 years and annually thereafter (87).

Wide local excision with postoperative irradiation may ultimately have a local recurrence rate of 30 percent or more, although it approximates 10 to 20 percent in recent reports (81). In a follow-up study of 17 patients treated in this manner, 18 percent subsequently developed invasive carcinoma that was fatal (61). The likelihood of multicentricity and occult microinvasion in nonpalpable tumors has been shown to be greatest for intraductal carcinoma with comedonecrosis, whereas it is least likely in association with micropapillary or cribriform carcinomas presenting as incidental findings. Therefore, some recommend more intensive treatment, including lymph node dissection, for the former while the latter may be treated by excision alone (89).

It must be recognized that the assessment of the adequacy of the surgical margins of excision may be inaccurate because of multicentricity of involvement. Reliance upon the presence of mammographic microcalcifications to guide the extent of the biopsy may overlook foci of nonnecrotic intraductal carcinoma (68). Factors that must be considered in assigning therapy are the extent of the carcinoma, the ease of follow-up physical examination of the breast, the density of the breast on mammography, the patient's family history, and the patient's ability to comply with a follow-up schedule. The patient's age and the absence of grossly detectable carcinoma also may be factors. The cumulative risk for the future development of carcinoma is less in elderly patients (64).

Multicentricity of intraductal carcinoma is defined as the occurrence of foci of carcinoma in more than one quadrant of the breast. Separate foci of carcinoma in the same quadrant are termed multifocal. Multicentricity cannot be assessed with excisional biopsy specimens. In a serial subgross study with mammographic correlation of 53 mastectomies, Lagios et al. (70) noted an incidence of multicentricity of 32 percent. Furthermore, 21 percent of these patients had occult foci of invasive carcinoma in the involved breast. This latter group had grossly detectable intraductal carcinoma exceeding 2.5 cm in diameter. A higher incidence of multicentricity was noted by Schwartz et al. (88), who found such foci in 41 percent of breasts with nonpalpable intraductal carcinoma measuring less than 2.5 cm in diameter.

The presence of extensive intraductal carcinoma in grossly normal breast adjacent to an invasive neoplasm in the excisional biopsy specimen has been related to the presence of intraductal carcinoma in the remainder of the breast (67). Therefore, it is not surprising that the presence of multiple foci of intraductal carcinoma in the grossly normal breast adjacent to an invasive neoplasm is a predictor for an increased risk of recurrence following wide local excision of the neoplasm and subsequent irradiation (66). This is especially true if the growth pattern is that of comedonecrosis (71). The presence of comedonecrosis has been shown to be a predictor of local recurrence after local treatment for intraductal carcinoma (60).

When carcinoma is confined to the duct system, without violation of the basement membrane, axillary lymph node involvement is unlikely (60,86). However, it is difficult to exclude with certainty the possibility of stromal invasion in the case of multiple foci of carcinoma, when large regions are involved or when the presence of considerable periductal fibrosis or elastosis makes assessment of stromal invasion difficult. In this situation low axillary dissection may be appropriate. Axillary node dissection may be omitted if there is only a small area of intraductal carcinoma that lacks foci of indeterminate stromal invasion and is associated with uninvolved margins of surgical excision (90).

In contrast to LCIS, the risk of subsequent invasive carcinoma in the contralateral breast following the diagnosis of intraductal carcinoma is relatively small, occurring in only 3.4 percent of patients in one large series (93).

REFERENCES

Lobular Carcinoma In Situ and Atypical Hyperplasia

1. Alpers CE, Wellings SR. The prevalence of carcinoma in situ in normal and cancer-associated breasts. Hum Pathol 1985;16:796–807.

2. Andersen JA. Lobular carcinoma in situ: a long-term follow-up in 52 cases. Acta Pathol Microbiol Immunol Scand [A] 1974;82:519–33.

3. _____. Lobular carcinoma in situ of the breast with ductal involvement. Frequency and possible influence on prognosis. Acta Pathol Microbiol Immunol Scand [A] 1974;82:655–62.

4. _____. Multicentric and bilateral appearance of lobular carcinoma in situ of the breast. Acta Pathol Microbiol Immunol Scand [A] 1974;82:730–4.

5. _____, Vendelboe ML. Cytoplasmic mucous globules in lobular carcinoma in situ. Diagnosis and prognosis. Am J Surg Pathol 1981;5:251–5.

6. Baum M, Brinkley DM, Dossett JA, et al. Control trial of tamoxifen and adjuvant agent in management of early breast cancer. Lancet 1983;1:257–69.

7. Breslow A, Brancaccio ME. Intracellular mucin production by lobular breast carcinoma cells. Arch Pathol Lab Med 1976;100:620–1.

8. Bussolati G. Actin-rich (myoepithelial) cells in lobular carcinoma in situ of the breast. Virchows Arch [Cell Pathol] 1980;32:165–76.

9. Carter D, Smith RR. Carcinoma in situ of the breast. Cancer 1977;40:1189–93.

10. Farrow JH. Current concepts in the detection and treatment of the earliest of the early breast cancers. Cancer 1970;25:458–79.

11. Fechner RE. Epithelial alterations in extralobular ducts of breasts with lobular carcinoma. Arch Pathol 1972;93:164–71.

12. Fechner RE. Lobular carcinoma in situ in sclerosing adenosis. A potential source of confusion with invasive carcinoma. Am J Surg Pathol 1981;5:233–9.

13. Foote FW Jr, Stewart FW. Lobular carcinoma in situ. A rare form of mammary cancer. Am J Pathol 1941;17:491–6.

14. Frantz VK, Pickren JW, Melcher GW, Auchincloss H Jr. Incidence of chronic cystic disease in so-called "normal breasts." A study based on 225 postmortem examinations. Cancer 1951;4:762–83.

15. Gad A, Azzopardi JG. Lobular carcinoma of the breast: a special variant of mucin secreting carcinoma. J Clin Pathol 1975;28:711–6.

16. Haagensen CD. Lobular neoplasia (lobular carcinoma in situ). In: Diseases of the breast. 3rd ed. Philadelphia: WB Saunders, 1986:192–241.

17. _____, Lane N, Lattes R, Bodian C. Lobular neoplasia (so-called lobular carcinoma in situ) of the breast. Cancer 1978;42:737–69.

18. _____, Lane N, Lattes R. Neoplastic proliferation of the epithelium of the mammary lobules: adenosis, lobular neoplasia and small cell carcinoma. Surg Clin North Am 1972;52:497–524.

19. Hutter RV, Foote FW Jr, Farrow JH. In situ lobular carcinoma of the female breast, 1939-1968. In: Breast cancer: early and late. Chicago: Year Book Medical Publishers, Inc, 1970:201–26.

20. _____, Snyder RE, Lucas JC, Foote FW Jr, Farrow JH. Clinical and pathologic correlation with mammographic findings in lobular carcinoma in situ. Cancer 1969;23:826–39.

21. Kramer WM, Rush BF Jr. Mammary duct proliferation in the elderly. A histopathologic study. Cancer 1973;31:130–7.

22. Lewison EF, Finney GG Jr. Lobular carcinoma in situ of the breast. Surg Gynecol Obstet 1968;126:1280–6.

23. Morris DM, Walker AP, Coker DC. Lack of efficacy of xeromammography in preoperatively detecting lobular carcinoma in situ of the breast. Breast Cancer Res Treat 1981;1:365–8.

24. Nesland JM, Johannessen JV. Malignant breast lesions. J Submicrosc Cytol 1982;14:553–75.

25. Newman W. In situ lobular carcinoma of the breast. Ann Surg 1963;151:591–9.

26. Nielsen M, Thomsen JL, Primdahl S, Dyreborg U, Andersen JA. Breast cancer and atypia among young and middle-aged women: a study of 110 medicolegal autopsies. Br J Cancer 1987;56:814–9.

27. Ozzello L. Ultrastructure of intraepithelial carcinomas of the breast. Cancer 1971;28:1508–15.

28. Page DL, Anderson TJ. Diagnostic histopathology of the breast. New York: Churchill Livingstone, 1987.

29. Pope TL Jr, Fechner RE, Wilhelm MC, Wanebo HJ, De Paredes ES. Lobular carcinoma in situ of the breast: mammographic features. Radiology 1988;168:63–6.

30. Powles TJ, Hardy JR, Ashley SE, et al. Chemoprevention of breast cancer. Breast Cancer Res Treat 1989; 14:23–31.

31. Rosen PP. Axillary lymph node metastases in patients with occult noninvasive breast carcinoma. Cancer 1980;46:1298–306.

32. _____. Lobular carcinoma in situ and intraductal carcinoma of the breast. In: McDivitt RW, Oberman HA, Ozzello L, Kaufman N, eds. The breast. Baltimore: Williams and Wilkins, 1984:59–105.

33. _____. The pathological classification of human mammary carcinoma: past, present and future. Ann Clin Lab Sci 1979;9:144–56.

34. _____, Kosloff C, Lieberman PH, Adair F, Braun DW Jr. Lobular carcinoma in situ of the breast. Detailed analysis of 99 patients with average follow-up of 24 years. Am J Surg Pathol 1978;2:225–51.

35. _____, Lesser ML, Senie RT, Duthie K. Epidemiology of breast carcinoma IV: age and histologic tumor type. J Surg Oncol 1982;19:44–51.

36. _____, Saigo PE, Braun DW Jr. Predictors of recurrence in stage I (T1N0M0) breast carcinoma. Ann Surg 1981;193:15–25.

37. _____, Senie RT, Farr GH, Schottenfeld D, Ashikari R. Epidemiology of breast carcinoma: age, menstrual status, and exogenous hormone usage in patients with lobular carcinoma in situ. Surgery 1979;85:219–24.

38. _____, Tench W. Lobules in the nipple. Frequency and significance for breast cancer treatment. Pathol Annu 1985;20(Pt 2):317–22.

39. Shah JP, Rosen PP, Robbins GF. Pitfalls of local excision in the treatent of carcinoma of the breast. Surg Gynecol Obstet 1973;136:721–5.

40. Smart CR, Myers MH, Gloeckler LA. Implications from SEER data on breast cancer management. Cancer 1978;41:787–9.

41. Sunshine JA, Moseley HS, Fletcher WS, Krippaehne WW. Breast carcinoma in situ. A retrospective review of 112 cases with minimum 10 year follow-up. Am J Surg 1985;150:44–51.

42. Tobon H, Price HM. Lobular carcinoma in situ. Some ultrastructural observations. Cancer 1972;30:1082–91.

43. Urban JA. Biopsy of the "normal" breast in treating breast cancer. Surg Clin North Am 1969;49:291–301.

44. Warner NE. Lobular carcinoma of the breast. Cancer 1969; 23:840–6.

45. Wheeler JE, Enterline HT, Roseman JM, et al. Lobular carcinoma in situ of the breast: long term follow-up. Cancer 1974;34:554–63.

46. Zippel HH, Henatsch HJ, Kunze WP. Morphometric and cytophotometric investigations of lobular neoplasia of the breast with ductal involvement. J Cancer Res Clin Oncol 1979;93:265–74.

Intraductal Carcinoma and Atypical Hyperplasia

47. Azzopardi JG. Benign and malignant proliferative epithelial lesions of the breast: a review. Eur J Cancer Clin Oncol 1983;19:1717–20.

48. _____. Problems in breast pathology. Philadelphia: WB Saunders, 1979;192–203.

49. Betsill WL Jr, Rosen PP, Lieberman PH, Robbins GF. Intraductal carcinoma. Long-term follow-up after treatment by biopsy alone. JAMA 1978;239:1863–7.

50. Black MM, Barclay TH, Cutler SJ, Hankey BF, Asire AJ. Association of atypical characteristics of benign breast lesions with subsequent risk of breast cancer. Cancer 1972;29:338–43.

51. _____, Chabon AB. In situ carcinoma of the breast. Pathol Annu 1969;5:185–210.

52. Cook MG, Rohan TE. The patho-epidemiology of benign proliferative epithelial disorders of the female breast. J Pathol 1985;146:1–15.

53. Crissman JD, Visscher DW, Kubus J. Image cytophotometric DNA analysis of atypical hyperplasias and intraductal carcinomas of the breast. Arch Pathol Lab Med 1990;114:1249–53.

54. Cross AS, Azzopardi JG, Krausz T, Van Norden S, Polak JM. A morphological and immunocytochemical study of a distinctive variant of ductal carcinoma in situ of the breast. Histopathology 1985;9:21–37.

55. Davis HH, Simons M, Davis JB. Cystic disease of the breast: relationship to carcinoma. Cancer 1964; 17:957–78.

56. Dupont WD, Page DL. Relative risk of breast cancer varies with time since diagnosis of atypical hyperplasia. Hum Pathol 1989;20:723–5.

57. _____, Page DL. Risk factors for breast cancer in women with proliferative breast disease. N Engl J Med. 1985;312:145–51.

58. Eusebi V, Foschini MP, Cook MG, Berrino F, Azzopardi JG. Long-term follow-up of in situ carcinoma of the breast with special emphasis on clinging carcinoma. Semin Diagn Pathol 1989;6:165–73.

59. Fisher ER, Brown R. Intraductal signet ring carcinoma. A hitherto undescribed form of intraductal carcinoma of the breast. Cancer 1985;55:2533–7.

60. _____, Sass R, Fisher B, Wickerham L, Paik SM. Pathologic findings from the National Surgical Adjuvant Breast Project (protocol 6): I. Intraductal carcinoma (DCIS). Cancer 1986;57:197–208.

61. Gallagher WJ, Koerner FC, Wood WC. Treatment of intraductal carcinoma with limited surgery: long-term follow-up. J Clin Oncol 1989;7:376–80.

62. Giri DD, Dundas SA, Nottingham JF, Underwood JC. Oestrogen receptors in benign epithelial lesions and intraduct carcinomas of the breast: an immunohistological study. Histopathology 1989;15:575–84.

63. Guerry P, Erlandson RA, Rosen PP. Cystic hypersecretory hyperplasia and cystic hypersecretory duct carcinoma of the breast. Pathology, therapy, and follow-up of 39 patients. Cancer 1988;61:1611–20.

64. Gump FE, Jicha DL, Ozzelo L. Ductal carcinoma in situ (DCIS): a revised concept. Surgery 1987;102;790–5.

65. Haagensen CD. Diseases of the breast. 3rd ed. Philadelphia: WB Saunders, 1986:782.

66. Harris JR, Connolly JL, Schnitt SJ, et al. The use of pathologic features in selecting the extent of a surgical resection necessary for breast cancer patients treated by primary radiation therapy. Ann Surg 1985;201:164–9.

67. Holland R, Connolly JL, Gelman R, et al. The presence of an extensive intraductal component following a limited excision correlates with prominent residual disease in the remainder of the breast. J Clin Oncol 1990;8:113–8.

68. _____, Hendriks JH, Verbeek AL, Mravunac M, Stekhoven JH. Extent, distribution and mammographic/histological correlations of breast ductal carcinoma in situ. Lancet 1990;335:519–22.

69. Lagios MD, Margolin FR, Westdahl PR, Rose MR. Mammographically detected duct carcinoma in situ. Frequency of local recurrence following tylectomy and prognostic effect of nuclear grade on local recurrence. Cancer 1989;63:618–24.

70. _____, Westdahl PR, Margolin FR, Rose MR. Duct carcinoma in situ. Relationship of extent of noninvasive disease to the frequency of occult invasion, multicentricity, lymph node metastases, and short-term treatment failures. Cancer 1982;50:1309–14.

71. Lindley R, Bulman A, Parsons P, Phillips R, Henry K, Ellis H. Histologc features predictive of an increased risk of early local recurrence after treatment of breast cancer by local tumor excision and radical radiotherapy. Surgery 1989;105:13–20.

72. Lodato RF, Maguire HC, Greene MI, Weiner DB, LiVolsi VA. Immunohistochemical evaluation of c-erbB-2 oncogene expression in ductal carcinoma in situ and atypical ductal hyperplasia of the breast. Mod Pathol 1990;3:449–54.

73. Meyer JS. Cell kinetics of histologic variants of in situ breast carcinoma. Breast Cancer Res Treat 1986; 7:171–80.

74. Nielsen M, Jensen J, Andersen J. Precancerous and cancerous breast lesions during lifetime and at autopsy. A study of 83 women. Cancer 1984;54:612–5.

75. Ozzello L, Santipak P. Epithelial-stromal junction of intraductal carcinoma of the breast. Cancer 1970; 26:1186–98.

76. Page DL, Dupont WD, Rogers LW, Landenberger M. Intraductal carcinoma of the breast: follow-up after biopsy only. Cancer 1982;49:751–8.

77. _____, Dupont WD, Rogers LW, Rados MS. Atypical hyperplastic lesions of the female breast. A long-term follow-up study. Cancer 1985;55:2698–708.

77a. _____, Rogers LW. Combined histologic and cytologic criteria for the diagnosis of mammary atypical ductal hyperplasia. Hum Pathol 1992;23(10):1095–7.

78. _____, Vander Zwaag R, Rogers LW, Williams LT, Walker WE, Hartmann WH. Relation between component parts of fibrocystic disease complex and breast cancer. JNCI 1978;61:1055–63.

79. Parfrey NA, Doyle CT. Elastosis in benign and malignant breast disease. Hum Pathol 1985;16:674–6.

80. Raju U, Crissman JD, Zarbo RJ, Gottlieb C. Epitheliosis of the breast. An immunohistochemical characterization and comparison to malignant intraductal proliferations of the breast. Am J Surg Pathol 1990; 14:939–47.

81. Recht A, Danoff BS, Solin LJ, et al. Intraductal carcinoma of the breast: results of treatment with excisional biopsy and irradiation. J Clin Oncol 1985;3:1339–43.

82. Rosai J. Borderline epithelial lesions of the breast. Am J Surg Pathol 1991;15:209–21.

83. Rosen PP. "Borderline" breast lesions [Letter]. Am J Surg Pathol 1991;15:1100–2.

84. _____, Braun DW Jr, Kinne DE. The clinical significance of pre-invasive breast carcinoma. Cancer 1980;46:919–25.

85. _____, Scott M. Cystic hypersecretory duct carcinoma of the breast. Am J Surg Pathol 1984;8:31–41.

86. _____, Senie R, Schottenfeld D, Ashikari R. Noninvasive breast carcinoma. Frequency of unsuspected invasion and implications for treatment. Ann Surg 1979;189:377–82.

87. Schnitt SJ, Silen W, Sadowsky NL, Connolly JL, Harris JR. Ductal carcinoma in situ (intraductal carcinoma) of the breast. N Engl J Med 1988;318:898–903.

88. Schwartz GF, Patchefsky AS, Feig SA, Shaber GS, Schwartz AB. Multicentricity of non-palpable breast cancer. Cancer 1980;45;2913–6.

89. _____, Patchefsky AS, Finkelstein SD, et al. Nonpalpable in situ ductal carcinoma of the breast. Predictors of multicentricity and microinvasion and implications for treatment. Arch Surg 1989;124:29–32.

90. Silverstein MJ, Rosser RJ, Gierson ED, et al. Axillary lymph node dissection for intraductal breast carcinoma—is it indicated? Cancer 1987;59:1819–24.

91. Tavassoli FA, Norris HJ. A comparison of the results of long-term follow-up for atypical intraductal hyperplasia and intraductal hyperplasia of the breast. Cancer 1990; 65:518–29.

92. Tham KT, Dupont WD, Page DL, Gray GF Jr, Rogers LW. Micro-papillary hyperplasia with atypical features in female breast, resembling gynecomastia. In: Fenoglio-Preiser CM, Wolff M, Rilke F, eds. Progress in surgical pathology, Vol. 10. New York: Field & Wood, 1989:101–9.

93. Webber BL, Heise H, Neifeld JP, Costa J. Risk of subsequent contralateral breast carcinoma in a population of patients with in-situ breast carcinoma. Cancer 1981;47:2928–32.

94. Wellings SR. Development of human breast cancer. Adv Cancer Res 1980;31:287–314.

95. _____, Jensen HM, Marcum RG. An atlas of subgross pathology of the human breast with special reference to possible precancerous lesions. JNCI 1975; 55:231–73.

INVASIVE CARCINOMA

INVASIVE DUCTAL CARCINOMA

The largest group of malignant mammary tumors, constituting 65 to 80 percent of mammary carcinomas, is defined by exclusion in the WHO classification of breast tumors (112): "Invasive ductal carcinoma is the most frequently encountered malignant tumour of the breast, not falling into any of the other categories of invasive mammary carcinoma." This includes lesions characterized variously as duct carcinoma with productive fibrosis, scirrhous carcinoma, and carcinoma simplex. A generic term sometimes employed is invasive duct carcinoma, not otherwise specified (NOS). This useful designation recognizes the distinction between these tumors and the many other specific forms of duct carcinoma, such as tubular, medullary, metaplastic, colloid, and adenoid cystic carcinoma.

Invasive duct carcinoma includes tumors that express in part, rather than purely, one or more characteristics of the specific types of breast carcinoma. There can be limited microscopic foci of tubular, medullary, papillary, or mucinous differentiation. In one detailed review of 1000 carcinomas, approximately one third characterized as invasive duct carcinoma, expressed one or more combined features (22). Tumors combining invasive duct and lobular carcinoma and invasive duct carcinoma with associated Paget disease are also included in this category. The relatively favorable prognosis associated with specific histologic types only applies to those tumors composed entirely or in very large part of the designated pattern.

The growth pattern of the intraductal component is often reflected in the structure of the invasive carcinoma. Tubular carcinoma almost always arises from orderly micropapillary or cribriform intraductal carcinomas, which feature cytologically low-grade nuclei. The intraductal component of medullary carcinoma is typically solid with poorly differentiated nuclei. Moderately differentiated invasive duct carcinoma (NOS) most often originates from cribriform or papillary intraductal components. Invasive cribriform carcinoma is a subtype of invasive duct carcinoma with a prominent cribriform structure. Invasive lesions that are entirely cribriform

and those with a mixture of cribriform and tubular components are relatively low grade and have a very good prognosis. If less well-differentiated elements are present in the tumor, the prognosis is not as favorable. Invasive poorly differentiated duct carcinoma (NOS) tends to develop from solid or comedo intraductal carcinoma. Comedonecrosis may occur in invasive areas, duplicating the intraductal pattern.

Clinical Presentation. There are no clinical features specifically associated with invasive duct carcinoma. The lesions occur throughout the age range of breast carcinoma, most commonly in the mid to late fifties. The underlying invasive carcinoma associated with Paget disease of the nipple is almost always of the duct type.

Gross Findings. Invasive duct carcinoma invariably forms a solid tumor. The consistency and appearance of the cut surface vary considerably depending on the composition of the lesion. Cystic change is extremely uncommon but may be a manifestation of necrosis. Tumors with a relatively abundant scirrhous or fibrotic stroma are extremely firm to hard with a grey to white surface. When there is considerable elastosis of the stroma, a yellow tinge may be observed. Chalky white streaks in the tumor tissue are usually indicative of necrosis, calcification, or elastosis.

The measured gross size of a mammary carcinoma is one of the most significant prognostic variables. Numerous studies have shown that survival generally decreases with increasing tumor size and that there is a coincidental rise in the rate of axillary node metastases (1,89). Measurement of size is generally reported in terms of the greatest diameter.

The majority of invasive duct carcinomas can be assigned on the basis of gross tumor configuration to one of two groups: stellate (spiculated, infiltrative, radial, serrated) (fig. 243) and circumscribed (rounded, pushing, encapsulated, smooth) (fig. 244). Approximately one third of the tumors have grossly circumscribed margins; a minority have indistinct borders and cannot be described in these terms. In general, the gross appearance of the tumor duplicates the configuration visualized by mammography. However, tumors that appear to have circumscribed margins grossly or

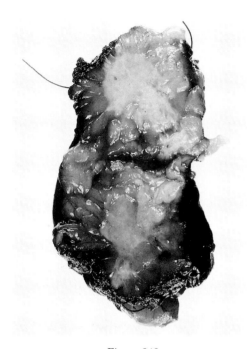

Figure 243
STELLATE INVASIVE DUCT CARCINOMA
Gross appearance of a transected tumor showing the spiculated infiltrative margin.

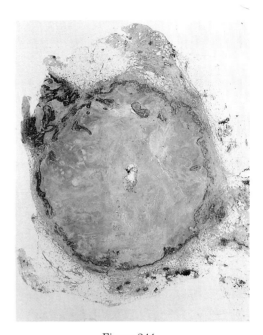

Figure 244
CIRCUMSCRIBED INVASIVE DUCT CARCINOMA
Macrophotograph showing rounded well-defined borders. There is extensive central necrosis.

mammographically may exhibit an invasive growth pattern when studied microscopically. Fisher et al. (22) found microscopically invasive margins in slightly more than half of carcinomas described as grossly circumscribed. Infiltrative tumors tend to be larger when detected (13,49) and are more likely to have axillary lymph node metastases than those with circumscribed margins (30,49). Tumors with a stellate configuration in which there is focal necrosis have an especially poor prognosis (13).

Microscopic Findings. Grading of carcinomas is an estimate of differentiation. Unless otherwise indicated, grading is usually limited to the invasive portion of the tumor.

Nuclear grading is a cytologic evaluation of the structural features of tumor nuclei, comparing them with the nuclei of normal mammary epithelial cells. Since nuclear grading does not involve an assessment of the growth pattern of the tumor, it is applicable to all types of mammary carcinoma. The most widely employed system for nuclear grading, introduced by Black et al. (11), is usually reported in terms of three categories: well differentiated (grade 3) (fig. 245), intermediate (grade 2),

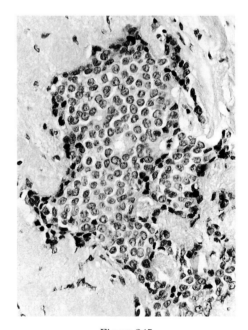

Figure 245
NUCLEAR GRADE
Well-differentiated cytologic appearance of low-grade carcinoma featuring small, round, uniform nuclei lacking nucleoli. (Fig. 12-12A from Rosen PP. The pathology of invasive breast carcinoma. In: Harris JR, Hellman S, Henderson IC, Kinne DW, eds. Breast diseases. 2nd ed. Philadelphia: JB Lippincott, 1991.)

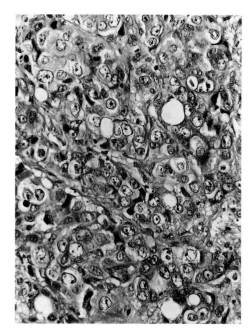

Figure 246
NUCLEAR GRADE
Poorly differentiated nuclei shown here are large, pleomorphic, and have prominent nucleoli. (Fig. 12-12B from Rosen PP. The pathology of invasive breast carcinoma. In: Harris JR, Hellman S, Henderson IC, Kinne DW, eds. Breast diseases. 2nd ed. Philadelphia: JB Lippincott, 1991.)

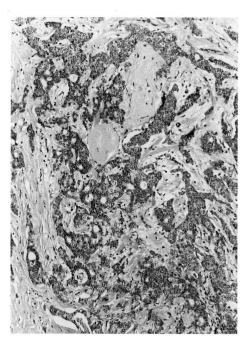

Figure 248
HISTOLOGIC GRADE
Intermediate differentiation characterized by gland formation in connected tumor masses. (Fig. 12-3B from Rosen PP. The pathology of invasive breast carcinoma. In: Harris JR, Hellman S, Henderson IC, Kinne DW, eds. Breast diseases. 2nd ed. Philadelphia: JB Lippincott, 1991.)

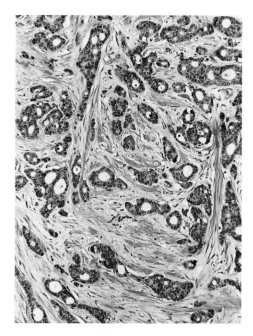

Figure 247
HISTOLOGIC GRADE
Well-differentiated pattern retains a tendency to form tubules and glands.

and poorly differentiated (grade 1) (fig. 246). By convention, numerical designations used for nuclear grading are in a reverse sequence to those of histologic grading. It has been suggested that the numerical designations employed for nuclear grading be changed to conform with those used in histologic grading (22).

Histologic grading takes into consideration the growth pattern of invasive ductal carcinomas as well as cytologic features of differentiation (12). The parameters measured are the extent of tubule formation, nuclear hyperchromasia, and mitotic rate. The histologic grade is usually expressed in three categories: well differentiated (grade I) (fig. 247), intermediate (grade II) (fig. 248), and poorly differentiated (grade III) (fig. 249).

The histologic and nuclear grades of a given tumor coincide in most invasive duct carcinomas. Studies have repeatedly demonstrated that patients with high-grade or poorly differentiated invasive duct carcinoma have a significantly higher frequency of axillary lymph node metastases, tumor

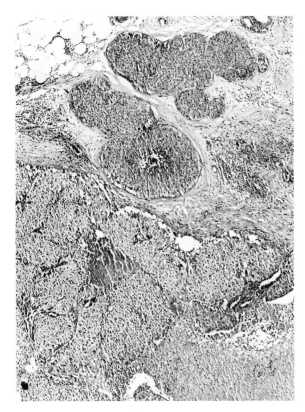

Figure 249
HISTOLOGIC GRADE
Poorly differentiated carcinoma growing as solid areas of tumor virtually devoid of gland formation. Note adjacent intraductal carcinoma.

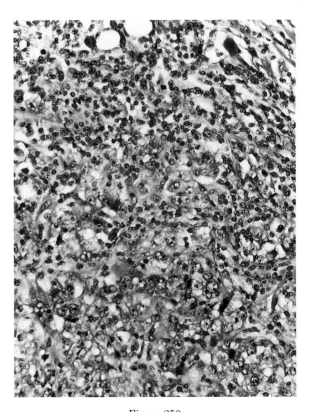

Figure 250
LYMPHOPLASMACYTIC INFILTRATION
Invasive duct carcinoma with marked lymphoplasmacytic reaction.

recurrences, and death from metastatic disease than do women with low-grade tumors (4,10–12, 40,79,95). Nuclear and histologic grade have been shown to be significant predictors of prognosis among patients stratified by stage of disease, especially among those without axillary lymph node metastases (stage I) (17,40,50,79). The absence of tubule formation is a particularly unfavorable histologic feature when combined with poorly differentiated nuclear cytology. Histologic grade is significantly related not only to the frequency of recurrence and death, but also to disease-free interval and overall length of survival (24) regardless of clinical stage. High-grade carcinomas result in early treatment failures while later recurrences are observed among low-grade tumors.

The prognostic significance of lymphoplasmacytic infiltration in the stroma within and around invasive duct carcinomas has been the subject of

considerable interest and some controversy. The reaction consists mainly of mature lymphocytes with a variable admixture of plasma cells. When plasma cells predominate the tumors are usually medullary carcinomas. A moderate to marked lymphoplasmacytic reaction occurs in a small proportion of nonmedullary invasive duct carcinomas (fig. 250) (22,79). A subset of these tumors with some but not all the features of medullary carcinoma, referred to as atypical medullary carcinoma, generally have a slightly more favorable prognosis than infiltrating duct carcinomas generally, but the difference is not statistically significant (73). The majority of nonmedullary duct carcinomas with a prominent lymphocytic reaction tend to be poorly differentiated and have a circumscribed rather than infiltrative contour. Some investigators have found that carcinomas with a lymphoplasmacytic "host response" have a relatively favorable prognosis (2,10); others have found no significant difference or even a

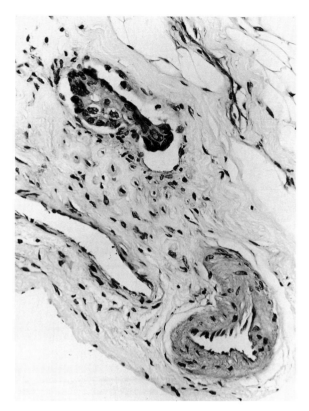

Figure 251
LYMPHATIC TUMOR EMBOLI
Cluster of carcinoma cells in a thin-walled endothelial-lined space next to small blood vessels. (Fig. 1B from Rosen PP. Tumor emboli in intramammary lymphatics in breast carcinoma. Pathologic criteria for diagnosis and clinical significance. Pathol Annu 1983;18(Pt 2):215–32.)

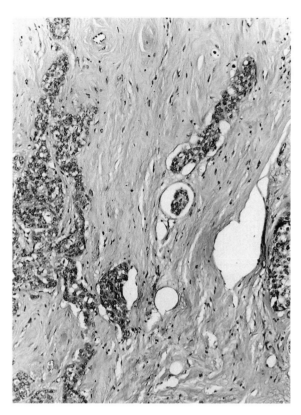

Figure 252
SHRINKAGE ARTEFACT
Within a carcinoma, artefactual spaces caused by tissue shrinkage simulate the appearance of lymphatic tumor emboli. (Fig. 4A from Rosen PP. Tumor emboli in intramammary lymphatics in breast carcinoma. Pathologic criteria for diagnosis and clinical significance. Pathol Annu 1983;18(Pt 2):215–32.)

less favorable outcome (17,79,81). Studies of the lymphocyte subgroups infiltrating mammary carcinomas indicate that they are largely of the T lymphocyte type (9,41,110). The intensity of mast cell infiltration in the substance or at the periphery of an invasive breast carcinoma is not significantly related to prognosis (23).

Lymphatic tumor emboli in the breast surrounding a carcinoma are unfavorable prognostic findings. Lymphatics are here defined as vascular channels lined by endothelium without supporting smooth muscle or elastica (fig. 251). Most do not contain red blood cells but some blood capillaries are included in this definition. Artefactual spaces are commonly formed around nests of tumor cells within an invasive carcinoma as a result of tissue shrinkage during processing (figs. 252, 253). Because it is very difficult to distinguish these arte-

facts from true lymphatic spaces, assessment for lymphatic invasion (LI) is most reliably accomplished in breast parenchyma adjacent to or well beyond the invasive tumor margin (76). Efforts to identify intratumoral lymphatic spaces by using immunoperoxidase reagents associated with endothelial cells (factor VIII and blood group antigens) have met with only limited success (53,82). False-negative immunohistochemical results can usually be recognized in extratumoral breast tissue, but the fact that they occur means these reagents are not reliable for detecting lymphatic emboli within a tumor. The prognostic significance of intratumoral lymphatic emboli has not been determined.

Extratumoral lymphatic tumor emboli in the breast are found in approximately 25 percent of invasive duct carcinomas. The majority of these

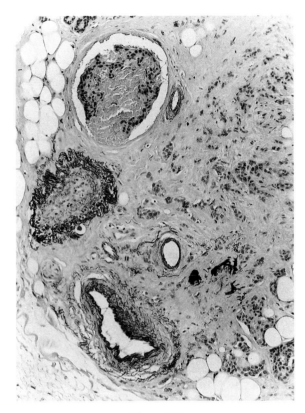

Figure 253
SHRINKAGE ARTEFACT
Partly necrotic carcinoma above is in a space created by shrinkage in the tissue. Endothelial cells are absent and the configuration of the tumor virtually duplicates the shape of the perimeter of the space. Elastic tissue in the walls of two blood vessels has been highlighted by the elastic van Gieson stain. The central vessel is thrombosed but contains no apparent tumor.

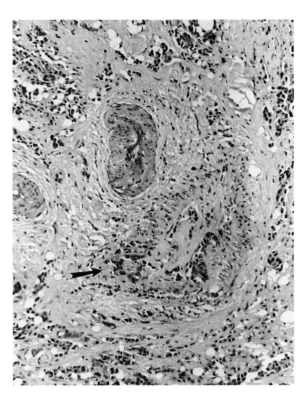

Figure 254
BLOOD VESSEL INVASION
Hematoxylin and eosin stained section with triangular structure (arrow) suggesting a blood vessel invaded by carcinoma next to an artery. (Figures 254 and 255 are from the same patient.)

patients also have axillary lymph node metastases and it has not yet been determined whether the presence of LI alters their prognosis. Lymphatic tumor emboli are found in the breast surrounding invasive duct carcinomas in 10 to 15 percent of patients who have pathologically negative lymph nodes. Several studies have shown that LI is prognostically unfavorable in node-negative patients treated by mastectomy (8,66,76,79,81) especially in women with T1N0M0 disease. In a 10-year follow-up study of 378 patients treated for T1N0M0 carcinoma, 33 percent of 30 women with LI died of disease. Death due to breast carcinoma was observed in 10 percent of the 348 women who did not have LI (79). Recurrences in node-negative patients

with peritumoral lymphatic emboli tend to occur more than 5 years after diagnosis and are almost always at systemic rather than local sites. Lymphatic tumor emboli do not predispose to local recurrence in node-negative patients treated by mastectomy but are associated with breast recurrence after breast conservation treatment, especially in women who are not irradiated.

Blood vessel invasion is defined as penetration by tumor into the lumen of an artery or vein (fig. 254). These vascular structures can be identified by the presence of a smooth muscle wall supported by elastic fibers demonstrated by special histochemical procedures (e.g., orcein or Verhoeff van Gieson stains) that selectively stain elastic tissue (fig. 255). Elastin fibers deposited around ducts that contain intraductal carcinoma in an invasive tumor create an appearance very similar to vascular invasion. Since larger vascular components in the breast usually consist of a

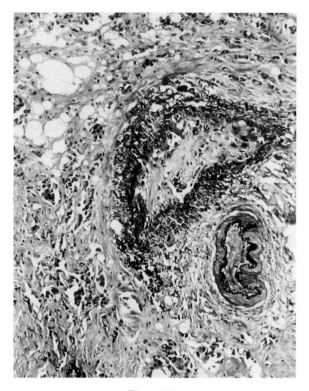

Figure 255
BLOOD VESSEL INVASION
Section consecutive with figure 254 is stained for elastic tissue which accentuates the elastica of the vein involved by carcinoma and an artery below.

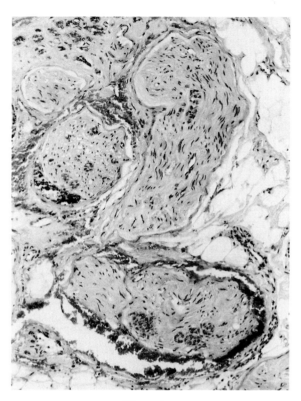

Figure 256
PERINEURAL INVASION
Carcinoma growing around and within nerves.

paired artery and vein, vascular invasion should only be diagnosed with confidence when tumor is within one or both of a pair of vessels demonstrated by an elastic fiber stain.

The reported frequency of blood vessel invasion varies from 4.7 to 47.2 percent (7,22,25,79–81,108). These widely divergent observations reflect differences in the methods of identification. Some report that blood vessel invasion denotes a poorer prognosis in node-positive patients (66) or only in those with two or more positive lymph nodes (110). Others conclude that this finding is prognostically significant only in the absence of axillary lymph node metastasis (7).

Blood vessel invasion was identified in 47 of 362 (13 percent) T1N0M0 patients treated by mastectomy and followed up for 10 years (79). Recurrence of carcinoma was more frequent when blood vessel invasion was present (26 percent) than in its absence (16 percent) and death due to disease occurred more often; differences in recur-

rence and death rates were not statistically significant however. In another study, blood vessel invasion was found in 23 of 117 (16 percent) stage II T1 tumors (T1N1M0) (80), and deaths due to metastatic breast carcinoma occurred with significantly greater frequency among these women (P <0.03), whether they had a single positive lymph node or two or more affected nodes.

Perineural invasion can be found in approximately 10 percent of invasive carcinomas (fig. 256). It occurs in high-grade tumors, frequently associated with lymphatic tumor emboli, and does not have independent prognostic significance.

A variety of patterns have been described in the connective tissue stroma formed in and around invasive duct carcinomas. Tumors vary considerably with respect to the quantity and qualitative characteristics of their stroma. Extremes are represented by very cellular variants of invasive duct carcinoma that contain virtually no fibrous stroma and scirrhous carcinoma characterized by marked collagenization.

Attempts to assess the character or composition of stroma in invasive duct carcinomas have focused on the amount of elastic tissue present. Stromal elastic fibers can be detected using the same stains employed to demonstrate the elastic components in blood vessels (orcein or Verhoeff van Gieson stains). The frequency of the most extreme or marked degrees of elastosis described in recent reports varied from 17 to 23 percent while from 12 to 55 percent of tumors were characterized by little or no elastosis (22,70). Abundant elastosis is significantly associated with estrogen receptor positivity (70). The significance of elastosis as an independent prognostic variable remains controversial. While marked elastosis has been described as a favorable prognostic feature (85,92), some investigators found that elastosis did not correlate with prognosis (70,74), or that abundant elastosis had a negative effect on outcome (29).

The pattern and amount of intraductal carcinoma have been evaluated as prognostic variables in patients with invasive duct carcinoma. Tumors vary in the relative proportions of intraductal and invasive components from those with only microscopic invasion to lesions composed entirely of invasive carcinoma. Silverberg and Chitale (86) observed a trend to decreased nodal metastases and a more favorable prognosis when the intraductal component in the tumor was relatively more abundant. In another study, little or no intraductal carcinoma was detected in sections from 72 percent of 974 tumors and 11 percent were described as composed of at least 66 percent intraductal carcinoma (22). These authors noted that lesions with a prominent intratumor intraductal component also tended to have intraductal carcinoma outside the main tumor with multicentric foci of carcinoma in other quadrants of the breast. The distribution of intraductal carcinoma in and around the primary tumor influences the risk for recurrence after lumpectomy and radiation therapy (84) but does not influence the risk for systemic recurrence in women treated by mastectomy (78). The risk for recurrence after lumpectomy alone or lumpectomy and radiation is highest among patients with comedo intraductal carcinoma.

Immunohistochemical Markers. When examined by immunohistochemical methods, the frequency of carcinoembryonic antigen (CEA) positivity varies considerably, with different laboratories reporting 34 percent (90), 50 percent (105), 65 percent (35), and 90 percent (54) positive reactivity. In most studies, the presence or absence of CEA in the primary tumor has proven to have little or no prognostic value (28,35,54, 75,90,105).

The prognostic significance of other marker substances that can be detected in breast carcinoma cells by immunohistochemical methods also remains somewhat uncertain. Beta-HCG has been found in 12 (103) to 18 percent (54) of carcinomas. Generally, most tumors have only a few scattered immunoreactive cells (54,103) which are otherwise morphologically indistinguishable from beta-HCG–negative cells (54,103). No significant relation has been observed between this pattern of beta-HCG reactivity, tumor type, stage, other prognostic indicators, or disease-free survival.

Pregnancy specific beta-1 glycoprotein (SP-1) is a normal placental protein that may be found in the serum and neoplastic tissue of patients with various cancers including mammary carcinoma (32,48,54,105). Immunohistochemical studies have found that 37 percent (105), 40 percent (48), and 56 percent (54) of carcinomas were SP-1 positive. Kuhajda et al. (48) found a higher frequency of axillary node metastases among patients with SP-1 positive tumors, with the difference statistically significant when the primary tumor was 3 cm or less in diameter. Lee et al. (54) found that patients who survived disease free for 10 or more years were more likely to have SP-1 reactive tumors than those with recurrences, but the differences were not statistically significant.

Placental lactogen, another ectopic placental protein associated with breast carcinoma (54,103) has been detected immunohistochemically in 30 percent of carcinomas (54). It is not significantly associated with the grade or type of carcinoma or with prognosis.

Alpha-lactalbumin (ALA) reactivity has been found in 56 (54) to 75 percent (51) of breast carcinomas. ALA expression is not significantly related to histologic grade (51,54), menstrual status (52), or prognosis. Tumors positive for estrogen and progesterone receptors are more likely to be ALA positive than are tumors positive for only one of these receptors (51).

The loss of blood group isoantigen expression has been associated with progression to invasion and metastases in early stages of carcinoma of the urinary bladder. Preservation of isoantigen expression comparable to the patient's AB blood group is observed in 26 to 37 percent of breast carcinomas (52,54). At least 75 percent of carcinomas demonstrate expression of H antigen, the precursor substrate of A and B antigens when tested with an antibody to *Ulex europaeus* I lectin. One group of investigators found no significant relationship between the presence or absence of isoantigen expression and prognosis (52,54). Others correlated the proportion of tumor cells reactive with two lectins, *Helix pomatia* and *Ulex europaeus*, with survival (21). Significantly reduced recurrence-free and overall survival were found in patients whose tumors had more than 50 percent of cells staining for either lectin.

S-100 protein, a calcium-binding protein, initially thought to be specific for neural tissues and neoplasms, has been found expressed in a wide variety of other tissues, including mammary carcinomas (19,64). Overall, approximately 50 percent of breast carcinomas contain S-100 reactive cells, including infiltrating duct carcinomas (45 percent). Immunoreactivity for S-100 in mammary carcinoma cells has not been significantly associated with differentiation, stage, or prognosis (19).

For the most part neoplastic cells express intermediate cytoskeletal filaments (IF) corresponding to their cell of origin. Cytokeratins are IF associated with epithelial cells or epithelial neoplasms while vimentin is regarded as primarily a property of mesodermal cells and mesenchymal tumors. However, vimentin has been detected in metaplastic components of mammary carcinomas that have a sarcomatous appearance microscopically and in epithelial cells in infiltrating duct carcinomas (71,72). Vimentin has been significantly associated with a higher growth fraction as measured with the Ki-67 antibody. There is a direct relationship between vimentin immunoreactivity and histologic grade but an inverse correlation with estrogen receptor level. Tumor size and axillary node status are not significantly related to vimentin positivity. These observations suggest that vimentin expression may be an independent indicator of prognosis (71).

Oncogenes. Insight into genetic changes involved in the development and progression of malignant neoplasms has been gained from the study of oncogenes. In some neoplastic systems transformation has been associated with structural change in normal genes (proto-oncogenes) induced by certain retroviruses. Numerous studies indicate that transformation may be the direct result of oncogenes or a consequence of amplified expression of proto-oncogenes through alterations in controls—promoter and enhancer elements of gene expression.

Some studies of proto-oncogene alterations (amplification or deletion) in DNA extracted from breast carcinomas have shown that patients with tumors exhibiting these changes presented with a more advanced stage of disease that was more likely to recur (15). Immunohistochemical reagents have been developed to examine tissues for oncogene expression. This involves monoclonal antibodies directed at specific protein products (oncoproteins) encoded by transforming oncogenes. Data obtained by this method suggest that oncogene expression may influence prognosis.

One group of oncogenes that has been evaluated extensively histologically are members of the *ras* family. Mutations of the *ras* proto-oncogene have been found in 10 to 30 percent of breast carcinomas. An even greater proportion of breast carcinomas exhibit enhanced or amplified expression of *ras* mRNA.

Monoclonal antibodies to the p21 protein products of *ras* oncogenes have been used in immunohistochemical studies. These proteins, involved in GTP binding, are located in the cell membrane where they participate in transduction of proliferative stimuli at the cell surface (43). No long-term follow-up studies have demonstrated that *ras* p21 expression influences prognosis. Failure to observe consistent correlations with prognostic variables may be due to several factors, including differing antibodies employed by various investigators, quality of the tissues related to storage or fixation, and variations in methodology (109).

The c-*erb*B-2(HER2/*neu*) proto-oncogene, a member of the tyrosine kinase oncogene family, codes for a transmembrane glycoprotein similar to the epidermal growth factor receptor (16). In human tissues, amplification of c-*erb*B-2(HER2/*neu*) was found to be associated with adenocarcinomas, especially mammary carcinoma (44,114,116). Amplification greater than 2- to 3-fold has been reported in up to 40 percent of breast carcinomas (87). Analysis of recurrence-free and overall survival revealed a significantly less favorable outcome among the node-positive women with 5-fold or greater amplification (87,88). Amplification was not found to have a significant association with relapse or survival among node-negative patients. Other investigators have failed to detect a significant relationship between c-*erb*B-2 (HER2/*neu*) amplification and prognostic factors or prognosis. Ali et al. (3) reported that c-*erb*B-2 (HER2/*neu*) was not significantly related to relapse-free or overall survival after univariate and multivariate analysis.

With the availability of techniques to evaluate oncogene amplification in DNA extracted from paraffin blocks, it is possible to carry out long-term retrospective studies. Tsuda et al. (96) studied paraffin-embedded formalin-fixed tissue from 176 patients with 10 years of follow-up. Among 164 women treated by mastectomy, disease-free survival was significantly reduced in patients with c-*erb*B-2(HER2/*neu*) amplification. The unfavorable effect on survival was greatest in cases with more than 4-fold amplification. When stratified by axillary node status, significantly reduced disease-free survival associated with amplification was found in patients with axillary metastases but not among those with negative lymph nodes. Multivariate analysis revealed that amplification of c-*erb*B-2(HER2/*neu*) was a statistically significant independent prognostic indicator, second only to lymph node status among the variables analyzed.

The availability of an antibody to the c-*erb*B-2 (HER2/*neu*) protein has made it possible to study expression of the protein directly in tissue sections by immunohistochemical procedures. Pathologic correlation with histopathologic features of primary carcinomas was reported by Gusterson et al. (33,34). Membrane staining, regarded as evidence of c-*erb*B-2(HER2/*neu*) reactivity, was found in 16 percent of 137 invasive duct carcinomas, 44 percent of intraductal carcinomas (33,74), particularly comedo and micropapillary lesions, and in 83 percent of Paget disease (5,6). Axillary node metastases exhibited the same staining pattern as the primary tumor. Staining for c-*erb*B-2(HER2/*neu*) protein was not significantly related to axillary node status. They also reported that the presence or absence of membrane staining was not predictive of overall or disease-free survival. Van de Vijver et al. (99) agreed that immunohistochemical reactivity was not significantly related to axillary node status, histologic grade of duct carcinomas, age at diagnosis, or relapse-free survival after adjustment for tumor size. However, Wright et al. (113) reported that only lymph node status was a stronger predictor of prognosis than c-*erb*B-2(HER2/*neu*) staining. After a median follow-up of 24 months patients with c-*erb*B-2 (HER2/*neu*) positive tumors had a shorter disease-free and overall survival rate. When stratified by nodal status, disease-free survival was reduced significantly by positive staining among those with lymph node metastases but not among node-negative patients. Overall survival was significantly lower in c-*erb*B-2(HER2/*neu*) positive patients regardless of nodal status.

Amplification of other oncogenes has also been correlated with breast cancer prognosis. Varley et al. (100) found amplification of c-*myc* in 7 of 41 carcinomas (17 percent); in another tumor with overexpression there was rearrangement of the c-*myc* gene. Patients with altered c-*myc* gene expression had a significantly shorter disease-free and overall survival rate. A low frequency of c-*myc* amplification (4 percent) was also reported by Tsuda et al. (96) who examined DNA extracted from formalin-fixed paraffin-embedded tissue. Disease-free and overall survival were significantly reduced in these patients.

Amplification of the proto-oncogene *int*-2 has been found in 13 percent of breast carcinomas accompanied in virtually all cases by coamplification of *hst*-1 (96). Amplification of *hst*-1/*int*-2 was significantly associated with reduced disease-free survival but appeared to be unrelated to TNM stage or lymph node status.

Proliferative Rate. *Thymidine labeling.* The proliferative proportion of cells in DNA synthesis determined by the thymidine labeling index (TLI) has been shown to correlate significantly with prognosis (26,61,97). High TLI has been associated with a higher frequency of recurrence, earlier recurrence, and shorter survival after recurrence (61). This is independent of stage at diagnosis (67,47) but may not be a better guide to prognosis than histologic grade (97).

Flow cytometry. Flow cytometry provides a simple and precise method for determining proliferative fraction (S-phase fraction), which is reported to be equivalent to thymidine labeling index (60). It has been observed that proliferative activity reflected in the S-phase fraction (SPF) is correlated with ploidy to the extent that diploid carcinomas usually have a lower SPF than aneuploid lesions (63,93). Tumors with a high SPF tend to be estrogen receptor negative (63,67,68). Ploidy and SPF have been found to correlate with the histologic differentiation of duct carcinomas and with nuclear or cytologic differentiation (63,67,68). While some investigators reported that ploidy or SPF did not correlate with nodal status at the time of initial treatment (58), others found that SPF was higher in node-positive than node-negative tumors (18,37).

Numerous studies have been published relating cell cycle kinetics and ploidy determined by flow cytometry to breast carcinoma prognosis using paraffin-embedded archival tissue (37,42), stored frozen tissue (14,18), or fresh tumor samples (60). The subject has been summarized in a comprehensive review by Visscher et al. (102). Results have not always been consistent, due in part to variations in methodology. Within the limits of the available follow-up, published reports indicate that the overall disease-free survival of patients with diploid tumors is somewhat better than that of patients with aneuploid tumors, although many authors have not found the difference to be statistically significant. The same effect has been seen when patients are stratified by lymph node status with the unfavorable influence of aneuploidy more prominent among women with lymph node metastases, especially when four or more lymph nodes are affected.

The prognostic significance of SPF has been evaluated by flow cytometry in several studies. Hedley et al. (37) found that node-positive patients had a better prognosis if the SPF of the primary tumor was below the mean SPF of all positive node tumors. The effect was most pronounced in patients with four or more involved nodes. Multivariate analysis indicated that the effect was dependant on tumor grade and that SPF was not an independent factor. Conversely, Kallioniemi et al. (42) reported that SPF was strongly correlated with prognosis as an independent factor in patients with stage II and III lesions. Deaths due to

disease occurred more frequently in patients with above median SPF. In an analysis of node-negative patients, Clark et al. (14) found that SPF was a significant prognostic factor in patients with diploid tumors but not in those with aneuploid lesions. Patients with diploid tumors and high SPF had a significantly reduced disease-free survival rate when compared to those with diploid tumors and low SPF. These differences were also reflected in overall survival. The disease-free survival of women with diploid-high SPF tumors was not significantly different from that of patients with aneuploid tumors grouped together regardless of SPF.

Immunohistochemical markers of growth rate. Bromodeoxyuridine (BrdU), a thymidine analog, is incorporated into DNA during the S-phase of the cell cycle. Uptake of BrdU after in vivo administration to patients or by in vitro incubation of biopsies can be measured in tissue sections by an immunohistochemical procedure that employs an anti-BrdU antibody (31). The results are comparable to those obtained by thymidine labeling (31,36). The in vitro labeling does not require radioactive reagents, and it can be completed in considerably less time than is necessitated by autoradiography of ^{3}H-thymidine labeled tissues. However, prospective long-term follow-up studies have yet to be reported in breast cancer patients. The development of an immunohistochemical procedure applicable to paraffin sections may make BrdU more useful clinically.

Ki-67 is a mouse monoclonal antibody to nuclear components of a cell line derived from Hodgkin disease. The antibody reacts with a nuclear antigen expressed in proliferating cells throughout the cell cycle that is not detectable in quiescent cells (27). It has been shown that there is a close correlation in most tumors between the Ki-67 growth fraction and estimates of S-phase by flow cytometry (106), the thymidine labeling index (TLI) (44), and the immunohistochemical detection of BrdU incorporation into nuclei (83). Ki-67 reactivity does not correlate well with the stage of the primary tumor as reflected in size or lymph node status and it appears to be an independent prognostic variable (6,55,59,109).

Proliferating cell nuclear antigen (PCNA), also termed cyclin, is a protein that plays an essential role in DNA synthesis (107). Antibodies prepared to PCNA have shown a direct correlation to immunostaining with Ki-67 in a number of tumor systems. Increased immunostaining for PCNA in noncancerous tissues surrounding carcinomas suggests that PCNA expression may be regulated by paracrine or autocrine growth factors.

Nuclear Morphometry. Nuclear morphometry provides a method for obtaining quantitative measurements of the size and shape of tumor cell nuclei. Among the parameters commonly recorded are nuclear diameter, nuclear area, and nuclear perimeter. Careful counts of mitotic activity are obtained. Measurements can be made using histologic sections (5) or aspiration cytology smears (91, 115). Prognostic correlations have been made with the nuclear morphometry of the primary tumor (5, 91,115) as well as with morphometric features of tumor cell nuclei in axillary node metastases (56). The morphometric feature that most often has a statistically significant association with prognosis is nuclear area (5,56,91,98). Nuclear diameter, a parameter included in the calculation of area, is also significantly related to prognosis (115), as is frequency of mitoses (5). Inverse relationships are observed between mean nuclear area, mean nuclear diameter, mitotic index, and prognosis. Concurrent assessment of nuclear and histologic grading prove prognostically significant (5,56).

Prognosis and Treatment. While many of the detailed factors discussed in this chapter may be considered in the assessment of prognosis for individual patients, the strongest determinant of outcome for women with invasive duct carcinoma is the pathologic stage at diagnosis. In most series, stage is described in terms of the TNM system. Data from randomized clinical trials comparing patients treated by breast conserving surgery, axillary dissection, and radiotherapy to mastectomy and axillary dissection have revealed no significant differences in survival results between these treatment modalities for women with T1N0M0 and T1N1M0 disease (101).

Among node-negative patients, the 10-year disease-free survival is approximately 80 percent for women with a T1N0 tumor, decreasing to about 70 percent for T2N0 and to 60 percent for T3N0 patients (77). A particularly favorable outcome of 90 percent disease-free survival has been reported in T1N0 patients who have tumors 1 cm or less in diameter (77).

When axillary lymph node metastases are present, outcome is influenced by the number of involved nodes as well as by primary tumor size. The most significant differences have been found when patients with one to three involved lymph nodes are separated from those with four or more nodal metastases. This stratification is particularly important for patients with T1N1 stage disease. For those with T1N1 (1-3+) stage, disease-free survival was about 74 percent at 10 years in the era prior to adjuvant chemotherapy. In the T1N1 (4+) group, 10-year disease-free survival after surgery alone has been about 50 percent (77). Among patients with T2N1 disease treated by surgery alone, the number of involved lymph nodes is also a prognostic discriminant with 10-year disease-free survival ranging from about 40 percent in T2N1 (1-3+) to about 20 percent for women with T2N1 (4+) disease (62). About 10 percent of women with T3N1 tumors survive 10 years disease free.

Data accumulated since the widespread use of adjuvant chemotherapy indicate an improvement in disease-free survival for node-negative patients (39). Many of these studies have not been in progress long enough to report 10-year results, but after 5 years survival appears to be improved by about 20 percent in women older than 50 years treated with tamoxifen and by 26 percent for women younger than 50 years treated with combination chemotherapy (20). Results from several trials have also shown that survival may be improved and the frequency of recurrence reduced by 10 to 15 percent when node-negative patients with T1N0 tumors larger than 1 cm and those with T2N0 and T3N0 tumors receive systemic adjuvant therapy (38,65).

INVASIVE LOBULAR CARCINOMA

The WHO classification of breast tumors (161) states that invasive lobular carcinoma is "composed of uniform cells resembling those of lobular carcinoma in situ and usually having a low mitotic rate." Furthermore:

> The cells grow typically in a single-file, linear arrangement, or appear individually embedded in fibrous tissue.... Infiltrating cells are often arranged concentrically around ducts, in a target-like pattern. Identification of remnants of lobular carcinoma in situ aids in the diagnosis. Tumour cells may appear in signet-ring shapes owing to distension with mucus. Other growth patterns have been described, e.g. tubulo-lobular and solid.

The term lobular carcinoma was established in 1941 with publication of the classic paper on this carcinoma by Foote and Stewart (131). A desmoplastic stromal reaction, linear arrangement of the carcinoma cells (the so-called "Indian file pattern"), and their tendency to grow in a circumferential fashion around ducts and lobules ("targetoid" growth) were the "peculiar" diagnostic features emphasized by these authors. When the diagnosis is based strictly on the criteria of Foote and Stewart, invasive lobular carcinoma usually constitutes 3 to 5 percent of the invasive carcinomas in most series (138,150, 152). With less restrictive diagnostic criteria, the disease frequency increases to 10 to 14 percent of invasive carcinomas (123,146,158).

Clinical Presentation. Invasive lobular carcinoma occurs throughout most of the age range of breast carcinoma in adult women (28 to 86 years). Various studies have placed the median age at diagnosis between 45 and 56 years (118,122,123, 127,128,150,152). It is relatively more common among women older than 75 years (11 percent) than in women 35 years or younger (153).

The presenting symptom in almost all cases is a mass with ill-defined margins. In some patients, the only evidence of the neoplasm is vague thickening or fine diffuse nodularity of the breast. Invasive lobular carcinoma is not prone to form calcifications but they may be present coincidentally in benign proliferative lesions such as sclerosing adenosis. Consequently, the detection of these tumors by mammography depends largely on the recognition of a mass. Infiltrating lobular carcinoma does not have a specific or characteristic mammographic appearance.

Patients are reported to have a relatively high frequency of bilateral carcinoma. The wide range of overall bilaterality that has been described (6 to 47 percent) has been influenced by how the data have been tabulated. Prior and concurrent contralateral carcinomas have been described in 6 to 28 percent of cases (122,124,128,143,150,152). The reported incidence of subsequent contralateral carcinoma ranges from 1.0 (124,139) to 2.38 (125) cases per 100 women per year. There is some evidence that the frequency of bilaterality is higher in patients with classic invasive lobular carcinoma than in patients with variant subtypes (122,125).

Although early studies suggested that invasive lobular carcinoma was exceptionally estrogen re-

ceptor rich, this has not been substantiated in subsequent analyses of larger groups of patients (144). However, particularly high levels of estrogen receptor were found in 12 cases of the alveolar variant of invasive lobular carcinoma, with amounts ranging from 336 to 1,495 fmol/mg cytosol protein (125,155). The majority of these lesions also had high levels of progesterone receptors.

Gross Findings. Tumor size ranges from occult, grossly inapparent lesions of microscopic dimensions to tumors that diffusely involve the entire breast. The median and average sizes of measurable tumors are not significantly different from the dimensions of invasive duct carcinomas. Typically, invasive lobular carcinoma forms a firm to hard tumor with irregular borders. In some cases, the excised specimen may not be visibly abnormal and only slightly firm to palpation although substantial involvement by tumor is evident microscopically.

Another gross manifestation of invasive lobular carcinoma is the formation of innumerable fine, hard nodules which feel like tiny pebbles or grains of sand in the breast parenchyma. These foci mimic sclerosing adenosis grossly and microscopically.

Microscopic Findings. Foote and Stewart (130) summarized their definition of the microscopic characteristics of invasive lobular carcinoma with the observation that

> ...the infiltrating portions of lobular carcinoma typically reveal thread-like strands of tumor cells rather loosely dispersed throughout a fibrous stroma.

At the cytologic level, the tumor cells were described as "small or medium-sized," "rather uniform in their staining properties," and exhibiting relatively little "irregularity." The presence of "central mucoid globules" in the tumor cells was cited as a helpful diagnostic feature.

Foote and Stewart's description has been widely accepted as defining the "classic" pattern of this type of carcinoma. The tumor cells exhibit a lack of cohesion and have a tendency to form slender strands arranged in a linear fashion (Indian file pattern) (figs. 257, 258). For the most part, the strands are no more than one or two cells across. Broader bands of cells constitute the trabecular growth pattern. In the targetoid or "bull's eye" pattern the tumor cells are arranged in concentric rings around ducts and lobules (fig. 259).

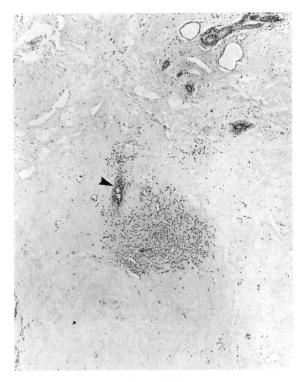

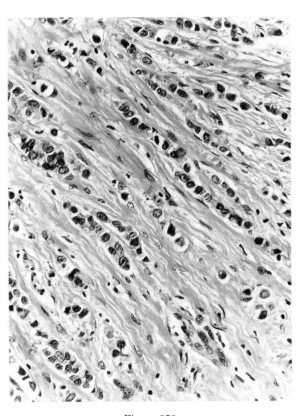

Figure 257
INVASIVE LOBULAR CARCINOMA
Microscopic appearance of a minute focus of carcinoma around a small duct (arrow) surrounded by normal mammary tissue. Numerous similar foci were found in all quadrants of the breast.

Figure 258
INVASIVE LOBULAR CARCINOMA
Linear "classic" growth pattern. (Fig. 5-6B from Rosen PP. Tumors of the breast: based on the preceedings of the 53rd Annual Anatomic Pathology Slide Seminar of the American Society of Clinical Pathologists. Chicago: American Society of Clinical Pathologists, 1987:37.)

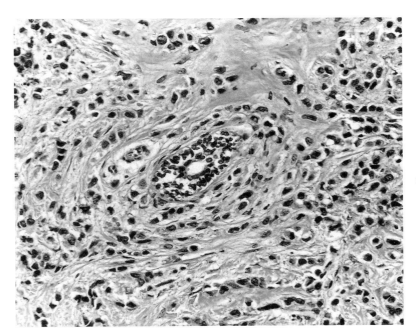

Figure 259
INVASIVE LOBULAR CARCINOMA
Tumor cells with "classic" pattern arranged around duct in "bull's eye" fashion.

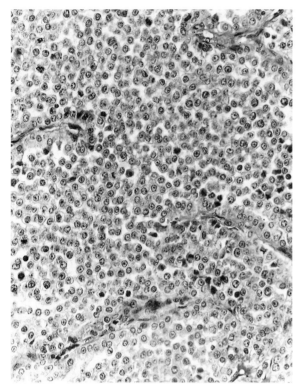

Figure 260
INVASIVE LOBULAR CARCINOMA
This tumor has a solid growth pattern that superficially resembles malignant lymphoma. Note the linear arrangement of tumor cells in some areas. (Fig. 3 from Di Costanzo D, Rosen PP, Gareen I, Franklin S, Lesser M. Prognosis in infiltrating lobular carcinoma. An analysis of "classical" and variant tumors. Am J Surg Pathol 1990;14:12–23.)

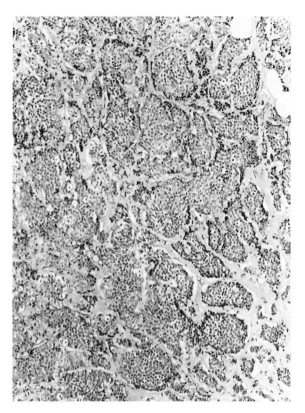

Figure 261
INVASIVE LOBULAR CARCINOMA
Alveolar pattern characterized by tumor cells arranged in discrete rounded aggregates separated by fibrous stroma.

It is not unusual to see an invasive carcinoma in which 100 percent of the microscopic fields fulfill the foregoing histologic criteria for invasive lobular carcinoma. However, many of the tumors composed largely of classic invasive lobular carcinoma have minor components in which the identical cells exhibit other growth patterns. The diagnosis of classic invasive lobular carcinoma is appropriate for tumors in which at least 70 percent of the lesion has a "single-file" growth pattern (152).

Tumors with the cytologic features of invasive lobular carcinoma with substantial elements of nonlinear growth have been referred to as "variant" forms. *Solid, tubulolobular,* and *alveolar variants* have been described. In the solid form tumor cells are "arranged in irregularly shaped solid nests...sometimes in continuity with a single file pattern of cytologically identical cells" (fig. 260) (127). Tubulolobular carcinomas are composed of small tubules as well as cords of tumor cells growing in the linear arrangement of classic invasive lobular carcinoma (129). The alveolar pattern has been defined as "a more-or-less globular aggregate of 20 or more cells, as seen in two planes, the cells being similar to those seen in other parts of the tumour" (fig. 261) (146).

The rarity of this entire group of tumors and the relatively small numbers of the several variant lesions hinder attempts to define and compare them. A series of 230 patients with stage I and II invasive lobular carcinoma included 176 women with classic lesions and 54 (23 percent) with variant growth patterns (122). Except for a younger age at diagnosis of classic lesions, no clinical differences were found when patients with classic and variant lesions were compared. Women with classic invasive lobular carcinoma

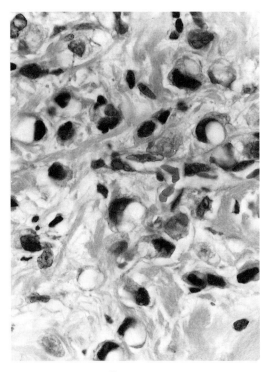

Figure 262
INVASIVE LOBULAR CARCINOMA
Signet ring cells.

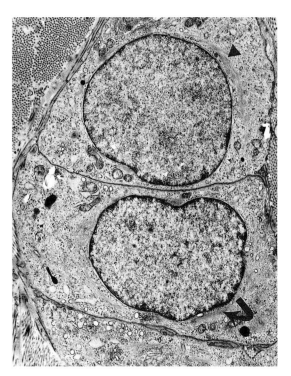

Figure 263
INVASIVE LOBULAR CARCINOMA
Electron micrograph showing carcinoma cells in a line
surrounded by collagen above and below. Note bundles of
cytokeratin filaments (arrows) and absence of basement membranes (X8000).

had significantly more frequent ductular extensions and a stronger trend to multicentricity
manifested by greater frequencies of bilaterality
as well as gross and microscopic multifocality.

The reported frequency of lobular carcinoma in
situ (LCIS) in association with invasive lobular
carcinoma of the classic type varies considerably.
Newman (34) found LCIS in 72 of 73 (98 percent)
cases. DiCostanzo et al. (122) detected LCIS associated with 65 percent of 176 classic infiltrating
lobular carcinomas and 57 percent of 54 variant
tumors. In other smaller series a LCIS component
was found in 31 (122) to 87 percent (123) of the cases.

The cytology of cells that comprise invasive
lobular carcinoma has received considerable attention. The cytologic types found in lobular
carcinoma in situ may also be present in invasive
lobular carcinoma. Classic invasive lobular carcinoma is usually described as consisting of
small, uniform cells with round nuclei and inconspicuous nucleoli. A variable proportion of cells
have intracytoplasmic lumina containing
sialomucins demonstrable with the mucicarmine and Alcian blue stains (119,132). When the

secretion is prominent, the cells have a signet
ring configuration (fig. 262) but with the aforementioned stains it is often possible to demonstrate small amounts of secretion in many non–
signet ring cells. Most so-called signet ring cell
carcinomas are forms of invasive lobular carcinoma (119,122,132,158) but similar cells are also
found in invasive duct carcinomas.

Grimelius-positive cells have been described
in a minority of invasive lobular carcinomas,
generally in tumors with a variant growth pattern (148). Dense core granules of a "neurosecretory" type have also been detected by electron
microscopy (19,32). Small cell (oat cell) neuroendocrine carcinoma of the breast may be a variant
of invasive lobular carcinoma (140,159).

Electron microscopic studies have yielded
variable ultrastructural findings in infiltrating
lobular carcinoma (126,147,148,156). In some
cases the cells have pale or clear organelle-poor
cytoplasm (fig. 263). Intracytoplasmic lumina are
often present (figs. 264, 265). Cells with darker,

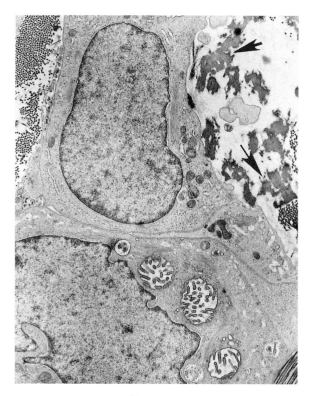

Figure 264
INVASIVE LOBULAR CARCINOMA
Intracytoplasmic lumens lined by microvilli are present in the cell below. The stroma contains elastic tissue (arrows) as well as collagen (X7000).

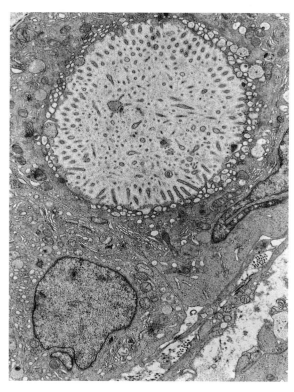

Figure 265
INVASIVE LOBULAR CARCINOMA
An intracytoplasmic lumen showing numerous microvilli. Perinuclear mucigen granules are evident (X7000).

irregular nuclei and organelle-rich cytoplasm may be myoid infiltrating lobular carcinoma (fig. 266). The cells of this histologic variant have deeply eosinophilic or amphophilic cytoplasm and resemble myoblasts (122). Neoplastic cells in the alveolar form of infiltrating lobular carcinoma have organelle-poor cytoplasm with oval, pale nuclei and inconspicuous nucleoli (148). Large cell variants with the classic growth pattern are referred to as pleomorphic or histiocytoid lobular carcinoma (fig. 267).

The diagnosis of invasive lobular carcinoma may be suspected in a fine-needle aspirate (151). The sample is usually sparsely cellular; small cells with scanty, inconspicuous cytoplasm are dispersed singly or in small groups on the slide. Signet ring cell forms may be found. Linear or Indian file arrays of tumor cells are a characteristic feature.

Prognosis and Treatment. Invasive lobular carcinoma can metastasize via lymphatics or by hematogenous dissemination. Axillary lymph

node metastases derived from invasive lobular carcinoma of the classic type may be distributed largely in sinusoids, sparing lymphoid areas. When lymph node involvement is sparse, the distinction between tumor cells and histiocytes may be difficult.

Reactive changes in histiocytes in the sinusoids of lymph nodes may resemble metastatic lobular carcinoma. Marked sinus histiocytosis sometimes duplicates the "sinus catarrh" pattern of metastatic lobular carcinoma. Signet ring cell sinus histiocytosis, a rare non-neoplastic reactive change of unknown etiology, is especially difficult to distinguish from metastatic lobular carcinoma (134). Cytoplasmic staining with PAS that is abolished with diastase and a weakly positive mucicarmine reaction can be found in signet ring cell histiocytes. These cells are not immunoreactive with cytokeratin markers for epithelial cells and they are variably reactive for histiocytic markers. Immunohistochemical studies for

173

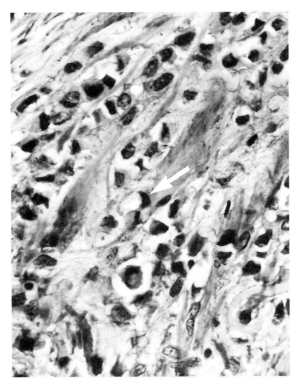

Figure 266
INVASIVE LOBULAR CARCINOMA
The tumor cells that have pleomorphic, hyperchromatic nuclei resemble myoblasts in the myoid form of invasive lobular carcinoma. A signet ring cell is indicated by the arrow.

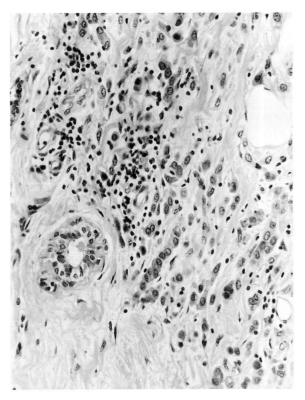

Figure 267
INVASIVE LOBULAR CARCINOMA
Mixed with lymphocytes, the tumor cells of the histiocytoid variant with vesicular nuclei and abundant cytoplasm shown here resemble histiocytes.

cytokeratin or epithelial membrane antigen frequently demonstrate many more carcinoma cells than routine histologic sections. Difficulty in distinguishing metastatic lobular carcinoma from histiocytes has been described in sites other than lymph nodes (117). Isolated tumor cells in the bone marrow may resemble hematopoietic elements (160) and in this setting immunohistochemical studies have proven especially useful (121).

Central nervous system metastases usually occur as carcinomatous meningitis in the form of diffuse leptomeningeal infiltration (136,157). Intra-abdominal metastases tend to involve the serosal surfaces, retroperitoneum (136,141), or ovaries (133). Diffuse spread in the uterus and ovaries with ovarian enlargement creates the features of Krukenberg tumor with clinical and pathologic findings indistinguishable from those of metastatic gastric carcinoma (136,137,141,162). A strongly positive immunohistochemical stain for estrogen receptor suggests metastatic breast car-

cinoma, but low levels of estrogen receptor have been found in gastric carcinoma cells. No significant differences have been found in the distribution of metastases between patients with the classic and variant patterns of invasive lobular carcinoma (122).

There are relatively few studies on the prognosis of patients with invasive lobular carcinoma (118,122,123,125,150,152). The disease-free survival of stage I patients followed for 5 to 10 years ranged from 72 to 86 percent and was not notably different from the survival of patients with invasive duct carcinoma.

Three series included enough patients to compare the prognosis of patients with classic and variant types of invasive lobular carcinoma. Of 103 woman studied by Dixon et al. (123), the combined group of patients with all types of lobular carcinoma had a significantly more favorable prognosis than women with invasive duct carcinomas.

Patients with classic invasive lobular carcinoma had a more favorable prognosis than those with variant forms. However, these results are inconclusive because the patients with duct carcinoma and classic and variant forms of invasive lobular carcinoma were not stratified by stage and most did not have an axillary dissection.

Analysis of 171 patients with invasive lobular carcinoma by du Toit et al. (125) revealed that patients with the classic subtype had a slightly better prognosis than those with alveolar and solid variants. The best prognosis was observed in patients with tubulolobular carcinoma, with a 13 percent recurrence rate. Recurrences developed in 40 to 57 percent of patients with classic and variant types of infiltrating lobular carcinoma. These results are difficult to assess since patients were not stratified by stage and were not treated in a consistent manner. Primary surgery consisted of "simple mastectomy, subcutaneous mastectomy or a lumpectomy followed by whole breast irradiation" and "lymph node status was determined by a triple node biopsy technique" rather than by conventional axillary dissection.

DiCostanzo et al. (122) studied 230 patients with stage I and II invasive lobular carcinoma treated by mastectomy and axillary dissection. They compared 176 women with classic invasive lobular carcinoma to 54 with variant histologic patterns (10 solid, 14 alveolar, 30 mixed). The groups did not differ significantly in tumor size, nodal status, or TNM stage. Median survival time and time to recurrence were similar in the two groups. When compared to patients with classic invasive lobular carcinoma, each of the variant subsets showed a trend to more frequent recurrence and death due to disease, but none of the differences was statistically significant. In a further analysis, women with classic invasive lobular carcinoma were compared with patients matched for age, tumor size, and nodal status with invasive duct carcinoma (122). Stage I patients with classic lesions had a significantly better disease-free survival rate (P=0.02). No significant difference in survival was found when stage II patients were compared.

These studies have not shown a consistent difference in prognosis of patients with invasive duct carcinoma and invasive lobular carcinoma when stage at diagnosis is taken into consideration. Most studies seem to indicate that pa-

tients with classic invasive lobular carcinoma have a better prognosis than those with variant forms as a group. No reproducible differences in prognosis have been demonstrated among patients with different variant lesions.

The important determinants of prognosis and treatment are primary tumor size and nodal status. Mastectomy with axillary dissection remains the standard primary treatment for most patients, although some reports of treatment by breast conservation with radiotherapy have appeared (142, 145,154). Kurtz et al. (142) found that local failure in the breast after 5 years was more frequent in patients with invasive lobular carcinoma (13.5 percent) than after treatment of invasive duct carcinoma (8.8 percent) but the difference was not statistically significant. Virtually all recurrences were at some distance from the primary tumor or multifocal. The 5-year actuarial survival rates were 100 percent and 77 percent for node-negative and node-positive patients, respectively. Schnitt et al. (154) reported that the 5-year actuarial risk for local recurrence was nearly identical for patients with invasive lobular (12 percent) and duct carcinomas (11 percent). The local recurrence rate for invasive lobular carcinoma was greater than the recurrence rate for patients with invasive duct carcinoma that lacked an extensive intraductal component (5 percent) but less than the 23 percent recurrence rate encountered for duct carcinoma with extensive intraductal carcinoma. In these studies, all recurrences were in the vicinity of the initial primary tumor.

TUBULAR CARCINOMA

This form of mammary duct carcinoma has been described in the WHO classification of breast tumors as (182):

> ...a highly differentiated invasive carcinoma whose cells are regular and arranged in well-defined tubules typically one layer thick and surrounded by an abundant fibrous stroma....Tubular carcinoma should not be confused with invasive ductal carcinomas with gland-like structures whose cells are less well differentiated.

The term "tubular" refers to the microscopic feature that defines the lesion, namely the formation of neoplastic tubules that closely resemble normal breast ductules (172). Other diagnostic terms sometimes applied to this tumor, "orderly" and "well-differentiated" carcinoma (180), are best used for the larger group of low-grade duct carcinomas in which tubular carcinoma constitutes the best differentiated extreme.

Pure tubular carcinomas constitute less than 2 percent of all breast carcinomas (166,167,179), although they are seen with increasing frequency as a result of the widespread use of mammography. Eight percent of invasive carcinomas 1 cm or less in diameter detected in the Breast Cancer Detection Demonstration Projects were of the tubular variety (164). Isolated examples of tubular carcinoma of the male breast have been reported (177,178) but these lesions constitute much less than 1 percent of male breast carcinomas (174).

Clinical Presentation. Among women, the age at diagnosis ranges from 24 to 83 years (177,178,180). The median age tends to be in the mid to late 40s (44 to 49 years), slightly younger than for breast carcinoma in general. Most patients report recent onset but occasionally a palpable lesion has been present for a substantial period before biopsy. Superficial tumors are fixed to the skin, producing retraction signs in about 15 percent of cases. Tubular carcinoma usually occurs in peripheral portions of the breast but uncommon examples have been detected arising from the major lactiferous ducts in the nipple or in the subareolar region.

Patients with pure tubular carcinoma tend to be younger than patients with mixed duct and tubular types, but no other consistent clinical differences have been reported (167,179). In one study, tubular carcinoma was associated with a 40 percent frequency of positive family history of breast carcinoma among first degree relatives (175) but others did not find this association. When studied by immunohistochemistry, tubular carcinomas are estrogen receptor positive (176).

Gross Findings. Most tubular carcinomas are 2 cm or less in diameter, but have been as large as 4 cm (177–179). In one series, the median size of 90 pure tubular carcinomas was 0.8 cm while only 52 percent of mixed tubular carcinomas were 1 cm or less. The median size of mixed lesions was 1.1 cm.(177).

When bisected, tubular carcinoma is often stellate and the cut surface retracts, becoming depressed in relation to the surrounding noncarcinomatous tissue. The gross appearance is similar to that of benign lesions such as sclerosing papillomatosis ("radial scar") (163).

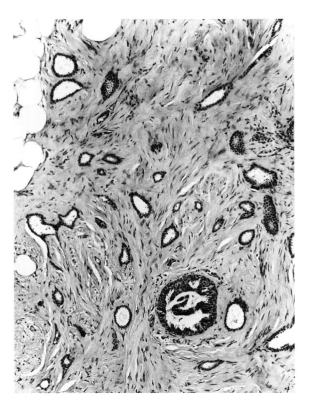

Figure 268
TUBULAR CARCINOMA

Typical pattern features haphazardly arranged glands of varying size invading fat separated by collagenous stroma. Note angular contours of many neoplastic glands and micropapillary intraductal carcinoma in the lower center. (Fig. 12-3A from Rosen PP. The pathology of invasive breast carcinoma. In: Harris JR, Hellman S, Henderson IC, Kinne DW, eds. Breast diseases. 2nd ed. Philadelphia: JB Lippincott, 1991.)

Microscopic Findings. Microscopically, tubular carcinoma is composed of small glands or tubules which resemble ductules in the non-neoplastic mammary parenchyma (figs. 268, 269). The overall configuration tends to be stellate and has ill-defined margins. Stroma between the glands appears different from stroma in the surrounding breast due to increased cellularity, collagenization, or abundant elastic tissue (168,181). However, elastosis is not a specific diagnostic feature since it also occurs in other types of carcinoma and in some benign lesions (163).

The glands in tubular carcinoma are composed, for the most part, of a single layer of neoplastic epithelial cells. They may have virtually any shape and have a haphazard distribution. In very orderly tumors the lesion may be

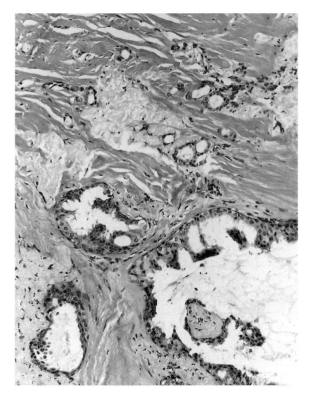

Figure 269
TUBULAR CARCINOMA
Very orderly micropapillary intraductal carcinoma and dense collagenized stroma with elastosis separating small round glands.

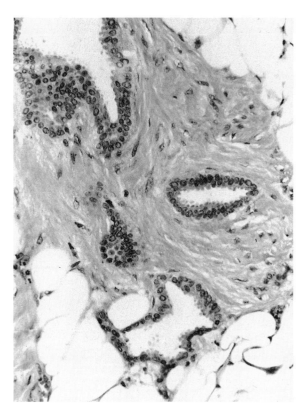

Figure 270
TUBULAR CARCINOMA
Angular glands composed of cells with round to oval basally oriented nuclei. Cytoplasmic "snouts" are evident at the luminal border.

composed of round or oval glands of relatively uniform caliber. More often, the glands have irregular shapes and angular contours (fig. 270).

The distinction between tubular carcinoma and sclerosing adenosis can be a challenging diagnostic problem (fig. 271). The proliferative pattern of sclerosing adenosis is lobulocentric and at low magnification it is almost always possible to perceive individual altered lobules in the lesion. Tubular carcinoma does not have a lobulocentric configuration although it can be multicentric. Individual foci of sclerosing adenosis are composed of elongated and largely compressed glands with interlacing spindled myoepithelial cells. Varying numbers of round, oval, or angular glands with open lumens are usually dispersed in these proliferative foci. Proliferation of myoepithelial cells is a regular feature of sclerosing adenosis while these cells are absent in tubular carcinoma. Both lesions may be present in fat. Tubular carcinoma invades

fat while lobules altered by sclerosing adenosis are sometimes located in fat and, therefore, appear to infiltrate it.

Histochemical studies have documented the presence of basement membranes around the glands in sclerosing adenosis and their absence in tubular carcinoma (figs. 272, 273). It is usually sufficient to use the periodic acid–Schiff or reticulin stains (171). Laminin, type IV collagen, and basement membrane proteoglycan were not detected in one series of nine tubular carcinomas (169).

The cells in tubular carcinoma glands appear to be relatively homogeneous. They are cuboidal or columnar with round or oval hyperchromatic nuclei that tend to be basally oriented. Nucleoli are inconspicuous or inapparent. Mitoses are rarely seen. "Apocrine" type cytoplasmic "snouts" are commonly present at the luminal cell border. The cytoplasm is usually amphophilic, infrequently clear, and rarely eosinophilic.

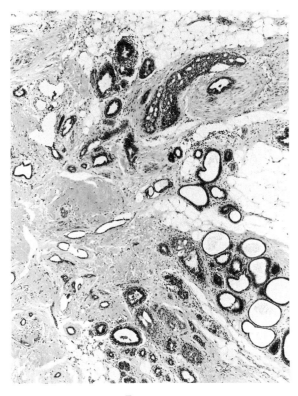

Figure 271
RADIAL SCLEROSING LESION
Angular glands in the sclerotic center can be mistaken for tubular carcinoma. Duct hyperplasia and microcysts at the periphery are not features of tubular carcinoma.

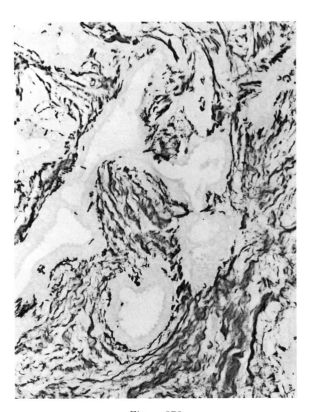

Figure 272
TUBULAR CARCINOMA
Reticulin stain demonstrating abundant reticulin fibers in stroma between tubular carcinoma glands. Reticulin fibers do not form a distinct continuous basement membrane around the neoplastic glands.

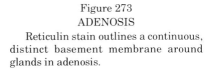

Figure 273
ADENOSIS
Reticulin stain outlines a continuous, distinct basement membrane around glands in adenosis.

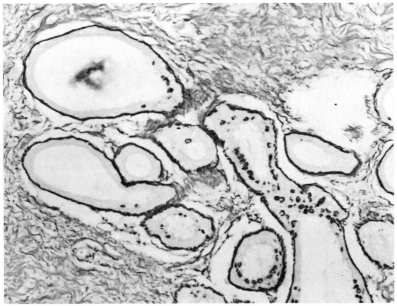

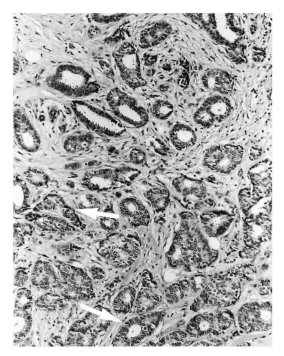

Figure 274
"MIXED" TUBULAR CARCINOMA
Glands below have a complex proliferative pattern that obscures the lumen (arrows). Above, glands have a tubular structure.

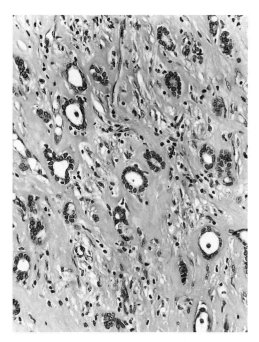

Figure 275
TUBULOLOBULAR CARCINOMA
This portion of the tumor consists of round and angular glands in collagenous stroma. (Figures 275 and 276 are from the same patient.)

A diagnosis of tubular carcinoma is made when at least 75 percent of the tumor exhibits the tubular growth pattern. When tubular components are not abundant enough to fulfill this quantitative criterion the lesion is described as a *mixed tubular carcinoma* or *duct carcinoma with tubular features* (fig. 274). These tumors form a heterogeneous group with respect to the proportion of the tubular component and also in regard to the degree of differentiation of the nontubular element. Mixed tubular carcinomas should be described according to the appearance of the nontubular component. Though rare, these tumors can have elements of invasive lobular carcinoma as well as tubular carcinoma; this combined pattern has been termed *tubulolobular carcinoma* (figs. 275, 276).

Calcifications are reportedly found microscopically in at least 50 percent of tubular carcinomas. They may be distributed in the neoplastic glands or in the stroma but are most often found in the intraductal carcinoma component which has been described in 60 to 84 percent of tubular carcinomas (167,177,178,180). It is possible to find intraductal

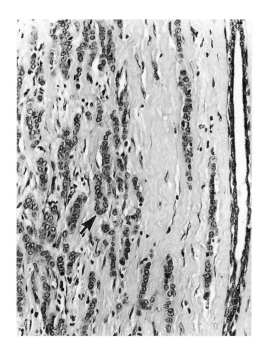

Figure 276
TUBULOLOBULAR
CARCINOMA
Another area in the carcinoma shown in figure 275 with the linear growth pattern of invasive lobular carcinoma. Traces of gland formation are evident (arrow).

179

carcinoma in almost all tubular carcinomas, typically with papillary or cribriform patterns or a mixture of the two (177). Coexistent lobular carcinoma in situ has been found in 0.7 to 23 percent of patients with tubular carcinoma (167,177,178). It is usually present in the immediate vicinity of the invasive tubular lesion but has also been found separately in the same breast or in the contralateral breast. Foci of atypical lobular hyperplasia are also not unusual.

Tubular carcinoma does not elicit a marked lymphocytic reaction. Perineural invasion is uncommon (fig. 277) while blood vessel invasion and lymphatic tumor emboli are virtually never seen.

Tubular carcinoma is usually a unicentric lesion in patients who present with a single mass detected by palpation or by mammography. When studied pathologically, a small number of patients have multifocal lesions growing as seemingly separate foci in one or more quadrants. These do not appear to be intramammary metastases since there is no associated lymphatic tumor emboli and intraductal carcinoma is often present in the carcinomatous areas. The frequency and prognostic significance of this uncommon multifocal variant has not been fully evaluated. Although several studies have described multifocal carcinoma in patients with tubular carcinoma, these additional areas rarely have a tubular pattern. In one study, 20 of 120 (16.7 percent) patients treated by mastectomy had tubular carcinoma remaining at the biopsy site, 6 (5 percent) had a second separate infiltrating carcinoma, 4 (3.3 percent) had multifocal intraductal carcinoma, and 3 (2.5 percent) had lobular carcinoma in situ (177).

The reported frequency of contralateral carcinoma varies from less than 1 to 38 percent (167,175) with two other studies reporting frequencies of 10 percent and 12 percent (177,178). Most contralateral tumors have been described as infiltrating duct carcinomas. Bilateral tubular carcinoma is uncommon (179).

Electron microscopy typically demonstrates uniform cells that usually form a single layer but may be slightly stratified within the neoplastic glands. Myoepithelial cells are scarce or not seen (170). Observations regarding the basal lamina have not been consistent but it is generally described as absent, incompletely formed, or discontinuous (173). Where the basal lamina is incom-

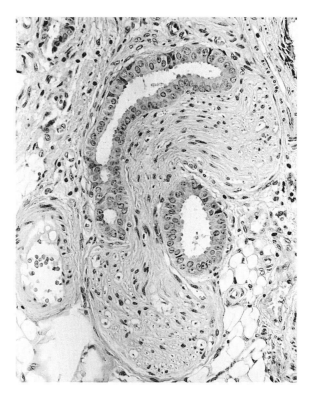

Figure 277
TUBULAR CARCINOMA
Perineural invasion with neoplastic glands wrapped around a nerve.

plete or absent one may find cytoplasmic protrusions of tumor cells into the stroma. Micro-villi are seen at the luminal cell surface. Cells are joined by numerous desmosomes and well-formed terminal bars. The cytoplasm contains mitochondria, rough endoplasmic reticulum, tonofilaments that may have a perinuclear distribution, and occasional cytoplasmic lumina. Collagen and elastic fibers are present in the stroma.

Prognosis and Treatment. The diagnosis of tubular carcinoma may be suggested by the findings in a specimen obtained by fine-needle aspiration (165), but excisional biopsy is necessary to confidently establish the diagnosis. The prognosis is favorable when tumors consist of at least 75 percent tubular elements (166,168,177–179). The average frequency of axillary lymph node metastases resulting from such lesions is 9 percent (177–179). Affected lymph nodes are usually in the low axilla (level I) and only rarely are more than three involved (177). Metastases in lymph nodes tend to have a tubular growth pattern (fig. 278). Axillary

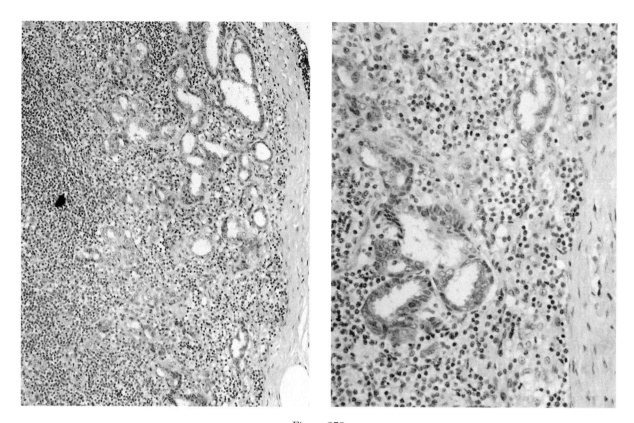

Figure 278
TUBULAR CARCINOMA
A. Metastatic carcinoma in an axillary lymph node. B. Tubular pattern is evident in this figure.

lymph node metastases have been found in up to 29 percent of patients with mixed tubular carcinomas.

The majority of the patients with pure and mixed tubular carcinomas described in the literature have been treated by modified or radical mastectomy. Review of seven follow-up studies describing a total of 341 women with pure tubular carcinoma, reveals that 12 (3.5 percent) had recurrences; 6 in the same breast following simple excision and 6 after mastectomy. Three of these patients originally had axillary lymph node metastases. Two had local recurrence, three had systemic metastases, and the sixth had "persistent carcinoma." Death due to metastatic mammary carcinoma in several patients with bilateral carcinoma has been attributable to a less well-differentiated contralateral carcinoma when one breast had a tubular carcinoma (177). Recurrences have been reported in up to 32 percent of patients with mixed tubular carcinoma and 6 to 28 percent of these patients died (167,179).

Patients with unifocal pure tubular carcinoma are candidates for breast conservation therapy. It would be prudent to employ radiation as an adjunct in view of the reported instances of recurrence in the breast after excisional treatment. Low axillary dissection should be performed in patients with a tubular carcinoma larger than 1 cm, when there are multifocal invasive lesions, or if there are other indications that suggest axillary node metastases. In view of the extremely favorable prognosis of tubular carcinoma, there is no evidence that systemic adjuvant therapy would prove beneficial except possibly for women with axillary metastases or if there is also a less well-differentiated carcinoma in the ipsilateral or contralateral breast. Patients with mixed tubular carcinomas should receive treatment appropriate for an infiltrating duct carcinoma of the grade of the nontubular component as determined by tumor size and stage.

MEDULLARY CARCINOMA

Medullary carcinoma is defined in the WHO classification of breast tumors (216) as a "well circumscribed carcinoma composed of poorly differentiated cells with scant stroma and prominent lymphoid infiltration."

Clinical Presentation. Medullary carcinomas constituted less than 5 percent and up to 7 percent of tumors in several series (187,204, 206,208). They are relatively more frequent among women in Japan than women in the United States (199,209) and possibly among black than white women in the United States (185,197,200), although a significant racial association is not always seen (204,207,214). Patients tend to be relatively young; at least 10 percent of carcinomas diagnosed in women 35 years of age or less are medullary carcinomas. The mean age in several series ranged from 46 to 54 years (207,211,213).

Medullary carcinomas have circumscribed margins, a firm consistency, and are easily mistaken clinically or radiologically for fibroadenomas, especially in young women. When arising in the axillary tail, they are difficult to distinguish clinically from metastatic carcinoma in a lymph node. Bilateral carcinoma has been found in 3 to 18 percent of patients with medullary carcinoma in one breast (195,204,213,214) but synchronous or metachronous medullary carcinoma involving both breasts is uncommon. Multicentricity, defined as microscopic foci of carcinoma outside the primary quadrant, is found in not more than 10 percent of cases (195,204).

Ipsilateral axillary lymph nodes tend to be enlarged even when there are no nodal metastases. This is due to a lymphoplasmacytic infiltrate, germinal center hyperplasia, and sinus histiocytosis. Consequently, the average number of axillary lymph nodes found grossly in the axillary dissection is greater than for other types of carcinoma.

Gross Findings. The size distribution of medullary carcinomas is not appreciably different from that of infiltrating duct carcinomas, which constitute about 75 percent of breast carcinomas; the median size is 2 to 3 cm. Grossly, medullary carcinoma is usually a moderately firm discrete tumor. Peripheral fibrosis may suggest encapsulation. Some small tumors may have poorly circumscribed borders (207) due to an intense lympho-

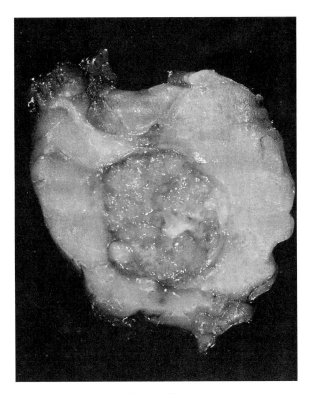

Figure 279
MEDULLARY CARCINOMA
Cut surface of a bisected tumor revealing the sharply defined margin. A bosselated contour and internal nodularity are apparent.

plasmacytic reaction that extends into adjacent breast tissue well beyond the immediate perimeter of the tumor. Some nonmedullary infiltrating carcinomas are as well circumscribed as the typical medullary carcinoma.

Inspection of the cut surface usually reveals a lobulated or nodular internal structure (fig. 279). The pale brown to grey tumor tissue is softer than the average breast carcinoma. Hemorrhage and necrosis are not uncommon and the extent of necrosis is directly related to tumor size. As necrosis increases, the tumor develops cystic foci.

Microscopic Findings. It is necessary to adhere to strict morphologic criteria if the diagnosis of medullary carcinoma is to be associated with a relatively favorable prognosis (201,204,207,214). Medullary carcinoma is defined by a constellation of histopathologic features initially described by Foote and Stewart (188). When most but not all of the components are present, the tumor may be termed atypical. Definitive histopathologic features

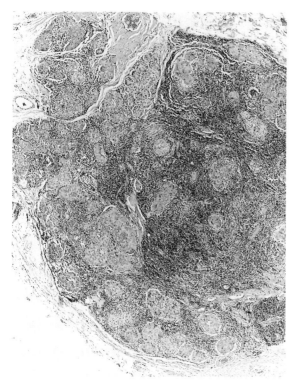

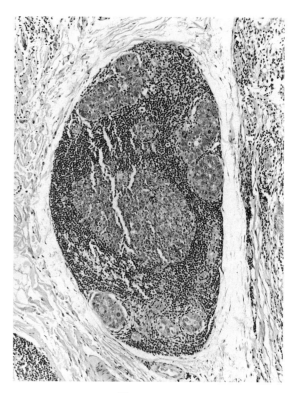

Figure 280
MEDULLARY CARCINOMA
Most of a small tumor is seen in this low magnification view. Characteristic features are circumscription, nodular internal architecture, and the dense lymphoplasmacytic infiltrate between islands of carcinoma cells and at the margin. (Fig. 12-10D from Rosen PP. The pathology of invasive breast carcinoma. In: Harris JR, Hellman S, Henderson IC, Kinne DW, eds. Breast diseases. 2nd ed. Philadelphia: JB Lippincott, 1991.)

Figure 281
MEDULLARY CARCINOMA
Lymphocytic infiltrate in a lobule at the periphery of a medullary carcinoma. The epithelia of a central terminal duct and of acinar glands have been replaced by medullary carcinoma cells. (Fig. 12-10E from Rosen PP. The pathology of invasive breast carcinoma. In: Harris JR, Hellman S, Henderson IC, Kinne DW, eds. Breast diseases. 2nd ed. Philadelphia: JB Lippincott, 1991.)

include a prominent lymphoplasmacytic reaction, circumscription, a syncytial growth pattern, poorly differentiated nuclear grade, and high mitotic rate (fig. 280).

The lymphoplasmacytic reaction must be intense enough to be "graded" at least as intermediate on a 3-point scale. The mononuclear infiltrate must involve at least 75 percent of the periphery and be present diffusely in the substance of the tumor. Usually the internal lymphoplasmacytic infiltrate is limited to the fibrovascular stroma, but on rare occasions the tumor can be largely devoid of stroma and the lymphoplasmacytic infiltrate mingles intimately with carcinoma cells. It is difficult to distinguish this later type of tumor from metastatic carcinoma in a lymph node. The lymphoplasmacytic reaction encompasses ducts and lobules in the surrounding

breast occupied by in situ carcinoma as well as nearby ducts and lobules not containing carcinoma (fig. 281). The infiltrate may be composed almost entirely of lymphocytes or plasma cells but usually there is a mixture of the two. Neutrophils, eosinophils, and monocytes are never the dominant cell types. Rarely, the lymphocytic infiltrate gives rise to germinal centers within and around the tumor.

Microscopic circumscription is defined by the appearance of the border of the infiltrating carcinoma, not by the periphery of the surrounding lymphoplasmacytic reaction. In medullary carcinoma the edge of the tumor should have a smooth, rounded contour that appears to push aside, rather than infiltrate, the breast. Consequently, glandular or fatty breast tissue should not be found within the invasive portion of the tumor.

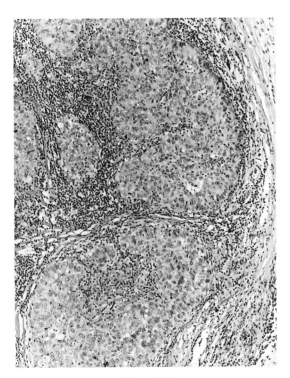

Figure 282
MEDULLARY CARCINOMA
Carcinoma cells with a syncytial growth pattern form masses separated by stroma with a dense lymphocytic infiltrate. (Fig. 12-10B from Rosen PP. The pathology of invasive breast carcinoma. In: Harris JR, Hellman S, Henderson IC, Kinne DW, eds. Breast diseases. 2nd ed. Philadelphia: JB Lippincott, 1991.)

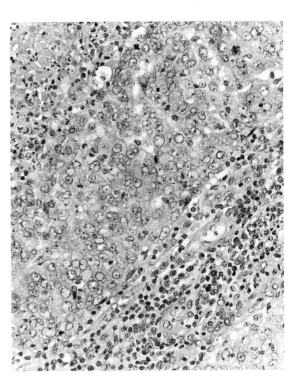

Figure 283
MEDULLARY CARCINOMA
A band of carcinoma cells with a syncytial arrangement demonstrating poorly differentiated nuclei. Necrosis of the carcinoma is evident in the upper left corner. A mixed lymphoplasmacytic reaction is seen in the stroma in the lower right corner.

If most of the tumor growth (variously defined as 75 percent or more of the histologically sampled areas) is arranged in broad irregular sheets or islands the pattern is syncytial (figs. 282, 283). This pattern often resembles a poorly differentiated epidermoid carcinoma. A tumor that is otherwise characteristic may be accepted as a medullary carcinoma if it has minor components of trabecular, glandular, alveolar, or papillary growth. It has been reported that overall and relapse-free survival are directly related to the extent of the syncytial component, with poorer prognosis with less than 75 percent syncytial pattern (202).

Poorly differentiated nuclear grade and high mitotic rate are interrelated characteristics of medullary carcinoma. Typically, the tumor cells have pleomorphic nuclei with coarse chromatin and prominent nucleoli (186).

A number of other microscopic features may be found. The presence of one or more of these secondary histopathologic characteristics is helpful to confirm a diagnosis of medullary carcinoma, but none must be present to establish it.

Intraductal carcinoma is found at the periphery of many medullary carcinomas as well as the epithelium of lobules (lobular extension of duct carcinoma) thereby creating foci of in situ carcinoma in the lobules (fig. 284). Cytologically, these ducts and lobules contain cells with the same poorly differentiated nuclei as the invasive portion of the medullary carcinoma. Expansile growth of in situ carcinoma in ducts and lobules leads to the formation of secondary peripheral tumor nodules responsible for the grossly nodular appearance of medullary carcinomas.

Metaplastic changes occur in a minority of medullary carcinomas, usually only focally (fig. 285). Squamous metaplasia has been found in 16 percent, often with necrosis (207), while osseous, cartilaginous, and spindle cell metaplasia are much less common.

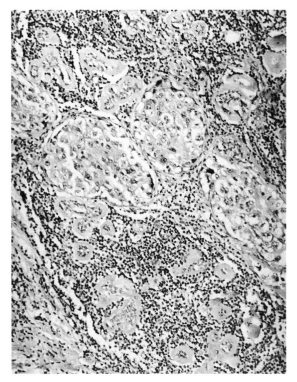

Figure 284
MEDULLARY CARCINOMA
A lobule at the periphery of a medullary carcinoma with in situ carcinoma in some acinar units. Note thick basement membranes that define acinar glands in this otherwise atrophic lobule. The basement membrane change is not specific for medullary carcinoma.

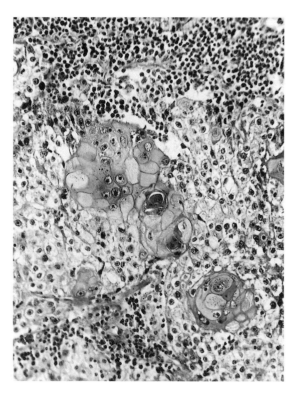

Figure 285
MEDULLARY CARCINOMA
Keratin pearl formation in focal areas of squamous metaplasia. Note solid growth pattern of carcinoma cells which tend to have distinct cell borders in regions of squamous metaplasia. Intense lymphocytic reaction is present in the stroma.

Ultrastructural Findings. Electron microscopy has not yielded consistent findings (183,189) or findings sufficiently specific to be regarded as diagnostic for medullary carcinoma. Intracytoplasmic lumens lined by microvilli are much less frequent than in other types of carcinoma. Light and dark cells, differing in cytoplasmic density, have been described by most authors; the dark cells tend to have more organelles, especially rough endoplasmic reticulum (189). Cells containing tonofilaments may be evidence of squamous differentiation. There do not appear to be distinctive ultrastructural differences between the tumor cells of medullary and atypical medullary carcinomas (189).

Immunohistochemistry. Immunohistochemical studies have shown that IgG cells predominate in medullary carcinomas and in infiltrating duct carcinomas (190–192). Lymphocytes infiltrating medullary and nonmedullary carcinomas are predominantly peripheral T lymphocytes (184,215). There are no significant differences in the distribution of antigenic phenotypes of lymphocytes between medullary and infiltrating duct carcinomas (184).

Atypical Medullary Carcinoma. Atypical medullary carcinoma describes carcinomas that resemble medullary carcinoma but lack all of the necessary features (figs. 286, 287). The growth pattern of the carcinoma must be at least 75 percent syncytial and not more than two other histologic features of medullary carcinoma may be altered to be termed atypical. Structural variations that characterize atypical medullary carcinoma include focal invasive growth at the periphery of the tumor, diminished lymphoplasmacytic reaction, well-differentiated nuclear cytology, few mitoses, and conspicuous glandular or papillary growth. Tumors with more than two of

185

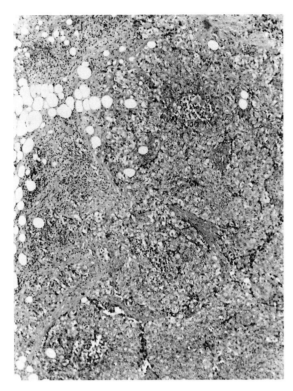

Figure 286
ATYPICAL MEDULLARY CARCINOMA
At low magnification it is apparent that this carcinoma invades the fat and that it does not have a microscopically circumscribed margin. Fat cells are evident in the substance of the tumor.

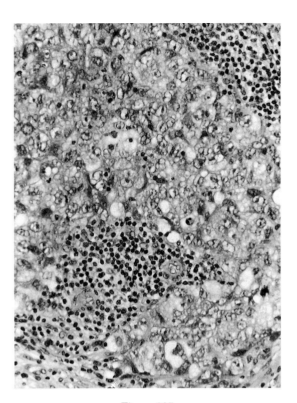

Figure 287
ATYPICAL MEDULLARY CARCINOMA
Medullary features seen at high magnification are poorly differentiated nuclei, syncytial growth pattern, and lymphoplasmacytic stromal infiltrate.

these aberrant features are best classified as infiltrating duct carcinomas (figs. 288, 289) (207,214).

Prognosis and Treatment. Overall, a high proportion of patients with medullary carcinoma remain disease free after treatment by modified or radical mastectomy. Successful treatment by lumpectomy and primary radiotherapy has also been reported (194). Moore and Foote (198) stated that only 11.5 percent of their patients with medullary carcinoma died of the tumor within 5 years despite the fact that 42 percent of the patients had axillary lymph node metastases. Several years later Richardson (206) confirmed Moore and Foote's observations. The 5-year disease-free survival of their 99 patients was 78 percent, with death due to disease in only 10 percent. Longer follow-up revealed a 95 percent 20-year disease-free survival rate for stage I patients in this series and 61 percent for stage II women (187). Later studies that refined the diagnostic criteria for

medullary carcinoma also confirmed the favorable prognosis of this type of tumor (204,207, 214). The outcome for patients with atypical medullary carcinoma was slightly better than for those with infiltrating duct carcinoma but the difference did not prove to be statistically significant. The major contribution of the term atypical medullary carcinoma has been to draw attention to the existence of a subset of infiltrating duct carcinomas that may be misdiagnosed as medullary carcinoma.

Patients with medullary carcinoma tend to have a lower overall frequency of axillary lymph node metastases than patients with atypical medullary or infiltrating duct carcinoma (204, 207,214). When nodal metastases are present, they usually involve no more than three lymph nodes (204,207). Stage II medullary carcinoma patients have a more favorable prognosis than comparable patients with nonmedullary carcinoma. Tumor size and node status are significant

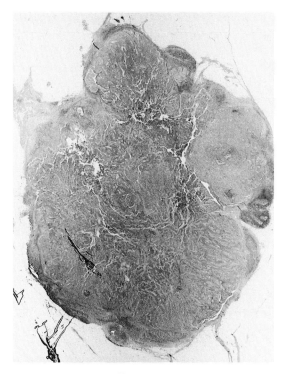

Figure 288
INFILTRATING DUCT CARCINOMA
This circumscribed, nodular carcinoma has a sparse lymphocytic infiltrate, limited to approximately one quarter of the margin between the 12 o'clock and 3 o'clock axes. India ink used to mark the margin in the lower left corner has spread into the adjacent tumor tissue causing the black crescentic artefact.

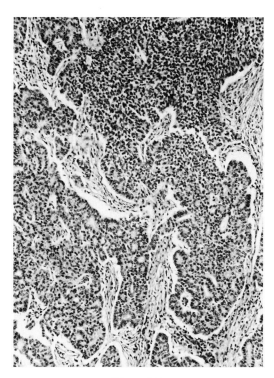

Figure 289
INFILTRATING DUCT CARCINOMA
Histologic section of the tumor reveals cells with well-differentiated small nuclei arranged in syncytial and cribriform patterns. Stromal lymphoplasmacytic infiltrate is sparse.

determinants of disease-free survival since the prognosis of patients with node-negative medullary carcinoma is particularly favorable (a disease-free survival of 90 percent or better) if the tumor is not larger than 3 cm in diameter (207,210). The survival results for stage II, T1N1M0 medullary carcinoma have also been exceptionally good at 20 years of follow-up (210). Patients whose tumors are larger than 3 cm with four or more involved lymph nodes have high recurrence rates that are not appreciably different from the recurrence rates of patients with infiltrating duct carcinoma.

More than 90 percent of medullary carcinomas are estrogen and progesterone receptor negative biochemically (203,212) and immunohistochemically (205). Medullary carcinoma has one of the highest growth rates among breast carcinomas (196) and the tumors are typically aneuploid or polyploid (193).

MUCINOUS CARCINOMA

As defined in the WHO classification of breast tumors (244), mucinous carcinoma contains "large amounts of extracellular epithelial mucous, sufficient to be visible grossly, and recognizable microscopically surrounding and within tumour cells." Other terms used to identify this tumor include *gelatinous, colloid, mucous,* and *mucoid carcinoma*.

When the diagnosis is restricted to tumors consisting of pure or nearly pure mucinous carcinoma, not more than 2 percent of mammary carcinomas fall into this category (218,233,241,242). Focal mucinous differentiation may be found in up to 2 percent of other carcinomas and if these tumors are also classified as mucinous carcinoma, the reported frequency of the tumor may be as high as 3.6 percent (227). The term *infiltrating duct carcinoma with focal mucinous carcinoma* is preferable for tumors with mixed histologic patterns. Pure mucinous carcinomas are described as tumors that are "virtually pure" (231), with at least 50 percent growing in a mucinous pattern and with extracellular mucin constituting at least 33 percent of the lesion (233). A widely accepted standard requires that at least 75 percent of the tumor have a mucinous growth pattern.

Clinical Presentation. Mucinous carcinoma occurs throughout the age range of breast carcinoma. The mean age of women with pure mucinous carcinoma is greater than those with nonmucinous carcinoma (238,241,242), constituting about 7 percent of carcinomas in women 75 years or older and only 1 percent in those younger than 35 years (237).

The initial symptom is a mass in the majority of patients. Fixation to the skin and chest wall occurs with large lesions. Only a few pure mucinous carcinomas have calcifications. The tumor usually appears as a circumscribed mass lesion on mammography.

The average duration of symptoms prior to biopsy and diagnosis tends to be 3 months or less (241), but some elderly patients who have large lesions may delay seeking treatment for considerably longer. About 60 percent of pure mucinous carcinomas are estrogen receptor positive (230,240). Similar patterns of estrogen receptor immunoreactivity have been observed in nonargyrophilic and argyrophilic mucinous carcinomas and in mixed mucinous carcinomas (240).

Gross Findings. Pure mucinous carcinomas measure from less than 1 cm to more than 20 cm in diameter, with a size distribution similar to that of breast carcinomas generally. A nationwide study of Danish breast cancer patients found that 84 percent of pure mucinous carcinomas were smaller than 5 cm (233). In a series from Finland, a greater proportion of mixed (48 percent) than of pure (22 percent) mucinous carcinomas were larger than 5 cm (242). Among Japanese women, 53.6 percent of mucinous carcinomas were 2 cm or less (T1) and 37.8 percent were 2.1 to 5.0 cm (T2).

The consistency of pure mucinous carcinoma varies somewhat depending upon the amount of fibrous stroma in the lesion. When stroma is sparse, the tumor feels soft and gelatinous. The cut surface is typically moist and glistening, even in relatively fibrotic tumors (fig. 290). Most pure mucinous carcinomas have a circumscribed gross margin often accentuated by a peripheral

red to purple zone of congested parenchyma. Cystic degeneration has been reported in relatively large tumors.

Microscopic Findings. Pure mucinous carcinoma is characterized by the accumulation of abundant extracellular mucin around invasive tumor cells (fig. 291). The relative proportions of mucin and neoplastic epithelium vary from one case to another but the distribution in any one tumor tends to be constant. Numerous sections may be required to detect sparse tumor cells in mucinous carcinomas composed almost entirely of extracellular mucin (figs. 292, 293). In one study, the proportion of extracellular mucin relative to carcinomatous epithelium varied from slightly less than 40 percent to up to 99.8 percent, with a mean of 83.5 ±14.3 percent (227). Infiltrating duct carcinomas with focal mucinous features had a lower mean proportion of extracellular mucin (68.3 ±16.6 percent), with the distribution ranging from 32 to 97 percent (figs. 294, 295).

Mucinous carcinoma should be distinguished from the benign mucocele-like tumor composed of cysts lined by cuboidal and columnar cytologically benign epithelium and extravasated mucin that does not contain neoplastic cells (figs. 296, 297) (236). The resultant picture resembles the mucocele of salivary gland origin commonly found in the oral cavity. The epithelium in the typical mucocele-like tumor is largely flat or cuboidal but columnar and focal papillary elements may be present. Detached epithelial cells are not found in the secretion within cysts or when it is discharged into the stroma.

Ro et al. (235) described a group of mucocele-like tumors with foci of more extensive epithelial proliferation, including atypical hyperplasia, intraductal carcinoma, and focal invasive mucinous carcinoma. The secretion in various mucocele-like tumors and mucinous carcinomas had similar immunohistochemical properties and the authors proposed that mucocele-like tumor and mucinous carcinoma may be two extremes of a spectrum of lesions. While available evidence suggests that some mucinous carcinomas resemble and may arise from mucocele-like tumors, the majority arise from conventional forms of intraductal carcinoma.

Mucinous carcinomas are variants of invasive duct carcinoma. Intraductal carcinoma is found associated with approximately 75 percent of the lesions, generally at the periphery. The intraductal

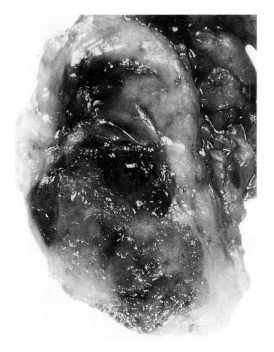

Figure 290
MUCINOUS CARCINOMA
Small circumscribed tumor with gelatinous appearance.

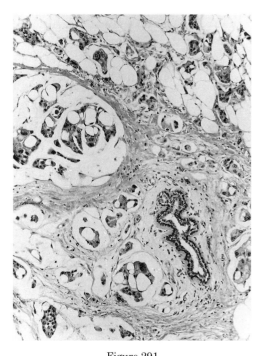

Figure 291
MUCINOUS CARCINOMA
Clusters of tumor cells in mucinous secretion surround a duct.

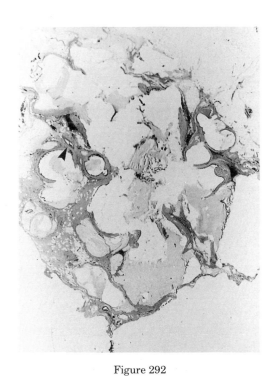

Figure 292
MUCINOUS CARCINOMA
Multilobulated lesion in which the epithelial component was very sparse. Arrow indicates intraductal carcinoma. (Figures 292 and 293 are from the same patient.)

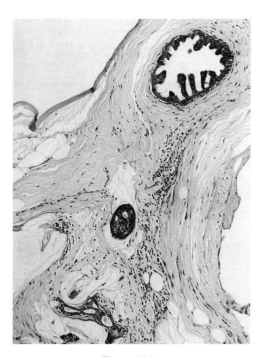

Figure 293
MUCINOUS CARCINOMA
Micropapillary intraductal carcinoma and cluster of invasive tumor cells surrounded by mucin.

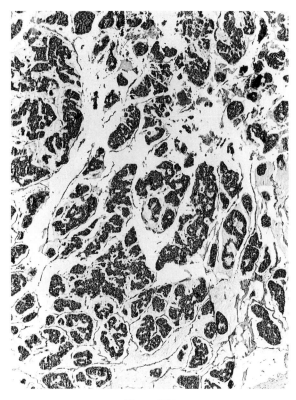

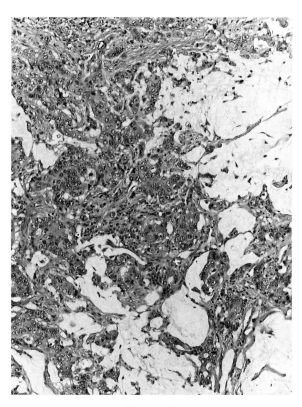

Figure 294
MUCINOUS CARCINOMA
Carcinoma cells arranged in alveolar and festoon patterns surrounded by mucinous secretion. Lesions with less mucin relative to epithelium should be classified as mixed mucinous carcinomas.

Figure 295
MIXED MUCINOUS CARCINOMA
Solid, poorly differentiated carcinoma accompanied by extracellular mucin. (Fig. 12-12C from Rosen PP. The pathology of invasive breast carcinoma. In: Harris JR, Hellman S, Henderson IC, Kinne DW, eds. Breast diseases. 2nd ed. Philadelphia: JB Lippincott, 1991.)

Figure 296
MUCOCELE-LIKE TUMOR
Multilobulated tumor composed of mucin-containing cysts. (Fig. 2A from Rosen PP. Mucocele-like tumors of the breast. Am J Surg Pathol 1986;10:464–9.)

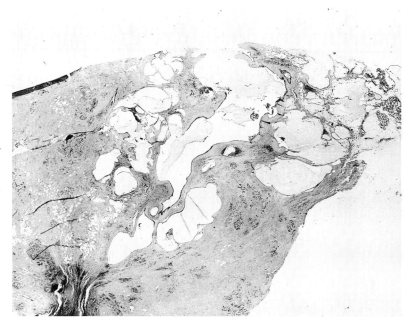

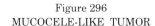

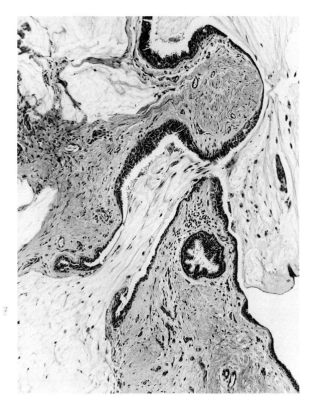

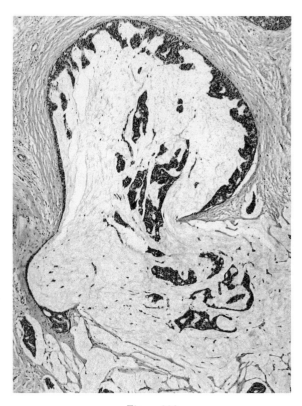

Figure 297
MUCOCELE-LIKE TUMOR
Site of rupture in cyst showing mucinous material extruded into the stroma. Mild epithelial hyperplasia is apparent. Tumor cells were not seen in the secretion or invading the stroma. (Fig. 1B from Rosen PP. Mucocele-like tumors of the breast. Am J Surg Pathol 1986;10:464–9.)

Figure 298
MUCINOUS CARCINOMA
Micropapillary intraductal carcinoma giving rise to invasive mucinous carcinoma.

component can have any pattern of intraductal carcinoma (cribriform, papillary, micropapillary, comedo) (fig. 298). Occasionally, mucinous differentiation is evident in the intraductal component. One of the most uncommon variants of this pattern is a form of cystic papillary carcinoma (226), in which multiple cysts are distended with mucin and lined by papillary carcinoma. "Mucin leakage" into the stroma surrounding cysts resembles the mucin extravasation seen in mucocele-like tumors. In the absence of intraductal carcinoma it is not possible to determine microscopically whether the lesion is a metastatic tumor or if it is primary in the breast.

Tumor cells are arranged in a variety of patterns in the mucinous secretion. Usually the epithelial arrangement duplicates the pattern of associated intraductal carcinoma. These configurations include tumor cells in strands, alveolar nests, and

papillary clusters as well as larger sheets that may have cribriform areas or focal comedonecrosis. Tubule and gland formation are uncommon. Calcifications are most often found in mucinous carcinomas that have papillary or comedo patterns.

The ploidy of mucinous carcinomas has been studied by flow cytometry (243). Pure mucinous carcinomas are virtually all diploid (25 of 26 or 96 percent). Only 42 percent (8 of 19) of mixed mucinous carcinomas were diploid, with the majority described as aneuploid.

The fine-needle aspirate from mucinous carcinoma reveals isolated cells and small clusters in a background of mucin. Occasionally, myxoid material from an edematous fibroadenoma results in an aspirate that resembles mucinous carcinoma. A fine-needle aspiration sample, however, is not reliable for distinguishing between mucocele-like tumor, pure mucinous carcinoma, and infiltrating duct carcinoma with a mucinous component (219).

191

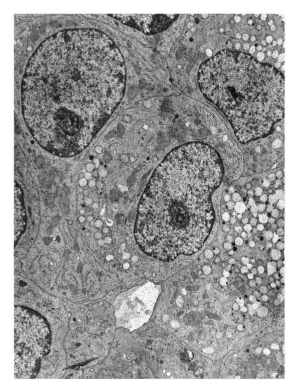

Figure 299
MUCINOUS CARCINOMA
Mucigen granules are present in the cytoplasm (X5400).

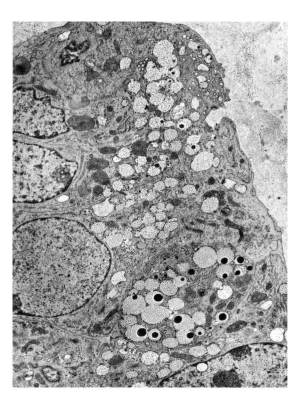

Figure 300
MUCINOUS CARCINOMA
Mucigen granules are present between tumor cell nuclei (left) and extracellular mucin (right). Some mucigen granules contain dense spherules (X5400).

Histochemistry and Electron Microscopy. The amount of intracellular mucin in mucinous carcinomas is variable. Often, only a small proportion of the tumor cells can be shown to contain mucin by histochemical procedures but intracellular mucin can be demonstrated readily by electron microscopy (figs. 299, 300) (217,220,223). Disruption of cells containing mucin results in discharge and extracellular accumulation of the secretion (217, 224). Some lesions have prominent signet ring cells. Argyrophilic granules have been detected in 25 to 50 percent of mucinous carcinomas (220, 233,234,242); these occur more frequently in elderly women and the tumor cells often grow in clumps, sheets, or trabeculae sometimes suggesting an endocrine growth pattern (figs. 301, 302). The granules can contain immunohistochemically detectable serotonin, somatostatin, and gastrin (225). In two studies, the presence of argyrophilic granules was not prognostically significant in pure mucinous tumors or in infiltrating duct carcinomas with focal mucinous differentiation (222,233).

Prognosis and Treatment. The relatively favorable prognosis commonly ascribed to mucinous carcinoma is supported by many studies (231, 241–243,245), although few investigators have been able to assemble substantial numbers of patients. Differences in the definition of the tumor and in reporting make it difficult to combine data from published series.

When compared with patients who have mucinous carcinoma containing infiltrating duct carcinoma components and those who have infiltrating duct carcinoma, women with pure mucinous carcinoma have a better relapse-free survival 5 and 10 years after mastectomy (231,232,238,241,245). Pure mucinous carcinomas tend to be smaller than tumors with a mixed pattern and these patients have a lower frequency of axillary lymph node metastases (227,231–233,241,242). In the past two decades, the reported frequency of negative axillary lymph nodes in patients with pure mucinous carcinoma ranged from 71 to 97 percent as compared to

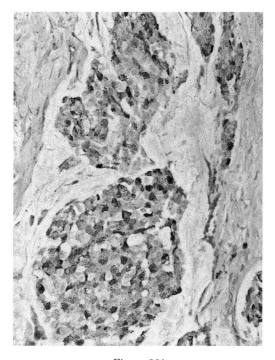

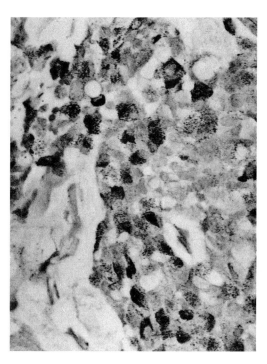

Figure 301
MUCINOUS CARCINOMA
WITH ENDOCRINE DIFFERENTIATION
Groups of carcinoma cells surrounded by extracellular mucin contain argyrophilic granules (Grimelius stain). (Figures 301 and 302 are from the same patient.)

Figure 302
MUCINOUS CARCINOMA
WITH ENDOCRINE DIFFERENTIATION
Magnified view of the tumor in figure 301 showing clumps of fine black argyrophilic granules. The tumor cells were immunoreactive for chromogranin (Grimelius stain).

50 percent for mixed mucinous carcinomas. Major prognostic factors that are relevant for most types of breast carcinoma also apply to pure mucinous carcinoma (231,242). Recurrence is least likely with relatively small tumors and when there are no lymph node metastases. The presence or absence of argyrophilic granules was not of prognostic importance in one series (242).

Five-year survival figures after the treatment of pure mucinous carcinoma by mastectomy have been 84 percent disease free (233), 87 percent disease free (231), and 100 percent disease free (241). Komaki et al. (227) described a 90 percent 10-year survival and 60 percent for those with mixed duct and mucinous carcinoma. In another report, the 15-year disease-free survival was 85 percent and 63 percent for pure mucinous and mixed mucinous-duct carcinoma patients, respectively (242).

Late systemic recurrences have been described after mastectomy (221,238,239,245). In one series, with a mean follow-up of 16 years, 27 percent of 41 patients with pure mucinous carcinoma died of breast carcinoma, with 42 percent of the deaths occurring 12 years or more after diagnosis (238). Clayton (221) found that the median survival of patients who died of mucinous carcinoma was 11.3 years after mastectomy. Intervals to recurrence of 25 (229) and 30 years (239) have been reported.

Most patients with pure and mixed mucinous-duct carcinoma have been treated by radical or modified radical mastectomy. Some elderly women were treated by local excision or simple mastectomy. Many patients who choose breast conservation treatment also have radiation therapy. Combined data from two institutions included 10 patients with mucinous carcinoma who remained disease free after excision and radiotherapy, with a median follow-up of 79 months (228). Until more patients have been evaluated with longer follow-up, the role of radiation therapy and breast conservation for the treatment of mucinous carcinoma remains uncertain.

CARCINOMA WITH METAPLASIA

Less than 5 percent of mammary adenocarcinomas undergo metaplastic change into a nonglandular growth pattern. The extent of metaplasia varies from a few microscopic foci in an otherwise typical mammary carcinoma to complete replacement of glandular growth by the metaplastic tumor pattern. Squamous metaplasia was present in 3.7 percent of 1,665 invasive carcinomas reviewed by Fisher et al. (248). Heterologous metaplasia was detected in 26 of 12,045 (0.2 percent) breast cancers in another study (253). Some lesions have been described as "mixed tumors," an unfortunate and confusing reference to tumors of the salivary glands that are predominantly benign. Others are referred to as carcinosarcomas. This latter term is best reserved for malignant neoplasms in which the carcinomatous and sarcomatous elements can be traced separately to epithelial and mesenchymal origins, such as carcinoma arising in a malignant cystosarcoma.

Clinical Presentation. The range of age at diagnosis and the clinical features of metaplastic mammary carcinoma are not appreciably different from those of invasive mammary carcinoma (251,253,255,260). The first symptom is typically a palpable tumor. There is no predilection for bilaterality. The patient usually describes rapid growth and short duration prior to diagnosis (256). The tumors tend to have circumscribed contours radiologically. With few exceptions, metaplastic mammary carcinomas have been estrogen receptor negative (261,262).

Gross Findings. The reported size of metaplastic mammary carcinomas ranges from 1 to 21 cm (251,253,260). The mean or median size (3 to 4 cm) tends to be greater than that of ordinary carcinomas. The tumors are described as solid, firm to hard, nodular, and circumscribed (fig. 303), but cystic areas can be found in squamous metaplasia (fig. 304) (256,261).

Microscopic Findings. Breast carcinomas with metaplasia are largely poorly differentiated

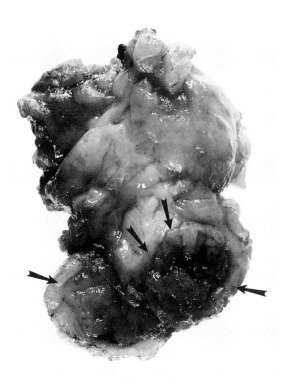

Figure 303
METAPLASTIC CARTILAGINOUS CARCINOMA
Circumscribed contour is evident in the lower half of the specimen in this view of a bisected tumor. Margin of tumor indicated by arrows.

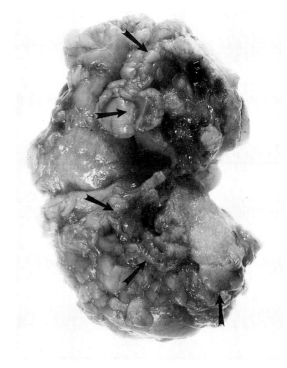

Figure 304
METAPLASTIC SQUAMOUS CARCINOMA
Two halves of a bisected tumor are shown. Cystic degeneration is evident on the right. Margin of tumor indicated by arrows.

duct carcinomas (253). Metaplasia has been reported in medullary carcinoma (258), tubular or well-differentiated duct carcinoma (251,253), infiltrating lobular carcinoma (251), and mucinous carcinoma (251). It has been customary to subdivide metaplastic carcinomas into squamous and heterologous or pseudosarcomatous types. This distinction is somewhat arbitrary since some tumors exhibit both types of growth.

The most common metaplastic pattern is focal squamous metaplasia in an otherwise typical invasive duct carcinoma (fig. 305). The metaplastic component usually constitutes less than 10 percent of the tumor. A spectrum of squamous differentiation may be found ranging from mature keratinizing epithelium to poorly differentiated carcinoma with spindle cell, pseudosarcomatous areas (fig. 306). Spindle cell is a variant of carcinoma with squamous metaplasia in which most or virtually all of the neoplasm has assumed a pseudosarcomatous growth pattern (246,249,

256). Extensive sampling is necessary to locate squamous differentiation and foci of intraductal or invasive adenocarcinoma (figs. 307, 308).

Heterologous metaplasia is most commonly encountered as bone or cartilage that may appear histologically benign or malignant (250–252,254). It is usually found in association with poorly differentiated heterologous areas composed of round or spindle cells. Myxoid change, a common feature of these undifferentiated elements, may also be found in transitional zones between adenocarcinoma and chondroid metaplasia (figs. 309, 310). Rhabdomyoid, adipose, and angiosarcomatous metaplasia have also been seen. Carcinomas with heterologous metaplasia tend to retain distinct adenocarcinoma components (figs. 311–316).

Matrix-producing carcinoma, a variant of heterologous metaplastic carcinoma, is an "overt carcinoma with direct transition to a cartilaginous and/or osseous stromal matrix without an

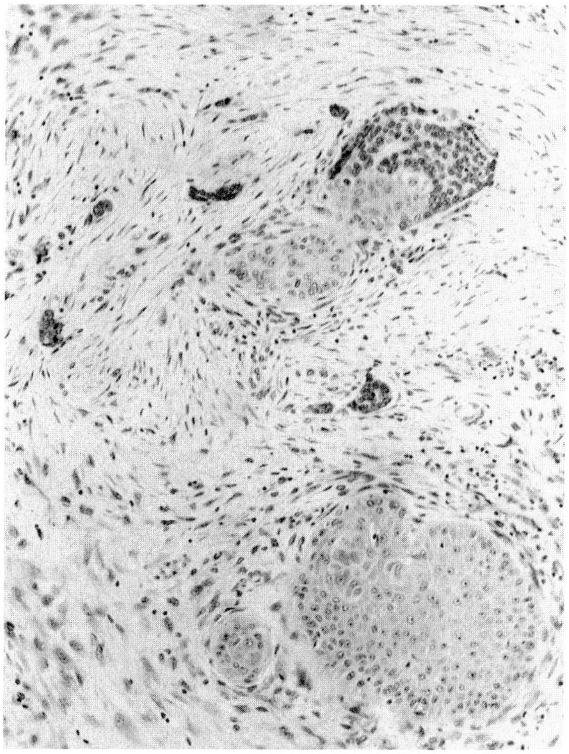

Figure 305
METAPLASTIC CARCINOMA
Well-differentiated epidermoid carcinoma and poorly differentiated adenocarcinoma merge with the spindle cell component. (Figures 305–309 are from the same patient.)

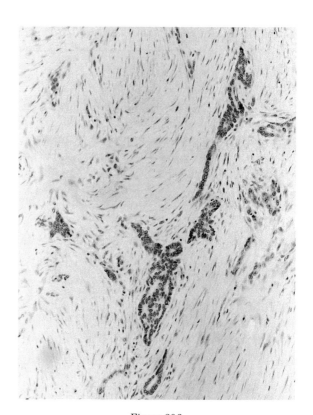

Figure 306
METAPLASTIC CARCINOMA
Adenocarcinoma with a tubular pattern in the metaplastic spindle cell component.

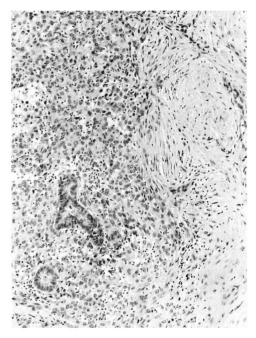

Figure 307
METAPLASTIC CARCINOMA
Carcinomatous glands surrounded by undifferentiated round cell neoplastic proliferation that merges with the less cellular spindle cell element.

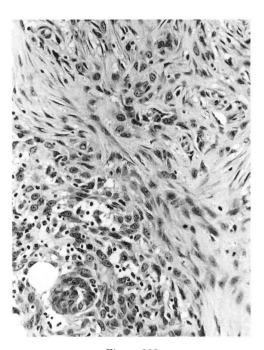

Figure 308
METAPLASTIC CARCINOMA
Magnified view of an area similar to figure 329 showing transition from adenocarcinoma to spindle cell pattern.

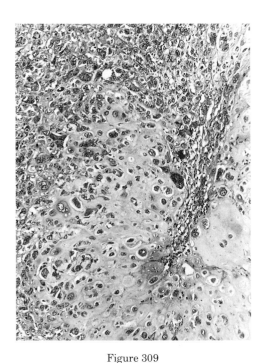

Figure 309
METAPLASTIC CARCINOMA
Chondroid metaplasia in an anaplastic portion of a carcinoma.

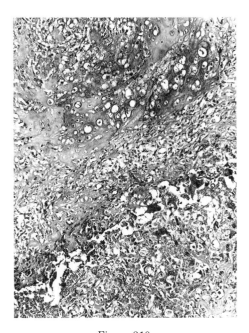

Figure 310
METAPLASTIC CARCINOMA
Chondroid (above) and osseous (below) metaplasia. (Figure 12-15 from Rosen PP. The pathology of invasive breast carcinoma. In: Harris JR, Hellman S, Henderson IC, Kinne DW, eds. Breast diseases. 2nd ed. Philadelphia: JB Lippincott, 1991.) (Figures 310 and 311 are from the same patient.)

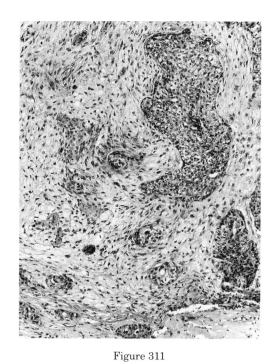

Figure 311
METAPLASTIC CARCINOMA
Poorly differentiated carcinoma with traces of squamous metaplasia giving rise to spindle cell component.

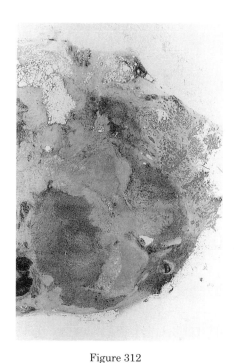

Figure 312
METAPLASTIC CARCINOMA
Overview of the tumor showing invasive adenocarcinoma at the upper right margin. Most of the neoplasm consisted of solid pseudosarcomatous metaplastic elements with serpiginous areas of necrosis that appear pale. (Figures 312–316 are from the same patient.)

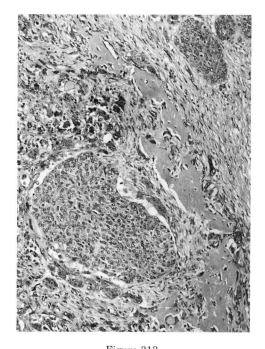

Figure 313
METAPLASTIC CARCINOMA
A zone of osteoid separates two areas of poorly differentiated carcinoma.

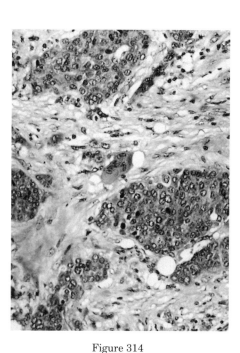

Figure 314
METAPLASTIC CARCINOMA
Osteoclast-like giant cell in the stroma associated with the carcinoma component.

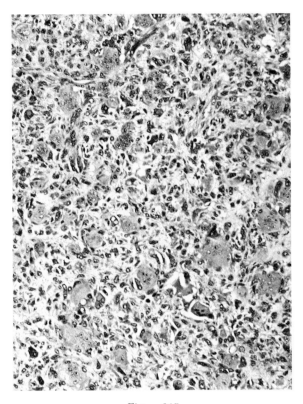

Figure 315
METAPLASTIC CARCINOMA
Portion of the tumor that resembles giant cell tumor of bone because it contains many osteoclast-like giant cells.

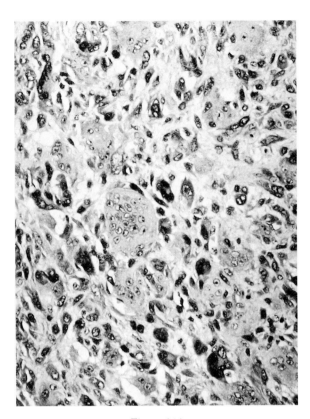

Figure 316
METAPLASTIC CARCINOMA
Magnified view of lesion shown in figure 315.

intervening spindle cell zone or osteoclastic cells" (figs. 317–320) (261). Many of these tumors have areas of mucinous carcinoma. Although mucin positivity is demonstrated in carcinomatous areas, the cartilage forming cells do not contain mucin. The cartilaginous matrix has histochemical properties of a sulfated acid mucopolysaccharide consistent with chondroitin sulfate. The carcinoma cells stain positively for keratin, epithelial membrane antigen (EMA), and S-100 with virtually no reactivity for vimentin. Metaplastic cells in the osseous and cartilaginous matrix stain diffusely for S-100 and vimentin, with variable reactivity for keratin and EMA.

Metastases derived from a metaplastic carcinoma may consist entirely of adenocarcinoma, entirely of metaplastic elements, or a mixture of these components (figs. 321–323). A minority of axillary metastases contain heterologous elements but they are expressed with greater fre-

quency in local recurrences on the chest wall and in visceral metastases (253,256). When metaplastic foci occur in metastatic deposits they tend to duplicate at least some of the components found in the primary tumor. It is also possible for squamous metaplastic changes to develop within axillary node metastases, although corresponding metaplasia cannot be detected in the primary tumor even after generous sampling.

Low-grade adenosquamous carcinoma is an unusual variant of metaplastic duct carcinoma (259) and is typically smaller than other varieties (1.5 to 3.4 cm, average 2.3 cm). The tumors are hard, yellow or tan, with grossly ill-defined infiltrative borders (fig. 324). Microscopically, they consist of small glandular structures with variable amounts of epidermoid differentiation in a collagenous stroma (fig. 325). There is a tendency to grow between or around ducts and lobules, particularly at the periphery of the lesion. Squamous metaplasia varies from syringoma-like differentiation to

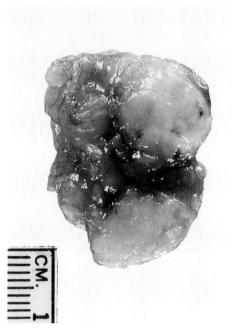

Figure 317
MATRIX PRODUCING METAPLASTIC CARCINOMA
Grossly the bisected tumor is circumscribed and has bulging mucoid surfaces.

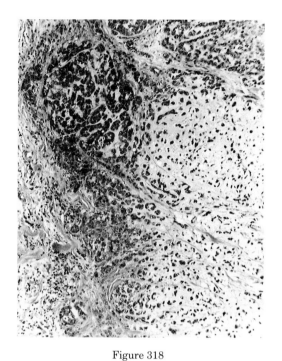

Figure 318
MATRIX PRODUCING METAPLASTIC CARCINOMA
Junction between poorly differentiated carcinoma arranged in lobulated fashion around the periphery of areas exhibiting chondromyxoid metaplasia. (Figures 318 and 319 are from the same patient.)

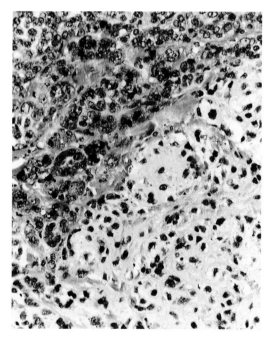

Figure 319
MATRIX PRODUCING METAPLASTIC CARCINOMA
Magnified view of lesion in figure 318.

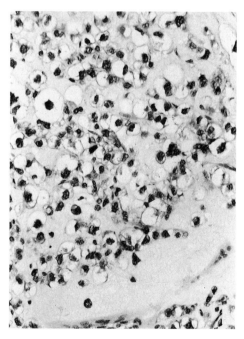

Figure 320
MATRIX PRODUCING METAPLASTIC CARCINOMA
Chondroid appearance of matrix metaplasia.

199

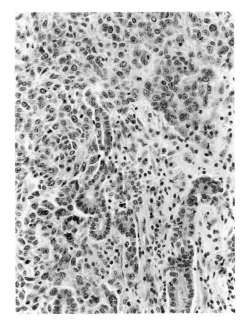

Figure 321
METAPLASTIC CARCINOMA
Adenocarcinoma with transition to undifferentiated component, an intermediate step in conversion to spindle cell metaplasia. (Figures 321–324 are from the same patient.)

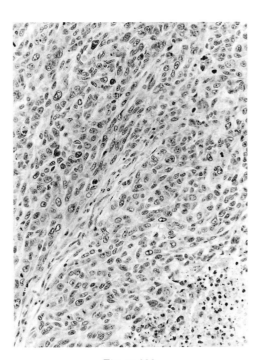

Figure 322
METAPLASTIC CARCINOMA
Spindle cell metaplasia in the tumor shown in figure 321. Both pictures are from the primary tumor.

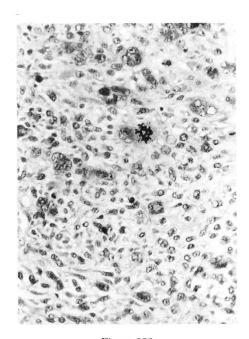

Figure 323
RECURRENT METAPLASTIC CARCINOMA
Chest wall recurrence 4 years after mastectomy for the tumor shown in figures 321 and 322. This tumor with anaplastic giant cells retains some of the spindle cell elements seen in the primary tumor. The patient had postoperative chest wall radiation and this lesion was initially interpreted as an irradiation-induced sarcoma.

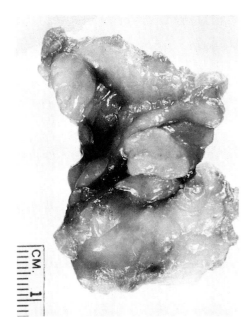

Figure 324
LOW-GRADE ADENOSQUAMOUS CARCINOMA
The tumor forms a circumscribed mass surrounded by fatty breast tissue.

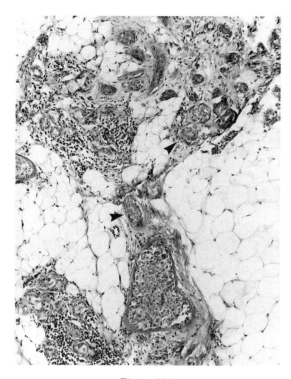

Figure 325
LOW-GRADE ADENOSQUAMOUS CARCINOMA
Intraductal carcinoma in a large duct below and in smaller branches (arrows) giving rise to adenosquamous carcinoma. (Figures 325–327 are from the same patient.)

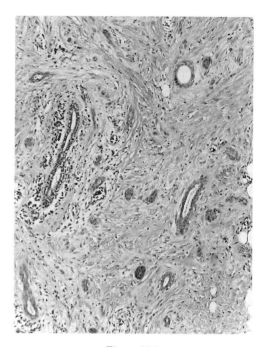

Figure 326
LOW-GRADE ADENOSQUAMOUS CARCINOMA
Invasive ductular elements with syringomatous features in dense collagenous stroma around a duct.

inconspicuous foci in largely glandular lesions (figs. 326–330). Keratinizing cysts are uncommon. Small osteocartilaginous foci have been encountered in two cases (259).

Immunohistochemistry. Immunohistochemical studies to elucidate the relationship between epithelial and heterologous elements in metaplastic carcinomas have been inconclusive (fig. 331). The usefulness of immunohistochemical markers is complicated by the reported coexpression of cytokeratin and vimentin in nonmetaplastic breast carcinomas (257). Some authors have observed coexpression of epithelial (cytokeratin, EMA) and mesenchymal (vimentin) associated markers in the spindle cell elements of metaplastic carcinomas (247,260). Others who failed to find coexpression reported vimentin reactivity in epithelial and spindle cells with cytokeratin expression only in the epithelial elements (255,256). Focal or rare EMA immunoreactivity was observed in the spindle cells of 21 percent of 48 lesions studied (260). Metaplastic carcinomas only rarely

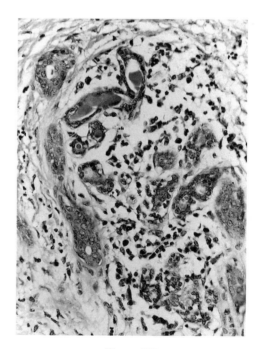

Figure 327
LOW-GRADE ADENOSQUAMOUS CARCINOMA
Magnified view of neoplastic ductules in and around a lobule.

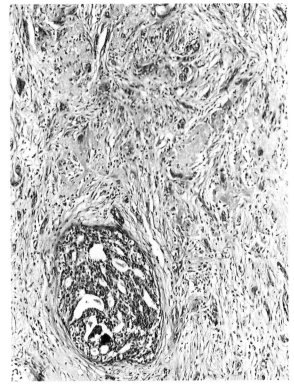

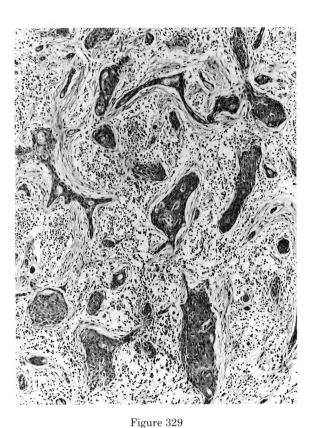

Figure 328
LOW-GRADE ADENOSQUAMOUS CARCINOMA
Intraductal carcinoma below surrounded by metaplastic fibrocollagenous neoplasm that contains small tubular elements. (Figures 328–330 are from the same patient.)

Figure 329
LOW-GRADE ADENOSQUAMOUS CARCINOMA
Irregular islands of carcinoma that exhibit epidermoid differentiation giving rise to slender syringomatous tubular elements. The lymphocytic stromal infiltrate is unusual in such tumors. (Fig.2A from Rosen PP, Ernsberger D. Low-grade adenosquamous carcinoma. A variant of metaplastic mammary carcinoma. Am J Surg Pathol 1987;11:351–8.)

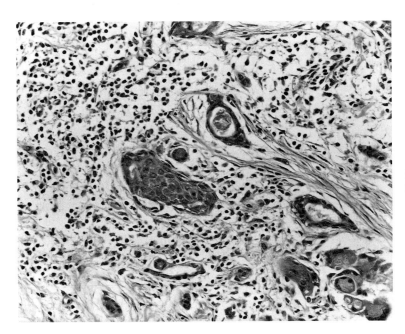

Figure 330
LOW-GRADE
ADENOSQUAMOUS CARCINOMA
Magnified view of an area similar to figure 329 showing secretion in neoplastic ductules.

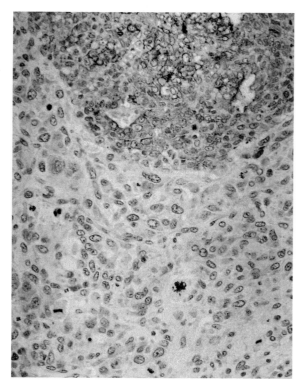

Figure 331
METAPLASTIC CARCINOMA
Poorly differentiated carcinoma above is immunoreactive for cytokeratin but the spindle cell pseudosarcomatous element below is unreactive (avidin-biotin, hematoxylin).

exhibit nuclear immunoreactivity for estrogen and progesterone receptors.

Electron Microscopy. Electron microscopy has usually supported the epithelial origin of heterologous elements by revealing that many ultrastructural characteristics are shared by the various cell types in the tumor. Most studies report cells with ultrastructural features intermediate between the epithelial and metaplastic elements (248,250,252–254). Myoepithelial cells are detectable to a variable extent, occasionally constituting a significant part of the lesion (260,262), and they may be the cellular component that undergoes metaplastic change.

Prognosis and Treatment. Five relatively large studies consisting of 22 to 40 cases provided sufficient data to assess prognosis (251,253,256, 261,262). Stage was stratified in only one study, which revealed declining survival with advancing stage (253). Size correlated with outcome in another study since patients with tumors smaller than 4 cm had a relatively favorable prognosis (256).

Prognostic data thus far have been based on patients treated by mastectomy, usually with axillary dissection. Mammary recurrence has been described in two of three patients after initial treatment by local excision for heterologous metaplastic carcinoma (253). The effect of primary irradiation and adjuvant chemotherapy on metaplastic carcinoma has not been determined. The relationship between the type of metaplasia and prognosis is uncertain because it has been difficult to assemble enough of these uncommon lesions to stratify them by stage.

The frequency of positive axillary nodes associated with heterologous metaplastic carcinoma, including so-called matrix-producing tumors, ranges from 6 (262) to 25 percent (253). Disease-free survival, generally reported for 5 or more years of follow-up, ranges from 38 (251,253) to 65 percent (262). Axillary lymph node metastases were reported in 11 (261) to 54 percent (251) of patients with squamous/spindle cell metaplastic carcinoma. Two studies reported 5-year survivals of 64 percent (261) and 65 percent (251) and in a third series 42 percent remained disease free (256). Very few patients with low-grade adenosquamous carcinoma have developed metastases in the axillary lymph nodes or systemic metastases. However, about 50 percent of women treated only by excisional biopsy have had recurrences in the same breast requiring mastectomy 1 to 3.5 years later.

It appears that heterologous metaplasia probably has a negative impact on prognosis, perhaps due to the poorly differentiated nature of these carcinomas. Squamous metaplasia does not seem to influence prognosis but extensive spindle cell metaplasia associated with squamous foci probably also has an adverse influence on outcome.

SQUAMOUS CELL CARCINOMA

Squamous cell carcinoma of the breast is a form of metaplastic carcinoma. The term is reserved for tumors composed entirely of keratinizing squamous carcinoma cells, with or without spindle cell components.

Clinical Presentation. There are no clinical features specific for squamous cell carcinoma of the breast. The reported age of diagnosis, 31 to 83 years, is within the range of breast carcinoma generally (265,273,274). In one review, the average age of 20 patients was 57 years; half of them

203

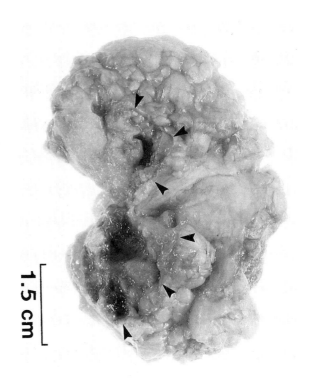

Figure 332
SQUAMOUS CARCINOMA
Gross appearance of a bisected 2 cm partially cystic tumor. Arrows indicate borders beyond which specimen consists of lobulated fibrofatty breast tissue.

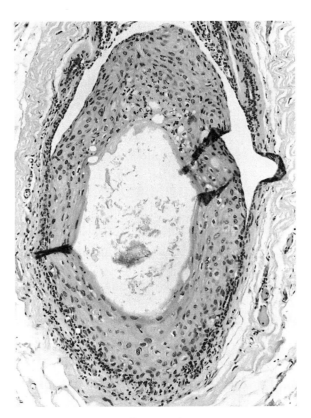

Figure 333
SQUAMOUS METAPLASIA
Squamous metaplasia arising in duct epithelium. Maturation with keratinization and cyst formation are evident centrally.

were 60 years or older (273). Large tumors may extend into and ulcerate the skin or be fixed to the chest wall. Extension to the skin may make it difficult to distinguish microscopically between origin in the skin and secondary involvement by a primary mammary lesion. Calcifications in necrotic squamous tissue can be seen radiographically but no specific mammographic findings have been reported (270,275). Most of these tumors have been estrogen receptor negative (273,274) although one tumor was estrogen and progesterone receptor positive (264).

Gross Findings. Reported size varies from 1 to 10 cm, with nearly half of the cases 5 cm or more in diameter. Tumors larger than 2 cm tend to develop cystic degeneration centrally (fig. 332).

Microscopic Findings. Before rendering a diagnosis of primary squamous cell carcinoma of the breast it is important to consider that the lesion may be metastatic from an extramammary primary (267,273). Common sources of metastatic

squamous carcinoma in the breast are the lung, esophagus, uterine cervix, and urinary bladder. It is possible to recognize squamous cell carcinoma in an aspiration cytology specimen (264). However, the distinction between a primary tumor and metastatic squamous cell carcinoma cannot be made by this method and may even be difficult in histologic sections.

Benign squamous metaplasia probably precedes squamous cell carcinoma in most cases (figs. 333, 334). Squamous metaplasia develops in hyperplastic mammary ducts (271), in papillomas (268,272), in the lining of cysts (270), and in inflammatory lesions such as infarcts of the parenchyma.

Squamous cell carcinomas of the breast resemble similar carcinomas that arise in other sites. The lesions tend to produce abundant keratin, which may contain keratohyalin granules. Ultrastructural and immunohistochemical studies have confirmed the squamous character of the tissue (276).

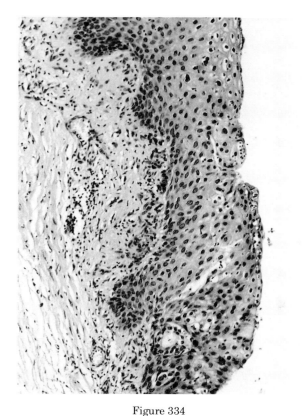

Figure 334
SQUAMOUS METAPLASIA
Portion of the lining of a cyst composed of metaplastic squamous epithelium. (Courtesy of Dr. S. Shousha, London, U.K.)

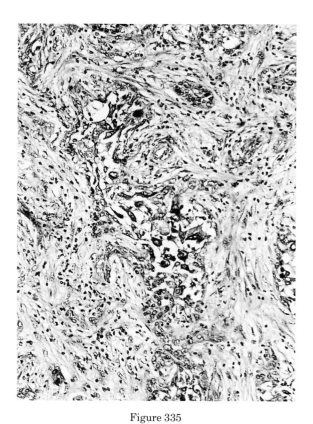

Figure 335
SQUAMOUS CARCINOMA
Invasive squamous carcinoma showing transition to spindle cell metaplastic components and early acantholytic change in the epithelial areas.

Conversion of the squamous pattern to spindle cell pseudosarcomatous growth is present in many mammary squamous cell carcinomas but is usually quite focal and inconspicuous (fig. 335). Occasionally a tumor is composed mostly or entirely of the spindle cell component (263,269). Extensive sampling to detect in situ or invasive epithelial elements and immunohistochemical studies may be necessary for diagnosis. A needle or incisional biopsy is likely to be interpreted as sarcoma.

Acantholytic change has been described (figs. 336–338). These tumors also often have prominent spindle cell areas. Degenerative spongiotic and acantholytic changes in the squamous component result in a pattern similar to a vascular neoplasm. The epithelial nature of the tumor can be demonstrated with immunohistochemical re-agents for keratin and EMA in the absence of demonstrable factor VIII and actin (266).

Prognosis and Treatment. Most patients are treated by mastectomy and axillary dissection sometimes followed by radiation or chemotherapy. The prognosis after this treatment does not differ appreciably from that of patients with breast carcinoma generally. Despite the relatively large size of these tumors most patients do not have axillary lymph node metastases. Among reported cases, 8 of 16 women with negative axillary lymph nodes were alive and free of disease 1 to 12 years later, 2 died of other causes, and 6 died of metastatic carcinoma 4 to 30 months after diagnosis. Two patients with axillary lymph node metastases died 6 and 17 months after treatment; 2 others were alive without recurrence 16 months and 6 years after diagnosis.

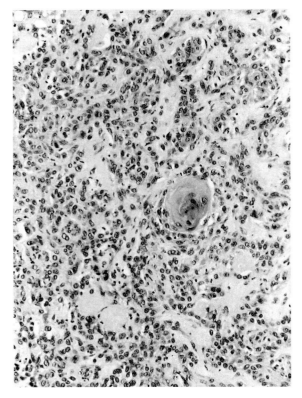

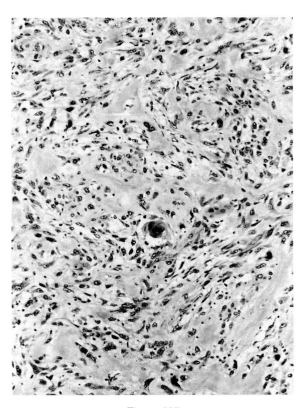

Figure 336
SQUAMOUS CARCINOMA
Keratin pearl surrounded by invasive poorly differentiated squamous carcinoma in which there is loss of cohesion
that occurs in acantholytic carcinoma. (Figures 336–338 are
from the same patient.)

Figure 337
SQUAMOUS CARCINOMA
Loss of virtually all epithelial features is evident, leaving
only spindle cell metaplastic elements surrounding the remnants of a keratin pearl.

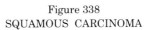

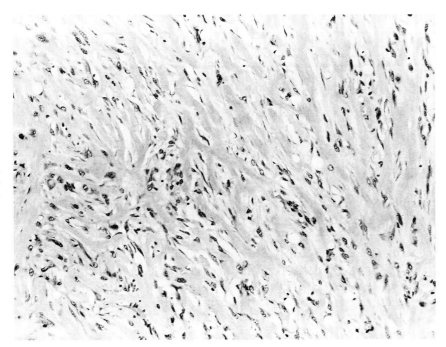

Figure 338
SQUAMOUS CARCINOMA
Collagenization is often prominent in the most pronounced spindle cell areas. Spaces among neoplastic cells create an appearance
that may be mistaken for a vascular neoplasm.

CARCINOMA WITH OSTEOCLAST-LIKE GIANT CELLS

Since the first series in 1979 (277), fewer than 100 mammary carcinomas with osteoclast-like giant cells have been reported (288,290,294). They constitute 0.5 to 1.2 percent of breast carcinomas (287,288).

Clinical Presentation. The initial manifestation is usually a mass. Patients range in age from 28 to 88 years; average age at diagnosis is about 53 years (277,287,291). The lesion has been found in all quadrants but most often in the upper outer quadrant. Mammographically, the well-circumscribed margin of most tumors suggests a benign lesion such as a cyst or fibroadenoma (287).

Gross Findings. The tumors tend to be well-defined, fleshy, and firm. The gross appearance is striking. When bisected the tumor is dark brown or red-brown (fig. 339). The color may suggest heavily pigmented metastatic malignant melanoma, but it tends to be brown rather than black. Reported diameters range from 0.5 to 10 cm, with the majority measuring 3 cm or less.

Microscopic Findings. Most of these lesions are moderately or poorly differentiated invasive duct carcinomas. Uncommon examples of tubular (288,294), infiltrating lobular (277), squamous (285), papillary (277), mucinous (291), and metaplastic (294) carcinomas with osteoclast-like giant cells have been reported. The giant cells are located around the edges of carcinomatous glands and in the glandular lumens. Extravasated red blood cells and hemosiderin are present in the highly vascular stroma (figs. 340–342). Fibroblastic reaction, collagenization, and lymphocytic infiltration are variably present. Metaplastic spindle, squamous, or osseous foci in these tumors may be evidence that they are variant forms of metaplastic carcinoma (277,289,294).

Fine-needle aspiration specimens contain inflammatory cells, erythrocytes, and tumor cells intermixed with multinucleated giant cells. The giant cells do not exhibit phagocytosis of red blood cells or cellular debris (280,281,286).

Mammary carcinoma with osteoclast-like giant cells should be distinguished from other mammary neoplasms that contain giant cells, including carcinomas with anaplastic neoplastic giant cells (284). Osteoclast-like giant cells are found in meta-

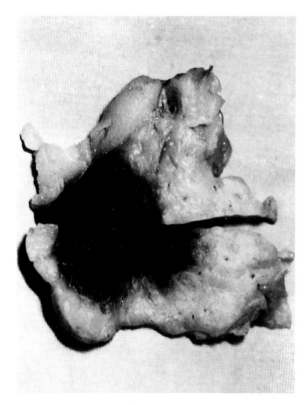

Figure 339
CARCINOMA WITH
OSTEOCLAST-LIKE GIANT CELLS
Gross photograph of a transected tumor that had the dark red color of clotted blood when fresh and appeared dark brown after formalin fixation.

plastic carcinomas with osseous and cartilaginous differentiation. While this may be a variant of metaplastic carcinoma (295), it is appropriate to regard mammary carcinoma with osteoclast-like giant cells as a distinct entity until the clinicopathologic characteristics of the lesion have been fully defined. Megakaryocytes in foci of myeloid metaplasia in the breast (282) might be mistaken for osteoclast-like giant cells but these lesions have abundant myeloid elements in various stages of maturation, a feature not found in carcinomas with osteoclast-like giant cells. Granulomatous foci present in inflammatory conditions such as sarcoidosis or coexistent with carcinoma also contain giant cells (279,292).

Electron Microscopy and Immunohistochemistry. Electron microscopic and immunohistochemical studies have demonstrated that the giant cells are of mesenchymal origin (284, 287,290,291,293,294). Strong acid phosphatase

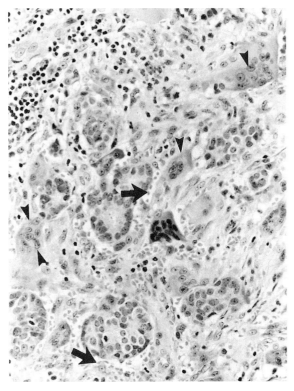

Figure 340
CARCINOMA WITH
OSTEOCLAST-LIKE GIANT CELLS
Islands of carcinoma cells lie in stroma that contains multinucleated giant cells (arrow heads), erythrocytes (arrows), and lymphocytes.

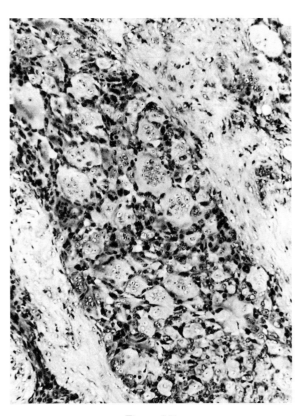

Figure 341
CARCINOMA WITH
OSTEOCLAST-LIKE GIANT CELLS
In this neoplasm, carcinoma cells mingle with multinucleated giant cells in the invasive component of the tumor (Figures 341 and 342 are from the same patient.)

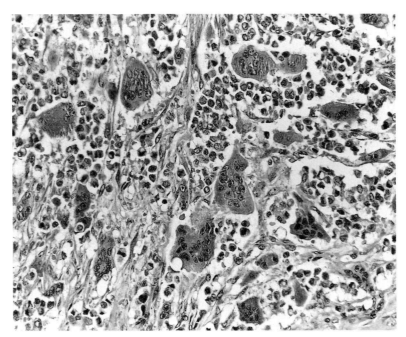

Figure 342
CARCINOMA WITH
OSTEOCLAST-LIKE GIANT CELLS
Infiltrating lobular carcinoma with giant cells. (Fig. 12-17 from Rosen PP. The pathology of invasive breast carcinoma. In: Harris JR, Hellman S, Henderson IC, Kinne WD, eds. Breast diseases. 2nd ed. Philadelphia: JB Lippincott, 1991.)

reactivity (283,288,294), the positive esterase reaction (281), absence of alkaline phosphatase staining, and other histochemical features (291) are indicative of a morphologic similarity to histiocytic cells and osteoclasts of bone (283). Athanasou et al. (278) carried out in vitro functional studies of osteoclast-like giant cells isolated from mammary carcinomas and concluded that the giant cells are macrophages with osteoclastic functional capabilities.

Prognosis and Treatment. Axillary lymph node metastases are reported in approximately one third of cases. Osteoclast-like giant cells are found in some, but not all, metastases in axillary lymph nodes or other sites (277,287). Osteoclast-like multinucleated giant cells have been observed within intralymphatic tumor emboli (fig. 343). Nearly two thirds of reported patients are alive and well although follow-up rarely is beyond 5 years (288,294). The tumors have low levels of estrogen receptor but many have high progesterone receptor levels (287,294). Primary treatment is usually mastectomy with axillary dissection.

PAPILLARY CARCINOMA

About 1 to 2 percent of breast carcinomas in women can be classified as papillary (299-301, 303,304); this is slightly greater in males. The World Health Organization classification of breast tumors (324) defines papillary carcinoma as:

> ...a rare carcinoma whose invasive pattern is predominantly in the form of papillary structures. The same architecture is usually displayed in the metastases. Frequently foci of intraductal papillary growth are recognizable.

The relationship between benign and malignant papillary tumors of the breast has long been a controversial subject (317). Most follow-up studies have confirmed the low "precancerous" potential of intraductal papillomas, especially when solitary. The data from many of these reports are summarized in Table 2. Overall, less than 5 percent of patients have developed breast carcinoma following excision of a papilloma and nearly half of the subsequent cancers were detected in the opposite breast. A solitary papilloma that has been excised and not found to contain carcinoma or severe atypical hyperplasia is not a precancerous lesion; the risk of detecting carcinoma subsequently in the same breast is low. An increased risk, however, has

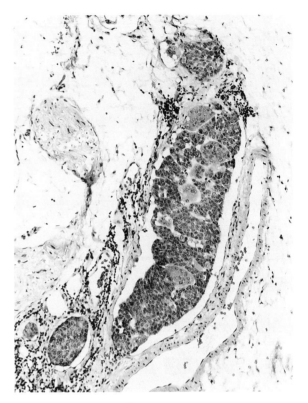

Figure 343
CARCINOMA WITH
OSTEOCLAST-LIKE GIANT CELLS
Intravascular tumor embolus containing multinucleated giant cells. (Fig. 12-18 from Rosen PP. The pathology of invasive breast carcinoma. In: Harris JR, Hellman S, Henderson IC, Kinne WD, eds. Breast diseases. 2nd ed. Philadelphia: JB Lippincott, 1991.)

been associated with the prior excision of a breast mass consisting of multiple papillomas. To some extent this reflects a tendency in some studies to include orderly papillary carcinomas in the group of papillomas.

In some cases, the close proximity of mammary carcinoma and a papilloma is such that they must be regarded as parts of a single lesion. Mingling of the two processes is evidence of carcinoma arising in a papilloma. Usually, the carcinomatous component is in situ (intraductal). Papillary tumors that have progressed to invasion less often contain areas of papilloma.

Clinical Presentation. The mean reported age of patients with cystic papillary carcinoma ranges from 63 to 67 years. In one series, the mean age of women with noncystic papillary carcinoma was 57 years and papillary carcinoma

Table 2

**INTRADUCTAL PAPILLOMA AND CARCINOMA:
A SELECTED LITERATURE REVIEW**

Reference	No. Cases Biopsied	No. of Carcinomas
Kilgore (307)	57	8 (6 ipsi, 2 contra)
Lewison (309)	23	0
Haagensen (305)	76	0
Snyder (320)	30	0
Hendrick (306)	207	2 (2 contra)
Kraus (308)	19	0
Buhl-Jorgensen (297)	53	7 (3 ipsi, 3 contra, 1 bila)
Carter (298)	64	6 (2 ipsi, 3 contra, 1 bila)
Total	529	11 ipsi (2 percent) 10 contra (2 percent) 2 bilat (0.3 percent)

was found in 2 of 169 (1.2 percent) women who were at least 75 years old when breast carcinoma was diagnosed (318).

Nearly 50 percent of papillary carcinomas arise in the central part of the breast and, as a consequence, nipple discharge has been described in 22 to 34 percent of patients (299,304). Bleeding from the nipple occurs in more patients with papillary carcinoma than in those with a papilloma.

The average size clinically is 2 to 3 cm. Papillary carcinomas are usually estrogen and progesterone receptor rich (310,311) and they tend to have a low growth rate when measured by thymidine labeling (322). Flow cytometry has not been helpful in distinguishing between benign and malignant papillary tumors. All benign lesions were diploid in one study. Only one of 15 "borderline" lesions and 5 of 19 carcinomas were aneuploid (322).

Papillary carcinomas often appear as rounded, circumscribed lesions on mammography (302,319). The differential diagnosis includes fibroadenoma, benign cystic lesions, and medullary or mucinous carcinoma. An invasive component may be suspected when part of the contour lacks circumscription (302). Examination by ultrasound

can suggest a papillary tumor when a solid area is imaged in an otherwise cystic lesion (302,319).

Gross Findings. Papillary carcinomas are usually well circumscribed grossly and may even appear encapsulated. Bleeding into the tumor can impart a dark brown or hemorrhagic appearance but usually these lesions are described as tan or grey.

Cystic papillary carcinomas contain dark brown, partly clotted blood and detached degenerated papillary fragments of the tumor (fig. 344). Mural nodules of residual tumor can usually be found on the luminal surface or in the cyst wall (figs. 345–347).

Microscopic Findings. The term papillary should be employed to describe in situ (intraductal) and invasive carcinomas in which the microscopic pattern is predominantly frond-forming. Many papillary carcinomas have cystic areas but this is not necessary for the diagnosis (fig. 348). When cyst formation is minimal or absent, separate fronds may be inconspicuous. In some parts of the tumor the cell proliferation becomes so dense that basic papillary properties are obscured. Such a tumor is described as having a solid papillary pattern (fig. 349).

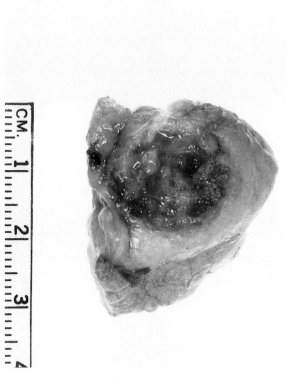

Figure 344
PAPILLARY CARCINOMA
Circumscribed, partly cystic lesion that contains rounded fleshy papillary nodules.

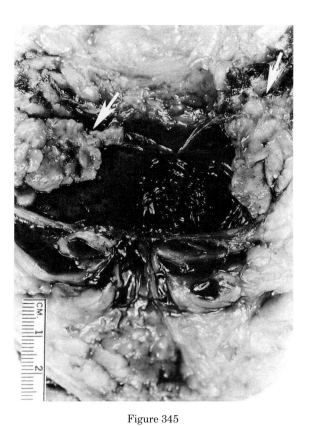

Figure 345
PAPILLARY CARCINOMA
Large cystic lesion filled with blood. Arrows indicate nodules of papillary carcinoma protruding into the lumen from the surface of the cyst. (Fig. 2A from Schaefer G, Rosen PP, Lesser ML, Kinne DW, Beattie EJ Jr. Breast carcinoma in elderly women: pathology, prognosis, and survival. Pathol Annu 1984;19(Pt 1):195–219.) (Figures 345–347 and 352 are from the same patient.)

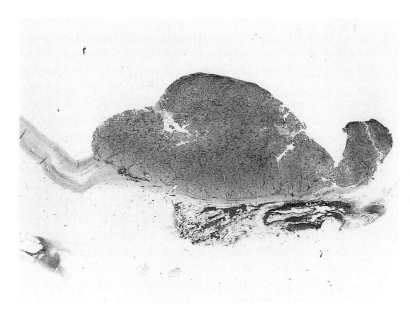

Figure 346
PAPILLARY CARCINOMA
Mural nodule of papillary carcinoma in cystic lesion. (Fig. 2B from Schaefer G, Rosen PP, Lesser ML, Kinne DW, Beattie EJ Jr. Breast carcinoma in elderly women: pathology, prognosis, and survival. Pathol Annu 1984;19(Pt 1):195–219.)

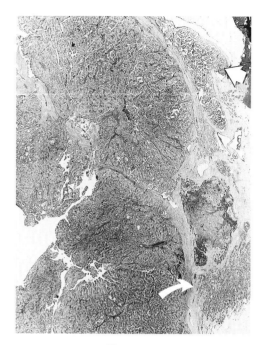

Figure 347
PAPILLARY CARCINOMA

Part of the cystic tumor in figure 345 showing a solid mural nodule. Papillary intraductal carcinoma beyond the cyst wall (straight arrow) and invasion (hooked arrow). (Fig. 2C from Schaefer G, Rosen PP, Lesser ML, Kinne DW, Beattie EJ Jr. Breast carcinoma in elderly women: pathology, prognosis, and survival. Pathol Annu 1984;19(Pt 1):195–219.)

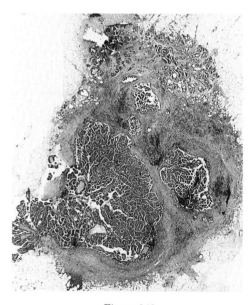

Figure 348
PAPILLARY CARCINOMA

Cross section of most of a papillary carcinoma composed of compact fronds. Invasive component is present above (Figures 348, 353, and 365 are from the same patient.)

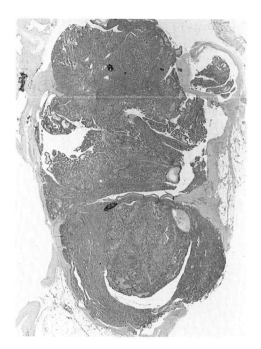

Figure 349
PAPILLARY CARCINOMA

Solid variant with relatively inconspicuous frond-forming areas in the center.

Neoplastic papillae are found within the body or central portion of a papillary carcinoma and are usually also formed in ducts at the periphery of the lesion. When the interpretation of an orderly papillary tumor presents a challenging diagnostic problem, surrounding ducts should be examined for foci of papillary, cribriform, or comedocarcinoma.

The distinction between a papilloma and noninvasive intraductal papillary carcinoma is determined by the cytology and microscopic structure of the lesion. There are no simple rules and in many cases the diagnosis is a judgement reached after assessing all the features. In 1962 Kraus and Neubecker (308) set forth often quoted criteria for distinguishing benign from malignant papillary tumors. The histologic characteristics are summarized in Table 3. The application of these criteria is complicated by numerous exceptions and structural variations.

In carcinoma, the papillae are composed of strands of cells arranged in varying patterns that include micropapillary or filiform, cribriform, trabecular, and solid (figs. 350–352). This epithelial proliferation gives rise to a complex series of secondary and tertiary arborizing branches.

Table 3

CRITERIA OF KRAUS AND NEUBECKER*
FOR THE DIAGNOSIS OF PAPILLARY BREAST LESIONS

Histologic Feature	Papilloma	Papillary Carcinoma
1. Cell types	Epithelial/myoepithelial	Epithelial
2. Chromasia	Normochromatic nuclei	Hyperchromatic nuclei
3. Apocrine metaplasia	Present	Absent
4. Glandular pattern	Complex	Cribriform
5. Stroma	Prominent; fibrosis with epithelial entrapment	Delicate or absent; stroma invaded in invasive lesions
6. Adjacent ducts	Hyperplasia	Intraductal carcinoma
7. Sclerosing adenosis	Sometimes present in breast	Usually absent

* Kraus and Neubecker (308). See text for detailed discussion and interpretation of these criteria.

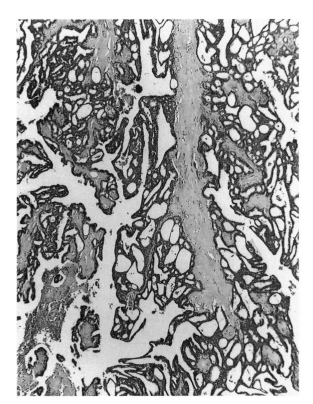

Figure 350
PAPILLARY CARCINOMA
Complex cribriform, papillary, and micropapillary pattern.

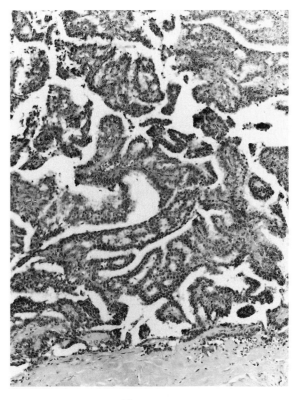

Figure 351
PAPILLARY CARCINOMA
Cribriform and papillary growth pattern. (Fig. 12-13A from Rosen PP. The pathology of invasive breast carcinoma. In: Harris JR, Hellman S, Henderson IC, Kinne DW, eds. Breast diseases. 2nd ed. Philadelphia: JB Lippincott, 1991.)

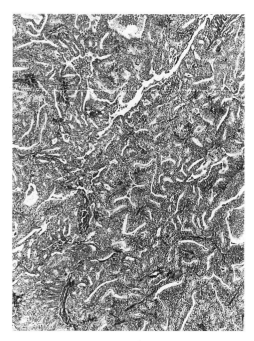

Figure 352
PAPILLARY CARCINOMA
Compact, complex papillary pattern.

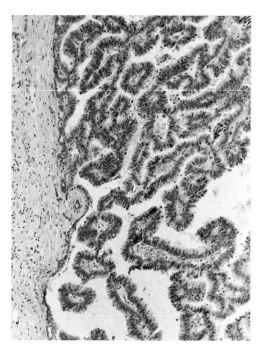

Figure 354
PAPILLARY CARCINOMA
Columnar cells with crowded, variably-staining nuclei covering the papillary fibrovascular fronds. (Figures 354, 355, and 360 are from the same patient.)

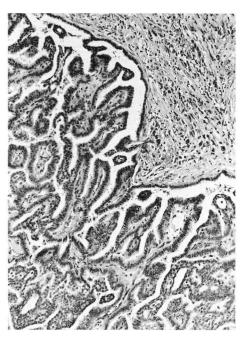

Figure 353
RESIDUAL PAPILLOMA
IN PAPILLARY CARCINOMA

Orderly growth pattern of residual papilloma in a carcinomatous lesion. Note basal orientation of crowded nuclei. The finding of foci such as this is evidence that carcinoma sometimes arises in a papilloma.

Connections and fusion of these papillae contribute to the formation of complex patterns of glandular spaces and solid areas within the lesion. Supporting fibrovascular stroma is present in virtually all papillary carcinomas but it tends to be inconspicuous and less evenly distributed than in benign papillary lesions.

The epithelial cells in papillary intraductal carcinoma grow in a less orderly fashion than in papillomas and tend to be packed closely together (fig. 353). Nuclei are characteristically hyperchromatic regardless of cytologic grade and there is usually a high nuclear-cytoplasmic ratio (figs. 354–356). Mitotic figures are variably present and more numerous in lesions that exhibit the most severe cytologic atypia. The cytoplasm is typically amphophilic but eosinophilic, and apocrine cells are found in a substantial number of lesions (fig. 357). Apocrine areas in a papillary carcinoma exhibit cytologic atypia consistent with the rest of the tumor and therefore differ from the bland foci of apocrine metaplasia commonly encountered in papillomas (fig. 358).

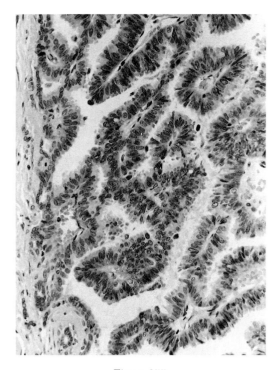

Figure 355
PAPILLARY CARCINOMA
Overlapping crowded nuclei with loss of basal polarity.

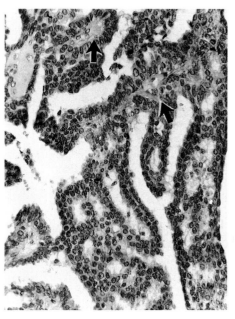

Figure 356
PAPILLARY CARCINOMA
Overgrowth of carcinomatous epithelium connecting inconspicuous papillary fronds that have fibrovascular stroma (arrows). (Fig. 12-13B from Rosen PP. The pathology of invasive breast carcinoma. In: Harris JR, Hellman S, Henderson IC, Kinne DW, eds. Breast diseases. 2nd ed. Philadelphia: JB Lippincott, 1991.)

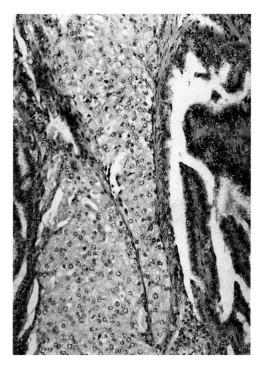

Figure 357
PAPILLARY CARCINOMA
Solid apocrine carcinomatous area in a papillary lesion.

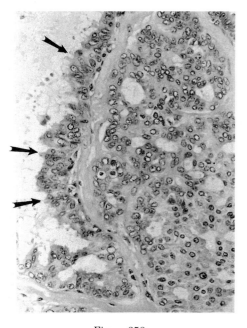

Figure 358
PAPILLARY CARCINOMA
Cribriform pattern in an apocrine papillary carcinoma. Note apocrine "snouts" on cells along the papillary frond (arrows).

215

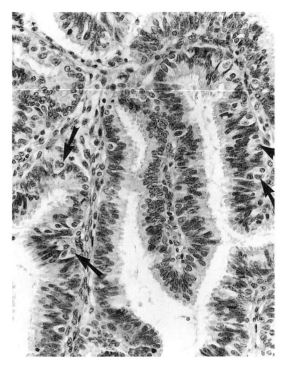

Figure 359
ATYPICAL HYPERPLASIA
IN PAPILLARY CARCINOMA
Myoepithelial cells are easily identified (arrows) in this atypical papillary proliferation that was part of a papillary tumor that had an extensive papillary carcinoma component.

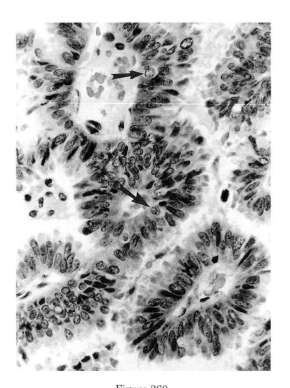

Figure 360
PAPILLARY CARCINOMA
Inconspicuous myoepithelial cells (arrows) in papillary carcinoma.

The cellular proliferation that forms a papillary duct carcinoma of the breast is composed of neoplastic epithelial cells. Myoepithelial cells, distributed relatively uniformly and proportionately within the epithelium in benign papillary lesions, are largely overgrown in papillary carcinomas (figs. 359, 360). However, they may not be entirely absent from a papillary carcinoma; the finding of myoepithelial cells in some parts of a papillary lesion is not inconsistent with a diagnosis of carcinoma (312,315,316). Usually myoepithelial cells are present in the areas of a papilloma that gave rise to a papillary carcinoma but tend to be inconspicuous or absent in the carcinomatous areas.

The diagnosis of an intraductal papillary carcinoma that has arisen in a papilloma is particularly difficult. These lesions typically retain areas of papilloma that appear benign or atypical as well as having foci of more cellular proliferation that lead to a diagnosis of carcinoma (figs. 359, 360). Small areas of papilloma in such lesions are of little

consequence and they should not impede recognition of the carcinomatous element. The diagnosis of papillary carcinoma can be "a 'shadow land' even for the most experienced pathologist" (321). "Borderline" papillary lesions often have modest or substantial areas of benign papillary proliferation as well as more cellular and atypical components. When the diagnosis of a discrete papillary tumor is uncertain and the surrounding breast does not have clear cut foci of intraductal carcinoma, the lesion is best regarded as an atypical papillary proliferation.

Immunohistochemical studies have been little help in evaluating difficult lesions. Results showed areas of papilloma negative for CEA but cytoplasmic CEA present in carcinomatous portions of the same papillary tumors (315,316). Actin-positive myoepithelial cells, however, were present only in areas of papilloma. The authors concluded that "CEA-positive myoepithelial cell-free carcinomatous areas can be anatomically associated with and even present inside the benign-looking papillary lesions." The observations were seen "as evidence

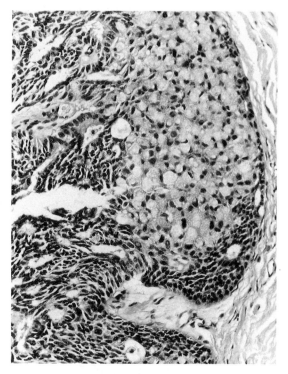

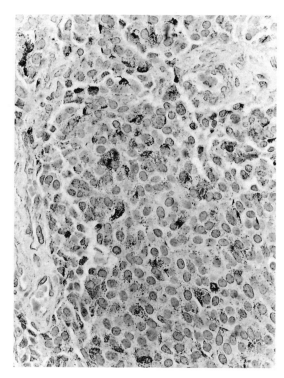

Figure 361
PAPILLARY CARCINOMA
Prominent intracytoplasmic mucin in an unusual solid variant of papillary carcinoma. (Figures 361 and 362 are from the same patient.)

Figure 362
PAPILLARY CARCINOMA
Neurosecretory-type granules demonstrated with the Grimelius stain. The tumor cells were also immunoreactive for chromogranin.

of a malignant transformation of intraductal papillomas, or less likely, of their 'cancerization' by ductal carcinoma." The cells in a minority of papillary carcinomas also contain Grimelius- and chromogranin-positive neurosecretory type cytoplasmic granules that have not been demonstrated by histochemical methods in papillomas.

There is also a broad range of mucin secretion demonstrable with the mucicarmine, Alcian blue, and periodic acid–Schiff stains. Most lesions have detectable mucin, although in the majority, positive mucin secretion is not prominent. A few, however, exhibit abundant and diffuse intracellular secretion (fig. 361). Such papillary carcinomas are prone to having Grimelius- and chromogranin-positive cytoplasmic neurosecretory-like granules (fig. 362). The microcalcifications found in most papillary carcinomas are usually distributed in the glandular portions of the lesion but they may also be found in the papillary stroma.

Three-dimensional reconstruction of the microscopic structure of papillary lesions has re-

vealed some differences between papillomas and papillary carcinomas (313,314). In papillomas and papillomatosis consisting of multiple microscopic intraductal papillomas, the luminal spaces between the proliferating epithelial cells form a complex but diffusely anastomosing continuous network of channels. In intraductal carcinomas, the luminal spaces tend to be separate without forming a continuous network. These elegant and painstaking studies have resulted in a more complete appreciation of the structural relationship between hyperplastic and carcinomatous papillary lesions. They have also provided independent evidence that multiple papillomas are more susceptible to the development of carcinoma than are solitary papillomas.

Electron microscopy generally confirms the light microscopic characteristics of papillary carcinoma and is not regarded as particularly helpful in evaluating difficult cases (296,323). Myoepithelial cells are more numerous in benign papillary lesions than in papillary carcinomas. Papillomas

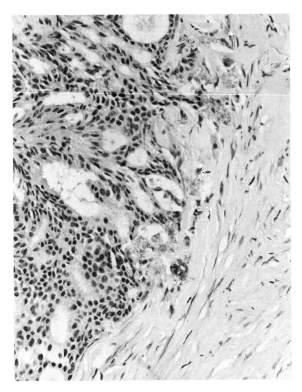

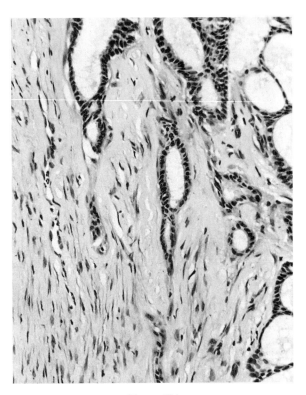

Figure 363
PAPILLARY CARCINOMA
Irregular border at the sclerotic margin of the tumor is not evidence of invasion. (Figures 363 and 364 are from the same patient.)

Figure 364
PAPILLARY CARCINOMA
Neoplastic glands trapped in the sclerotic reaction around a papillary carcinoma are not definitive evidence of invasion.

tend to have abundant well-formed microvilli at the luminal surfaces of epithelial cells while in some papillary carcinomas microvilli are less abundant, stunted, and poorly formed (296). Intracytoplasmic lumens have been described in papillary carcinoma (323).

The microscopic diagnosis of invasive papillary carcinoma may be difficult. Many papillary carcinomas are bounded by zones of fibrosis, recent or resolved hemorrhage, and chronic inflammation. Similar alterations may also occur within the lesion. Papillary or glandular clusters of epithelial cells routinely found within these areas present a particularly challenging problem for which there is no completely satisfactory answer (figs. 363, 364). Since the same pattern of epithelial dispersal occurs in sclerotic portions of benign papillary lesions, these foci are not considered evidence of invasion. The most reliable evidence of invasion is extension of tumor beyond the zone of reactive changes into the mammary parenchyma and fat (figs. 365, 366).

The growth patterns found in areas of invasive papillary carcinoma are variations on the structure of carcinoma in the in situ portion of the lesion (303). Cribriform, comedo, tubular, or mucinous foci may be present. Apocrine features can be seen in invasive papillary carcinoma.

Prognosis and Treatment. Whether cystic or solid, papillary carcinoma without invasion is a form of intraductal carcinoma. Patients with apparently noninvasive papillary carcinoma are subject to the same very low risk of obscure invasion that occurs with other types of intraductal carcinoma. Consequently, axillary node metastases are seen in less than 1 percent of cases. These patients are cured by mastectomy.

In a series of 18 patients with noninvasive cystic papillary carcinoma, 7 had simple mastectomies and 11 were treated by mastectomy with axillary dissection (299). None of the latter group had axillary metastases and there were no recurrences. Sixteen patients remained alive after an average of 83 months and 13 died of causes other than

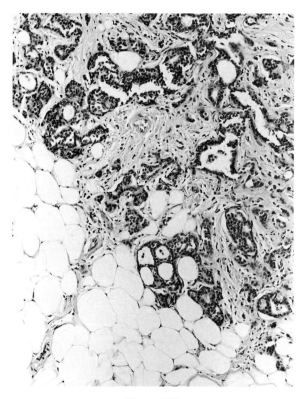

Figure 365
INVASIVE PAPILLARY CARCINOMA
Moderately differentiated invasive duct carcinoma invading fat that arose in a papillary carcinoma.

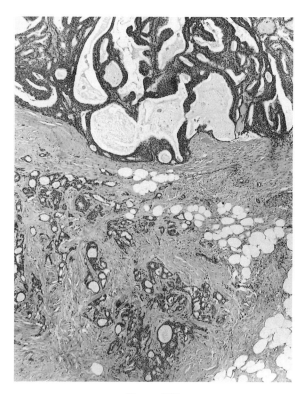

Figure 366
INVASIVE PAPILLARY CARCINOMA
Invasive duct carcinoma that arose from the noninvasive papillary component above.

breast carcinoma, having remained recurrence-free for an average of 65 months. Eleven other patients studied by the same authors were treated by excisional biopsy alone. Three of the 11 (27 percent) had subsequent recurrences in the ipsilateral breast. Two were invasive lesions detected 3 and 6 years later. The third patient was found to have recurrent noninvasive papillary carcinoma 3 years after her initial excisional therapy. There were no systemic recurrences. Invasive papillary carcinomas tend to be relatively large tumors due to the bulky, cystic component that is frequently present. The low frequency of axillary lymph node metastases (299,303) is consistent with the actual sizes of the invasive elements as well as the histologically low-grade character of most of the carcinomas. When axillary node metastases occur, they usually do not involve more than three lymph nodes (303). The papillary growth pattern of the primary tumor is often duplicated in metastatic

foci. The prognosis of patients with invasive papillary carcinoma is reportedly very favorable, even in women with axillary node metastases (303). Recurrences often become clinically apparent more than 5 years after diagnosis.

ADENOID CYSTIC CARCINOMA

The term adenoid cystic carcinoma was first applied to tumors of the breast by Geschickter in 1945 (332). Less than 0.1 percent of mammary carcinomas have an adenoid cystic growth pattern.

Clinical Presentation. Adenoid cystic carcinoma occurs in adult women throughout the age distribution of mammary carcinoma among patients between 25 and 80 years of age (325,331, 336,338,346,347,349,355), with a mean age of 50 to 63 years. Isolated cases have been encountered in men (336,347). There is no predilection to bilaterality but other types of carcinoma may develop in the contralateral breast (331,346,349) or elsewhere in the same breast (338).

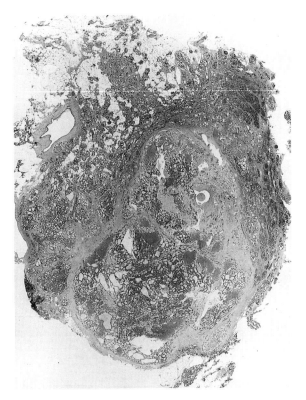

Figure 367
ADENOID CYSTIC CARCINOMA
Low magnification view of an entire tumor showing central nodule that appeared grossly circumscribed. More widely invasive elements extending into the breast are evident above, and there are cysts in the central nodule.

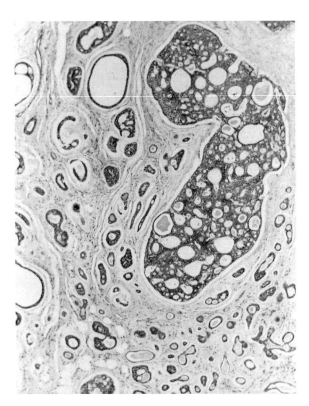

Figure 368
ADENOID CYSTIC CARCINOMA
Typical invasive growth pattern with intervening collagenous stroma. This patient was a 13-year-old boy.

Adenoid cystic carcinoma typically presents as a palpable discrete firm mass. Very few of these tumors have been detected by mammography and in some cases the mammogram was reportedly negative (349). Skin dimpling, ulceration, or peau d'orange have been reported in patients with superficial or large lesions. Nipple discharge is rarely a presenting symptom (349).

Most patients report that the tumor was detected shortly before seeking medical attention but intervals of 10 years or more have been described (347). In one series (349), duration prior to diagnosis ranged from 1 month to 9 years, median of 24 months; six tumors were present for a year or more before diagnosis.

Seven adenoid cystic carcinomas have been examined biochemically for hormone receptors (329,349,355). One lesion was positive for estrogen (15 fmol) and progesterone (17 fmol) receptors, five were negative for both, and one was positive for progesterone (19 fmol) and negative for estrogen receptors.

Gross Findings. Gross size of the lesions described in various reports has varied from 2 mm to 12 cm with the majority between 1 and 3 cm (325,346,349). Most appear circumscribed or nodular grossly (fig. 367). Cystic areas are not unusual (349). The lesions have been described as grey, pale yellow, tan, and pink.

Microscopic Findings. About 50 percent of adenoid cystic carcinomas have an invasive growth pattern microscopically with extension of the tumor into the surrounding breast parenchyma (fig. 368) (349). Perineural invasion is found in a minority of tumors. Lymphatic tumor emboli have been described at the periphery of one lesion (349). Shrinkage artifacts occur relatively often and may be mistaken for lymphatic tumor emboli.

Adenoid cystic carcinoma is composed of proliferating glands (adenoid component) and stromal or

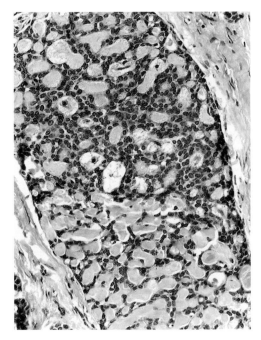

Figure 369
ADENOID CYSTIC CARCINOMA
Adenoid glandular elements are more abundant above while the lower portion consists exclusively of the cylindromatous component. (Fig. 12-16B from Rosen PP. The pathology of invasive breast carcinoma. In: Harris JR, Hellman S, Henderson IC, Kinne DW, eds. Breast diseases. 2nd ed. Philadelphia: JB Lippincott, 1991.)

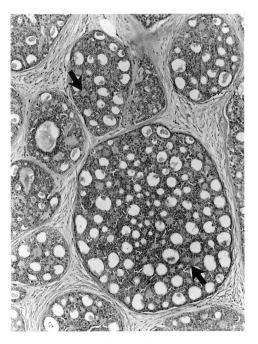

Figure 370
ADENOID CYSTIC CARCINOMA
Area with prominent cribriform growth pattern. Cylindromatous components are present (arrows). (Fig. 8A from Rosen PP. Adenoid cystic carcinoma of the breast. A morphologically heterogenous neoplasm. Pathol Annu 1989;24(Pt 2):237–54.)

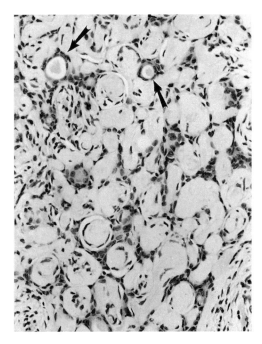

Figure 371
ADENOID CYSTIC CARCINOMA
Few glands (arrows) are seen in this area consisting almost entirely of the cylindromatous component.

basement membrane elements ("pseudo-glandular" or cylindromatous component) (fig. 369). These components are rarely distributed homogeneously in a given tumor (figs. 370, 371). Some areas consist only of the adenoid elements, creating a resemblance to cribriform carcinoma (334). Abundant stromal material in other parts of the tumor produces a pattern easily mistaken for scirrhous carcinoma. Adenoid cystic carcinoma can be diagnosed in a fine-needle aspiration specimen if adenoid glandular clusters and globules of cylindromatous material are present (343,344).

A variety of microscopic growth patterns may be present (345,348,349). These configurations have been described as cribriform, solid, glandular (tubular), reticular (trabecular), and basaloid. Adenomyoepitheliomatous and syringomatous areas are further evidence of structural diversity (349). Sebaceous differentiation was found in 14 percent of adenoid cystic carcinomas reviewed by Tavassoli and Norris (351). These authors also

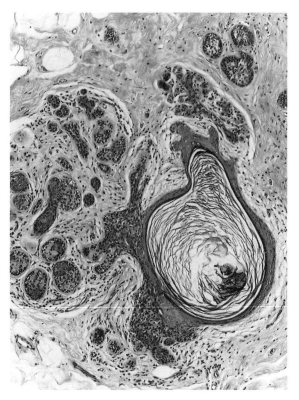

Figure 372
ADENOID CYSTIC CARCINOMA

Squamous metaplasia seen here in a terminal duct was also present in the invasive portion of this tumor. Note "in situ" involvement of intralobular ductules by adenoid cystic carcinoma. (Fig. 7D from Rosen PP. Adenoid cystic carcinoma of the breast. A morphologically heterogenous neoplasm. Pathol Annu 1989;24(Pt 2):237–54.)

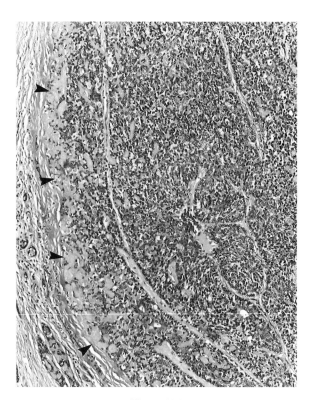

Figure 373
ADENOID CYSTIC CARCINOMA

"High-grade" variant with solid growth pattern and inconspicuous cylindromatous elements (arrows).

found foci of adenosquamous differentiation in a substantial number of cases (fig. 372).

Ro et al. (348) proposed stratifying adenoid cystic carcinomas into three grades on the basis of the proportion of solid growth within the lesion (I - no solid elements; II - less than 30 percent solid; III - more than 30 percent solid) (fig. 373). They found that tumors with a solid component (grades II and III) tended to be larger than those without a solid element (grade I) and were more likely to have recurrences. The only patient who developed metastatic adenoid cystic carcinoma had a grade III lesion.

Some conventional, less favorable forms of mammary carcinoma may be incorrectly diagnosed as adenoid cystic carcinoma (325,334,350). In one review, about half of the cases recorded by the Connecticut Tumor Registry were misclassi-

fied (350). Most of the errors resulted from including invasive duct and even multifocal intraductal carcinomas with a prominent cribriform component. Problems were also encountered in distinguishing adenoid cystic from papillary and mucinous carcinomas.

Collagenous spherulosis is a benign duct proliferation that must be considered in the differential diagnosis of adenoid cystic carcinoma (see p. 63) (327,349). It combines gland formation and acellular deposits (spherules) of stromal material among the epithelial cells. The spherule material often has an internal stellate or laminar structure, which differs from that ordinarily seen in adenoid cystic carcinoma. It contains elastin, PAS-positive material, and type IV collagen (326,333) indicative of the presence of a component of basal lamina material.

Histochemistry. Histochemical stains such as mucicarmine or Alcian blue ordinarily stain the secretion within glands while laminin and fibronectin, noncollagenous glycoproteins associated with basal lamina, can be demonstrated by immunohistochemistry in the cylindromatous elements (328,329). Fibronectin and laminin may be found in the basement membranes of ducts that contain intraductal cribriform carcinoma but neither is seen within the tumor itself (328). Glandular cells stain for EMA, keratin, and CEA (329,339) while basaloid cells are immunoreactive for vimentin (339).

Electron Microscopy. Ultrastructural studies reveal the same diverse cell types in mammary adenoid cystic carcinoma as are encountered in adenoid cystic carcinoma arising in the salivary glands and other organs (340). In addition to epithelial and myoepithelial cells (338,347,355), the tumors contain varying numbers of basaloid cells (351,355) as well as cells exhibiting sebaceous and adenosquamous differentiation (351).

Prognosis and Treatment. Currently, data on the prognosis of adenoid cystic carcinoma are based almost entirely on patients treated surgically (325,331,336,338,346–350,354). Mastectomy has been curative in virtually all cases. Chest wall recurrence was reported after simple mastectomy in one case (354) and there have been a few isolated instances of systemic metastases after mastectomy (341,343,346,352). All patients with metastases have had pulmonary involvement with recurrences in the lung being detected as late as 6 (330), 8 (343), 9 (341,343), 10 (346), and 12 years (330) after initial treatment. All of these patients had negative axillary lymph nodes. Axillary metastases were present at mastectomy in three other cases (348,352, 353). Each of these patients had pulmonary metastases and two reportedly died of metastatic mammary adenoid cystic carcinoma, although the diagnosis is not well documented in one of these cases (352). Other sites of metastases include bones, liver, and brain (335,337).

Recurrence in the breast has been described after treatment by local excision alone (346, 347,351) with the interval to recurrence varying from less than 1 year (347) to more than 20 years (342). Negative axillary lymph nodes were found in three cases when an axillary dissection was performed and the tumor was reportedly controlled by surgical removal in all seven cases of local recurrence in the breast.

SECRETORY CARCINOMA

This form of mammary carcinoma has been described in the WHO classification of breast tumors (375):

> A carcinoma with pale-staining cells showing prominent secretory activity of the type seen in pregnancy and lactation. PAS-positive material is present in the cytoplasm and in acinar-like spaces.

These tumors have been termed "juvenile carcinoma" because they were first identified in children. However, the majority of cases in later studies were reported in adults and, consequently, the term secretory is preferable to juvenile. The microscopic appearance of the lesion is the same regardless of patient age.

Clinical Presentation. Secretory carcinoma was first fully described in 1966 by McDivitt and Stewart (366) in seven patients whose ages ranged from 3 to 15 years, averaging 9 years. Oberman and Stephens (368) described a 25-year-old woman with two recurrences and Oberman (367) subsequently reported four more cases in adult women 22 to 73 years old. The median age of 19 patients studied at the Armed Forces Institute of Pathology (373) was 25 years (range 9 to 69 years); 14 were older than 20 years while 1 was a 9-year-old boy. At least 24 additional adult cases have been described (356,360,364,370–372) and there have been a number of reports of secretory carcinoma in children (357,358,359,361,363, 365,370) including a 6-year-old boy who had axillary node metastases. Affected boys are usually less than 10 years old although it was reported in a 24-year-old man (364). Secretory carcinoma is uncommon in perimenarchal girls 10 to 15 years of age.

In most cases the patient presented with a circumscribed mass. Subareolar lesions have been associated with nipple discharge. No clinical evidence of a hormonal abnormality has been described to explain the secretory properties of the tumor and secretory carcinoma has not been associated with pregnancy. Estrogen receptors have been negative in nine tumors (361, 370) and positive in one tumor examined by biochemistry or immunohistochemistry. Three tumors were positive and four were negative for progesterone receptors. Coexistence of juvenile papillomatosis and secretory carcinoma has been described in four

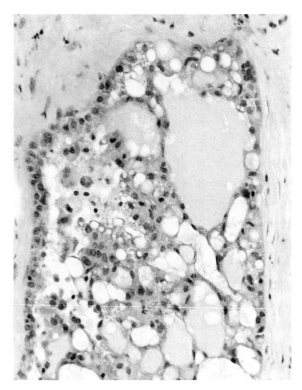

Figure 374
SECRETORY CARCINOMA
Intraductal component with microcystic features.

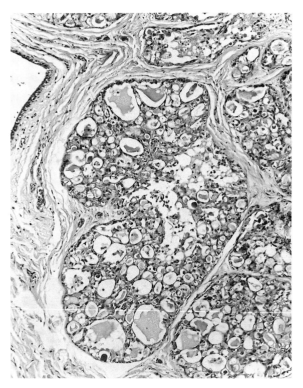

Figure 375
SECRETORY CARCINOMA
Microcystic growth pattern is evident in this multinodular lesion. (Fig. 12-19 from Rosen PP. The pathology of invasive breast carcinoma. In: Harris JR, Hellman S, Henderson IC, Kinne DW, eds. Breast diseases. 2nd ed. Philadelphia: JB Lippincott, 1991.)

patients (361,369), three of whom had the lesions concurrently in the same breast.

Gross Findings. There is usually a circumscribed, firm mass which may be lobulated. The tumor may have infiltrative margins. Tumors tend to be 3 cm or less in diameter, with larger lesions up to 12 cm found mainly in adults.

Microscopic Findings. Secretory carcinoma has an intraductal component which is ordinarily papillary or cribriform but solid foci, and infrequently comedonecrosis, may be found (fig. 374). These features are duplicated in the invasive components, which tend to have papillary, microcystic, and cribriform patterns. Microcalcifications are rarely seen in neoplastic glands or in the stroma.

Tumor cells, glands, and microcystic spaces contain abundant secretion, which is usually pale pink or amphophilic with a vacuolated or "bubbly" appearance (figs. 375–377). The secretion is positive with the mucicarmine and PAS reactions. Positive staining for alpha-lactalbumin has been reported (356,370). Ultrastructurally, secre-

tion has been found in membrane-bound secretory vacuoles within the cytoplasm of tumor cells and in intracytoplasmic lumina (fig. 378). Cytologically, the tumor cells have abundant, pale to clear, amphophilic cytoplasm and small, round, cytologically low-grade nuclei. Portions of the lesion may infrequently have more granular or eosinophilic cytoplasm and a nuclear cytology suggesting apocrine carcinoma (fig. 379).

Prognosis and Treatment. In the majority of patients secretory carcinoma has a low-grade clinical course and a favorable prognosis. Most children and adults have been treated by mastectomy, but a few have been free of disease 7 to 15 years after excisional biopsy alone (366,368). Axillary metastases have been described (356,358, 359,362–364,373,374), but they rarely involve more than three lymph nodes. The risk of nodal involvement is at least as great in children as it

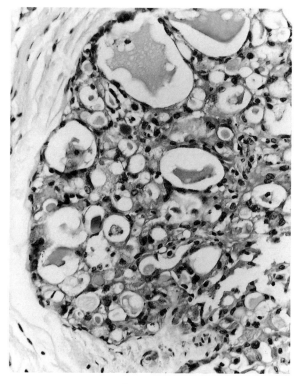

Figure 376
SECRETORY CARCINOMA
Secretion evident in microcysts of varying size tends to shrink toward the center of the lumen. In larger microcysts, secretion may have a scalloped border. Some tumor cells have vacuolated or clear cytoplasm.

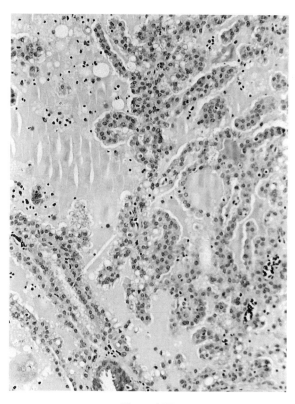

Figure 377
SECRETORY CARCINOMA
This lesion has a prominent papillary structure. Note abundant extracellular secretion and "bubbly" cytoplasm in the papillary clusters of cells. (Fig. 3 from Rosen PP, Cranor ML. Secretory carcinoma of the breast. Arch Pathol Lab Med 1991;115:141–4.)

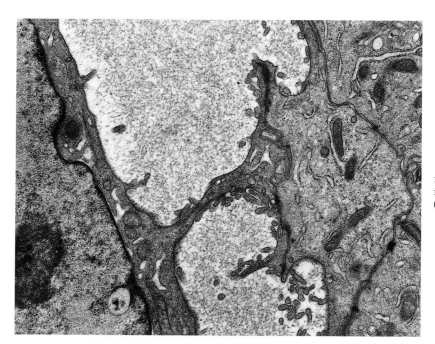

Figure 378
SECRETORY CARCINOMA
The cytoplasm contains large irregular vacuoles lined in part by microvilli. A nucleus is seen on the left (X12800).

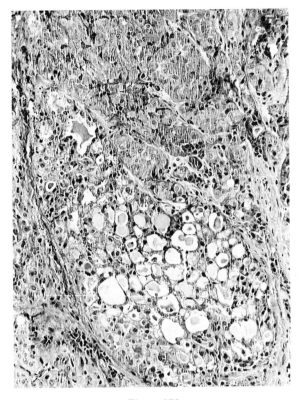

Figure 379
SECRETORY CARCINOMA
Combined pattern with typical microcystic component below and solid growth above composed of cells with apocrine cytology.

is in adults. A recent literature review found positive nodes in 5 of 18 (27 percent) childhood cases (363). Recurrence in the breast after excision alone has been described by several authors (357,358,364,366,368,370,372–374). One 28-year-old patient treated initially by excision alone developed multifocal recurrent disease in the breast accompanied by metastases in four axillary lymph nodes (370).

Surgical biopsy is necessary for the diagnosis of secretory carcinoma, although the lesion may be suspected in a fine-needle aspiration specimen (360). Local excision is the preferred initial treatment in children. Consideration should be given to preserving the breast bud in prepubertal patients. In postmenarchal children, wide local excision may suffice for small lesions but quadrantectomy may be necessary to obtain negative margins around larger tumors. Axillary dissection is indicated if clinical examination

suggests nodal involvement. There is no evidence that radiation therapy is beneficial in adults after excisional biopsy and no data are available to support the use of adjuvant systemic therapy in children or adults since very few patients have received this treatment (364,374).

CYSTIC HYPERSECRETORY CARCINOMA

This variant of duct carcinoma, described in 1984 (378), warrants separate discussion because it has unusual pathologic features. Cystic hypersecretory hyperplasia is a benign proliferative lesion that resembles cystic hypersecretory carcinoma (377). The latter is not cited in the WHO classification of breast tumors published in 1982 (379).

Clinical Presentation. The patients are distributed throughout most of the age range of breast carcinoma with the youngest 34 and the oldest 79 years. The mean age in the largest series was 56 years (377). The presenting symptom has usually been a mass or other palpable abnormality. Mammography in one case revealed a prominent ductal pattern and an irregular density in the breast (376). Among 10 tumors studied biochemically, 8 had negative levels of estrogen and progesterone receptors while 2 were positive for both.

Gross Findings. The tumors have measured from 1 to 10 cm in diameter. The lesions are firm but usually not hard. Many of these tumors are a shade of brown or grey-brown, and numerous cysts, measuring up to 1.5 cm, are apparent within the lesion (fig. 380). Secretion within cysts has been described as gelatinous or resembling thyroid colloid. It is not possible to distinguish cystic hypersecretory carcinoma from cystic hypersecretory hyperplasia grossly. An invasive component associated with the carcinoma produces a noncystic mass.

Microscopic Findings. Microscopically, there are many cystically dilated ducts that contain eosinophilic secretion bearing a striking resemblance to thyroid colloid (fig. 381). The homogeneous secretion is virtually acellular and retracted from the surrounding epithelium, producing a scalloped margin. There are no appreciable differences in the character of the secretion between cystic hypersecretory carcinoma and hyperplasia. Positive reactions for CEA,

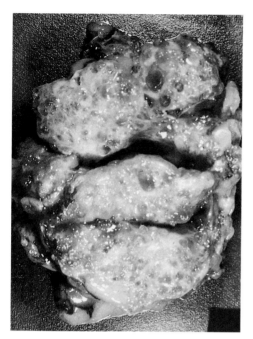

Figure 380
CYSTIC HYPERSECRETORY CARCINOMA
Gross appearance of a tumor that measured 8 x 5.5 x 2.5 cm. The lesion was described as "multicystic, yellow-brown and appeared to be representative of thyroid parenchyma." (Fig. 1 from Rosen PP, Scott M. Cystic hypersecretory duct carcinoma of the breast. Am J Surg Pathol 1984;8:31–41.)

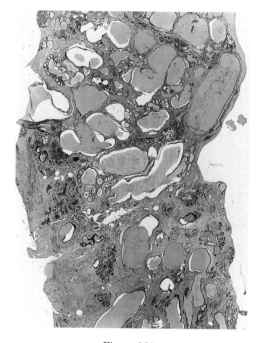

Figure 381
CYSTIC HYPERSECRETORY CARCINOMA
At low magnification cysts are prominent and ducts containing carcinoma are inconspicuous in the intervening stroma.

alpha-lactalbumin, PAS, and mucin have been observed while the cyst contents are consistently negative for thyroglobulin. Disruption of cysts results from spillage of cyst contents which elicits an intense inflammatory reaction consisting of lymphocytes and histiocytes.

Many of the cysts in cystic hypersecretory lesions are lined by inconspicuous flat cells or a single layer of cuboidal or columnar cells (fig. 382). When this is the only epithelial pattern, the lesion is regarded as cystic hypersecretory hyperplasia (377). The cells in such lesions have uniform, cytologically bland nuclei and eosinophilic cytoplasm. Atypical features include epithelial crowding, hyperchromasia, and enlargement of nuclei which may contain nucleoli (figs. 383, 384). Epithelial crowding of cells in atypical cystic hypersecretory hyperplasia may result in small mounds or buds of cells protruding into the lumen.

In cystic hypersecretory carcinoma, the epithelium of some cysts and ducts has proliferated in the form of micropapillary intraductal carcinoma

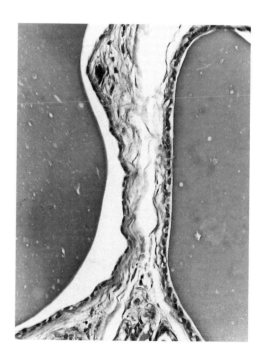

Figure 382
CYSTIC HYPERSECRETORY LESION
Cysts lined by flat cuboidal epithelium contain homogeneous secretion. Such cysts can be found in cystic hypersecretory hyperplasia or carcinoma.

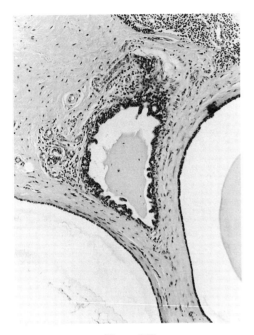

Figure 383
CYSTIC HYPERSECRETORY HYPERPLASIA
WITH ATYPIA
Ducts between the cysts have crowded epithelium.

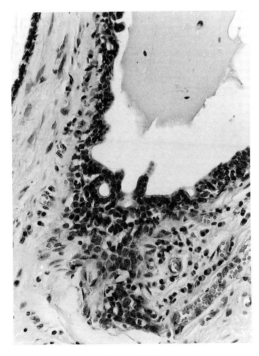

Figure 384
CYSTIC HYPERSECRETORY
HYPERPLASIA WITH ATYPIA
Duct shown in figure 383 with epithelial buds. Traces of
the myoepithelial layer are evident.

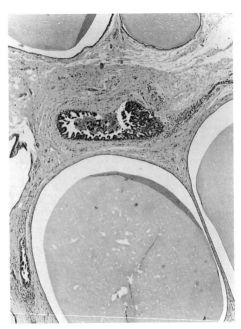

Figure 385
CYSTIC HYPERSECRETORY CARCINOMA
Micropapillary intraductal carcinoma in the stroma between cysts. (Fig. 12-20 from Rosen PP. The pathology of invasive breast carcinoma. In: Harris JR, Hellman S, Henderson IC, Kinne DW, eds. Breast diseases. 2nd ed. Philadelphia: JB Lippincott, 1991.)

(figs. 385–387). The epithelial proliferation ranges from short, knobby epithelial tufts to complex branching fronds that may extend across the duct lumen. The so-called "Roman arch" or bridging pattern commonly seen in other forms of micropapillary carcinoma is uncommon in these lesions.

Cytologically, the cells have crowded and overlapping hyperchromatic nuclei and sparse cytoplasm. There is no secretion within the cytoplasm but frayed, irregular cell borders and cytoplasmic blebs are seen.

Invasive cystic hypersecretory carcinoma consists of cystic hypersecretory intraductal carcinoma accompanied by an invasive component (fig. 388). These invasive carcinomas have all been poorly differentiated duct carcinomas with a solid growth pattern (figs. 389, 390). Light microscopy has disclosed little or no secretory activity within the cells. Metastatic foci in the axillary lymph nodes of one patient had small cystic foci that contained eosinophilic secretion (fig. 391) (377).

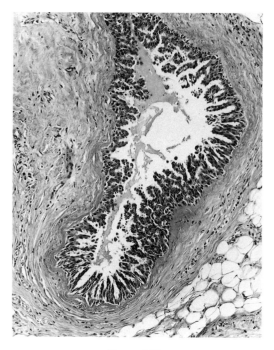

Figure 386
CYSTIC HYPERSECRETORY CARCINOMA
Micropapillary intraductal carcinoma and sparse secretion that is retracted from the epithelium.

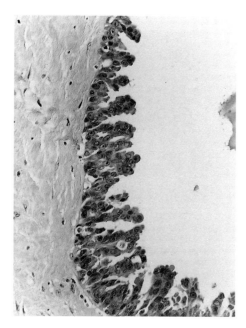

Figure 387
CYSTIC HYPERSECRETORY CARCINOMA
Micropapillary intraductal carcinoma. Secretion is not evident in the cytoplasm of tumor cells which have a hobnail configuration. In this section individual nuclei appear relatively "clear" with small, discrete nucleoli.

Electron Microscopy. Electron microscopy has been performed in only one case (377). The affected ductules were lined by epithelial cells largely devoid of surface microvilli (fig. 392), surrounded by myoepithelial cells. No polarization of secretory vesicles or inclusions was seen. Large secretory granules that contained sparse, fine granular material were limited to the basal cytoplasm. Ductular lumens contained amorphous or finely granular material. Mucinous carcinoma differs from cystic hypersecretory carcinoma in having abundant extracellular mucin and intracytoplasmic mucinogen granules.

Prognosis and Treatment. Excisional biopsy is required for definitive diagnosis and especially to distinguish cystic hypersecretory hyperplasia from cystic hypersecretory carcinoma. Little is known about the clinical course of this uncommon breast carcinoma. The finding of areas with typical features of cystic hypersecretory hyperplasia, sometimes with atypia, in association with cystic hypersecretory carcinoma, suggests that these processes are related. However, convincing evidence has not yet been presented. Follow-up of

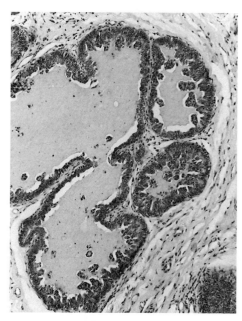

Figure 388
CYSTIC HYPERSECRETORY CARCINOMA
WITH INVASION
This part of the lesion has the typical micropapillary intraductal carcinoma pattern. (Figures 388, 389, and 391 are from the same patient.)

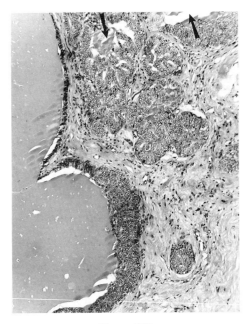

Figure 389
CYSTIC HYPERSECRETORY CARCINOMA
WITH INVASION
Note transition in cyst epithelium with the formation of a plaque of tumor cells below. The micropapillary pattern is partly obscured where carcinoma nearly fills ducts above but traces of retracted secretion remain (arrows). "Clear" nuclei are evident in tumor cells even at this magnification.

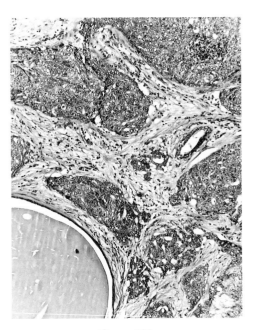

Figure 390
CYSTIC HYPERSECRETORY CARCINOMA
WITH INVASION
Islands of poorly differentiated carcinoma invading stroma adjacent to a cyst.

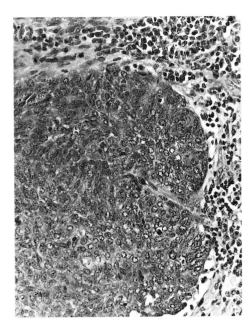

Figure 391
CYSTIC HYPERSECRETORY CARCINOMA
WITH INVASION
Metastatic carcinoma in a lymph node. Note "clear" nuclei.

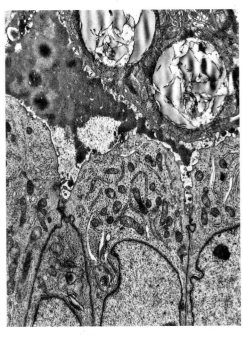

Figure 392
CYSTIC HYPERSECRETORY CARCINOMA
The dense secretion in the lumen above contains two lipid droplets. Note mitochondria and endoplasmic reticulum in the tumor cells (X8000). (Fig. 10 from Guerry P, Erlandson RA, Rosen PP. Cystic hypersecretory carcinoma. Cancer 1988;61:1611–20.)

eight patients with cystic hypersecretory hyperplasia revealed subsequent breast carcinoma in two cases (377). One woman developed a fatal contralateral invasive duct carcinoma that lacked cystic hypersecretory features. The other patient had intraductal carcinoma separate from cystic hypersecretory hyperplasia in a biopsy and residual cystic hypersecretory hyperplasia in the mastectomy specimen.

The clinical course of cystic hypersecretory intraductal carcinoma has thus far not differed from that of other forms of intraductal carcinoma. There have been no recurrences in women treated by mastectomy after a mean follow-up of 8 years, extending in one case to 23 years (377). All had negative lymph nodes. Two of four women with invasive cystic hypersecretory carcinoma had metastases in axillary lymph nodes and a third patient who presented with locally advanced or inflammatory carcinoma died of disease. Therapeutic options are similar to those available for other forms of duct carcinoma.

APOCRINE CARCINOMA

Apocrine glands are part of the odoriferous or accessory sex gland system. They are normally present in the skin, the ears (ceruminous glands), and eyelids (Moll glands). Cutaneous apocrine glands are particularly responsive to hormonal stimulation in a fashion analogous to the mammary gland. Axillary apocrine gland hyperplasia during pregnancy may occasionally produce palpable glandular enlargement that can be mistaken for ectopic breast tissue.

Embryologically, the breasts develop from the anlage that gives rise to apocrine glands but apocrine glands are not a constituent of the normal microscopic anatomy of the mammary gland. Mammary apocrine metaplasia is seen most frequently in the epithelium of simple cysts and hyperplastic ducts but can also be found in sclerosing adenosis, fibroadenomas, papillomas, and other benign proliferative abnormalities. When studied by histochemistry or by electron microscopy, apocrine cells formed by metaplasia are similar to the cells of normal apocrine glands (381,382,387,398,399,401).

Apocrine change may occur focally in mammary carcinomas but the diagnosis of apocrine carcinoma should be reserved for tumors in which all or nearly all of the epithelium is distinctly apocrine. The WHO classification of breast tumors (406) describes apocrine carcinoma as:

> ...composed predominantly of cells with abundant eosinophilic cytoplasm reminiscent of metaplastic apocrine cells...

This tumor has been referred to as oncocytic carcinoma and sweat gland carcinoma. However, the term sweat gland carcinoma should not be used for these lesions because apocrine glands are morphologically and functionally different from sweat glands. The observation that a cell derived from an apocrine carcinoma retains apocrine carcinoma characteristics in vitro is evidence that such carcinomas constitute a morphologically distinct tumor variant (402).

The frequency of apocrine carcinoma in different series varies from less than 1 percent to about 4 percent of mammary carcinomas. When rigorously defined, not more than 1 percent of carcinomas can be classified as apocrine. Some carcinomas described under the term "histiocytoid" are probably examples of apocrine carcinoma while others appear to be variants of lobular carcinoma (390,405).

Clinical Presentation. There are no striking differences in the clinical features of patients with apocrine and nonapocrine duct carcinomas. Most authors have observed no difference in the age distribution either (388,391,395,398).

Patients who have invasive apocrine carcinoma usually present with a mass. Pain, symptoms of Paget disease, nipple discharge, and other symptoms are relatively uncommon initial manifestations. Occasionally, intraductal apocrine carcinoma forms a mass but more often it is detected by mammography. The majority of the lesions are located in the upper outer quadrant. The stage at diagnosis of apocrine carcinoma is not appreciably different from nonapocrine carcinomas and the frequency of bilaterality is not exceptional. Only occasionally is nonapocrine carcinoma found in the contralateral breast (391).

Hormone receptor analyses of apocrine carcinomas have yielded conflicting results. In one series (398), six tumors were estrogen (ER) and progesterone (PR) receptor negative, despite the fact that all of the patients were postmenopausal. Others found that about half of the tumors were estrogen receptor positive and that about one third were progesterone receptor positive (380,390).

Testosterone metabolism is enhanced in apocrine carcinomas (397), androgen metabolites are concentrated in some apocrine secretions (394), and the growth of cutaneous apocrine glands can be stimulated by androgens (404).

Apocrine carcinoma of the male breast is uncommon (383,392). One unusual apocrine male mammary carcinoma had a glandular structure and psammoma bodies.

Gross Findings. Invasive apocrine carcinomas are firm to hard tumors that usually have infiltrating rather than circumscribed borders. The bisected tumor is generally grey to white. The tan to brown color associated with some cellular benign apocrine lesions is less evident in apocrine carcinomas. Comedonecrosis is sometimes present in intraductal lesions.

Microscopic Findings. Apocrine carcinomas have the same structure as other mammary carcinomas, differing only in the cytologic appearance of the cells. Apocrine features have been noted in mucinous (391,396), lobular (390), tubular (380,396,398), and medullary carcinomas (384).

The architecture of apocrine intraductal carcinoma is similar to that commonly found in nonapocrine intraductal carcinomas including comedo, micropapillary, solid, and cribriform patterns (figs. 393–398). Calcifications are frequently seen in the affected ducts regardless of the growth pattern. Periductal fibrosis and inflammation are common reactive changes around the ducts. "Foamy" histiocytes may be a prominent feature of the reactive process (403) and should not be mistaken for invasive carcinoma cells. In some cases intraductal apocrine carcinoma is found to arise in complex papillary lesions in which there is also a benign hyperplastic component.

Cytologic features that characterize intraductal and invasive apocrine carcinomas are manifested in the nuclei and cytoplasm (figs. 399, 400). The nuclei are enlarged and pleomorphic when compared to the nuclei of benign apocrine cells. They contain nucleoli that typically are large, prominent, and usually eosinophilic although they occasionally exhibit basophilia. Some apocrine carcinomas have pleomorphic, deeply basophilic nuclei in which little or no internal structure can be discerned. In these cells nucleoli are usually not evident. In most cases the cytoplasm exhibits eosinophilia that

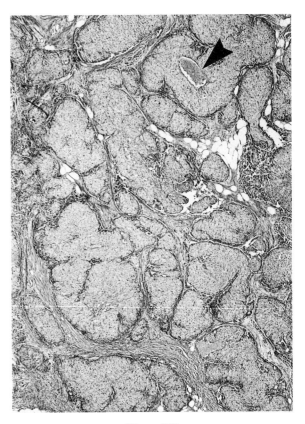

Figure 393
INTRADUCTAL APOCRINE CARCINOMA
Solid and comedo (arrow) growth patterns. Note overall pallor at this low magnification. (Fig. 5 from Abati AD, Kimmel M, Rosen PP. Apocrine mammary carcinoma. A clinicopathologic study of 72 cases. Am J Clin Pathol 1990;94: 371–7.) (Figures 393 and 394 are from the same patient.)

may be homogeneous or granular. Cytoplasmic vacuolization or clearing are features associated with atypical apocrine proliferations and are most prominent in apocrine carcinomas. Lymphatic tumor emboli may present with increased frequency in breast parenchyma around invasive apocrine carcinomas (388,400).

The finding of atypical apocrine cells in a fine-needle aspirate may suggest a diagnosis of apocrine carcinoma (393). However, caution should be exercised in the evaluation of such findings, especially when the aspirate is obtained from a mammographically detected nonpalpable lesion. Apocrine metaplasia in sclerosing adenosis and radial scars, which may be identified by mammography, is often atypical (386).

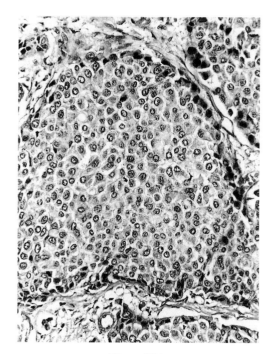

Figure 394
INTRADUCTAL APOCRINE CARCINOMA
Magnified view of tumor in figure 393.

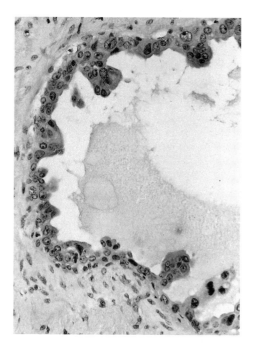

Figure 395
INTRADUCTAL APOCRINE CARCINOMA
Micropapillary growth pattern. (Figures 395 and 396 are
from the same patient.)

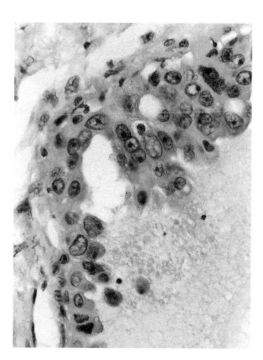

Figure 396
INTRADUCTAL APOCRINE CARCINOMA
In this lesion tumor cells have relatively dense, eosinophilic cytoplasm and pleomorphic nuclei that feature prominent nucleoli.

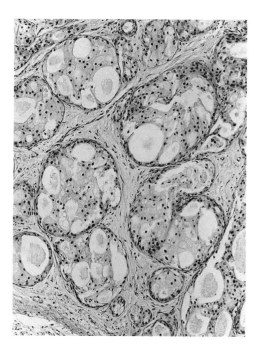

Figure 397
INTRADUCTAL APOCRINE
CARCINOMA
Cribriform pattern composed of cells with abundant, pale,
finely granular or vesicular cytoplasm with small uniform punc-
tate nuclei.

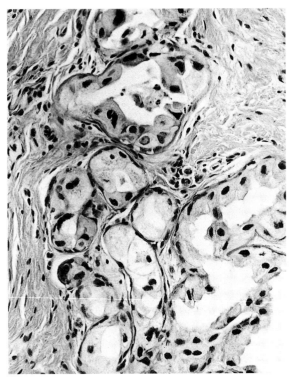

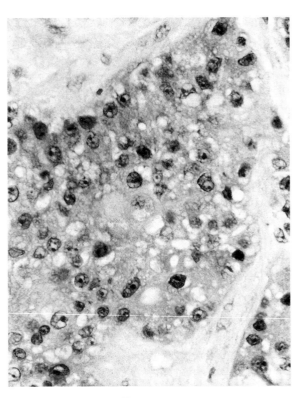

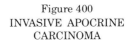

Figure 398
INTRADUCTAL APOCRINE CARCINOMA
Extension of duct carcinoma into terminal duct lobular epithelium is seen here. Tumor cells with pale, finely granular or vacuolated cytoplasm and pleomorphic hyperchromatic nuclei are evident in this variant.

Figure 399
INVASIVE APOCRINE CARCINOMA
Solid growth pattern. Note indistinct cell borders, vacuolated granular cytoplasm and vesicular nuclei with prominent nucleoli.

Figure 400
INVASIVE APOCRINE
CARCINOMA
Histiocytoid variant characterized by isolated cells that resemble histiocytes in desmoplastic stroma. This neoplasm can be confused with granular cell tumor.

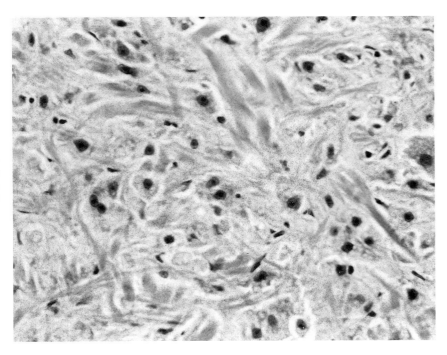

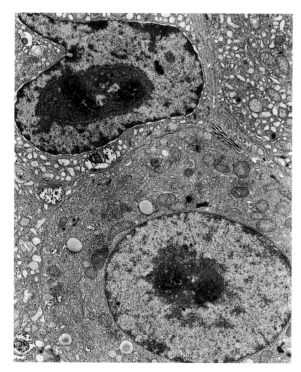

Figure 401
APOCRINE CARCINOMA
The cytoplasm contains numerous organelles including smooth endoplasmic reticulum and vesicular, rough endoplasmic reticulum. Note dense nucleoli (X7200).

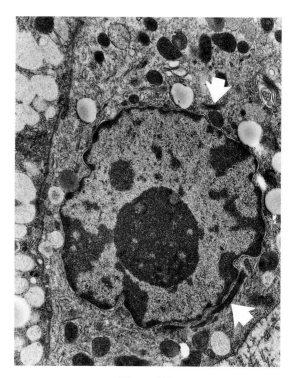

Figure 402
APOCRINE CARCINOMA
Numerous lipid droplets and lysosomes are present in addition to mitochondria. Arrows indicate cytokeratin filaments (X10800).

Immunohistochemistry. The tumor cells contain diastase-resistant periodic acid-Schiff–positive granules which also stain with toluidine blue and appear red with the trichrome stain. Cytoplasmic iron granules, a feature of benign apocrine cells, are variably present. Occasional cells may contain mucicarmine-positive secretion but most tumors are negative for mucin and alpha-lactalbumin (385,389).

Apocrine carcinomas tend to be immunoreactive for CEA (403), negative for S-100, and reactive for cytokeratins. Benign and malignant apocrine cells are strongly immunoreactive for gross cystic disease fluid protein-15 (GCDFP-15). This marker was positive in 55 percent of carcinomas including 75 percent of those with apocrine histologic features, 70 percent of intraductal carcinomas, and 90 percent of infiltrating lobular carcinomas that had signet ring cell features (390,396,398). Positive staining was found in only 23 percent of carcinomas that did not have apocrine features and in 5 percent of medullary carcinomas. Staining for GCDFP-15 has not been a useful predictor of prognosis (396).

Electron Microscopy. At the ultrastructural level, apocrine carcinoma cells contain abundant organelles including many mitochondria varying in size (399) and often having incomplete cristae and varying numbers of osmiophilic secretory granules (figs. 401–403) (390,398,403,407). Many tumor cells also contain empty vesicles of about the same size as the osmiophilic granules.

Prognosis and Treatment. The prognosis of apocrine carcinoma, whether intraductal or invasive, is determined mainly by conventional prognostic factors such as grade, tumor size, and nodal status (380,388,391,395). Apocrine differentiation should be mentioned as a descriptive feature of the lesion but presently it does not seem to be a determinant of prognosis or treatment. The observation that androgen metabolism is altered in apocrine carcinoma cells may prove therapeutically useful in the future (397).

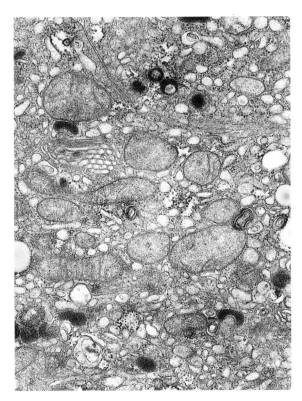

Figure 403
APOCRINE CARCINOMA
The cytoplasm is filled with numerous lysosomes, lipid droplets, dilated mitochondria, and vesicular endoplasmic reticulum.

CARCINOMA WITH ENDOCRINE FEATURES

Some mammary carcinomas synthesize substances, including hormones, not considered to be normal products of the breast. The capacity to produce ectopic hormones is considered endocrine or biochemical metaplasia. Breast carcinomas have been found to contain peptide hormones including human chorionic gonadotrophin (HCG) (445), calcitonin (426), adrenal corticotropic hormone (ACTH) (416), parathormone (433), and epinephrine (428), detectable not only by biochemical analysis but also morphologically by immunohistochemical study of the tumor tissue.

In a few unusual instances, the microscopic growth pattern simulates the structure of nonmammary neoplasms that commonly contain the hormone in question, resulting in coincidental structural as well as biochemical metaplasia. A striking example of this combined metaplasia

is mammary carcinoma with choriocarcinomatous differentiation (445). Here, areas that microscopically look like trophoblast are strongly reactive for the beta unit of HCG. Isolated carcinoma cells reactive immunohistologically for alpha- and beta-HCG can be found in 15 to 21 percent of ordinary infiltrating duct carcinomas that do not exhibit choriocarcinomatous metaplasia (431). These HCG-reactive cells are otherwise morphologically indistinguishable microscopically from surrounding carcinoma cells that are not immunoreactive for HCG. The presence of these occasional HCG-positive cells does not appear to have prognostic significance (431) and no functional effects have been described.

A more frequent form of biochemical and structural metaplasia occurs in mammary carcinomas containing argyrophilic cytoplasmic granules, detected by light microscopy employing histochemical techniques. In the argyrophil reaction (e.g., Grimelius stain) an exogenous reducing agent is added since some granules do not contain endogenous reducing substances. Because most cells with either argentaffin or argyrophilic granules are visualized with the argyrophil reaction, this is the preferable procedure. Breast neoplasms that contain argyrophilic granules have been argentaffin negative (414,423,437,441). The presence of these granules has conventionally been associated with neuroendocrine neoplasms such as carcinoid tumors of the intestine. The reported frequency of argyrophilia in female mammary carcinomas varies from 3 (446) to 25 percent (Table 4) (436). A few descriptions of argyrophil-positive tumors in men have been published (428,429,442,450). Scopsi et al. (448) reported finding argyrophilic cells in 28 of 134 (20.8 percent) male carcinomas.

Clinical Presentation. There are no specific clinical features associated with mammary carcinomas that exhibit structural and/or histochemical evidence of endocrine differentiation. The majority of the patients present with a palpable tumor. Systemic evidence of ectopic hormonal secretion has been absent in all but a few cases. Individual case reports have described patients with symptoms attributable to ectopic ACTH (416), parathormone (433), and epinephrine (428) secreted by mammary carcinomas.

Argyrophilia has been identified in breast carcinomas throughout the age distribution of that

Table 4

FREQUENCY OF ARGYROPHILIA IN FEMALE BREAST CARCINOMAS

Reference	No. Cases Studied	Argyrophilia No. (percent)
Santini et al. (446)	70	2 (3)
Partanen et al. (441)	90	3 (3.3)
Azzopardi et al. (409)	67	3 (4.5)
McCutcheon et al. (434)	42	3 (7)
Toyoshima (450)	253	27 (10.7)
Fetissof et al. (423)	92	19 (21)
Nesland et al. (436)	68	17 (25)
Total	682	74 (10.8)

disease: early thirties to late eighties (409,419, 423,437,450). An association between argyrophilia and positive, often very high levels of estrogen receptors determined biochemically has been described (412,414,437,450). In one series, the majority of argyrophilic tumors were also progesterone receptor positive (437).

Gross Findings. Argyrophilic mammary carcinomas have not exhibited specific gross pathologic features. The invasive tumors generally measure 1 to 5 cm in diameter with the majority between 1.5 and 3.0 cm. They are likely to be grossly circumscribed but some have invasive borders. Most have been solitary but in rare cases multiple foci of carcinoma were described in the breast (437).

Microscopic Findings. Many of the tumors that contain argyrophilic granules are infiltrating duct carcinomas with varying degrees of differentiation. Argyrophilic cells can be found in the intraductal as well as invasive portion of these tumors (figs. 404,405) (419,441). Argyrophilia has also been detected in other tumor types including tubular (434), intraductal (408,418), in situ lobular (449), infiltrating lobular (434,436, 441), mucinous (423,425,441), and papillary (442) carcinomas. Maluf et al. (432) described an unusual solid papillary variant of mucinous carcinoma that exhibited argyrophilic differentiation.

The reported frequency of argyrophilic infiltrating duct carcinomas varies from 15 (423) to 71 percent (437), and among infiltrating lobular carcinomas, 50 (423) to 100 percent (437) have reportedly been argyrophilic. A few examples of medullary (423,441), adenoid cystic (423), and apocrine (441) carcinomas did not contain detectable argyrophilic granules. An invasive small cell carcinoma with oat cell features and neuroendocrine differentiation was described in a single case report (451). Some argyrophilic granules have proven to contain mucin.

A number of argyrophilic cancers have "endocrine" growth patterns that resemble carcinoid tumors arising in other organs (fig. 406). The term *primary carcinoid tumor of the breast* was introduced in 1977 to describe these neoplasms (419). Carcinoid-like characteristics include the arrangement of tumor cells in nests and cords separated by bands of stroma, which may be highly vascular or densely collagenous areas with ribbon and papillary patterns, and microgland formation. Typically, the tumors are composed of small cells with poorly defined cell borders and hyperchromatic round to oval nuclei. The tumors are positive with the Grimelius stain (argyrophilic) and negative with the Fontana-Masson stain for argentaffin granules (fig. 407).

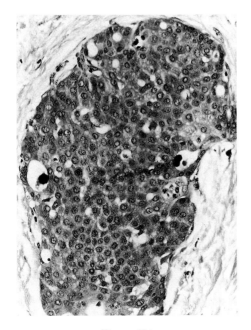

Figure 404
INTRADUCTAL CARCINOMA
WITH ENDOCRINE FEATURES
Intraductal carcinoma composed of small cells with uniform round nuclei and dense, deeply stained amphophilic cytoplasm. Some individual degenerating cells are evident. (Figures 404 and 405 are from the same patient.)

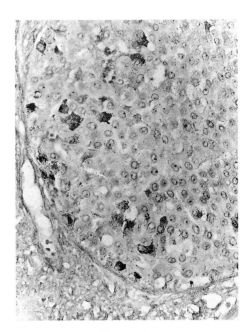

Figure 405
INTRADUCTAL CARCINOMA
WITH ENDOCRINE FEATURES
Isolated cells in the intraductal carcinoma contain fine black argyrophilic granules. The cells were immunoreactive for chromogranin (Grimelius stain).

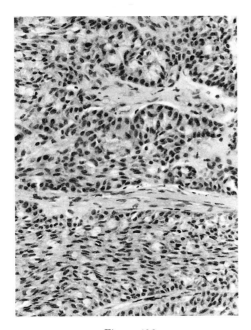

Figure 406
INVASIVE DUCT CARCINOMA
WITH ENDOCRINE FEATURES
Endocrine "ribbon" growth pattern in which some tumor cells have a spindle shape. (Figures 406 and 407 are from the same patient.)

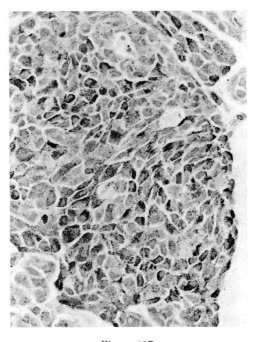

Figure 407
INVASIVE DUCT CARCINOMA
WITH ENDOCRINE FEATURES
Numerous cells contain fine argyrophilic Grimelius-positive granules. The tumor was immunoreactive for chromogranin.

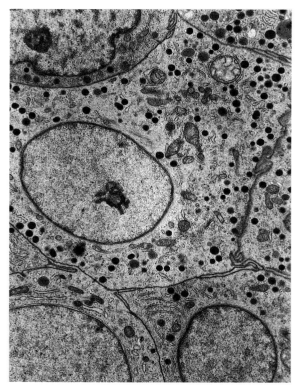

Figure 408
CARCINOMA WITH ENDOCRINE FEATURES
Dense core granules are distributed throughout the cytoplasm but they tend to concentrate near the cell membrane. Mitochondria and cytofilaments are evident (X2880).

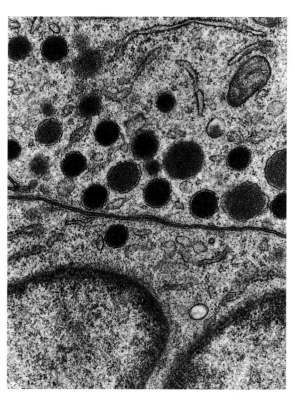

Figure 409
CARCINOMA WITH ENDOCRINE FEATURES
Dense core granules that measure 270 to 430 nm clustered near the cell membrane (X7200).

The concept of a primary carcinoid tumor of the breast has been the subject of considerable controversy (409,423,425,441,446,449,450). Although some argyrophilic mammary carcinomas have microscopic structural features of an endocrine neoplasm, others are microscopically indistinguishable from argyrophil-negative mammary carcinomas (447). Not all carcinomas with an endocrine growth pattern contain argyrophilic cells and it has not been possible to demonstrate polypeptide hormones or biogenic amines in most argyrophilic carcinomas (415,423,435). Despite the efforts of many investigators to find progenitor argyrophilic cells in normal mammary duct epithelium, such cells have rarely been detected, and then only in small numbers (411,424,425).

These and other observations have led most investigators to conclude that neoplasms with argyrophilic granules do not constitute a specific histopathologic category of female mammary carcinoma (415,436,437). These are variants of mammary adenocarcinoma in which neuroendocrine traits constitute structural and/or biochemical metaplasia presumed to result from altered gene expression or "genomic derepression" as a consequence of neoplastic transformation (441). A similar hypothesis has been proposed to explain the finding of neurosecretory granules in neoplasms in other organs, such as small cell carcinoma of the urinary bladder (417) and the lung (410).

Electron Microscopy, Immunohistochemistry, and Cytology. Neuroendocrine secretions are packaged in round dense core granules that typically measure between 100 and 400 nm, averaging about 250 nm (figs. 408, 409). It is not possible to determine the nature of the secretory product from the ultrastructural appearance of the granule. Dense core granules have been found in mammary carcinomas that were proven to produce clinically detectable ACTH (416) and norepinephrine (428).

239

Little success has been achieved in characterizing the secretory products within the dense core granules that contain chromogranin A and B (438). Nesland et al. (437) studied 22 carcinomas found to contain dense core granules by electron microscopy. Eighteen of the lesions contained argyrophilic granules when tested with the Grimelius stain. Nine of the 10 tumors immunoreactive for one or two neuropeptides were argyrophilic. Immunoelectron microscopy was carried out with the protein A–gold method (444) for neuropeptides (bombesin, somatostatin, vasoactive intestinal peptide (VIP), gastrin, ACTH) seen by light microscopic immunohistochemistry. No granules were marked at the ultrastructural level by these antisera. The only positive finding was scattered granules that exhibited reactivity for casein.

Attempts to demonstrate peptide hormones in argyrophilic tumor cells have yielded negative results in most cases. Chromogranin A, a specific marker of a component of neuroendocrine granules, has been detected in about 50 percent of female (412) and 14 percent of male argyrophilic carcinomas while 61 percent of male argyrophilic carcinomas contained chromogranin B (448). Synaptophysin, a marker associated with presynaptic vesicles in neuroendocrine cells, was found in 9 of a consecutive series of 100 carcinomas (439). Five of these tumors were argyrophilic. In the same series, somatostatin receptors were present in 17 tumors, including 7 with high receptor density. Five of these 7 tumors were argyrophilic and 6 were synaptophysin positive. Ultrastructural study demonstrated presynaptic clear vesicles in the cytoplasm of cells immunoreactive for synaptophysin (413,441). ACTH and HCG were demonstrated immunohistochemically in one tumor (427). The cytologic features of mammary endocrine carcinoma have been reported (430).

Prognosis and Treatment. Argyrophilic breast tumors are best diagnosed as mammary carcinomas with endocrine features. If ectopic hormones are detected, they should be specified. An example is "infiltrating duct carcinoma with endocrine features, argyrophil and ACTH positive." Endocrine differentiation should be confirmed with the chromogranin stain.

Relatively little information is available about prognosis. Nearly half of the patients have had axillary node metastases (409,412,419,437,441). While it appears that stage at diagnosis is the major determinant of prognosis (450), there have been no case controlled studies comparing patients who have mammary carcinoma with endocrine differentiation to age and stage matched control groups. One study limited to mucinous carcinomas, found that 23 of 75 tumors (31 percent) were argyrophilic with the Grimelius stain (420). These patients were more likely to have axillary node metastases (48 percent) than those with Grimelius-negative tumors (26 percent), as well as a higher frequency of recurrence and death due to breast carcinoma (65 percent versus 33 percent). In another study, however, the presence or absence of argyrophilic granules did not influence the prognosis of patients with mucinous carcinoma (443). Argyrophilia does not appear to affect the prognosis of male breast carcinoma (448).

At present, it appears that the choice of primary treatment for mammary carcinomas with argyrophilia should be determined by conventional clinical and pathologic parameters. Until further information becomes available, ectopic hormone production or endocrine differentiation have not been proven to be factors that significantly influence prognosis or treatment.

GLYCOGEN-RICH CARCINOMA

Extraction of the water soluble glycogen during histologic processing causes the cytoplasm of glycogen-rich carcinoma cells to appear vacuolated and optically clear in routine sections. Thirty-one cases have been described since the first in 1981 (452–457). Six of 439 (1.4 percent) cases of breast carcinoma in a population based study were glycogen-rich clear cell carcinoma (457).

Clinical Presentation. The patients ranged in age from 41 to 78 years. Most tumors measured between 2 and 5 cm, with the largest lesion 10 cm clinically (456). Two tumors were estrogen receptor positive and progesterone receptor negative (452,454) and one tumor was negative for estrogen and progesterone receptors (456).

Gross Findings. No specific gross features have been identified. A papillary component was noted grossly in one case (454).

Microscopic Findings. The lesions have the structural features of intraductal and infiltrating duct carcinoma. When present, the intraductal component has compact solid, comedo, or papillary growth patterns. The invasive tumor forms cords, solid nests, or papillary structures

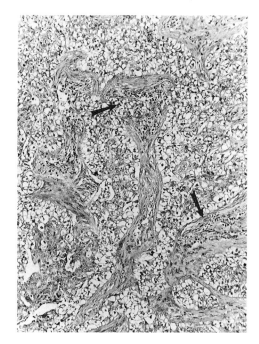

Figure 410
GLYCOGEN-RICH CARCINOMA
At low magnification the tumor is composed of sheets and broad bands of polygonal cells that have distinct cell borders, small nuclei, and clear cytoplasm. Lymphocytes and plasma cells are distributed in the fibrovascular stroma (arrows).

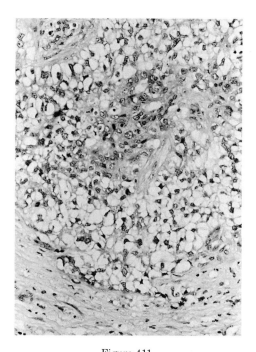

Figure 411
GLYCOGEN-RICH CARCINOMA
Clear cells surround a small group of tumor cells with less vesicular amphophilic cytoplasm.

(fig. 410). Clear cell glycogen-rich variants of tubular and medullary carcinoma have been noted (453). Lymphatic tumor emboli and perineural invasion have been reported.

Cytologically, the tumor cells tend to have sharply defined borders and polygonal rather than rounded contours. The cytoplasm is clear and, less often, finely granular or foamy (fig. 411). The central or eccentrically placed nuclei are hyperchromatic, sometimes exhibiting clumped chromatin and nucleoli. The cytoplasm gives a positive, diastase-labile reaction with the PAS stain (fig. 412). The cells are only focally Alcian blue or mucicarmine positive (455,456) and the oil red O stain for lipid is negative (5). In one case the tumor cells were immunoreactive for CEA, cytokeratin, and EMA but negative for alpha-lactalbumin, desmin, and vimentin (456). Electron microscopy reveals pools of nonmembrane-bound glycogen as well as smaller amounts of glycogen intermixed with cytoplasmic organelles (452,456). Glycogen-rich clear cell carcinomas are reported to be nondiploid and to have a high S-phase fraction (mean 19.2 percent) (457).

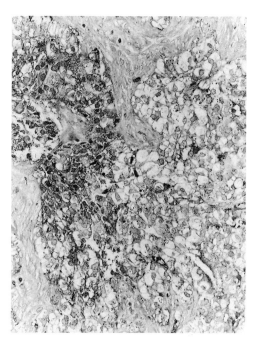

Figure 412
GLYCOGEN-RICH CARCINOMA
Formalin-fixed paraffin-embedded tissue stained with the periodic acid–Schiff reaction reveals abundant glycogen which appears as fine dark granules. Staining was abolished by pretreatment with diastase.

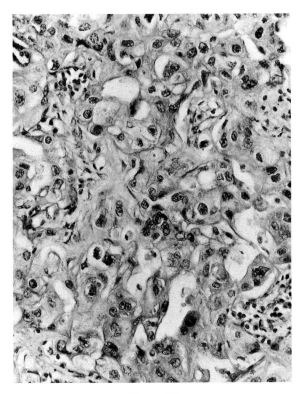

Figure 413
LIPID-RICH CARCINOMA
Polygonal carcinoma cells with distinct cell borders and variable cytoplasmic clearing. This tumor, obtained from an elderly woman, was oil red O positive.

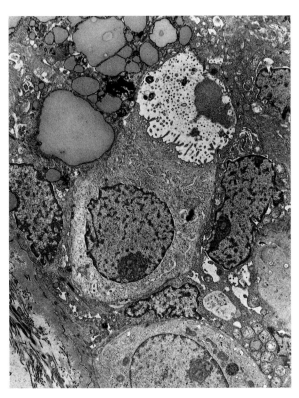

Figure 414
LIPID-RICH CARCINOMA
In this electron micrograph, the tumor cell in the center of the picture has a cytoplasmic lumen lined by microvilli and lipid droplets (upper right corner). Mitochondria are also present (arrow). A thickened basement membrane is evident in the lower left corner (X4320).

Prognosis and Treatment. Almost all patients have been treated by mastectomy and axillary dissection. More than half had metastatic tumor in the axillary lymph nodes. The prognosis is not favorable and may be worse than that of ordinary invasive duct carcinoma when compared on a stage-matched basis (453). In one series, 50 percent of the women treated by mastectomy died of metastatic mammary carcinoma 1 to 175 months (median 15 months) after diagnosis and one was alive with recurrent carcinoma 36 months after local excision and lymph node dissection (455). Except for one woman who underwent simple mastectomy without axillary dissection, all patients with recurrent or fatal disease had axillary node metastases. In another report, 5 of 6 women had axillary node metastases at the time of diagnosis and died of breast carcinoma within 7 years (457).

LIPID-RICH CARCINOMA

This rare variant of infiltrating duct carcinoma is composed of cells that contain abundant lipid (fig. 413) (458–460). The tumor cells have small, round, uniform nuclei and clear vacuolated cytoplasm, and are therefore similar to cells found in clear cell renal carcinoma. The presence of lipid can be demonstrated in frozen sections of fresh tissue, by electron microscopy, or in tissue prepared by processes that preserve cytoplasmic lipids (fig. 414).

The disease was first described by Aboumrad et al. (458) who estimated the frequency of lipid-rich carcinoma to be 1 percent. Ramos and Taylor (459) described 13 cases with the growth pattern of lipid-rich carcinoma seen in routine histologic sections but lipid was found in only 4 unfixed specimens. Eleven of 12 patients treated by radical mastectomy had axillary lymph node metastases. In a follow-up of less than 2 years, 6 patients died of metastatic disease, 2 were alive with recurrence, and the remainder were alive and disease free.

CRIBRIFORM CARCINOMA

Cribriform carcinoma is a well-differentiated variant of invasive duct carcinoma. Tumors with an invasive component growing largely in a cribriform pattern, often with a tubular carcinoma component, have been termed *classic cribriform carcinomas*. A diagnosis of *mixed invasive cribriform carcinoma* has been reserved for tumors in which less than 50 percent of the lesion is composed of cribriform areas, the remainder consisting of less well-differentiated non-cribriform components. Approximately 6 percent of invasive mammary carcinomas have a cribriform element with nearly equal proportions of "pure" and "mixed" lesions (462,464).

Clinical Presentation. One male and 113 female patients (ranging in age from 19 to 86 years) have been described (462,464,465). Venable et al. (464) found 16 classic and mixed cribriform carcinomas that were estrogen receptor positive and 11 (69 percent) that were also progesterone receptor positive.

Gross Findings. No distinctive gross pathologic features have been noted. In one study 7 of 35 (20 percent) patients with classic and 1 of 16 (6 percent) patients with a mixed cribriform carcinoma had grossly apparent multifocal invasive foci in the affected breast (462).

Microscopic Findings. The invasive component of cribriform carcinoma has the sieve-like growth pattern of conventional cribriform intraductal carcinomas (fig. 415). The round and angular masses of uniform, well-differentiated tumor cells are embedded in collagenous stroma. In some cases it may be difficult or impossible to distinguish between intraductal and invasive components of the lesion. When present, myoepithelial cells serve as a clue to intraductal carcinoma. Mucin-positive secretion is present in varying amounts within these lumens. Electron microscopy reveals luminal differentiation of tumor cells that have microvilli and are joined by tight junctions (465). Only a few scattered remnants of basal lamina are present. Neurosecretory-type granules have not been found (464,465).

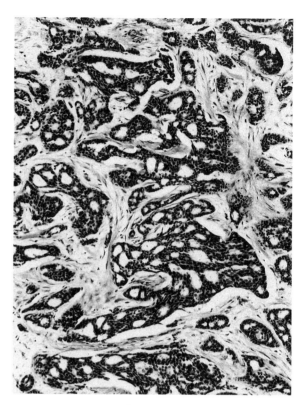

Figure 415
CRIBRIFORM CARCINOMA
Invasive duct carcinoma with a cribriform pattern characterized by extensive secondary lumen formation within angular masses of tumor cells.

In addition to the cribriform structure, a minority of tumors have tubular areas comprising up to 50 percent of the tumor (462,464). Page et al. (461) found tubular differentiation in 17 percent of classic tumors. When present, nodal metastases from classic tumors usually also have a cribriform structure while those derived from mixed tumors are more likely to have a less well-differentiated noncribriform pattern (462,464). Cribriform areas may also be found in adenoid cystic carcinomas when gland formation is more prominent than cylindromatous elements. They are part of the spectrum of adenoid cystic carcinoma (463) although the term *adenocystic* has been applied to such lesions (461). Cribriform carcinoma lacks the cylindromatous component that characterizes adenoid cystic carcinoma. An invasive carcinoma with tubular elements in which more than 25 percent of the invasive neoplasm has a cribriform pattern should be classified as a cribriform rather than a tubular carcinoma.

Prognosis and Treatment. Most patients have been treated by mastectomy and axillary dissection (462,464). Two studies concluded that patients with classic cribriform carcinoma are less likely to develop axillary lymph node metastases than women with mixed cribriform (462) or ordinary invasive duct carcinoma (464). No deaths due to classic cribriform carcinoma oc- curred among 34 patients with follow-up of 10 to 21 years (462), although one patient had recur- rence and another died of metastases from a contralateral carcinoma. Among 16 women with mixed cribriform carcinoma followed an average of 12.5 years, there were 6 deaths (38 percent) from breast carcinoma. Venable et al. (464) re- ported a disease-free survival of 100 percent among 45 patients with classic cribriform carci- noma followed for 1 to 5 years.

REFERENCES

Invasive Ductal Carcinoma

1. Adair F, Berg J, Joubert L, Robbins GF. Long-term follow-up of breast cancer patients: the 30-year report. Cancer 1974;33:1145–50.
2. Alderson MR, Hamlin I, Staunton MD. The relative significance of prognostic factors in breast carcinoma. Br J Cancer 1971;25:646–56.
3. Ali IU, Campbell G, Libereau R, Callahan R. Lack of evidence for the prognostic significance of c-*erb*B-2 amplification in human breast carcinoma. Oncogene Res 1988;3:139–46.
4. Andersen JA, Fischermann K, Hou-Jensen K, et al. Selection of high risk groups among prognostically favorable patients with breast cancer. An analysis of the value of prospective grading of tumor anaplasia in 1048 patients. Ann Surg 1981;194:1–3.
5. Baak JP, VanDop H, Kurver PH, Hermans J. The value of morphometry to classic prognosticators in breast cancer. Cancer 1985;56:374–82.
6. Barnard NJ, Hall PA, Lemoine NR, Kadar N. Prolifer- ative index in breast carcinoma determined in situ by Ki-67 immunostaining and its relationship to clinical and pathological variables. J Pathol 1987;152:287–95.
7. Bell JR, Friedell GH, Goldenberg IS. Prognostic signif- icance of pathologic findings in human breast carci- noma. Surg Gynecol Obstet 1969;129:258–62.
8. Bettelheim R, Penman HG, Thornton-Jones H, Neville AM. Prognostic significance of peritumoral vascular invasion in breast cancer. Br J Cancer 1984;50:771–7.
9. Bilik R, Mor C, Haraz B, Moroz C. Characterization of T-lymphocyte subpopulations infiltrating primary breast cancer. Cancer Immunol Immunother 1989;28:143–7.
10. Black MM, Barclay TH, Hankey BF. Prognosis in breast cancer utilizing histologic characteristics of the primary tumor. Cancer 1975;36:2048–55.
11. _____, Speer FD. Nuclear structure in cancer tissues. Surg Gynecol Obstet 1957;105:97–102.
12. Bloom HJ, Richardson WW. Histological grading and prognosis in breast cancer. A study of 1049 cases of which 359 have been followed for 15 years. Br J Cancer 1957;11:359–77.
13. Carter D, Pipkin RD, Shepard RH, Elkins RC, Abbey H. Relationship of necrosis and tumor border to lymph node metastases and 10-year survival in carcinoma of the breast. Am J Surg Pathol 1978;2:39–46.
14. Clark GM, Dressler LG, Owens MA, Pounds G, Olda- ker T, McGuire WL. Prediction of relapse or survival in patients with node-negative breast cancer by DNA flow cytometry. N Engl J Med 1989;320:627–33.
15. Cline MJ, Battifora H, Yokota J. Proto-oncogene abnor- malities in human breast cancer: correlations with anatomic features and clinical course of disease. J Clin Oncol 1987;5:999–1006.
16. Coussens L, Yang-Feng TL, Liao YC, et al. Tyrosine kinase receptor with extensive homology to EGF recep- tor shares chromosomal location with *neu* oncogene. Science 1985;230:1132–9.
17. Dawson PJ, Ferguson DJ, Karrison T. The pathological findings of breast cancer in patients surviving 25 years after radical mastectomy. Cancer 1982;50:2131–8.
18. Dressler LG, Seamer LC, Owens MA, Clark GM, McGuire WL. DNA flow cytometry and prognostic factors in 1331 frozen breast cancer specimens. Cancer 1988;61:420–7.
19. Dwarakanath S, Lee AK, DeLellis RA, Silverman MA, Frasca L, Wolfe HJ. S-100 protein sensitivity in breast carcinomas: a potential pitfall in diagnostic immuno- histochemistry. Hum Pathol 1987;18:1144–8.
20. Early Breast Cancer Trialists' Collaborative Group. Effects of adjuvant tamoxifen and of cytotoxic therapy on mortality in early breast cancer. N Engl J Med 1988;319:1681–92.
21. Fenlon S, Ellis IO, Bell J, Todd JH, Elston CW, Blamey RW. *Helix pomatia* and *Ulex europaeus* lectin binding in human breast carcinoma. J Pathol 1987;152:169–76.
22. Fisher ER, Gregorio RM, Fisher B, et al. The pathology of invasive breast cancer. A syllabus derived from find- ings of the National Surgical Adjuvant Breast Project (No.4). Cancer 1975;36:1–85.
23. _____, Sass R, Watkins G, et al. Tissue mast cells in breast cancer. Breast Cancer Res Treat 1985;5:285–91.
24. Freedman LS, Edwards DN, McConnell EM, Downham DY. Histological grade and other prognostic factors in relation to survival of patients with breast cancer. Br J Cancer 1979;40:44–55.

25. Friedell GH, Betts A, Sommers SC. The prognostic value of blood vessel invasion and lymphocytic infiltrates in breast carcinoma. Cancer 1965;18:164–6.

26. Gentili C, Sanfilippo O, Silvestrini R. Cell proliferation and its relationship to clinical features and relapse in breast cancers. Cancer 1981;48:974–9.

27. Gerdes J, Lemke H, Baisch H, Wacker HH, Schwab U, Stein H. Cell cycle analysis of cell proliferation-associated human nuclear antigen defined by the monoclonal antibody Ki-67. J Immunol 1984;133:1710–5.

28. Gilchrist KW, Kalish L, Gould VE, et al. Immunostaining for carcinoembryonic antigen does not discriminate for early recurrence in breast cancer. The ECOG experience. Cancer 1985;56:351–5.

29. Glaubitz LC, Bowen JH, Cox ED, McCarty KS. Elastosis in human breast cancer. Correlation with sex steroid receptors and comparison with clinical outcome. Arch Pathol Lab Med 1984;108:27–30.

30. Gold RH, Main G, Zippin C, Annes GP. Infiltration of mammary carcinoma as an indicator of axillary node metastasis. A preliminary report. Cancer 1972;29:35–40.

31. Gratzner HG. Monoclonal antibody to 5-bromo- and 5-iododeoxyuridine: a new reagent for detection of DNA replication. Science 1982;218:474–5.

32. Grudzinskas JG, Coombes RC, Ratcliffe JG, et al. Circulating levels of pregnancy specific beta 1 glycoprotein in patients with testicular, bronchogenic and breast carcinomas. Cancer 1980;45:102–3.

33. Gusterson BA, Machin LG, Gullick WJ, et al. C-*erb*B-2 expression in benign and malignant breast disease. Br J Cancer 1988;58:453–7.

34. _____, Machin LG, Gullick WJ, et al. Immunohistochemical distribution of c-*erb*B-2 in infiltrating and in situ breast cancer. Int J Cancer 1988;42:842–5.

35. Halter SA, Fraker LD, Parmenter M, Dupont WD. Carcinoembryonic antigen expression and patient survival in carcinoma of the breast. Oncology 1984;41:297–302.

36. Hamada S. A double labeling technique combining ^{3}H-thymidine autoradiography with BrdUrd immunocytochemistry [Letter]. Acta Histochem Cytochem 1985; 18:267–70.

37. Hedley DW, Rugg CA, Gelber RD. Association of DNA index and S-phase fraction with prognosis of nodes positive early breast cancer. Cancer Res 1987;47:4729–35.

38. Henderson IC, Hayes DF, Parker, LM, et al. Adjuvant systemic therapy for patients with node-negative tumors. Cancer 1990; 65:2132–47.

39. Himel HN, Liberati A, Gelber R, et al. Adjuvant chemotherapy for breast cancer. A pooled estimate based on published randomized control trials. JAMA 1986; 256:1148–59.

40. Hopton DS, Thorogood J, Clayden AD, MacKinnon D. Histological grading of breast cancer: significance of grade on recurrence and mortality. Eur J Surg Oncol 1989;15:25–31.

41. Horny HP, Horst HA. Lymphoreticular infiltrates in invasive ductal breast cancer. A histological and immunohistological study. Virchows Arch [A] 1986;409:275–86.

42. Kallioniemi OP, Hietanen T, Mattila J, Lehtinen M, Lauslahti K, Koivula T. Aneuploid DNA content and high S-phase fraction of tumor cells are related to poor prognosis in patients with primary breast cancer. Eur J Cancer Clin Oncol 1987;23:277–82.

43. Kamata T, Feramisco JR. Epidermal growth factor stimulates guanine nucleotide binding activity and phosphorylation of ras oncogene proteins. Nature 1984;310:147–50.

44. Kamel OW, Franklin WA, Ringus JC, Meyer JS. Thymidine labeling index and Ki-67 growth fraction in lesions of the breast. Am J Pathol 1989;134:107–13.

45. King CR, Kraus MH, Aaronson SA. Amplification of a novel v-*erb*B-related gene in a human mammary carcinoma. Science 1985;229:974–6.

46. Kister SJ, Sommers SC, Haagensen CD, Cooley E. Re-evaluation of blood-vessel invasion as a prognostic factor in carcinoma of the breast. Cancer 1966;19:1213–6.

47. Klintenberg C, Stål O, Nordenskjöld B, Wallgren A, Arjvidsson S, Skoog L. Proliferative index, cytosol estrogen receptor and axillary node status as prognostic predictors in human mammary carcinoma. Breast Cancer Res Treat 1986;7(Suppl):99–106.

48. Kuhajda FP, Bohn H, Mendelsohn G. Pregnancy-specific beta-1 glycoprotien (SP-1) in breast carcinoma. Pathologic and clinical considerations. Cancer 1984;54:1392–6.

49. Lane N. Goksel H, Salerno RA, Haagensen CD. Clinicopathologic analysis of the surgical curability of breast cancers. A minimum ten-year study of a personal series. Ann Surg 1961;153:483–98.

50. Le Doussal V, Tubiana-Hulin M, Friedman S, Hacene K, Spyratos F, Brunet M. Prognostic value of histologic grade nuclear components of Scarff-Bloom-Richardson (SBR). An improved score modification based on a multivariate analysis of 1262 invasive ductal carcinomas. Cancer 1989;64:1914–21.

51. _____, Zangerle PF, Collette J, et al. Immunohistochemical detection of alpha-lactalbumin in breast lesions. Eur J Cancer Clin Oncol 1984;20:1069–78.

52. Lee AK, DeLellis RA, Rosen PP, et al. ABH blood group isoantigen expression in breast carcinomas—an immunohistochemical evaluation using monoclonal antibodies. Am J Clin Pathol 1985;83:308–19.

53. _____, DeLellis RA, Wolfe HJ. Intramammary lymphatic invasion in breast carcinomas. Evaluation using ABH isoantigens as endothelial markers. Am J Surg Pathol 1986;10:589–94.

54. _____, Rosen PP, DeLellis RA, et al. Tumor marker expression in breast carcinomas and relationship to prognosis. An immunohistochemical study. Am J Clin Pathol 1985;85:687–96.

55. Lelle RJ, Heidenreich W, Stauch G, Gerdes J. The correlation of growth fractions with histologic grading and lymph node status in human mammary carcinoma. Cancer 1987;59:83-8.

56. Mæhle BO, Thoresen S, Skjærven R, Hartveit F. Mean nuclear area and histological grade of axillary node tumor in breast cancer, related to prognosis. Br J Cancer 1982;46:95–100.

57. Mansour EG, Hastert M, Park CH, Koehler KA, Petrelli M. Tissue and plasma carcinoembryonic antigen in early breast cancer. A prognostic factor. Cancer 1983;51:1243–8.

58. McDivitt RW, Stone KR, Craig B, Palmer JO, Meyers JS, Bauer WC. A proposed classification of breast cancer based on kinetic information: derived from a comparison of risk factors in 168 primary operable breast cancers. Cancer 1986;57:269–76.

59. McGurrin JF, Doria MI Jr, Dawson PJ, Karrison T, Stein H, Franklin WA. Assessment of tumor cell kinetics by immunohistochemistry in carcinoma of breast. Cancer 1987;59:1744–50.

60. Meyer JS, Coplin MD. Thymidine labeling index, flow cytometric S-phase measurement, and DNA index in human tumors. Am J Clin Pathol 1988;89:586–95.

61. _____, Prey MU, Babcock DS, McDivitt RW. Breast carcinoma cell kinetics, morphology, stage and host characteristics. A thymidine labelling study. Lab Invest 1986;54:41–51.

62. Moon TE, Jones SE, Bonadonna G, et al. Development and use of a natural history data base of breast cancer studies. Am J Clin Oncol 1987;10:396–403.

63. Moran RE, Black M, Alpert L, Straus MJ. Correlation of cell-cycle kinetics, hormone receptors, histopathology, and nodal status in human breast cancer. Cancer 1984;54:1586–90.

64. Nakajima T, Watanabe S, Sato Y, Kameya T, Hirota T, Shimasato Y. An immunoperoxidase study of S-100 protein distribution in normal and neoplastic tissues. Am J Surg Pathol 1982;6:715–26.

65. NIH Consensus Conference. Treatment of early-stage breast cancer. JAMA 1991;265:391–5.

66. Nime FA, Rosen PP, Thaler HT, Ashikari R, Urban JA. Prognostic significance of tumor emboli in intramammary lymphatics in patients with mammary carcinoma. Am J Surg Pathol 1977;1:25–30.

67. Olszewski W, Darzynkiewicz Z, Rosen PP, Schwartz MK, Melamed MR. Flow cytometry of breast carcinoma: I. Relation of DNA ploidy level to histology and estrogen receptor. Cancer 1981;48:980–4.

68. _____, Darzynkiewicz Z, Rosen PP, Schwartz MK, Melamed MR. Flow cytometry of breast carcinoma. II. Relation of tumor cell cycle distribution to histology and estrogen receptor. Cancer 1981;48:985–8.

69. Parl FF, Dupont WD. A retrospective cohort study of histologic risk factors in breast cancer patients. Cancer 1982;50:2410–6.

70. Rasmussen BB, Pedersen BV, Thorpe SM, Rose C. Elastosis in relation to prognosis in primary breast carcinoma. Cancer Res 1985;45:1428–30.

71. Raymond WA, Leong AS. Vimentin—a new prognostic parameter in breast carcinoma. J Pathol 1989;158:107–14.

72. _____, Leong AS. Co-expression of cytokeratin and vimentin intermediate filament proteins in benign and neoplastic breast epithelium. J Pathol 1989;157: 299–306.

73. Ridolfi RL, Rosen PP, Port A, Kinne D, Miké V. Medullary carcinoma of the breast. A clinicopathologic study with 10 year follow-up. Cancer 1977;40:1365–85.

74. Robertson AJ, Brown RA, Cree IA, MacGillivray JB, Slidders W, Beck JS. Prognostic value of measurement of elastosis in breast carcinoma. J Clin Pathol 1981; 34:738–43.

75. Robertson JF, Ellis IO, Bell J, et al. Carcinoembryonic antigen immunohistochemistry in primary breast carcinoma. Cancer 1989;64:1638–45.

76. Rosen PP. Tumor emboli in intramammary lymphatics in breast carcinoma: pathologic criteria for diagnosis and clinical significance. Pathol Annu 1983;18(Pt 2):215–32.

77. _____, Groshen S, Saigo PE, Kinne DW, Hellman S. A long-term follow-up study of survival in stage I (T1N0M0) and stage II (T1N1M0) breast carcinoma. J Clin Oncol 1989;7:355–66.

78. _____, Kinne DW, Lesser M, Hellman S. Are prognostic factors for local control of breast cancer treated by primary radiotherapy significant for patients treated by mastectomy? Cancer 1986;57:1415–20.

79. _____, Saigo PE, Braun DW Jr, Weathers E, DePalo, A. Predictors of recurrence in stage I (T1N0M0) breast carcinoma. Ann Surg 1981;193:15–25.

80. _____, Saigo PE, Braun DW, Weathers E, Kinne DW. Prognosis in stage II (T1N1M0) breast cancer. Ann Surg 1981;194:576–84.

81. Roses DF, Bell DA, Flotte TJ, Taylor R, Ratech H, Dubin N. Pathologic predictors of recurrence in stage 1 (T1N0M0) breast cancer. Am J Clin Pathol 1982;78:817–20.

82. Saigo PE, Rosen PP. The application of immunohistochemical stains to identify endothelial-lined channels in mammary carcinoma. Cancer 1987;59:51–4.

83. Sasaki K, Matsumura K, Tsuji T, Shinozaki F, Takahashi M. Relationship between labeling indices of Ki-67 and BrdUrd in human malignant tumors. Cancer 1988;62:989–93.

84. Schnitt SJ, Connolly JL, Harris JR, Hellman S, Cohen RB. Pathologic predictors of early local recurrence in stage I and II breast cancer treated by primary radiation therapy. Cancer 1984;53:1049–57.

85. Shivas AA, Douglas JG. The prognostic significance of elastosis in breast carcinoma. J R Coll Surg Edinb 1972;17:315–20.

86. Silverberg SG, Chitale AR. Assessment of significance of proportions of intraductal and infiltrating tumor growth in ductal carcinoma of the breast. Cancer 1973;32:830–7.

87. Slamon DJ, Clark GM, Wong SG, Levin WJ, Ullrich A, McGuire WL. Human breast cancer: correlation of relapse and survival with amplification of the HER-2/*neu* oncogene. Science 1987;235:177–82.

88. _____, Godolphin W, Jones LA, et al. Studies of the HER-2/*neu* proto-oncogene in human breast and ovarian cancer. Science 1989;244:707–12.

89. Smart CR, Myers MH, Gloeckler LA. Implications from SEER data on breast cancer management. Cancer 1978;41:787–9.

90. Smith SR, Howell A, Minawa A, Morrison JM. The clinical value of immunohistochemically demonstrable CEA in breast cancer: a possible method of selecting patients for adjuvant chemotherapy. Br J Cancer 1982;46:757–64.

91. Stenkvist B, Bengtsson E, Eriksson O, Jarkrans T, Nordin B. A morphometric expression of differentiation in fine-needle biopsies of breast cancer. Cytometry 1981;1:292–5

92. Tamura S, Enjoji M. Elastosis in neoplastic and non-neoplastic tissues from patients with mammary carcinoma. Acta Pathol Jpn 1988;38:1537–46.

93. Taylor IW, Musgrove EA, Friedlander ML, Foo MS, Hedley DW. The influence of age on the DNA ploidy levels of breast tumors. Eur J Cancer Clin Oncol 1983;19:623–8.

94. Teel P, Sommers SC. Vascular invasion as a prognostic factor in breast carcinoma. Surg Gynecol Obstet 1964;118:1006–8.

95. Thoresen S. Histological grading and clinical stage at presentation in breast carcinoma. Br J Cancer 1982;46:457–8.

96. Tsuda H, Hirohashi S, Shimosato Y, et al. Correlation between long-term survival in breast cancer patients and amplification of two putative oncogene-coamplification units: *hst*-1/*int*-2 and c-*erb*B-2/ear-1. Cancer Res 1989;49:3104–8.

97. Tubiana M, Pejovic MH, Chavaudra N, Contesso G, Malaise EP. The long-term prognostic significance of the thymidine labelling index in breast cancer. Int J Cancer 1984;33:441–5.

99. van de Vijver MJ, Peterse JL, Mooi WJ, et al. Neu-protein overexpression in breast cancer. Association with comedo-type ductal carcinoma in situ and limited prognostic value in stage II breast cancer. N Engl J Med 1988;319:1239–45.

98. Van der Linden HC, Baak JP, Lindeman J, Hermans J, Meyer CJ. Morphometry and breast cancer. II. Characterization of breast cancer cells with high malignant potential in patients with spread to lymph nodes: preliminary results. J Clin Pathol 1986;39:603–9.

100. Varley JM, Swallow JE, Brammar WJ, Whittaker JL, Walker RA. Alterations to either c-erbB-2 (neu) or c-myc proto-oncogenes in breast carcinomas correlate with poor short-term prognosis. Oncogene 1987;1:423–30.

101. Veronesi U, Banfi A, Salvadori B, et al. Breast conservation is the treatment of choice in small breast cancer: long-term results of a randomized trial. Eur J Cancer 1990;26:668–70.

102. Visscher DW, Zarbo RJ, Greenawald KA, Crissman JD. Prognostic significance of morphologic parameters and flow cytometric DNA analysis in carcinoma of the breast. Pathol Annu 1990;25(Pt 1):171–210.

103. Wachner R, Wittekind C, Von Kleist S. Immunohistological localization of beta-HCG in breast carcinomas. Eur J Cancer Clin Oncol 1984;20:679–84.

104. Walker RA. Demonstration of carcinoembryonic antigen in human breast carcinomas by the immunoperoxidase technique. J Clin Pathol 1980;33:356–60.

105. _____. Differentiation of human breast carcinomas: an immunohistological study of appropriate and inappropriate protein production. J Pathol 1981;135:87–95.

106. _____, Camplejohn RS. Comparison of monoclonal antibody Ki-67 reactivity with grade and DNA flow cytometry of breast carcinomas. Br J Cancer 1988;57:281–3.

107. Waseem NH, Lane DP. Monoclonal antibody analysis of the proliferating cell nuclear antigen (PCNA). Structural conservation and the detection of a nucleolar form. J Cell Sci 1990;96(Pt 1):121–9.

108. Weigand RA, Isenberg WM, Russo J, Brennan MJ, Rich MA. Blood vessel invasion and axillary lymph node involvement as prognostic indicators for human breast cancer. Cancer 1982;50:962–9.

109. Weikel W, Beck T, Mitze M, Knapstein PG. Immuno-histochemical evaluation of growth fractions in human breast cancers using monoclonal antibody Ki-67. Breast Cancer Res Treat 1991;18:149–54.

110. Whiteside TL, Miescher S, Hurlimann J, Moretta L, Von Fliedner V. Clonal analysis and in situ characterization of lymphocytes infiltrating human breast carcinomas. Cancer Immunol Immunother 1986;23:169–78.

111. Wick MR. Immunohistologic detection of ras oncogene products. Specific or spurious? [Editorial] Arch Pathol Lab Med 1989;113:13–5.

112. World Health Organization. Histological typing of breast tumours. 2nd ed. International Histological Classification of Tumours No. 2. Geneva: World Health Organization, 1981:19.

113. Wright C, Angus B, Nicholson S, et al. Expression of c-erbB-2 oncoprotein: a prognostic indicator in human breast cancer. Cancer Res 1989;49:2087–90.

114. Yokota J, Yamamoto T, Toyoshima K, et al. Amplification of the c-erbB-2 oncogene in human adenocarcinomas in vivo. Lancet 1986;1:765–7.

115. Zajdela A, De LaRiva LS, Ghossein NA. The relation of prognosis to the nuclear diameter of breast cancer cells obtained by cytologic aspiration. Acta Cytol 1979;23:75–80.

116. Zhou D, Battifora H, Yokota J, Yamamoto T, Cline MJ. Association of multiple copies of the c-erbB-2 oncogene with spread of breast cancer. Cancer Res 1987;47:6123–5.

Invasive Lobular Carcinoma

117. Allenby PA, Chowdhury LN. Histiocytic appearance of metastatic lobular breast carcinoma. Arch Pathol Lab Med 1986;110:759–60.

118. Ashikari R, Huvos AG, Urban JA, Robbins GF. Infiltrating lobular carcinoma of the breast. Cancer 1973;31:110–6.

119. Breslow A, Brancaccio ME. Intracellular mucin production by lobular breast carcinoma cells. Arch Pathol Lab Med 1976;100:620–1.

120. Davis RP, Nora PF, Kooy RG, Hines JR. Experience with lobular carcinoma of the breast. Emphasis on recent aspects of management. Arch Surg 1979;114:485–8.

121. Dearnaley DP, Sloane JP, Ormerod MG, et al. Increased detection of mammary carcinoma cells in marrow smears using antisera to epithelial membrane antigen. Br J Cancer 1981;44:85–90.

122. DiCostanzo D, Rosen PP, Gareen I, Franklin S, Lesser M. Prognosis in infiltrating lobular carcinoma. An analysis of "classical" and variant tumors. Am J Surg Pathol 1990;14:12–23.

123. Dixon JM, Anderson TJ, Page DL, Lee D, Duffy SW. Infiltrating lobular carcinoma of the breast. Histopathology 1982;6:149–61.

124. _____, Anderson TJ, Page DL, Lee D, Duffy SW, Stewart HJ. Infiltrating lobular carcinoma of the breast: an evaluation of the incidence and consequence of bilateral disease. Br J Surg 1983;70:513–6.

125. Du Toit RS, Locker AP, Ellis IO, Elston CW, Nicholson RI, Blamey RW. Invasive lobular carcinomas of the breast—the prognosis of histopathological subtypes. Br J Cancer 1989;60:605–9.

126. Eusebi V, Pich A, Macchiorlatti E, Bussolati G. Morphofunctional differentiation in lobular carcinoma of the breast. Histopathology 1977;1:301–14.

127. Fechner RE. Histologic variants of infiltrating lobular carcinoma of the breast. Hum Pathol 1975;6:373–8.

128. _____. Infiltrating lobular carcinoma without lobular carcinoma in situ. Cancer 1972;29:1539–45.

129. Fisher ER, Gregorio RM, Redmond C, Fisher B. Tubulolobular invasive breast cancer: a variant of lobular invasive cancer. Hum Pathol 1977;8:679–83.

130. Foote FW Jr, Stewart FW. A histologic classification of carcinoma of the breast. Surgery 1946;19:74–99.

131. _____, Stewart FW. Lobular carcinoma in situ: a rare form of mammary cancer. Am J Pathol 1941;17:491–6.

132. Gad A, Azzopardi JG. Lobular carcinoma of the breast: a special variant of mucin-secreting carcinoma. J Clin Pathol 1975;28:711–6.

133. Gagnon Y, Tètu B. Ovarian metastases of breast carcinoma. A clinicopathologic study of 59 cases. Cancer 1989;64:892–8.

134. Gould E, Perez J, Albores-Saavedra J, Legaspi A. Signet ring cell sinus histiocytosis. A previously unrecognized histologic condition mimicking metastatic adenocarcinoma in lymph nodes. Am J Clin Pathol 1989;92:509–12.

135. Gould VE, Chejfec G. Case 13: lobular carcinoma of the breast with secretory features. Ultrastruct Pathol 1980;1:151–6.

136. Harris M, Howell A, Chrissohou M, Swindell RI, Hudson M, Sellwood RA. A comparison of the metastatic pattern of infiltrating lobular carcinoma and infiltrating duct carcinoma of the breast. Br J Cancer 1984;50:23–30.

137. Hartmann WH, Sherlock P. Gastroduodenal metastases from carcinoma of the breast. An adrenal steroid-induced phenomenon. Cancer 1961;14:426–31.

138. Henson D, Tarone R. A study of lobular carcinoma of the breast based on the Third National Cancer Survey in the United States of America. Tumori 1979;65:133–42.

139. Hislop TG, Ng V, McBride ML, Coldman AJ, Worth AJ. Incidence and risk factors for second breast primaries in women with lobular breast carcinoma. Breast Dis 1990;3:95–105.

140. Jundt G, Schulz A, Heitz PU, Osborn M. Small cell neuroendocrine (oat cell) carcinoma of the male breast. Virchows Arch [A] 1984;404:213–21.

141. Klein MS, Sherlock P. Gastric and colonic metastases from breast cancer. Am J Dig Dis 1972;17:881–6.

142. Kurtz JM, Jacquemier J, Torhorst JR, et al. Conservation therapy for breast cancers other than infiltrating ductal carcinoma. Cancer 1989;63:1630–5.

143. Lesser ML, Rosen PP, Kinne DW. Multicentricity and bilaterality in invasive breast carcinoma. Surgery 1982;91:234–40.

144. _____, Rosen PP, Senie RT, Duthie K, Menendez-Botet C, Schwartz MK. Estrogen and progesterone receptors in breast carcinoma: correlations with epidemiology and pathology. Cancer 1981;48:299–309.

145. Martin MA, Welling RE, Strobel SL. Infiltrating lobular carcinoma of the breast treated with segmental and modified radical mastectomy. J Surg Oncol 1989;41:117–20.

146. Martinez V, Azzopardi JG. Invasive lobular carcinoma of the breast: incidence and variants. Histopathology 1979;3:467–48.

147. Murad TM. Ultrastructure of ductular carcinoma of the breast (in situ and infiltrating lobular carcinoma). Cancer 1971;27:18–28.

148. Nesland JM, Holm R, Johannessen JV. Ultrastructural and immunohistochemical features of lobular carcinoma of the breast. J Pathol 1985;145:39–52.

149. Nesland JM, Holm R, Lunde S, Johannessen JV. Diagnostic problems in breast pathology: the benefit of ultrastructural and immunocytochemical analysis. Ultrastruct Pathol 1987;11:293–311.

150. Newman W. Lobular carcinoma of the female breast. Report of 73 cases. Ann Surg 1966;164:305–14.

151. Oertel YC. Fine needle aspiration of the breast. Stoneham, Mass: Butterworth, 1987:145–9.

152. Richter GO, Dockerty MB, Clagett OT. Diffuse infiltrating scirrhous carcinoma of the breast. Special consideration of the single-filing phenomenon. Cancer 1967;20:363–70.

153. Rosen PP, Lesser ML, Kinne DW. Breast carcinoma at the extremes of age: a comparison of patients younger than 35 years and older than 75 years. J Surg Oncol 1985;28:90–6.

154. Schnitt SJ, Connolly JL, Recht A, Silver B, Harris JR. Influence of infiltrating lobular histology on local tumor control in breast cancer patients treated with conservative surgery and radiotherapy. Cancer 1989;64:448–54.

155. Shousha S, Backhous CM, Alaghband-Zadeh J, Burn I. Alveolar variant of invasive lobular carcinoma of the breast. A tumor rich in estrogen receptors. Am J Clin Pathol 1986;85:1–5.

156. _____, Bull TB, Burn I. Alveolar variant of invasive lobular carcinoma of the breast: an electron microscopic study. Ultrastruct Pathol 1986;10:311–9.

157. Smith DB, Howell A, Harris M, Bramwell VH, Sellwood RA. Carcinomatous meningitis associated with infiltrating lobular carcinoma of the breast. Eur J Surg Oncol 1985;11:33–6.

158. Steinbrecher JS, Silverberg SG. Signet-ring cell carcinoma of the breast. The mucinous variant of infiltrating lobular carcinoma. Cancer 1976;37:828–40.

159. Wade PM Jr, Mills SE, Read M, Cloud W, Lambert MJ III, Smith RE. Small cell neuroendocrine (oat cell) carcinoma of the breast. Cancer 1983;52:121–5.

160. Warren RB. Infiltrating lobular carcinoma metastatic to bone marrow—an unusual morphologic pattern. Breast 1985;11:16–8.

161. World Health Organization. Histological typing of breast tumors. Tumori 1982;68:181–98.

162. Yoshida Y. Metastases and primary neoplasms of the stomach in patients with breast cancer. Am J Surg 1973;125:738–43.

Tubular Carcinoma

163. Andersen JA, Carter D, Linell F. A symposium on sclerosing duct lesions of the breast. Pathol Annu 1986;21(Pt 2):145–79.

164. Beahrs OH, Shapiro S, Smart C. Report of the working group to review the National Cancer Institute–American Cancer Society Breast Cancer Detection Demonstration Projects. JNCI 1979;62:640–709.

165. Bondeson L, Lindholm K. Aspiration cytology of tubular breast carcinoma. Acta Cytol 1990;34:15–20.

166. Carstens PH, Greenberg RA, Francis D, Lyon H. Tubular carcinoma of the breast. A long term follow-up. Histopathology 1985;9:271–80.

167. Cooper HS, Patchefsky AS, Krall RA. Tubular carcinoma of the breast. Cancer 1978;42:2334–42.

168. Egger H, Dressler W. A contribution to the natural history of breast cancer. 1. Duct obliteration with periductal elastosis in the centre of breast cancers. Arch Gynecol 1982;231:191–8.

169. Ekblom P, Miettinen M, Forsman L, Andersson LC. Basement membrane and apocrine epithelial antigens in differential diagnosis between tubular carcinoma and sclerosing adenosis of the breast. J Clin Pathol 1984;37:357–63.

170. Erlandson RA, Carstens PH. Ultrastructure of tubular carcinoma of the breast. Cancer 1972;29:987–95.

171. Flotte TJ, Bell DA, Greco MA. Tubular carcinoma and sclerosing adenosis: the use of basal lamina as a differential feature. Am J Surg Pathol 1980;4:75–7.

172. Foote FW Jr. Surgical pathology of cancer of the breast. In: Parsons WH, ed. Cancer of the breast. Springfield, Ill: Charles C. Thomas, 1959:37–8.

173. Harris M, Ahmed A. The ultrastructure of tubular carcinoma of the breast. J Pathol 1977;123:79–83.

174. Heller KS, Rosen PP, Schottenfeld D, Ashikari R, Kinne DW. Male breast cancer. A clinicopathologic study of 97 cases. Ann Surg 1978;188:60–5.

175. Lagios MD, Rose MR, Margolin FR. Tubular carcinoma of the breast: association with multicentricity, bilaterality, and family history of mammary carcinoma. Am J Clin Pathol 1980;73:25–30.

176. Masood S, Barwick KW. Estrogen receptor expression of the less common breast carcinomas [Abstract]. Am J Clin Pathol 1990;93:437.

177. McDivitt RW, Boyce W, Gersell D. Tubular carcinoma of the breast. Clinical and pathological observations concerning 135 cases. Am J Surg Pathol 1982;6:401–11.

178. Oberman HA, Fidler WJ Jr. Tubular carcinoma of the breast. Am J Surg Pathol 1979;3:387–95.

179. Peters GN, Wolff M, Haagensen CD. Tubular carcinoma of the breast. Clinical pathologic correlations based on 100 cases. Ann Surg 1981;193:138–49.

180. Taylor HB, Norris HJ. Well-differentiated carcinoma of the breast. Cancer 1970;25:687–92.

181. Tremblay G. Elastosis in tubular carcinoma of the breast. Arch Pathol 1974;98:302–7.

182. World Health Organization. Histological typing of breast tumours. 2nd ed. International Histological Classification of Tumours No. 2. Geneva: World Health Organization, 1981:19.

Medullary Carcinoma

183. Ahmed A. The ultrastructure of medullary carcinoma of the breast. Virchows Arch [A] 1980;388:175–86.

184. Ben-Ezra J, Sheibani K. Antigenic phenotype of the lymphocytic component of medullary carcinoma of the breast. Cancer 1987;59:2037–41.

185. Berg JW, Robbins GF. The histologic epidemiology of breast cancer. In: Breast cancer: early and late. Chicago: Year Book Medical Publishers, 1970:19–26.

186. Bloom HJ, Richardson WW. Histological grading and prognosis in breast cancer. A study of 1049 cases of which 359 have been followed for 15 years. Br J Cancer 1957;11:359–77.

187. _____, Richardson WW, Fields JR. Host resistance and survival in carcinoma of breast: a study of 104 cases of medullary carcinoma in a series of 1411 cases of breast cancer followed for 20 years. Br Med J 1970;3:181–8.

188. Foote FW Jr, Stewart FW. A histologic classification of carcinoma of the breast. Surgery 1946;19:74–99.

189. Harris M, Lessells AM. The ultrastructure of medullary, atypical medullary and non-medullary carcinomas of the breast. Histopathology 1986;10:405–14.

190. Hsu SM, Raine L, Nayak RN. Medullary carcinoma of breast: an immunohistochemical study of its lymphoid stroma. Cancer 1981;48:1368–76.

191. Ito T, Saga S, Nagayoshi S, et al. Class distribution of immunoglobulin-containing plasma cells in the stroma of medullary carcinoma of breast. Breast Cancer Res Treat 1986;7:97–103.

192. Jacquemier J, Robert-Vague D, Torrente M, Lieutaud R. Mise en evidence des immunoglobulines lymphoplasmocytaires et epitheliales dans les carcinomes infiltrants a stroma lymphoid et les carcinomes medullaires du sein. Arch Anat Cytol Pathol 1983;31:296–300.

193. Kallioniemi OP, Blanco G, Alavaikko M, et al. Tumour DNA ploidy as an independent prognostic factor in breast cancer. Br J Cancer 1987;56:637–42.

194. Kurtz JM, Jacquemier J, Torhorst J, et al. Conservation therapy for breast cancers other than infiltrating ductal carcinoma. Cancer 1989;63:1630–5.

195. Lesser ML, Rosen PP, Kinne DW. Multicentricity and bilaterality in invasive breast carcinoma. Surgery 1982;91:234–40.

196. Meyer JS, Friedman E, McCrate MM, Bauer WC. Prediction of early course of breast carcinomas by thymidine labeling. Cancer 1983;51:1879–86.

197. Mittra NK, Rush BF Jr, Verner E. A comparative study of breast cancer in the black and white populations of two inner-city hospitals. J Surg Oncol 1980;15:11–7.

198. Moore OS Jr, Foote FW Jr. The relatively favorable prognosis of medullary carcinoma of the breast. Cancer 1949;2:635–42.

199. Morrison AS, Black MM, Lowe CR, MacMahon B, Yuasa S. Some international differences in histology and survival in breast cancer. Int J Cancer 1973;11:261–7.

200. Natarajan N, Nemoto T, Mettlin C, Murphy GP. Race-related differences in breast cancer patients. Results of the 1982 National Survey of Breast Cancer by the American College of Surgeons. Cancer 1985;56:1704–9.

201. Pedersen LP, Holck S, Schiödt T, Zedeler K, Mouridsen HT. Inter- and intraobserver variability in the histopathological diagnosis of medullary carcinoma of the breast, and its prognostic implications. Breast Cancer Res Treat 1989;14:91–9.

202. _____, Schiödt T, Holck S, Zedeler K. The prognostic importance of syncytial growth pattern in medullary carcinoma of the beast. APMIS 1990;98:921–6.

203. Ponsky JL, Gliga L, Reynolds S. Medullary carcinoma of the breast: an association with negative hormonal receptors. J Surg Oncol 1984;25:76–8.

204. Rapin V, Contesso G, Mouriesse H, et al. Medullary breast carcinoma. A reevaluation of 95 cases of breast cancer with inflammatory stroma. Cancer 1988;61:2503–10.

205. Reiner A, Reiner G, Spona J, Schemper M, Holzner JH. Histopathologic characterization of human breast cancer in correlation with estrogen receptor status. A comparison of immunocytochemical and biochemical analysis. Cancer 1988;61:1149–54.

206. Richardson WW. Medullary carcinoma of the breast. A distinctive tumor type with a relatively good prognosis following radical mastectomy. Br J Cancer 1956;10:415–23.

207. Ridolfi RL, Rosen PP, Port A, Kinne D, Miké V. Medullary carcinoma of the breast: a clinicopathologic study with 10 year follow-up. Cancer 1977;40:1365–85.

208. Rosen PP. The pathological classification of human mammary carcinoma: past, present and future. Ann Clin Lab Sci 1979;9:144–56.

209. _____, Ashikari R, Thaler H, et al. A comparative study of some pathologic features of mammary carcinoma in Tokyo, Japan and New York, USA. Cancer 1977;39:429–34.

210. _____, Groshen S, Saigo PE, Kinne DW, Hellman S. A long-term follow-up study of survival in stage I (T1N0M0) and stage II (T1N1M0) breast carcinoma. J Clin Oncol 1989;7:355–66.

211. _____, Lesser ML, Senie RT, Duthie K. Epidemiology of breast carcinoma IV: age and histologic tumor type. J Surg Oncol 1982;19:44–51.

212. _____, Mendendez-Botet CJ, Nisselbaum JS, et al. Pathological review of breast lesions analyzed for estrogen receptor protein. Cancer Res 1975;35:3187–94.

213. Schwartz GF. Solid circumscribed carcinoma of the breast. Ann Surg 1969;169:165–73.

214. Wargotz ES, Silverberg SG. Medullary carcinoma of the breast: a clinicopathologic study with appraisal of current diagnostic criteria. Hum Pathol 1988;19:1340–6.

215. Winsten S, Tabachnick J, Young I. Immunoglobulin G (IgG) levels in breast tumour cytosols. Am J Clin Pathol 1985;83:364–6.

216. World Health Organization. Histological typing of breast tumors. Tumori 1982;68:181–98.

Mucinous Carcinoma

217. Ahmed A. Electron-microscopic observations of scirrhous and mucin-producing carcinomas of the breast. J Pathol 1974;112:177–81.

218. Beahrs OH, Shapiro S, Smart C, et al. Report of the working group to review the National Cancer Institute–American Cancer Society Breast Cancer Detection Demonstration Projects. JNCI 1979;62:640–709.

219. Bhargava V, Miller TR, Cohen MB. Mucocele-like tumors of the breast. Cytologic findings in two cases. Am J Clin Pathol 1991;95:875–7.

220. Capella C, Eusebi V, Mann B, Azzopardi JG. Endocrine differentiation in mucoid carcinoma of the breast. Histopathology 1980;4:613–30.

221. Clayton F. Pure mucinous carcinomas of breast: morphologic features and prognostic correlates. Hum Pathol 1986;17:34–8.

222. Coady AT, Shousha S, Dawson PM, Moss M, James KR, Bull TB. Mucinous carcinoma of the breast: further characterization of its three subtypes. Histopathology 1989;15:617–26.

223. Ferguson DJ, Anderson TJ, Wells CA, Battersby S. An ultrastructural study of mucoid carcinoma of the breast: variability of cytoplasmic features. Histopathology 1986;10:1219–30.

224. Harris M, Vasudev KS, Anfield C, Wells S. Mucin-producing carcinomas of the breast: ultrastructural observations. Histopathology 1978;2:177–88.

225. Hull MT, Warfel KA. Mucinous breast carcinomas with abundant intracytoplasmic mucin and neuroendocrine features: light microscopic, immunohistochemical and ultrastructural study. Ultrastruct Pathol 1987;11:29–38.

226. Komaki K, Sakamoto G, Sugano H, et al. The morphologic feature of mucus leakage appearing in low papillary carcinoma of the breast. Hum Pathol 1991;22:231–6.

227. _____, Sakamoto G, Sugano H, Morimoto T, Monden Y. Mucinous carcinoma of the breast in Japan. A prognostic analysis based on morphologic features. Cancer 1988;61:989–96.

228. Kurtz JM, Jacquemier J, Torhorst J, et al. Conservation therapy for breast cancers other than infiltrating ductal carcinoma. Cancer 1989;63:1630–5.

229. Lee M, Terry R. Surgical treatment of carcinomas of the breast. I. Pathological finding and pattern of relapse. J Surg Oncol 1983;23:11–5.

230. Lesser ML, Rosen PP, Senie RT, Duthie K, Menendez-Botet C, Schwartz MK. Estrogen and progesterone receptors in breast carcinoma: correlations with epidemiology and pathology. Cancer 1981;48:229–309.

231. Melamed MR, Robbins GF, Foote FW Jr. Prognostic significance of gelatinous mammary carcinoma. Cancer 1961;14:699–704.

232. Rasmussen BB. Human mucinous carcinomas and their lymph node metastases. A histological review of 247 cases. Pathol Res Pract 1985;180:377–82.

233. _____, Rose C, Christensen IB. Prognostic factors in primary mucinous breast carcinoma. Am J Clin Pathol 1987;87:155–60.

234. _____, Rosen C, Thorpe SM, Andersen KW, Houjensen K. Argyrophilic cells in 202 human mucinous breast carcinomas. Relation to histopathologic and clinical features. Am J Clin Pathol 1985;84:737–40.

235. Ro JY, Sneige N, Sahin AA, Silva EG, Del Junco GW, Ayala AG. Mucocele-like tumor of the breast associated with atypical duct hyperplasia or mucinous carcinoma. A clinicopathologic study of seven cases. Arch Pathol Lab Med 1991;115:137–40.

236. Rosen PP. Mucocele-like tumors of the breast. Am J Surg Pathol 1986;10:464–9.

237. _____, Lesser ML, Kinne DW. Breast carcinoma at the extremes of age: a comparison of patients younger than 35 years and older than 75 years. J Surg Oncol 1985;28:90–6.

238. _____, Wang T. Colloid carcinoma of the breast. Analysis of 64 patients with long-term follow-up [Abstract]. Am J Clin Pathol 1980;73:304.

239. Scharnhorst D, Huntrakoon M. Mucinous carcinoma of the breast: recurrence 30 years after mastectomy. South Med J 1988;81:656–7.

240. Shousha S, Coady AT, Stamp T, James KR, Alaghband-Zadeh J. Oestrogen receptors in mucinous carcinoma of the breast: an immunohistochemical study using paraffin wax sections. J Clin Pathol 1989;42:902–5.

241. Snyder M, Tobon H. Primary mucinous carcinoma of the breast. Breast 1977;3:17–20.

242. Toikkanen S, Kujari H. Pure and mixed mucinous carcinomas of the breast: a clinicopathologic analysis of 61 cases with long-term follow-up. Hum Pathol 1989;20:758–64.

243. _____, Eerola E, Ekfors TO. Pure and mixed mucinous breast carcinomas: DNA stemline and prognosis. J Clin Pathol 1988;41:300–3.

244. World Health Organization. Histological typing of breast tumors. Tumori 1982;68:181–98.

245. Wulsin JH, Schreiber JT. Improved prognosis in certain patterns of carcinoma of the breast. Arch Surg 1962;85:791–800.

Carcinoma with Metaplasia

246. Bauer TW, Rostock RA, Eggleston JC, Barol E. Spindle cell carcinoma of the breast: four cases and review of the literature. Hum Pathol 1984;15:147–52.

247. Ellis IO, Bell J, Ronan JE, Elston CW, Blamey RW. Immunocytochemical investigation of intermediate filament proteins and epithelial membrane antigen in spindle cell tumours of the breast. J Pathol 1988;154:157–65.

248. Fisher ER, Palekar AS, Gregorio RM, Paulson JD. Mucoepidermoid and squamous cell carcinomas of breast with reference to squamous metaplasia and giant cell tumors. Am J Surg Pathol 1983;7:15–27.

249. Gersell DJ, Katzenstein AL. Spindle cell carcinoma of the breast. A clinicopathologic and ultrastructural study. Hum Pathol 1981;12:550–61.

250. Gonzalez-Licea A, Yardley JH, Hartmann WH. Malignant tumor of the breast with bone formation. Studies by light and electron microscopy. Cancer 1967;20:1234–47.

251. Huvos AG, Lucas JC Jr, Foote FW Jr. Metaplastic breast carcinoma. NY State J Med 1973;73:1078–82.

252. Kahn LB, Uys CJ, Dale J, Rutherford S. Carcinoma of the breast with metaplasia to chondrosarcoma: a light and electron microscopic study. Histopathology 1978;2:93–106.

253. Kaufman MW, Marti JR, Gallager HS, Hoehn JL. Carcinoma of the breast with pseudosarcomatous metaplasia. Cancer 1984;53:1908–17.

254. Llombart-Bosch A, Peydro A. Malignant mixed osteogenic tumours of the breast. An ultrastructural study of two cases. Virchows Arch [A] 1975;366:1–14.

255. Meis JM, Ordóñez NG, Gallager HS. Sarcomatoid carcinoma of the breast: an immunohistochemical study of six cases. Virchows Arch [A] 1987;410:415–21.

256. Oberman HA. Metaplastic carcinoma of the breast. A clinicopathologic study of 29 patients. Am J Surg Pathol 1987;11:918–29.

257. Raymond WA, Leong AS. Co-expression of cytokeratin and vimentin intermediate filament proteins in benign and neoplastic breast epithelium. J Pathol 1989;157:299–306.

258. Ridolfi RL, Rosen PP, Port A, Kinne D, Miké V. Medullary carcinoma of the breast. A clinicopathologic study with 10 year follow-up. Cancer 1977;40:1365–85.

259. Rosen PP, Ernsberger D. Low-grade adenosquamous carcinoma. A variant of metaplastic mammary carcinoma. Am J Surg Pathol 1987;11:351–8.

260. Wargotz ES, Deos PH, Norris HJ. Metaplastic carcinomas of the breast. II. Spindle cell carcinoma. Hum Pathol 1989;20:732–40.

261. _____, Norris HJ. Metaplastic carcinomas of the breast. I. Matrix-producing carcinoma. Hum Pathol 1989;20:628–35.

262. _____, Norris HJ. Metaplastic carcinomas of the breast, IV. Squamous cell carcinoma. Cancer 1990; 65:272–6.

Squamous Cell Carcinoma

263. Bauer TW, Rostock RA, Eggleston JC, Baral E. Spindle cell carcinoma of the breast: four cases and review of the literature. Hum Pathol 1984;15:147–52.

264. Chen KT. Fine needle aspiration cytology of squamous cell carcinoma of the breast. Acta Cytol 1990;34:664–8.

265. Eggers JW, Chesney TM. Squamous cell carcinoma of the breast: a clinicopathologic analysis of eight cases and review of the literature. Hum Pathol 1984;15:526–31.

266. Eusebi V, Lamovec J, Cattani MG, Fedeli F, Millis RR. Acantholytic variant of squamous-cell carcinoma of the breast. Am J Surg Pathol 1986;10:855–61.

267. Farrand R, LaVigne R, Lokich J, et al. Epidermoid carcinoma of the breast. J Surg Oncol 1979;12:207–11.

268. Flint A, Oberman HA. Infarction and squamous metaplasia of intraductal papilloma: a benign breast lesion that may simulate carcinoma. Hum Pathol 1984;15:764–7.

269. Gersell DJ, Katzenstein AL. Spindle cell carcinoma of the breast: a clinicopathologic and ultrastructural study. Hum Pathol 1981;12:550–61.

270. Hasleton PS, Misch KA, Vasudev KS, George D. Squamous carcinoma of the breast. J Clin Pathol 1978;31:116–24.

271. Hurt MA, Dïaz-Arias AA, Rosenholtz MJ, Havey AD, Stephenson HE Jr. Posttraumatic lobular squamous metaplasia of breast. An unusual pseudocarcinomatous metaplasia resembling squamous (necrotizing) sialometaplasia of the salivary gland. Mod Pathol 1988;1:385–90.

272. Reddick RL, Jennette JC, Askin FB. Squamous metaplasia of the breast. An ultrastructural and immunologic evaluation. Am J Clin Pathol 1985;84:530–3.

273. Rostock RA, Bauer TW, Eggleston JC. Primary squamous carcinoma of the breast: a review. Breast 1984;10:27–31.

274. Shousha S, James AH, Fernandez MD, Bull TB. Squamous cell carcinoma of the breast. Arch Pathol Lab Med 1984;108:893–6.

275. Tashjian J, Kuni CC, Bohn LE. Primary squamous cell carcinoma of the breast: mammographic findings. Can Assoc Radiol J 1989;40:228–9.

276. Toikkanen S. Primary squamous cell carcinoma of the breast. Cancer 1981;48:1629–32.

Carcinoma with Osteoclast-like Giant Cells

277. Agnantis NT, Rosen PP. Mammary carcinoma with osteoclast-like giant cells. A study of eight cases with follow-up data. Am J Clin Pathol 1979;72:383–9.

278. Athanasou NA, Wells CA, Quinn J, Ferguson DP, Heryet A, McGee JO. The origin and nature of stromal osteoclast-like multinucleated giant cells in breast carcinoma: implications for tumor osteolysis and macrophage biology. Br J Cancer 1989;59:491–8.

279. Bässler R, Birke, F. Histopathology of tumour associated sarcoid-like stromal reaction in breast cancer. An analysis of 5 cases with immunohistochemical investigations. Virchows Arch [A] 1988;412:231–9.

280. Boccato P, Briani G, D'Atri C, Pasini L, Blandamura S, Bizzaro N. Spindle cell and cartilaginous metaplasia in breast carcinoma with osteoclast-like stromal cells. A difficult fine needle aspiration diagnosis. Acta Cytol 1988;32:75–8.

281. Bondeson L. Aspiration cytology of breast carcinoma with multinucleated reactive stromal giant cells. Acta Cytol 1984;28:313–6.

282. Brooks JJ, Krugman DT, Damjanov I. Myeloid metaplasia presenting as a breast mass. Am J Surg Pathol 1980;4:281–5.

283. Chilosi M, Bonetti F, Menestrina F, Lestani M. Breast carcinoma with stromal multinucleated giant cells [Letter]. J Pathol 1987;152:55–6.

284. Douglas-Jones AG, Barr WT. Breast carcinoma with tumor giant cells. Report of a case with fine needle aspiration cytology. Acta Cytol 1989;33:109–14.

285. Fisher ER, Palekar AS, Gregorio RM, Paulson JD. Mucoepidermoid and squamous cell carcinomas of breast with reference to squamous metaplasia and giant cell tumors. Am J Surg Pathol 1983;7:15–27.

286. Gupta RK, Wakefield SJ, Holloway LJ, Simpson JS. Immunocytochemical and ultrastructural study of the rare osteoclast-type carcinoma of the breast in a fine needle aspirate. Acta Cytol 1988;32:79–82.

287. Holland R, Van Haelst UJ. Mammary carcinoma with osteoclast-like giant cells. Additional observations on six cases. Cancer 1984;53:1963–73.

288. Ichijima K, Kobashi Y, Ueda Y, Matsuo S. Breast cancer with reactive multinucleated giant cells: report of three cases. Acta Pathol Jpn 1986;36:449–57.

289. Inauen W, Gloor FJ. Malignant giant cell tumor of the breast associated with infiltrating duct carcinoma. Virchows Arch [A] 1981;393:359–64.

290. McMahon RF, Ahmed A, Connoly CE. Breast carcinoma with stromal multinucleated giant cells—a light microscopic, histochemical and ultrastructural study. J Pathol 1986;150:175–9.

291. Nielsen BB, Kiaer HW. Carcinoma of the breast with stromal multinucleated giant cells. Histopathology 1985;9:183–93.

292. Oberman HA. Invasive carcinoma of the breast with granulomatous response. Am J Clin Pathol 1987;88:718–21.

293. Sugano I, Nagao K, Kondo Y, Nabeshima S, Murakami S. Cytologic and ultrastructural studies of a rare breast carcinoma with osteoclast-like giant cells. Cancer 1983;52:74–8.

294. Tavassoli FA, Norris HJ. Breast carcinoma with osteoclast-like giant cells. Arch Pathol Lab Med 1986;110:636–9.

295. Wargotz ES, Norris HJ. Metaplastic carcinomas of the breast: V. Metaplastic carcinoma with osteoclastic giant cells. Hum Pathol 1990;21:1142–50.

Papillary Carcinoma

296. Ahmed A. Ultrastructural aspects of human breast lesions. Pathol Annu 1980;15(Pt 2):411–43.

297. Buhl-Jørgensen SE, Fischermann K, Johansen H, Peterson B. Cancer risk in intraductal papilloma and papillomatosis. Surg Gynecol Obstet 1968;127:1307–12.

298. Carter D. Intraductal papillary tumors of the breast. A study of 76 cases. Cancer 1977;39:1689–92.

299. _____, Orr SL, Merino MJ. Intracystic papillary carcinoma of the breast after mastectomy, radiotherapy or excisional biopsy alone. Cancer 1983;52:14–9.

300. Czernobilsky B. Intracystic carcinoma of the female breast. Surg Gynecol Obstet 1967;124:93–8.

301. Devitt JE, Barr JR. The clinical recognition of cystic carcinoma of the breast. Surg Gynecol Obstet 1984;159:130–2.

302. Estabrook A, Asch T, Gump F, Kister SJ, Geller P. Mammographic features of intracystic papillary lesions. Surg Gynecol Obstet 1990;170:113–6.

303. Fisher ER, Palekar AS, Redmond C, Barton B, Fisher B. Pathologic findings from the National Surgical Adjuvant Breast Project (Protocol No. 4). VI. Invasive papillary cancer. Am J Clin Pathol 1980;73:313–22.

304. Haagensen CD. Diseases of the breast. 2nd ed. Philadelphia: WB Saunders Co, 1971:528–44.

305. _____, Stout AP, Phillips JS. The papillary neoplasms of the breast. I. Benign intraductal papilloma. Ann Surg 1951;133:18–36.

306. Hendrick JW. Intraductal papilloma of the breast. Surg Gynecol Obstet 1957;105:215–23.

307. Kilgore AR, Fleming R, Ramos MM. The incidence of cancer with nipple discharge and the risk of cancer in the presence of papillary disease of the breast. Surg Gynecol Obstet 1953;96:649–60.

308. Kraus FT, Neubecker RD. The differential diagnosis of papillary tumors of the breast. Cancer 1962;15:444–55.

309. Lewison EF, Lyons JG Jr. Relationship between benign breast disease and cancer. Arch Surg 1953;66:94–114.

310. Masood S, Barwick K. Estrogen receptor expression of the less common breast carcinomas [Abstract]. Am J Clin Pathol 1990;93:437.

311. Meyer JS, Bauer WC, Rao BR. Subpopulations of breast carcinoma defined by S-phase fraction, morphology and estrogen receptor content. Lab Invest 1978;39:225–35.

312. Murad TM, Swaid S, Pritchett P. Malignant and benign papillary lesions of the breast. Hum Pathol 1977;8:379–90.

313. Ohuchi N, Abe R, Kasai M. Possible cancerous change in intraductal papillomas of the breast. A 3-D reconstruction study of 25 cases. Cancer 1984;54:605–11.

314. _____, Abe R, Takahashi T, Tezuka F, Kyogoku, M. Three-dimensional atypical structure in intraductal carcinoma differentiating from papilloma and papillomatosis of the breast. Breast Cancer Res Treat 1985;5:57–65.

315. Papotti M, Eusebi V, Gugliotta P, Bussolati G. Immunohistochemical analysis of benign and malignant papillary lesions of the breast. Am J Surg Pathol 1983;7:451–61.

316. _____, Gugliotta P, Ghiringhello B, Bussolati G. Association of breast carcinoma and multiple intraductal papillomas: an histological and immunohistochemical investigation. Histopathology 1984;8:963–75.

317. Rosen PP. Arthur Purdy Stout and papilloma of the breast. Comments on the occasion of his 100th birthday. Am J Surg Pathol 1986;10(Suppl 1):100–7.

318. Schaefer G, Rosen PP, Lesser ML, Kinne DW, Beattie EJ Jr. Breast carcinoma in elderly women: pathology, prognosis, and survival. Pathol Annu 1984;19(Pt 1):195–219.

319. Schneider JA. Invasive papillary breast carcinoma: mammographic and sonographic appearance. Radiology 1989;171:377–9.

320. Snyder WH, Chaffin L. Main duct papilloma of the breast. Arch Surg 1955;70:680–5.

321. Stout AP. Diagnosis of benign, borderline and malignant lesions of the breast. In: Proceedings of the Second National Cancer Conference. Cincinnati: American Cancer Society, 1954:179–83.

322. Tiltman AJ. DNA ploidy in papillary tumours of the breast. S Afr Med J 1989;75:379–80.

323. Tsuchiya S, Takayama S, Higashi Y. Electron microscopy of intraductal papilloma of the breast. Ultrastructural comparison of papillary carcinoma with normal large duct. Acta Pathol Jpn 1983;33:97–112.

324. World Health Organization. Histological typing of breast tumours. 2nd ed. International Histological Classification of Tumours No. 2. Geneva: World Health Organization, 1981:19.

Adenoid Cystic Carcinoma

325. Anthony PP, James PD. Adenoid cystic carcinoma of the breast: prevalence, diagnostic criteria and histogenesis. J Clin Pathol 1975;28:647–55.

326. Clement PB. Collagenous spherulosis [Letter]. Am J Surg Pathol 1987;11:907.

327. _____, Young RH, Azzopardi JG. Collagenous spherulosis of the breast. Am J Surg Pathol 1987;11:411–7.

328. D'Ardenne AJ, Kirkpatrick P, Wells CA, Davies JD. Laminin and fibronectin in adenoid cystic carcinoma. J Clin Pathol 1986;39:138–44.

329. Düe W, Herbst WD, Loy V, Stein H. Characterization of adenoid cystic carcinoma of the breast by immunohistology. J Clin Pathol 1989;42:470–6.

330. Elsner B. Adenoid cystic carcinoma of the breast. Review of the literature. Pathol Eur 1970;5:357–64.

331. Friedman BA, Oberman HA. Adenoid cystic carcinoma of the breast. Am J Clin Pathol 1970;54:1–14.

332. Geschickter CF. Diseases of the breast: diagnosis, pathology, treatment. 2nd ed. Philadelphia: JB Lippincott, 1945:824.

333. Grignon DJ, Ro JY, Mackay BN, Ordóñez NG, Ayala AG. Collagenous spherulosis of the breast. Immunohistochemical and ultrastructural studies. Am J Clin Pathol 1989;91:386–92.

334. Harris M. Pseudoadenoid cystic carcinoma of the breast. Arch Pathol Lab Med 1977;101:307–9.

335. Herzberg AJ, Bossen EH, Walther PJ. Adenoid cystic carcinoma of the breast metastatic to the kidney. A clinically symptomatic lesion requiring surgical management. Cancer 1991;68:1015–20.

336. Hjorth S, Magnusson PH, Blomquiste PJ. Adenoid cystic carcinoma of the breast. Report of a case in a male and review of the literature. Acta Chir Scand 1977;143:155–8.

337. Koller M, Ram Z, Findler G, Lipshitz M. Brain metastasis: a rare manifestation of adenoid cystic carcinoma of the breast. Surg Neurol 1986;26:470–2.

338. Koss LG, Brannan CD, Ashikari R. Histologic and ultrastructural features of adenoid cystic carcinoma of the breast. Cancer 1970;26:1271–9.

339. Lamovec J, Us-Krašovec M, Zidar A, Kljun A. Adenoid cystic carcinoma of the breast: histologic, cytologic and immunohistochemical study. Semin Diagn Pathol 1989;6:153–64.

340. Lawrence JB, Mazur MT. Adenoid cystic carcinoma. A comparative pathologic study of tumors in salivary gland, breast, lung, and cervix. Hum Pathol 1982;13:916–24.

341. Lim SK, Kovi J, Warner OG. Adenoid cystic carcinoma of breast with metastasis: a case report and review of the literature. J Nat Med Assoc 1979;71:329–30.

342. Lusted D. Structural and growth patterns of adenoid cystic carcinoma of breast. Am J Clin Pathol 1970;54:419–25.

343. Nayer HR. Cylindroma of the breast with pulmonary metastases. Dis Chest 1957;31:324–7.

344. Oertel YC, Galblum LI. Fine needle aspiration of the breast. Diagnostic criteria. Pathol Annu 1983;18(Pt 1):375–407.

345. Orenstein JM, Dardick I, Van Nostrand AW. Ultrastructural similarities of adenoid cystic carcinoma and pleomorphic adenoma. Histopathology 1985;9:623–38.

346. Peters GN, Wolff M. Adenoid cystic carcinoma of the breast. Report of 11 new cases: review of the literature and discussion of biological behavior. Cancer 1982;52:680–6.

347. Qizilbash AH, Patterson MC, Oliveira KF. Adenoid cystic carcinoma of the breast. Light and electron microscopy and a brief review of the literature. Arch Pathol Lab Med 1977;101:302–6.

348. Ro JY, Silva EG, Gallager HS. Adenoid cystic carcinoma of the breast. Hum Pathol 1987;18:1276–81.

349. Rosen PP. Adenoid cystic carcinoma of the breast. A morphologically heterogeneous neoplasm. Pathol Annu 1989;24(Pt 2):237–54.

350. Sumpio BE, Jennings TA, Merino MJ, Sullivan PD. Adenoid cystic carcinoma of the breast. Data from the Connecticut Tumor Registry and a review of the literature. Ann Surg 1987;205:295–301.

351. Tavassoli FA, Norris HJ. Mammary adenoid cystic carcinoma with sebaceous differentiation. A morphologic study of the cell types. Arch Pathol Lab Med 1986;110:1045–53.

352. Verani RR, Van der Bel-Kahn J. Mammary adenoid cystic carcinoma with unusual features. Am J Clin Pathol 1973;59:653–8.

353. Wells CA, Nicoll S, Ferguson DJ. Adenoid cystic carcinoma of the breast: a case with axillary lymph node metastasis. Histopathology 1986;10:415–24.

354. Wilson WB, Spell JP. Adenoid cystic carcinoma of breast: a case with recurrence and regional metastases. Ann Surg 1967;166:861–4.

355. Zaloudek C, Oertel YC, Orenstein JM. Adenoid cystic carcinoma of the breast. Am J Clin Pathol 1984;81:297–307.

Secretory Carcinoma

356. Akhtar M, Robinson C, Ali MA, Godwin JT. Secretory carcinoma of the breast in adults. Light and electron microscopic study of three cases with review of the literature. Cancer 1983;51:2245–54.

357. Ben Romdhane K, Ben Ayed M, Labbane N, et al. Carcinome secretant juvenile du sein. A propos d'une observation chez une fille de 4 ans. Ann Pathol 1987; 7:227–30.

358. Botta G, Fessia L, Ghiringhello B. Juvenile milk protein secreting carcinoma. Virchows Arch [A] 1982;395: 145–52.

359. Byrne MP, Fahey MM, Gooselaw JG. Breast cancer with axillary metastasis in an eight and one-half-year-old girl. Cancer 1973;31:726–8.

360. d'Amore ES, Maisto L, Gatteschi MB, Toma S, Canavese G. Secretory carcinoma of the breast. Report of a case with fine needle aspiration biopsy. Acta Cytol 1986;30:309–12.

361. Ferguson TB Jr, McCarty KS Jr, Filston HC. Juvenile secretory carcinoma and juvenile papillomatosis: diagnosis and treatment. J Pediatr Surg 1987;22:637–9.

362. Hartman AW, Magrish P. Carcinoma of breast in children. Case report: six-year-old boy with adenocarcinoma. Ann Surg 1955;141:792–7.

363. Karl SR, Ballantine TV, Zaino R. Juvenile secretory carcinoma of the breast. J Pediatr Surg 1985;20:368–71.

364. Krausz T, Jenkins D, Grontoft O, Pollock DJ, Azzopardi JG. Secretory carcinoma of the breast in adults: emphasis on late recurrence and metastasis. Histopathology 1989;14:25–36.

365. Massë SR, Rioux A, Beauchesne C. Juvenile carcinoma of the breast. Hum Pathol 1981;12:1044–6.

366. McDivitt RW, Stewart FW. Breast carcinoma in children. JAMA 1966;195:388–90.

367. Oberman HA. Secretory carcinoma of the breast in adults. Am J Surg Pathol 1980;4:465–70.

368. _____, Stephens PJ. Carcinoma of the breast in childhood. Cancer 1972;30:420–74.

369. Rosen PP, Cranor ML. Secretory carcinoma of the breast. Arch Pathol Lab Med 1991;115:141–4.

370. _____, Holmes G, Lesser ML, Kinne DW, Beattie EJ. Juvenile papillomatosis and breast carcinoma. Cancer 1985;55:1345–52.

371. Roth JA, Discafani C, O'Malley M. Secretory breast carcinoma in a man. Am J Surg Pathol 1988;12:150–4.

372. Sullivan JJ, Magee HR, Donald KJ. Secretory (juvenile) carcinoma of the breast. Pathology 1977;9:341–6.

373. Tavassoli FA, Norris HJ. Secretory carcinoma of the breast. Cancer 1980;45:2404–13.

374. Tournemaine N, Audouin AF, Anguill C, Gordeeff S. Le carcinome secretoire juvenile. Cinq nouveaux cas chez des femmes d'age adulte. Arch Anat Cytol Pathol 1986;34:146–51.

375. World Health Organization. Histological typing of breast tumors. Tumori 1982;68:181–98.

Cystic Hypersecretory Carcinoma

376. Colandrea JM, Shmookler BM, O'Dowd GJ, Cohen MH. Cystic hypersecretory duct carcinoma of the breast. Report of a case with fine-needle aspiration. Arch Pathol Lab Med 1988;112:560–3.

377. Guerry P, Erlandson RA, Rosen PP. Cystic hypersecretory hyperplasia and cystic hypersecretory duct carcinoma of the breast. Pathology, therapy, and follow-up of 39 patients. Cancer 1988;61:1611–20.

378. Rosen PP, Scott M. Cystic hypersecretory duct carcinoma of the breast. Am J Surg Pathol 1984;8:31–41.

379. World Health Organization. Histological typing of breast tumors. Tumori 1982;68:181–98.

Apocrine Carcinoma

380. Abati AD, Kimmel M, Rosen PP. Apocrine mammary carcinoma. A clinicopathologic study of 72 cases. Am J Clin Pathol 1990;94:371–7.

381. Ahmed A. Apocrine metaplasia in cystic hyperplastic mastopathy. Histochemical and ultrastructural observations. J Pathol 1975;115:211–4.

382. Archer F, Omar M. Pink cell (oncocytic) metaplasia in a fibroadenoma of the human breast: electron-microscopic observations. J Pathol 1969;99:119–24.

383. Bryant J. Male breast cancer: a case of apocrine carcinoma with psammoma bodies. Hum Pathol 1981; 12:751–3.

384. Burt AD, Seywright MM, George WD. Mixed apocrine-medullary carcinoma of the breast. Report of a case with fine needle aspiration cytology. Acta Cytol 1987; 31:322–4.

385. Bussolati G, Cattani MG, Gugliotta P, Patriarca E, Eusebi V. Morphologic and functional aspects of apocrine metaplasia in dysplastic and neoplastic breast tissue. Ann NY Acad Sci 464:262–74.

386. Carter DJ, Rosen PP. Atypical apocrine metaplasia. Mod Pathol 1991;4:1–5.

387. Charles A. An electron microscopic study of the human axillary apocrine gland. J Anat 1959;93:226–32.

388. d'Amore ES, Terrier-Lacombe MJ, Travagli JP, Friedman S, Contesso G. Invasive apocrine carcinoma of the breast: a long term follow-up study of 34 cases. Breast Cancer Res Treat 1988;12:37–44.

389. Eisenberg BL, Bagnall JW, Harding CT III. Histiocytoid carcinoma: a variant of breast cancer. J Surg Oncol 1986;31:271–4.

390. Eusebi V, Betts C, Haagensen DE Jr, Gugliotta P, Bussolati G, Azzopardi JG. Apocrine differentiation in lobular carcinoma of the breast: a morphologic, immunologic, and ultrastructural study. Hum Pathol 1984;15:134–40.

391. Frable WJ, Kay S. Carcinoma of the breast. Histologic and clinical features of apocrine tumors. Cancer 1968; 21:756–63.

392. Haagensen CD. Diseases of the breast. 3rd ed. Philadelphia: WB Saunders Co, 1974:779–92.

393. Johnson TL, Kini SR. The significance of atypical apocrine cells in fine-needle aspirates of the breast. Diagn Cytopathol 1989;5:248–54.

394. Labows JN, Preti G, Hoelzle E, Leyden J, Kligman A. Steroid analysis of human apocrine secretion. Steroids 1979;34:249–58.

395. Lee BJ, Pack GT, Scharnagel I. Sweat gland cancer of the breast. Surg Gynecol Obstet 1933;56:975–96.

396. Mazoujian G, Bodian C, Haagensen DE Jr, Haagensen CD. Expression of GCDFP-15 in breast carcinomas. Relationship to pathologic and clinical factors. Cancer 1989;63:2156–61.

397. Miller WR, Telford J, Dixon JM, Shivas AA. Androgen metabolism and apocrine differentiation in human breast cancer. Breast Cancer Res Treat 1985;5:67–73.

398. Mossler JA, Barton TK, Brinkhous AD, McCarty KS, Moylan JA, McCarty KS Jr. Apocrine differentiation in human mammary carcinoma. Cancer 1980;46:2463–71.

399. Pier WJ Jr, Garancis JC, Kuzma JF. The ultrastructure of apocrine cells in intracystic papilloma and fibrocystic disease of the breast. Arch Pathol 1970;89:446–52.

400. Robbins GF, Shah J, Rosen P, Chu F, Taylor J. Inflammatory carcinoma of the breast. Surg Clin North Am 1974;54:801–10.

401. Roddy HJ, Silverberg SG. Ultrastructural analysis of apocrine carcinoma of the human breast. Ultrastruct Pathol 1980;1:385–93.

402. Shivas AA, Hunt CT. Cultural characteristics of an apocrine variant of human mammary carcinoma. Clin Oncol 1979;5:299–303.

403. Shousha S, Bull TB, Southall PJ, Mazoujian G. Apocrine carcinoma of the breast containing foam cells. An electron microscopic and immunohistochemical study. Histopathology 1987;11:611–20.

404. Wales NA, Ebling FJ. The control of apocrine glands of the rabbit by steroid hormones. J Endocrinol 1971;51:763–70.

405. Walford N, ten Velden J. Histiocytoid breast carcinoma: an apocrine variant of lobular carcinoma. Histopathology 1989;14:515–22.

406. World Health Organization. Histological typing of breast tumours. 2nd ed. International Histological Classification of Tumours No. 2. Geneva: World Health Organization, 1981:19.

407. Yates AJ, Ahmed A. Apocrine carcinoma and apocrine metaplasia. Histopathology 1988;13:228–31.

Carcinoma with Endocrine Features

408. Ashworth MT, Haqqani MT. Endocrine variant of ductal carcinoma in situ of breast: ultrastructural and light microscopical study. J Clin Pathol 1986;39:1355–9.

409. Azzopardi JG, Muretto P, Goddeeris P, Eusebi V, Lauweryns JM. Carcinoid tumors of the breast: the morphological spectrum of argyrophil carcinomas. Histopathology 1982;6:549–69.

410. Blobel GA, Gould VE, Moll R, et al. Coexpression of neuroendocrine markers and epithelial cytoskeletal proteins in bronchopulmonary neuroendocrine neoplasms. Lab Invest 1985;52:39–51.

411. Bussolati G, Gugliotta P, Sapino A, Eusebi V, Lloyd RV. Chromogranin-reactive endocrine cells in argyrophilic carcinomas ("carcinoids") and normal tissue of the breast. Am J Pathol 1985;120:186–92.

412. _____, Papotti M, Sapino A, Gugliotta P, Ghiringhello B, Azzopardi JG. Endocrine markers in argyrophilic carcinomas of the breast. Am J Surg Pathol 1987;11:248–56.

413. Capella C, Usellini L, Papotti M, et al. Ultrastructural features of neuroendocrine differentiated carcinomas of the breast. Ultrastruct Pathol 1990;14:321–34.

414. Chabon AB, Costales F. Estrogen receptor activity in primary argyrophil carcinoma of the breast. Diagn Gynecol Obstet 1980;2:93–7.

415. Clayton F, Sibley RK, Ordonez NG, Hanssen G. Argyrophilic breast carcinomas: evidence of lactational differentiation. Am J Surg Pathol 1982;6:323–33.

416. Cohle SD, Tschen JA, Smith FE, Lane M, McGavran MH. ACTH-secreting carcinoma of the breast. Cancer 1979;43:2370–6.

417. Cramer SF, Aikawa M, Cebelin M. Neurosecretory granules in small cell invasive carcinoma of the urinary bladder. Cancer 1981;47:724–30.

418. Cross AS, Azzopardi JG, Krausz T, Van Noorden S, Polak JM. A morphological and immunocytochemical study of a distinctive variant of ductal carcinoma in situ of the breast. Histopathology 1985;9:21–37.

419. Cubilla AL, Woodruff JM. Primary carcinoid tumor of the breast. A report of eight patients. Am J Surg Pathol 1977;1:283–92.

420. _____, Woodruff JM, Erlandson RA. Comparative clinicopathologic study of endocrine-like and ordinary mucinous carcinomas of the breast [Abstract]. Lab Invest 1984;50:14A.

421. Eusebi V, Azzopardi JG. Lobular endocrine neoplasia in fibroadenoma of the breast. Histopathology 1980;4:413–28.

422. Ferguson DJ, Anderson TJ. Distribution of dense core granules in normal, benign and malignant breast tissue. J Pathol 1985;147:59–65.

423. Fetissof F, Dubois MP, Arbeille-Brassart B, Lansac J, Jobard P. Argyrophilic cells in mammary carcinoma. Hum Pathol 1983;14:127–34.

424. Feyrter F, Hartmann G. Uber die carcinoide wachsform des carcinoma mammae, inbesondere das carcinoma solidum (gelatinosum) mammae. Frankf Z Pathol 1963;73:24–35.

425. Fisher ER, Palenkar AS. Solid and mucinous varieties of so-called mammary carcinoid tumors. Am J Clin Pathol 1979;72:909–16.

426. Hillyard CJ, Coombes RC, Greenberg PB, Galante LS, MacIntyre I. Calcitonin in breast and lung cancer. Clin Endocrinol 1976;5:1–8.

427. Juntti-Berggren L, Pitkänen P, Wilander E. Argyrophil endocrine cells with ACTH and HCG immunoreactivity in a carcinoma of the breast. Virchows Arch [Cell Pathol] 1983;43:37–42.

428. Kaneko H, Hojo H, Ishikawa S, Yamanouchi H, Sumida T, Saito R. Norepinephrine-producing tumors of bilateral breasts: a case report. Cancer 1978;41:2002–7.

429. _____, Sumida T, Sekiya M, Toshima M, Kobayashi H, Naito K. A breast carcinoid tumor with special reference to ultrastructural study. Acta Pathol Jpn 1982;32:327–32.

430. Lazarevic B, Rodgers JB. Aspiration cytology of carcinoid tumor of the breast. A case report. Acta Cytol 1983;27:329–33.

431. Lee AK, Rosen PP, DeLellis RA, et al. Tumor marker expression in breast carcinomas and relationship to prognosis. An immunohistochemical study. Am J Clin Pathol 1985;84:687–96.

432. Maluf HM, Zukerberg LR, Dickersin GR, Koerner FC. Spindle-cell argyrophilic mucin-producing carcinoma of the breast. Histological, ultrastructural, and immunohistochemical studies of two cases. Am J Surg Pathol 1991;15:677–86.

433. Mavligit GM, Cohen JL, Sherwood LM. Ectopic production of parathyroid hormone by carcinoma of the breast. N Engl J Med 1971;285:154–6.

434. McCutcheon J, Walker RA. The significance of argyrophilia in human breast carcinomas. Virchows Arch [A] 1987;410:369–74.

435. Min K. Argyrophilia in breast carcinomas: histochemical, ultrastructural and immunocytochemical study. Lab Invest 1983;48:58A–9A.

436. Nesland JM, Holm R, Johannessen JV. A study of different markers for neuroendocrine differentiation in breast carcinomas. Pathol Res Pract 1986;181:524–30.

437. _____, Memoli VA, Holm R, Gould VE, Johannessen JV. Breast carcinomas with neuroendocrine differentiation. Ultrastruct Pathol 1985;8:225–40.

438. Pagani A, Papotti M, Höfler H, Weiler R, Winkler H, Bussolati G. Chromogranin A and B gene expression in carcinomas of the breast. Correlation of immunocytochemical, immunoblot, and hybridization analyses. Am J Pathol 1990;136:319–27.

439. Papotti M, Macrï L, Bussolati G, Reubi JC. Correlative study on neuro-endocrine differentiation and presence of somatostatin receptors in breast carcinomas. Int J Cancer 1989;43:365–9.

440. _____, Macrï L, Finzi G, Capella C, Eusebi V, Bussolati G. Neuroendocrine differentiation in carcinomas of the breast: a study of 51 cases. Semin Diagn Pathol 1989;6:174–88.

441. Partanen S, Syrjänen J. Argyrophilic cells in carcinoma of the female breast. Virchows Arch [A] 1981;391:45–51.

442. Ramos CV, Boeshart C, Restrepo GL. Intracystic papillary carcinoma of the male breast. Arch Pathol Lab Med 1985;109:858–61.

443. Rasmussen BB, Rose C, Thorpe SM, Andersen KW, Hou-Jensen K. Argyrophilic cells in 202 human mucinous breast carcinomas. Relation to histopathologic and clinical features. Am J Clin Pathol 1985;84:737–40.

444. Roth J, Bendayan M, Orci L. Ultrastructural localization of intracellular antigens by the use of protein A-gold complex. J Histochem Cytochem 1978;26:1074–81.

445. Saigo PE, Rosen PP. Mammary carcinoma with "choriocarcinomatous" features. Am J Surg Pathol 1981;5:773–8.

446. Santini D, Bazzocchi F, Pileri S, et al. Mammary carcinoma with argyrophilic cells: an immunohistochemical and ultrastructural study. Tumori 1985;71:331–8.

447. Sariola H, Lehtonen E, Saxén E. Breast tumors with a solid and uniform carcinoid pattern. Ultrastructural and immunohistochemical study of two cases. Pathol Res Pract 1985;179:405–11.

448. Scopsi L, Andreola S, Saccozzi R, et al. Argyrophilic carcinoma of the male breast. A neuroendocrine tumor containing predominantly chromogranin B (secretogranin I). Am J Surg Pathol 1991;15:1063–71.

449. Taxy JB, Tischler AS, Insalaco SJ, Battifora H. "Carcinoid" tumor of the breast. A variant of conventional breast cancer? Hum Pathol 1981;12:170–9.

450. Toyoshima S. Mammary carcinoma with argyrophil cells. Cancer 1983;52:2129–38.

451. Wade PM, Mills SE, Read M, Cloud W, Lambert MJ III, Smith RE. Small cell neuroendocrine (oat cell) carcinoma of the breast. Cancer 1983;52:121–5.

Glycogen-Rich Carcinoma

452. Benisch B, Peison B, Newman R, Sobel HJ, Marquet E. Solid glycogen-rich clear cell carcinoma of the breast (a light and ultrastructural study). Am J Clin Pathol 1983;79:243–5.

453. Fisher ER, Tavares J, Bulatao IS, Sass R, Fisher B. Glycogen-rich, clear cell breast cancer: with comments concerning other clear cell variants. Hum Pathol 1985;16:1085–90.

454. Hull MT, Priest JB, Broadie TA, Ransburg RC, McCarthy LJ. Glycogen-rich clear cell carcinoma of the breast: a light and electron microscopic study. Cancer 1981;48:2003–9.

455. _____, Warfel KA. Glycogen-rich clear cell carcinomas of the breast. A clinicopathologic and ultrastructural study. Am J Surg Pathol 1986;10:553–9.

456. Sörensen FB, Paulsen SM. Glycogen-rich clear cell carcinoma of the breast: a solid variant with mucus. A light microscopic, immunohistochemical and ultrastructural study of a case. Histopathology 1987;11:857–69.

457. Toikkanen S, Joensuu H. Glycogen-rich clear cell carcinoma of the breast: a clinicopathologic and flow cytometric study. Hum Pathol 1991;22:81–3.

Lipid-Rich Carcinoma

458. Aboumrad MH, Horn RC Jr, Fine G. Lipid-secreting mammary carcinoma: report of a case associated with Paget's disease of the nipple. Cancer 1963;16:521–5.

459. Ramos CV, Taylor HB. Lipid-rich carcinoma of the breast. A clinicopathologic analysis of 13 examples. Cancer 1974;33:812–9.

460. Van Bogaert LJ, Maldague P. Histologic variants of lipid-secreting carcinoma of the breast. Virchows Arch [A] 1977;375:345–53.

Cribriform Carcinoma

461. Fisher ER, Gregorio RM, Fisher B, Redmond C, Vellios F, Sommers SC. The pathology of invasive breast cancer. A syllabus derived from findings of the National Surgical Adjuvant Breast Project (protocol no. 4) Cancer 1975;36:1–85.
462. Page DL, Dixon JM, Anderson TJ, Lee D, Stewart HJ. Invasive cribriform carcinoma of the breast. Histopathology 1983;7:525–36.
463. Rosen PP. Adenoid cystic carcinoma of the breast: a morphologically heterogenous neoplasm. Pathol Annu 1989;24(Pt 2):237–54.
464. Venable JG, Schwartz AM, Silverberg SG. Infiltrating cribriform carcinoma of the breast: a distinctive clinicopathologic entity. Hum Pathol 1990;21:333–8.
465. Wells CA, Ferguson DJ. Ultrastructural and immunocytochemical study of a case of invasive cribriform breast carcinoma. J Clin Pathol 1988;41:17–20.

UNUSUAL CLINICAL PRESENTATION OF CARCINOMA

CARCINOMA IN PREGNANCY AND LACTATION

Although carcinoma of the breast presenting during pregnancy or lactation is comparatively rare, it presents important therapeutic and prognostic problems. At one time it was thought that carcinoma arising in this setting was inherently more aggressive, with an exceptionally poor prognosis. However, the microscopic patterns of carcinoma in pregnancy are similar to those of age-matched nonpregnant patients (1); the more advanced stage at diagnosis can be attributed in some cases to delay in diagnostic intervention because the neoplasm is obscured by physiologic changes in the breast (3).

Few investigators have assessed the hormonal receptor status of these carcinomas (2,4). The majority of assays for both estrogen and progesterone receptors proved negative. It is unclear whether this is an intrinsic feature of the neoplasm or whether it relates to binding of higher levels of circulating estrogens, an increased number of available binding sites, or a combination of factors during pregnancy. The lack of response to ovarian ablation suggests that the tumors are truly receptor negative.

Therapeutic options are limited by pregnancy. Radiation of the breast should be avoided and there are concerns for the teratogenic effects of adjuvant chemotherapy, especially during the first trimester. Chemotherapeutic medications may be present in the breast milk and could be a hazard to the nursing newborn. The vascularity of the breast makes its surgical removal more complex. Suppression of lactation reduces vascularity but does not alter prognosis.

There have been only rare instances of metastasis of breast cancer to the placenta and no cases of metastasis to the fetus (5).

INFLAMMATORY CARCINOMA

Lee and Tannenbaum (20) proposed the currently used term inflammatory carcinoma in 1924. Although inflammatory carcinoma is not a specific histologic subtype of mammary carcinoma (33), some investigators include histopathologic findings among their diagnostic criteria.

Clinical Presentation. Clinical inflammatory changes associated with the initial presentation of the disease characterize *primary inflammatory carcinoma.* Recurrent carcinoma with inflammatory changes is referred to as *secondary inflammatory carcinoma.*

Primary inflammatory carcinoma features warm erythema of the mammary skin. The skin is thickened, especially at the edge of the erysipeloid area, with peau d'orange conspicuous over dependant portions of the breast (12,27). In advanced cases, skin changes may extend to the chest wall. The breast is usually diffusely indurated; a mass may be palpated but in some cases only cutaneous changes are initially evident. The diagnosis of inflammatory carcinoma requires that at least one third of the mammary skin be affected (18). Skin thickening is invariably seen on mammography. Within the breast, the only evidence of the condition is often diffuse increased parenchymal density (6). Thickening of the skin due to edema is not a specific radiologic feature since it can be found in patients with less advanced lesions that lack inflammatory features (12,31).

Cutaneous erythema localized to the skin overlying a large palpable tumor has been referred to as locally advanced breast cancer with an inflammatory component (26). The prognosis of patients with limited cutaneous changes is as grave as that of women with classic inflammatory carcinoma (26). Inflammatory carcinoma may be mistaken at first for a non-neoplastic inflammatory condition because of the rapid onset and pain described by the patient (20). A substantial number of patients present with enlarged axillary or supraclavicular lymph nodes (27). Patients with the clinical syndrome of rapidly progressing breast carcinoma described in Tunisia usually have inflammatory carcinoma (23).

The primary tumor is negative for estrogen and progesterone receptors in 62 to 100 percent of cases (24,25,30). When analyzed biochemically, skin biopsies are usually estrogen receptor negative (28). Immunohistochemical procedures make it possible to selectively examine the tumor; most are receptor negative by this

259

method but some tumor cells are estrogen receptor positive even when biochemical analysis was reportedly receptor negative.

One group of investigators found amplified expression of C-*erb*B-2(HER2/*neu*) proto-oncogene significantly more often in inflammatory (41 percent) than in noninflammatory (19 percent) breast carcinomas (17). Over-expression was not significantly related to histologic tumor grade. There was a trend toward more frequent amplified expression in cases with negative estrogen receptors or positive lymph nodes.

The majority of patients with secondary inflammatory carcinoma have axillary lymph node metastases when initially treated. Recurrent inflammatory carcinoma is characterized by the same discoloration and edema of the skin as primary inflammatory lesions. Clinical inflammatory changes can also be found associated with distant cutaneous recurrences (32), but they are not specific for mammary carcinoma since they have been reported in metastases from carcinoma of the pancreas, stomach, lung, and other sites (7,19).

Gross Findings. All patients with primary inflammatory carcinoma have an underlying invasive mammary carcinoma. The breast is often diffusely involved or a large tumor is described. Localized tumors measure 2 to 12 cm, averaging 6 cm in greatest diameter. The majority of the carcinomas are located in the central portion of the breast or occupy virtually the entire breast. The skin is thickened, averaging 4 mm, substantially more than the normal thickness of 1.0 to 1.5 mm (31).

Microscopic Findings. Primary inflammatory carcinomas are almost all poorly differentiated infiltrating duct carcinomas (27). Tumor emboli are usually seen throughout the breast, but can be inconspicuous in rare cases. Many of the vascular spaces devoid of red blood cells that contain tumor cells are considered to be lymphatics. Channels of similar structure and caliber containing erythrocytes and tumor emboli are also encountered.

A lymphoplasmactyic reaction may be present in the tumor or surrounding breast. The reactive infiltrate does not correlate with the severity and distribution of the clinical cutaneous manifestations of the disease. There is also no direct relationship between clinical findings and the number of lymphatic tumor emboli, or the extent of vascular distension. Neutrophils, eosinophils, or numerous mast cells are not a common feature in the breast or skin.

The diagnosis of carcinoma can be made easily by needle biopsy of the breast if there is an underlying palpable mass. When sampled, the skin typically displays the histologic features customarily associated with inflammatory carcinoma. The collagenous reticular dermal layer is broader than normal due to increased collagen and edema. Dilation of lymphatics tends to be prominent in the papillary and reticular dermis and intralymphatic tumor emboli can be found at either level (fig. 416). A lymphoplasmacytic reaction of varying intensity is localized around dilated lymphatic channels. The skin within and outside the zone of erythema and edema may appear histologically identical, with lymphatic tumor emboli detectable in areas that appear clinically uninvolved. Nodular or plaque-like extralymphatic dermal tumor infiltrates are uncommon. In some patients tumor may not be found in biopsies of the skin even if serial sections of the specimen have been prepared (12,13,21).

In secondary (recurrent) inflammatory carcinoma, microscopic examination of the skin usually reveals nodules and plaques of invasive carcinoma in the dermis, as well as intralymphatic tumor emboli, which at times may be inconspicuous or undetectable. Clinically, erythema and edema occur equally in the skin over and around palpable dermal tumor infiltrates regardless of the presence of dermal lymphatic tumor emboli.

A review of the primary lesions in patients who develop inflammatory recurrence suggested some predisposing features (27). All patients had infiltrating duct carcinomas including a disproportionately high number with apocrine cytology. Recurrence was occasionally found following treatment of papillary, medullary, and mucinous carcinomas. Although these patients did not exhibit the clinical signs of inflammatory carcinoma initially, parenchymal intralymphatic tumor emboli were seen in many of the mastectomy specimens.

"Occult" inflammatory carcinoma describes cutaneous and parenchymal lymphatic tumor emboli associated with the primary tumor in the absence of cutaneous signs that typify inflammatory carcinoma (21,29). Occult inflammatory carcinoma

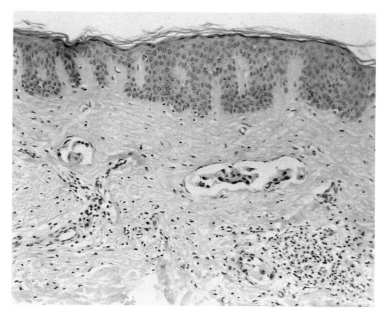

Figure 416
INFLAMMATORY CARCINOMA
Section of skin showing tumor emboli in dilated lymphatic spaces. Note scattered lymphocytic infiltrate in the dermis.

occurs in 1 to 2 percent of patients with invasive carcinomas that are not clinically inflammatory (21). The primary tumors tend to be central, larger than 4 cm, and often multicentric. The pathologic findings are not appreciably different than those of primary inflammatory carcinoma.

Prognosis and Treatment. Until the introduction of combined modality treatment, including intensive chemotherapy, less than 5 percent of patients survived 5 years (27). While one group of investigators suggested that inflammatory carcinoma patients with no detectable dermal lymphatic tumor emboli had a more favorable prognosis (13), others did not find this to be the case (11,14,21). Patients with occult inflammatory carcinoma may have a slightly less acute clinical course but ultimately not a better survival rate than women with classic primary inflammatory carcinoma.

Contemporary reports describe 5-year survivals ranging from 25 to 48 percent (11,14,16). While mastectomy alone was shown to be ineffective for inflammatory carcinoma (27), it is now an integral part of multimodality treatment programs. Mastectomy appears to be more effective for obtaining local control of the primary tumor when combined with radiation and/or chemotherapy (8,9,10,16,30).

Pathologic findings in the mastectomy specimen predict prognosis more accurately than the clinical assessment of response to treatment (14,15,22). Patients who exhibit a good response

clinically and pathologically appear to have the best prognosis. The number of involved lymph nodes is a particularly important prognostic factor since patients with the least extensive axillary involvement have the most favorable disease-free survival (22).

OCCULT CARCINOMA PRESENTING WITH AXILLARY LYMPH NODE METASTASES

Fewer than 1 percent of patients with mammary carcinoma present with a palpable axillary lymph node metastasis as the first sign (fig. 417) (35). In a series of 10,014 primary operable breast carcinoma patients treated at one institution, 35 (0.35 percent) had occult carcinoma presenting with axillary metastases. Among patients subjected to axillary dissection, the number of lymph nodes found to be involved histologically varied from 1 to as many as 65 (34,45,48).

Clinical Presentation. This presentation occurs throughout virtually the entire age distribution of breast carcinoma, from 30 to 83 years, with the mean and median age around 57 years (34,35,42,45). In studies, a nonmammary primary was ruled out by at least one of a variety of techniques that included chest X ray, bone scan, abdominal sonogram, scans of the liver and spleen, CT scans, gastrointestinal contrast studies, and intravenous pyelogram (35,42). Mammography

261

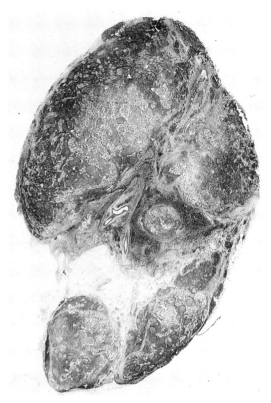

Figure 417
OCCULT CARCINOMA
Cross section of enlarged axillary lymph node from patient with no palpable primary tumor. Pale areas are metastatic carcinoma distributed throughout the lymph node. (Fig. 17-1 from Rosen PP. Tumors of the breast. Based on the proceedings of the 53rd Annual Anatomic Pathology Slide Seminar of the American Society of Clinical Pathologists. Chicago: ASCP Press, 1987:108.) (Figures 417 and 418 are from the same patient.)

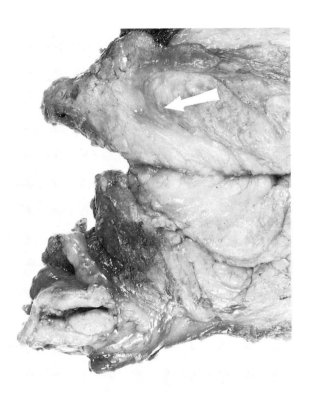

Figure 418
OCCULT CARCINOMA
Mastectomy specimen dissected to show a small primary tumor (arrow) and enlarged axillary lymph nodes (lower left).

performed in virtually all cases revealed abnormalities in 12 (34), 25 (45), 26.5 (35), and 35 percent (42,48) of patients examined. Some investigators have excluded patients with significant mammographic abnormalities from the syndrome of subclinical carcinoma presenting with axillary metastases (38,47). However, there is often no correlation between the location of the radiologic abnormality and the site at which a carcinoma is ultimately located (42). In a series of patients presenting with axillary metastases from subclinical carcinoma, about 8 percent were previously treated for contralateral carcinoma (34,35) or developed subsequent carcinoma in the contralateral breast (35,38).

Gross Findings. In most series, a documented primary was found in about 75 percent of patients (34,35,39,42,45,48). Although not clinically palpable, the majority of carcinomas were found upon gross examination of a mastectomy or excisional biopsy specimen (fig. 418). The lesions measured up to 6.5 cm (42,45) but most were 1 to 2 cm. The majority of the primary lesions occurred in the upper outer quadrant (34,42,45) and rarely in the central or subareolar regions or in the axillary tail.

About 30 percent of the primary carcinomas were not grossly evident (figs. 419, 420). These lesions were usually found in tissue that appeared grossly normal in multiple random sections of breast. Radiography of breast biopsies and mastectomies was not helpful in locating these minute primary tumors. The likelihood of finding a primary lesion in the breast is related to the thoroughness with which the tissue is studied. Patients not proven to have a primary breast carcinoma or a primary tumor at another site have a similar age distribution, similar lymph node findings, and comparable survival

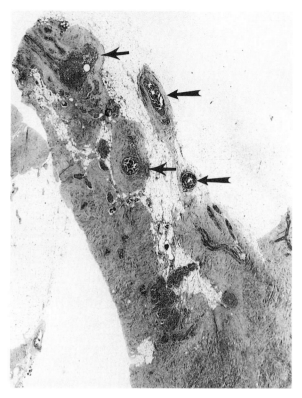

Figure 419
OCCULT CARCINOMA
Low-power view of an occult primary tumor. Ducts with intraductal carcinoma are evident (arrows). This lesion was not palpable clinically or in the mastectomy specimen. (Figures 419–422 are from the same patient.)

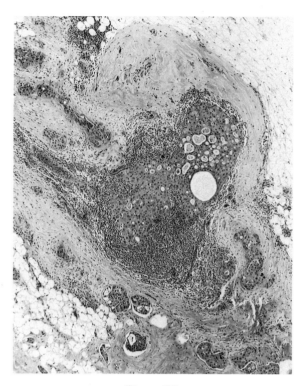

Figure 420
OCCULT CARCINOMA
Primary tumor with lymphocytic infiltration and fibrous stromal reaction that contains invasive carcinoma around a duct with intraductal carcinoma.

Table 5

LYMPH NODE PATHOLOGY IN PATIENTS WITH AND WITHOUT PRIMARY BREAST CARCINOMA

	With Primary (N=31)	Without Primary (N=12)
Large apocrine cells	20 (65%)	8 (67%)
Mammary carcinoma pattern	7 (23%)	1 (8%)
Mixed pattern	4 (13%)	3 (25%)

Adapted from Haupt et al. (42).

results as those with a demonstrated breast carcinoma. In one series, none of the 12 patients without a documented primary lesion in the breast was later shown to have an extramammary primary (42).

Microscopic Findings. Three patterns of metastatic adenocarcinoma are found in the lymph nodes (Table 5). About 65 percent of the lymph nodes contain infiltrates of relatively large apocrine cells diffusely distributed in the lymphoid tissue, as well as in sinusoids (figs. 421, 422). Little or no gland formation is evident in this type of metastasis, but mucicarmine-positive secretion can usually be demonstrated in at least a few cells. This cell type and pattern are sometimes suggestive of malignant melanoma and metastatic renal cell carcinoma may be considered when cytoplasmic clearing is prominent. When the tumor cells are dispersed singly or in small groups throughout a lymph node, the resulting pattern might be confused with diffuse large cell lymphoma (fig. 423).

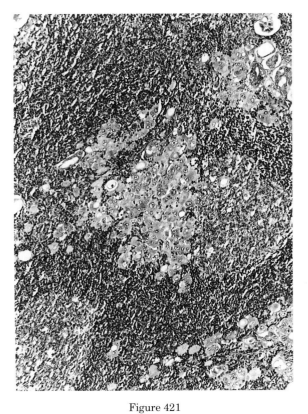

Figure 421
OCCULT CARCINOMA
Metastatic carcinoma in axillary lymph node composed of large, poorly differentiated tumor cells between germinal centers.

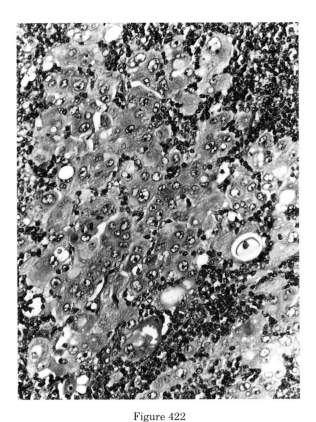

Figure 422
OCCULT CARCINOMA
Tumor cells have abundant eosinophilic cytoplasm and round to oval nuclei with prominent nucleoli.

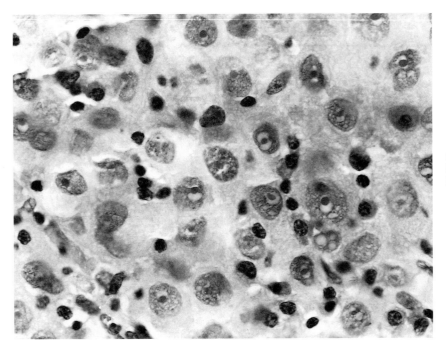

Figure 423
OCCULT CARCINOMA
Metastatic carcinoma cells dispersed among lymphocytes in a lymph node resembling large cell lymphoma.

About 20 percent of axillary lymph node metastases consist of adenocarcinoma with growth patterns similar to those more commonly encountered in primary tumors in the breast. These include cribriform, papillary, glandular, and comedo forms of invasive carcinoma. A scirrhous stromal reaction is rarely present. The remaining 15 percent of the lymph nodes contain mixtures of diffuse apocrine cells with the conventional patterns.

Approximately 50 percent of the lymph nodes in each of the three groups have some mucicarmine-positive cells. A positive result narrows the differential diagnosis substantially. It is not unusual to find mucin-positive cells limited to one of several lymph nodes. Other studies may be helpful if a diagnosis of adenocarcinoma is not apparent from the growth pattern and mucin stain. Immunohistochemical procedures for cytokeratin, epithelial membrane antigen, S-100 protein, alpha-lactalbumin, carcinoembryonic antigen, lymphoid markers, gross cystic disease fluid protein-15 (GCDFP-15), and other cellular constituents usually resolve the differential diagnosis. It is rarely necessary to employ electron microscopy (43). Estrogen and progesterone receptors may be analyzed in axillary node metastases biochemically and immunohistochemically (36,40, 43,45). The presence of one or both receptors in amounts regarded as positive is highly suggestive of, but not specific for, mammary carcinoma.

When adenocarcinoma is diagnosed in tissue removed from an axillary mass, this may be a metastasis or a primary tumor of axillary breast tissue. Because some primary lesions tend to accumulate lymphocytes, the distinction between medullary carcinoma and metastatic carcinoma in a lymph node can be a problem. A reticulin stain is useful in revealing the underlying architecture of ducts in a primary carcinoma or a lymph node obscured by metastatic tumor. A biopsy that includes more than one lymph node usually provides a sample of axillary tissue around the mass that can be studied for evidence of axillary breast tissue. If found, this is presumptive evidence in support of an axillary primary. However, it is necessary to find in situ carcinoma in conjunction with an invasive axillary lesion to make a diagnosis of axillary carcinoma with confidence.

In most cases, the histologic characteristics of the primary tumor and nodal metastases are similar. Nearly two thirds of the primary tumors have apocrine cytologic features. A striking characteristic of many of the primary lesions, particularly tumors too small to be palpable, is a prominent lymphocytic reaction in and around the lesion (42). This is especially conspicuous in cases in which the primary tumor appears by light microscopy to be largely or entirely in situ. Invasive duct carcinoma is the most common occult primary tumor identified in the breast but infiltrating lobular (34,41), medullary (37,43,46), mucinous (43), and papillary carcinoma have occasionally been described.

Prognosis and Treatment. Once it has been established that the excised lymph node contains metastatic adenocarcinoma consistent with a mammary origin and there is no clinical evidence of a nonmammary tumor, treatment should be based on the assumption that there is an invasive primary carcinoma in the ipsilateral breast. A random biopsy of the breast may be obtained before initiating therapy, but without localizing clinical or radiologic signs this procedure is unlikely to detect the primary lesion. The majority of patients described in reports published in the past three decades were treated by mastectomy, often supplemented by local irradiation or, more recently, chemotherapy. Mastectomy offers an opportunity to characterize and stage the primary tumor. Axillary dissection is effective for preventing recurrence in the axilla and provides information about the number of affected lymph nodes.

Breast conserving surgery coupled with axillary dissection has usually been followed by breast irradiation (35,44). In some reports, radiation was given to the breast and axilla after the diagnosis of carcinoma was established by excisional or needle biopsy of an enlarged axillary lymph node (38,47).

Available data indicate that these unusual stage II patients have a prognosis similar to and possibly better than stage II patients who present with a palpable breast carcinoma. Two follow-up studies from Memorial Hospital reported that 23 percent (35) and 25 percent (45) of patients died of breast carcinoma. In a smaller series, 9 percent (34) and 12 percent (42) of patients had recurrent carcinoma or died of the disease.

Data from two series compared the outcome of patients treated by mastectomy with those treated by breast preservation and radiation (35,45). In these studies survival rates were similar and few patients had recurrences in the breast. Others have reported breast recurrences in 23 percent of patients treated with mammary radiation, with a 5-year disease-free survival of 73 percent (38).

PAGET DISEASE OF THE NIPPLE

This condition is defined in the WHO report on the Histological Classification of Breast Tumours (79) as a

> ...lesion in which large pale-staining cells are present within the epidermis of the nipple predominantly in its deep half.... Paget disease of the nipple is almost invariably found to be associated with an intraductal carcinoma and less frequently with an invasive carcinoma.

Paget disease of the nipple is the result of intraepithelial spread from underlying intraductal carcinoma in virtually all cases. The intraductal carcinoma may occur in association with invasive carcinoma or may exist alone. Under exceptional circumstances, invasive carcinoma arising in the nipple or invading the nipple from a large underlying lesion may impinge on the epidermis in which there is Paget disease. This very unusual configuration suggests that direct extension from an underlying invasive carcinoma can result in Paget disease. There is no convincing evidence that Paget disease arises as a result of transformation of squamous cells into adenocarcinoma cells within the epidermis of the nipple. Considerable immunohistochemical data support evidence from conventional anatomic and histopathologic studies that Paget cells are derived from an underlying intraductal carcinoma. In particular, the distribution of CEA immunoreactive protein (62,78), casein (51), milk fat globule membrane antigens (60,78), lectins (59), cytokeratins (52,56,61,63,73), estrogen receptors (76), and apocrine gland epithelial antigens (62) are all indicative of a glandular origin.

Clinical Presentation. Paget disease shows no predilection for a particular age group and the age range in large series of patients is 26 to 88 years (49,52, 65,72). Paget disease may be limited to the nipple or extend to the areola, and in advanced cases the lesion also involves the skin surrounding the areola. Pain or itching are frequent complaints. Early changes include scaling and redness which may be mistaken for eczema or some other inflammatory condition. Ulceration, crusting, and serous or bloody discharge characterize more advanced cases.

Paget disease occurs in 1 to 2 percent of female patients with mammary carcinoma. The majority of these women have a clinically evident lesion. Ten to 28 percent of cases cause no clinical abnormality and are detected only in histologic sections of the nipple removed at mastectomy (68). There are no clinical or epidemiologic factors known to predispose patients to develop Paget disease.

Fifty to 60 percent of patients have a palpable tumor in the breast that exhibits Paget disease. An invasive carcinoma was detected in more than 90 percent of women with Paget disease accompanied by a mass (49,52); 45 to 66 percent had axillary lymph node metastases (49,52,65). In the absence of a clinically apparent tumor, invasive carcinoma occurs in no more than 40 percent of cases and axillary metastases have been reported in 5 (65) to 13 percent (49,52) of cases.

Fewer than 1 percent of reported cases of Paget disease occur in men (57) and less than 5 percent of male breast carcinomas are complicated by Paget disease (58), despite the fact that almost all carcinomas of the male breast are centrally located.

Gross Findings. Occasionally, enlarged lactiferous ducts can be detected if the excised nipple and underlying breast are examined carefully. Clinically palpable tumors have no specific gross pathologic features. A small percentage of women who present with Paget disease and have no tumor detected on clinical examination are found to have a grossly evident invasive carcinoma in the dissected mastectomy (74). An invasive tumor, if present, tends to be central, but peripheral tumors have been described (74).

Microscopic Findings. The diagnosis of Paget disease can be made from a wedge biopsy, a superficial "shave" biopsy of the epidermis, or a punch biopsy. It may be possible to recognize carcinoma cells cytologically in an imprint or scraping from the nipple surface but this material is not suitable for the specific diagnosis of Paget disease.

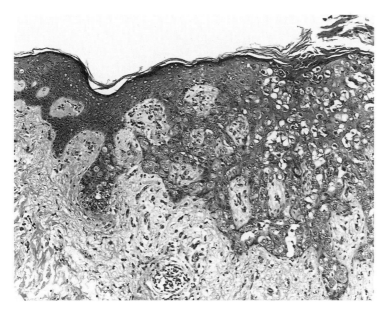

Figure 424
PAGET DISEASE
This low magnification view reveals Paget disease involving the entire thickness of the epidermis. Pseudoepitheliomatous hyperplasia and hyperkeratosis seen on the right are absent in the uninvolved epidermis on the left.

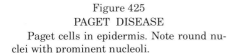

Figure 425
PAGET DISEASE
Paget cells in epidermis. Note round nuclei with prominent nucleoli.

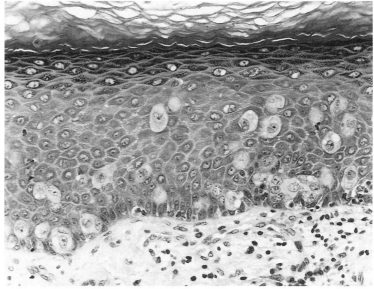

The characteristic histopathologic feature of this condition is the so-called Paget cell in the keratinizing epithelium of the nipple epidermis (fig. 424). These cells occur singly in superficial epidermal layers but tend to form clusters in the basal portions and have a distribution similar to that of junctional melanocytes in a nevus or melanoma. This resemblance to melanoma is further enhanced if the carcinoma cells take up melanin pigment released by epidermal cells (50,53). Isolated Paget cells appear to lie in vacuoles within the epidermis. They have more abundant cytoplasm than keratinocytes and it is usually pale or clear and may contain mucin secretion vacuoles. Nuclei of Paget cells characteristically have large nucleoli (fig. 425). Hyperplasia and hyperkeratosis of the epidermis commonly occur to some degree and this is occasionally severe enough to suggest pseudoepitheliomatous hyperplasia. The superficial, dermal stroma of the nipple is commonly infiltrated by a moderate to marked lymphocytic reaction.

An associated carcinoma has been found in the breast or nipple in more than 95 percent of the hundreds of cases of Paget disease described in the literature. These have virtually all been duct carcinomas with or without an invasive component. Rarely, these have been specialized forms of duct carcinoma (e.g., papillary or medullary) (49) or duct carcinoma arising in florid papillomatosis (adenoma) of the nipple (71). Paget disease of the nipple is not a manifestation of in situ lobular carcinoma.

Intraductal carcinoma associated with Paget disease characteristically has a comedo or solid growth pattern. In one series reported by Chaudary et al. (52), 25 of 32 (78 percent) mastectomy specimens had intraductal carcinoma beyond the subareolar area, and 8 patients had multicentric invasive foci. Intraductal carcinoma was limited to subareolar ducts in only two cases.

Invasive carcinoma associated with Paget disease does not have a specific histopathologic pattern. It is typically a poorly differentiated solid invasive carcinoma arising from affected ducts within the underlying breast parenchyma, although it can develop from a superficial or terminal portion of a lactiferous duct close to the site of Paget disease. In exceptional cases, invasion appears to come directly from Paget disease in the epidermis, there being no invasive carcinoma related to intraductal carcinoma in the nipple and breast.

Failure to detect an underlying carcinoma occurs in a small number of cases. Here, the carcinoma that gives rise to Paget disease originates from ductal epithelium at or very near the squamocolumnar junction of a lactiferous duct with growth limited to spread upward as Paget disease in the epidermis of the nipple (fig. 426).

Immunohistochemistry and Electron Microscopy. The histologic differential diagnosis of a lesion suspected to be Paget disease includes inflammatory conditions of the skin, clear cell change in epidermal cells (77), malignant melanoma, and such extremely uncommon lesions as squamous or basal cell carcinoma.

Clear cells in the epidermis are a non-neoplastic alteration of keratinocytes (fig. 427). The change tends to occur in isolated cells in the upper layers. These cells have small inconspicuous nuclei and consist largely of a vacuole that appears empty on routine sections. Mucin and

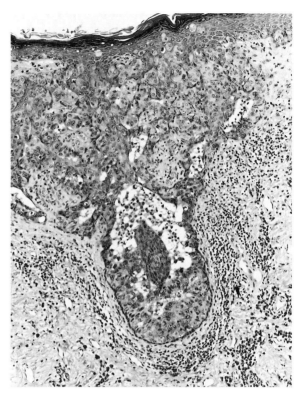

Figure 426
PAGET DISEASE
Terminal portion of a lactiferous duct at its junction with the epidermis. The duct contains comedo intraductal carcinoma and there is contiguous Paget disease in the epidermis. Rarely, this is the entire primary carcinoma complex and the underlying breast proves to be uninvolved.

other secretory substances detectable in Paget cells are absent.

The histopathologic distinction between melanoma and Paget disease may be exceedingly difficult in limited biopsy material. Some melanomas are devoid of pigment while Paget cells can incorporate melanin from epidermal cells. In many cases Paget cells do not contain mucin. Immunohistochemical studies are particularly helpful (Table 6). The demonstration of estrogen receptor in Paget cells excludes melanoma (76). Paget cells were reportedly positive for S-100 in 18 percent of lesions in one series (56), while S-100 is detectable in virtually all melanomas. The finding of immunoreactive CEA is useful since this is present in many mammary carcinomas and virtually always absent from melanomas (78). The neoplastic cells in Paget disease have histochemical and immunohistochemical

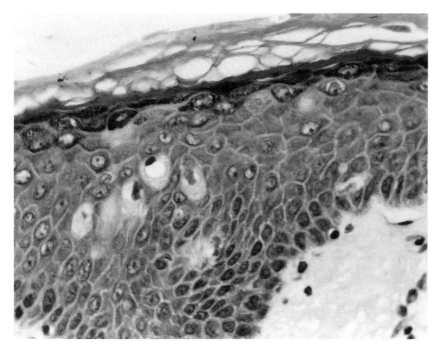

Figure 427
CLEAR CELL
KERATINOCYTES
These non-neoplastic altered squamous epithelial cells have pyknotic nuclei and vacuolated cytoplasm.

properties in common with adenocarcinomas growing within the breast. They are positive for epithelial membrane antigen (EMA) and human milk fat globule (78), low molecular weight cytokeratins (54kD and 57kD) (54,73), and CAM 5.2 (52,61). They are not reactive with antibodies to high molecular weight cytokeratins (66kD) that decorate the normal stratum corneum and neoplastic cells in epidermoid carcinoma or Bowen disease (73).

Immunoreactivity for the *ras* oncogene protein product p21 has been demonstrated in mammary and extramammary Paget disease (69). Strong immunoreactivity for the c-*erb*B-2 (HER2/*neu*) oncoprotein has been detected in 90 to 100 percent of mammary Paget disease samples (64,67) and 40 percent of cases of extramammary Paget disease (fig. 428) (64).

Prognosis and Treatment. Paget disease is a manifestation of mammary duct carcinoma. It does not constitute an independent disease process. Among patients treated by mastectomy, the prognosis of women who have Paget disease is determined by the extent of the associated carcinoma (49,65,72).

Until recently, Paget disease was regarded as a contraindication to breast conservation therapy. In 1969 Rissanen and Holsti (70) described eight patients with Paget disease treated by

Table 6

REACTIVITY OF ANTIBODY

Monoclonal Antibody	Paget Disease	Bowen Disease	Malignant Melanoma
S-100	±	-	+
CEA	±	-	-
EMA	+	-	-
HMFG	+	-	-
LMWCK (54kD)	+	+	+
HMWCK (66kD)	-	+	-
ER	±	-	-
c-*erb*B-2(HER2/*neu*)	+	?	?

CEA:	Carcinoembryonic Antigen
EMA:	Epithelial Membrane Antigen
HMFG:	Human Milk Fat Globule
LMWCK:	Low Molecular Weight Cytokeratin
HMWCK:	High Molecular Weight Cytokeratin
ER:	Estrogen Receptor

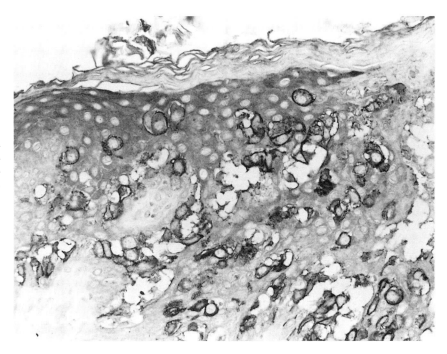

Figure 428
PAGET DISEASE
Immunoperoxidase stain for c-*erb*B-2(HER2/*neu*) oncoprotein revealing strong membrane immunoreactivity limited to Paget cells.

limited surgery and radiotherapy. Three developed recurrences and one ultimately died of breast carcinoma. Five patients treated by excision of the nipple-areola complex without radiation remained well for 30 to 69 months (average 50 months) (66). Three recurrences were reported after a median follow-up of 90 months (15 months to 20 years) in 20 patients who received radiation and breast conserving surgery for Paget disease (55). All recurrences were in the form of Paget disease and the lesions were controlled by mastectomy. Stockdale et al. (75) reported that primary radiotherapy was effective when Paget disease was not associated with a palpable tumor or mammographic abnormality.

CARCINOMA IN ECTOPIC BREAST

There are two general types of ectopic mammary tissue: supernumerary breasts and aberrant breast tissue (see p. 20). In most instances these are distinguishable anatomically but there are ambiguous situations in which the distinction is arbitrary.

Supernumerary breasts are subject to pathologic alterations that affect the normal breast. A supernumerary breast is usually a clinically evident mass of mammary glandular tissue along the embryologic milk line. Carcinoma has been described arising in axillary (81,82) and vulvar (80,84,88) breast tissue. Histologically, adenocarcinomas arising in supernumerary breast tissue have had a ductal growth pattern. Inflammatory carcinoma arising in the vulva was described in one patient (86), another had asynchronous bilateral mammary carcinomas and a separate mammary type adenocarcinoma in supernumerary vulvar breast tissue (83). Adenocarcinoma, metastatic from carcinoma that arose in supernumerary breast tissue, has been reported in ipsilateral axillary (81) and groin lymph nodes (80,88). In two cases, analysis of metastatic tumor in a lymph node revealed positive estrogen and progesterone receptor levels (80,88).

Treatment of carcinoma arising in supernumerary breast tissue generally consists of wide local excision and regional lymphadenectomy. Mastectomy is not indicated if origin in supernumerary axillary breast tissue can be documented. Vulvar lesions are managed by partial vulvectomy and ipsilateral groin dissection. Many of these carcinomas have had an aggressive clinical course with systemic metastases reported with axillary (81) and vulvar lesions (88).

Aberrant breast is a microscopic condition that is by definition anatomically separate from the duct system of the breast and differs in this

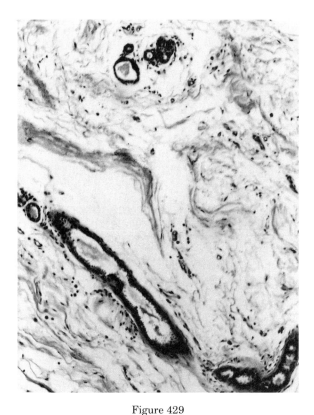

Figure 429
ABERRANT BREAST TISSUE
In the postmenopausal patient, atrophic aberrant breast ductules may be difficult to distinguish from skin appendage gland ducts. (Figures 429 and 430 are from the same patient.)

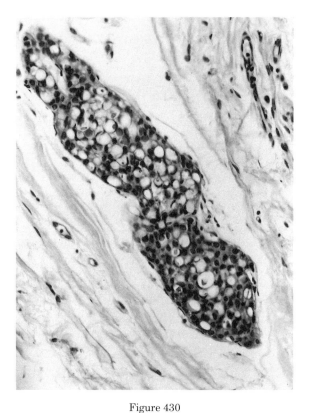

Figure 430
CARCINOMA IN ABERRANT
BREAST TISSUE
In situ carcinoma with prominent signet ring cell features in aberrant breast duct.

respect from peripheral extensions of the breast (85). Microscopically, aberrant and peripheral breast tissue are histologically indistinguishable, consisting of isolated mammary ductules and lobules in fibro-fatty subcutaneous tissue (fig. 429). A diagnosis of carcinoma arising in aberrant breast tissue can be made if intraductal or invasive carcinoma is found in subcutaneous mammary glandular parenchyma beyond the normal extent of the breast (fig. 430). In the absence of in situ changes and glandular parenchyma, the histologic appearance of invasive carcinoma is indistinguishable from carcinoma of sweat gland origin or metastatic carcinoma. Since estrogen receptor protein has been de-

tected in some carcinomas of sweat gland origin, including about one third of eccrine carcinomas, as well as in eccrine hidradenomas, this procedure is not reliable for distinguishing these tumors from mammary carcinomas (89). Carcinoma originating in aberrant breast tissue has been described in the clavicular and anterior axillary regions, over the sternum, and in the upper abdominal skin outside the distribution of the milk lines (87). Treatment may consist of wide excision usually accompanied by regional lymph node dissection, although the choice of the lymph node group most likely to be involved by metastases may be difficult.

REFERENCES

Carcinoma in Pregnancy and Lactation

1. Gallenberg MM, Loprinzi CL. Breast cancer and pregnancy. Semin Oncol 1989;16:369–76.
2. Holdaway IM, Mason BH, Kay RG. Steroid hormone receptors in breast tumors presenting during pregnancy or lactation. J Surg Oncol 1984;25:38–41.
3. Maz MH, Klamer TW. Pregnancy and breast cancer. South Med J 1983;76:1088–90.
4. Nugent P, O'Connell TX. Breast cancer and pregnancy. Arch Surg 1985;120:1221–4.
5. Potter JF, Schoeneman M. Metastasis of maternal cancer to the placenta and fetus. Cancer 1970;25:380–8.

Inflammatory Carcinoma

6. Berger SM. Inflammatory carcinoma of the breast. AJR 1962;88:1109–16.
7. Brownstein MH, Helwig EB. Spread of tumors to the skin. Arch Dermatol 1973;107:80–6.
8. Brun B, Otmezguine Y, Feuilhade F, et al. Treatment of inflammatory breast cancer with combination chemotherapy and mastectomy versus breast conservation. Cancer 1988;61:1096–103.
9. Chevallier B, Asselain B, Kunlin A, Veyret C, Bastit P, Graic Y. Inflammatory breast cancer. Determination of prognostic factors by univariate and multivariate analysis. Cancer 1987;60:897–902.
10. Crowe J, Hakes T, Rosen PP, Kinne DW, Robbins GF. Changing trends in the management of inflammatory breast cancer: a clinical-pathological review of 69 patients. Am J Clin Oncol 1985;8:21.
11. Donegan WL, Padrta B. Combined therapy for inflammatory breast cancer. Arch Surg 1990;125:578–82.
12. Droulias CA, Sewell CW, McSweeney MB, Powell RW. Inflammatory carcinoma of the breast. A correlation of clinical, radiologic and pathologic findings. Ann Surg 1976;184:217–22.
13. Ellis DL, Teitelbaum SL. Inflammatory carcinoma of the breast. A pathologic definition. Cancer 1974;33:1045–7.
14. Fastenberg NA, Martin RG, Buzdar AU, et al. Management of inflammatory carcinoma of the breast. A combined modality approach. Am J Clin Oncol 1985;8:134–41.
15. Feldman LD, Hortobagyi GN, Buzdar AU, Ames FC, Blumenschein GR. Pathological assessment of response to induction chemotherapy in breast cancer. Cancer Res 1986;46:2578–81.
16. Fields JN, Perez CA, Kuske RR, Fineberg BB, Bartlett N. Inflammatory carcinoma of the breast: treatment results of 107 patients. Int J Radiat Oncol Biol Phys 1989;17:249–55.
17. Guérin M, Gabillot M, Mathieu MC, et al. Structure and expression of c-erbB-2 and EGF receptor genes in inflammatory and non-inflammatory breast cancer: prognostic significance. Int J Cancer 1989;43:201–8.
18. Haagensen CD. Inflammatory carcinoma. In: Diseases of the breast. 2nd ed. Philadelphia: WB Saunders Co, 1971:576–84.
19. Hazelrigg DC, Rudolph AH. Inflammatory metastatic carcinoma. Arch Dermatol 1977;113:69–70.
20. Lee BJ, Tannenbaum NE. Inflammatory carcinoma of the breast: a report of twenty-eight cases from the breast clinic of Memorial Hospital. Surg Gynecol Obstet 1924;39:580–95.
21. Lucas FV, Perez-Mesa C. Inflammatory carcinoma of the breast. Cancer 1978;41:1595–605.
22. McCready DR, Hortobagyi GN, Kau SW, Smith TL, Buzdar AU, Balch GM. The prognostic significance of lymph node metastases after preoperative chemotherapy for locally advanced breast cancer. Arch Surg 1989;124:21–5.
23. Mourali N, Muenz LR, Tabbane F, Belhassen S, Bahi J, Levine PH. Epidemiologic features of rapidly progressing breast cancer in Tunisia. Cancer 1980;46:2741–6.
24. Noguchi S, Miyauchi K, Nishizawa Y, Koyama H, Terasawa T. Management of inflammatory carcinoma of the breast with combined modality therapy including intraarterial infusion chemotherapy as an induction therapy. Long-term follow-up results of 28 patients. Cancer 1988;61:1483–91.
25. Paradiso A, Tommasi S, Brandi M, et al. Cell kinetics and hormonal receptor status in inflammatory breast carcinoma. Comparison with locally advanced disease. Cancer 1989;64:1922–7.
26. Piera JM, Alonso MC, Ojeda MB, Biete A. Locally advanced breast cancer with inflammatory component: a clinical entity with a poor prognosis. Radiother Oncol 1986;7:199–204.
27. Robbins GF, Shah J, Rosen P, Chu F, Taylor J. Inflammatory carcinoma of the breast. Surg Clin North Am 1974;54:801–10.
28. Rosen PP, Menendez-Botet CJ, Senie RT, Schwartz MK, Schottenfeld D, Farr GH. Estrogen receptor protein (ERP) and the histopathology of human mammary carcinoma. In: McGuire ML, ed. Hormones, receptors and breast cancer. New York: Raven Press, 1978:71–83.
29. Saltzstein SL. Clinically occult inflammatory carcinoma of the breast. Cancer 1974;34:382–8.
30. Schäfer P, Alberto P, Forni M, Obradovic D, Pipard G, Krauer F. Surgery as part of a combined modality approach for inflammatory breast carcinoma. Cancer 1987;59:1063–7.
31. Shukla HS, Hughes LE, Gravelle IH, Satir A. The significance of mammary skin edema in noninflammatory breast cancer. Ann Surg 1979;189:53–7.
32. Tschen EH, Apisarnthanarax P. Inflammatory metastatic carcinoma of the breast. Arch Dermatol 1981;177:120–1.
33. World Health Organization. Histological typing of breast tumors. 2nd ed. International Histological Classification of Tumours, No.2. Geneva: World Health Organization, 1981:21.

Occult Carcinoma Presenting with Axillary Lymph Node Metastases

34. Ashikari R, Rosen PP, Urban JA, Senoo T. Breast cancer presenting as an axillary mass. Ann Surg 1976;183:415–7.

35. Baron PL, Moore MP, Kinne DW, Candela FC, Osborne MP, Petrek JA. Occult breast cancer presenting with axillary metastases: updated management. Arch Surg 1990;125:210–4.

36. Bhatia SK, Saclarides TJ, Witt TR, Bonomi PD, Anderson KM, Economou SG. Hormone receptor studies in axillary metastases from occult breast cancers. Cancer 1987;59:1170–2.

37. Breslow A. Occult carcinoma of second breast following mastectomy. JAMA 1973;226:1000–1.

38. Campana F, Fourquet A, Ashby MA, et al. Presentation of axillary lymphadenopathy without detectable breast primary (T0N1b breast cancer): experience at Institut Curie. Radiother Oncol 1989;15:321–5.

39. Feuerman L, Attie JN, Rosenberg B. Carcinoma in axillary lymph nodes as an indicator of breast cancer. Surg Gynecol Obstet 1962;114:5–8.

40. Grundfest S, Steiger E, Sebek B. Metastatic axillary adenopathy. Use of estrogen receptor protein as an aid in diagnosis. Arch Surg 1978;113:1108–9.

41. Halsted WS. The results of radical operation for the cure of carcinoma of the breast. Ann Surg 1907;46:1–19.

42. Haupt HM, Rosen PP, Kinne DW. Breast carcinoma presenting with axillary lymph node metastases. An analysis of specific histopathologic features. Am J Surg Pathol 1985;9:165–75.

43. Inglehart JD, Ferguson BJ, Shingleton WW, et al. An ultrastructural analysis of breast carcinoma presenting as isolated axillary adenopathy. Ann Surg 1982;196:8–13.

44. Kemeny MM, Rivera DE, Terz JJ, Benfield JR. Occult primary adenocarcinoma with axillary metastases. Am J Surg 1986;152:43–7.

45. Rosen PP, Kimmel M. Occult breast carcinoma presenting with axillary lymph node metastases: a follow-up study of 48 patients. Hum Pathol 1990;21:518–23.

46. Smith GM. Occult carcinoma of the breast. Br Med J 1971;4:598–9.

47. Vilcoq JR, Calle R, Ferme F, Veith F. Conservative treatment of axillary adenopathy due to probable subclinical breast cancer. Arch Surg 1982;117:1136–8.

48. Westbrook KC, Gallager H. Breast carcinoma presenting as an axillary mass. Am J Surg 1971;122:607–11.

Paget Disease of the Nipple

49. Ashikari R, Park K, Huvos AG, Urban JA. Paget's disease of the breast. Cancer 1970;26:680–5.

50. Azzopardi JG, Eusebi V. Melanocyte colonization and pigmentation of breast carcinoma. Histopathology 1977;1:21–30.

51. Bussolati G, Pich A, Alfani V. Immunofluorescence detection of casein in human mammary dysplastic and neoplastic tissues. Virchows Arch [A] 1975;365:15–21.

52. Chaudary MA, Millis RR, Lane EB, Miller NA. Paget's disease of the nipple: a ten-year review including clinical, pathological and immunohistochemical findings. Breast Cancer Res Treat 1986;8:139–46.

53. Culberson JD, Horn RC Jr. Paget's disease of the nipple: review of 25 cases with special reference to melanin pigmentation of "Paget cells." Arch Surg 1956;72:224–31.

54. Fisher ER, Sass R, Fisher B, Wickerham L, Paik SM. Pathologic findings from the National Surgical Adjuvant Breast Project (protocol 6). I. Intraductal Carcinoma (DCIS). Cancer 1986;57:197–208.

55. Fourquet A, Campana F, Vielh P, Schlienger P, Jullien D, Vilcoq JR. Paget's disease of the nipple without detectable breast tumor: conservative management with radiation therapy. Int J Radiat Oncol Biol Phys 1987;13:1463–5.

56. Gillett CE, Bobrow LG, Millis RR. S100 protein in human mammary tissue—immunoreactivity in breast carcinoma, including Paget's disease of the nipple, and value as a marker of myoepithelial cells. J Pathol 1990;160:19–24.

57. Gupta S, Khanna NN, Khanna S, Gupta S. Paget's disease of the male breast: a clinicopathologic study and a collective review. J Surg Oncol 1983;22:151–6.

58. Heller KS, Rosen PP, Schottenfeld D, Ashikari R, Kinne DW. Male breast cancer: a clinicopathologic study of 97 cases. Ann Surg 1978;188:60–5.

59. Hyun KH, Nakai M, Kawamura K, Mori K. Histochemical studies of lectin binding patterns in keratinized lesions, including malignancy. Virchows Arch [A] 1984;402:337–51.

60. Imam A, Yoshida SO, Taylor CR. Distinguishing tumour cells of mammary from extramammary Paget's disease using antibodies to two different glycoproteins from human milk-fat-globule membrane. Br J Cancer 1988;58:373–8.

61. Jones RR, Spaull J, Gusterson B. The histogenesis of mammary and extramammary Paget's disease. Histopathology 1989;14:409–16.

62. Kariniemi AL, Forsman L, Wahlström T, Vesterinen E, Andersson L. Expression of differentiation antigens in mammary and extramammary Paget's disease. Br J Dermatol 1984;110:203–10.

63. _____, Ramaekers F, Lehto VP, Virtanen I. Paget cells express cytokeratins typical of glandular epithelia. Br J Dermatol 1985;112:179–83.

64. Keatings L, Sinclair J, Wright C, et al. C-erbB-2 oncoprotein expression in mammary and extramammary Paget's disease: an immunohistochemical study. Histopathology 1990;17:243–7.

65. Kister SJ, Haagensen CD. Paget's disease of the breast. Am J Surg 1970;119:606–9.

66. Lagios MD, Westdahl PR, Rose MR, Concannon S. Paget's disease of the nipple. Alternative management in cases without or with minimal extent of underlying breast carcinoma. Cancer 1984;54:545–51.

67. Lammie GA, Barnes DM, Millis RR, Gullick WJ. An immunohistochemical study of the presence of c-erbB-2 protein in Paget's disease of the nipple. Histopathology 1989;15:505–14.

68. Mendez-Fernandez MA, Henly WS, Geis RC, Schoen FJ, Hausner RJ. Paget's disease of the breast after subcutaneous mastectomy and reconstruction with a silicone prosthesis. Plast Reconstr Surg 1980;65:683–5.

69. Mori O, Hachisuka H, Nakano S, Sasai Y, Shiku H. Expression of *ras* p21 in mammary and extramammary Paget's disease. Arch Pathol Lab Med 1990; 114:858–61.

70. Rissanen PM, Holsti P. Paget's disease of the breast: the influence of the presence or absence of an underlying palpable tumor on the prognosis and on the choice of treatment. Oncology 1969;23:209–16.

71. Rosen PP, Caicco JA. Florid papillomatosis of the nipple: a study of 51 patients including nine with mammary carcinoma. Am J Surg Pathol 1986;10:87–101.

72. Salvadori B, Fariselli G, Saccozzi R. Analysis of 100 cases of Paget's disease of the breast. Tumori 1976; 62:529–35.

73. Shah KD, Tabibzadeh SS, Gerber MA. Immunohistochemical distinction of Paget's diseases from Bowen's disease and superficial spreading melanoma with the use of monoclonal cytokeratin antibodies. Am J Clin Pathol 1987;88:689–95.

74. Sievers DB, Huvos AG, Beattie EJ Jr, Ashikari H, Urban JA. Paget's disease of the nipple. Clin Bull (Mem Sloan-Kettering Cancer Center) 1973;3:141–5.

75. Stockdale AD, Brierley JD, White WF, Folkes A, Rostom AY. Radiotherapy for Paget's disease of the nipple: a conservative alternative. Lancet 1989;2:664–6.

76. Tani EM, Skoog L. Immunocytochemical detection of estrogen receptors in mammary Paget cells. Acta Cytol 1988;23:825–8.

77. Toker C. Clear cells of the nipple epidermis. Cancer 1970;25:601–10.

78. Vanstapel MJ, Gatter KC, De Wolf-Peeters C, Millard PR, Desmet VJ, Mason DY. Immunohistochemical study of mammary and extra-mammary Paget's disease. Histopathology 1984;8:1013–23.

79. World Health Organization. Histological typing of breast tumors. Tumori 1982;68:181–98.

Carcinoma in Ectopic Breast

80. Cho D, Buscema J, Rosenshein NB, Woodruff JD. Primary breast cancer of the vulva. Obstet Gynecol 1985;66:79S–81S.

81. Cogswell HD, Czerny EW. Carcinoma of aberrant breast of axilla. Am Surg 1961;27:388–90.

82. De Cholnoky T. Accessory breast tissue in the axilla. NY State J Med 1951;51:2245–8.

83. Guerry RL, Pratt-Thomas HR. Carcinoma of supernumerary breast of vulva with bilateral mammary cancer. Cancer 1976;38:2570–4.

84. Hendrix RC, Behrman SJ. Adenocarcinoma arising in a supernumerary mammary gland in the vulva. Obstet Gynecol 1956;8:238–41.

85. Hicken NF. Mastectomy: clinical and pathological study demonstrating why most mastectomies result in incomplete removal of the mammary gland. Arch Surg 1940;40:6–14.

86. Hoogerland DL, Buchler DA. Inflammatory carcinoma of the vulva. Gynecol Oncol 1979;8:240–5.

87. Petrek J, Rosen PP, Robbins GF. Carcinoma of aberrant breast tissue. Clin Bull 1980;10:13–5.

88. Simon KE, Dutcher JP, Runowicz CD, Wiernik PH. Adenocarcinoma arising in vulvar breast tissue. Cancer 1988;62:2234–8.

89. Swanson PE, Mazoujian G, Mills SE, Campbell J, Wick MR. Immunoreactivity for estrogen receptor protein in sweat gland tumors. Am J Surg Pathol 1991;15:835–41.

BREAST TUMORS IN CHILDREN

Most of the lesions seen in this age group are not unique to children or adolescents, although their frequency differs somewhat from older patients. In girls, the most common abnormality is a solitary fibroadenoma, while fibrocystic changes are comparatively rare. In boys, the most prevalent cause of breast enlargement is gynecomastia. For the most part, the characteristics of lesions not particularly associated with this age group will be described elsewhere in this Fascicle.

JUVENILE PAPILLOMATOSIS

This clinicopathologic entity is characterized by a discrete mammary lesion that simulates a fibroadenoma clinically, yet microscopically consists of intraductal hyperplasia accompanied by numerous cysts and other benign proliferative changes (14). The median age at diagnosis is around 20 years of age but juvenile papillomatosis occurs occasionally in women in the third to fifth decades of life. Juvenile papillomatosis is usually unilateral and unicentric but in rare instances multicentric or bilateral lesions are encountered.

The tumors may vary from 1 to 8 cm, averaging 4 cm in diameter. They appear grossly circumscribed but not encapsulated. No microscopic components are uniquely associated with this lesion. Numerous dilated ducts, usually containing fluid, result in grossly evident cysts as large as 1 cm in diameter (fig. 431). This prominent finding occasioned the appellation "Swiss cheese disease" in the original report. Of equal prominence is pronounced intraductal papillary epithelial proliferation, which may be solid or have epithelial bridges extending across the duct lumen, resulting in a complex growth pattern (fig. 432).

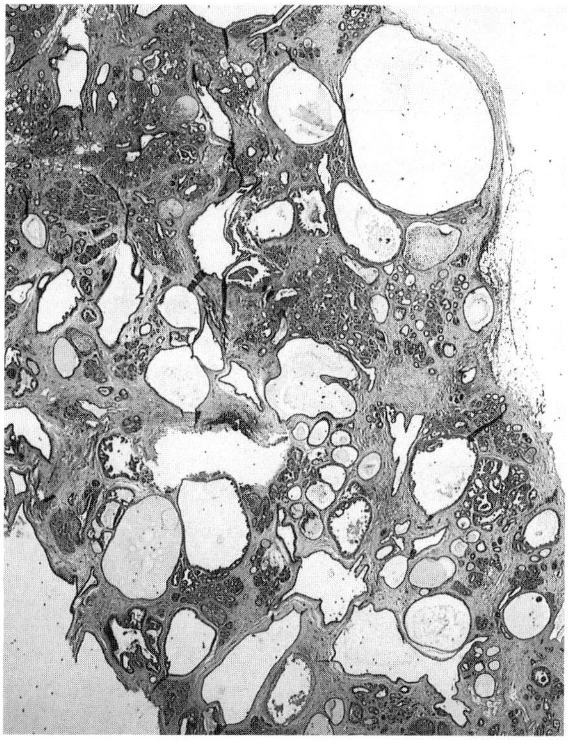

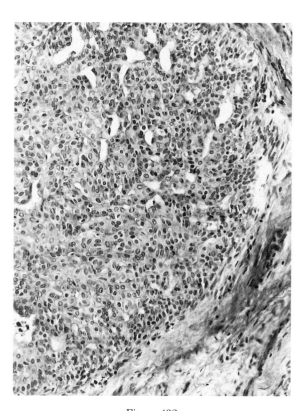

Figure 431
JUVENILE PAPILLOMATOSIS
Multiple cystically dilated ducts dominate the appearance of the lesion at low magnification.

Figure 432
JUVENILE PAPILLOMATOSIS
An ectatic duct contains hyperplastic epithelium forming irregular slits and lumens. Myoepithelial cell hyperplasia is present.

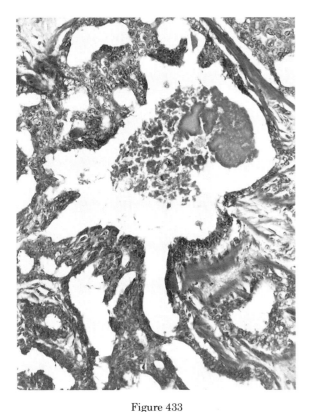

Figure 433
JUVENILE PAPILLOMATOSIS
Intraductal epithelial proliferation with necrosis. The hyperplastic process involves only a portion of the duct.

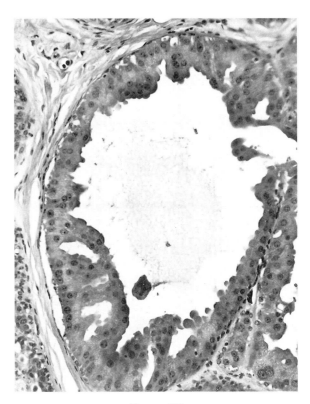

Figure 434
JUVENILE PAPILLOMATOSIS
Apocrine metaplasia of hyperplastic intraductal epithelium.

The epithelium and myoepithelium participate in the hyperplastic process. Rarely, comedonecrosis is present in ducts with solid intraductal hyperplasia that lack cytologic features of intraductal carcinoma (fig. 433). The presence of occasional mitoses may cause further confusion. The intraductal epithelial hyperplasia is atypical in approximately 10 percent of cases (15).

Cystic and papillary apocrine metaplasia of the proliferating epithelium is a prominent microscopic finding (fig. 434). In some instances the apocrine intraductal hyperplasia may be the most noteworthy microscopic finding. In addition, the dilated ducts often contain aggregates of foamy histiocytes (fig. 435). Prominent fibrosis may be present as well as foci of sclerosing adenosis and, occasionally, radial sclerosing lesions (fig. 436). The gross circumscription of the lesion distinguishes it from fibrocystic changes that are typically diffuse and uncommon in the breasts of women under 25 years old. Similarly, juvenile

papillomatosis should be distinguished from cyst formation in a fibroadenoma since the latter lesion lacks features such as duct hyperplasia. Noncystic fibroadenomas sometimes coexist with juvenile papillomatosis.

Studies have not revealed an increased incidence of subsequent carcinoma but the follow-up intervals have not been long enough to draw firm prognostic conclusions. More than 25 percent of the patients have a family history of breast carcinoma and in rare cases, carcinoma has been reported to coexist with juvenile papillomatosis (4,17).

In a recent study of 41 patients with juvenile papillomatosis, followed for a minimum of 10 years, 4 subsequently developed carcinoma and a fifth had a synchronous secretory carcinoma in the contralateral breast (16). The 4 patients with subsequent carcinoma had a positive family history for carcinoma of the breast and each had bilateral, multifocal, recurrent juvenile papillomatosis. None of the patients with unilateral, unicentric, nonrecurrent involvement developed carcinoma.

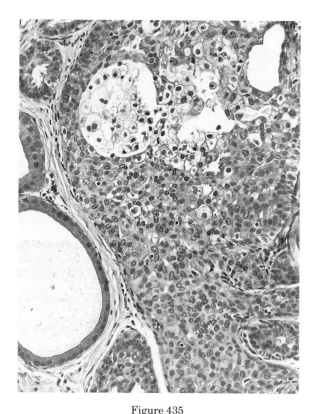

Figure 435
JUVENILE PAPILLOMATOSIS
Aggregates of foam cells amid hyperplastic intraductal epithelium.

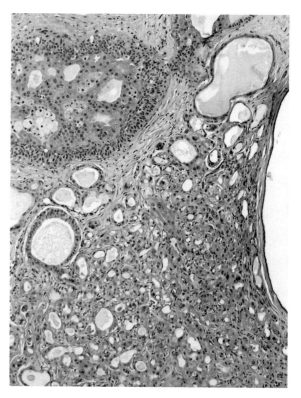

Figure 436
JUVENILE PAPILLOMATOSIS
Part of an area of sclerosing adenosis with apocrine metaplasia of ductal epithelium adjacent to cystically dilated ducts. Hyperplastic epithelium with apocrine metaplasia fills some ducts.

Treatment consists of excision and careful follow-up with regular physical examination by a physician as well as monthly self-examination. Mammography should be instituted when the patient reaches an appropriate age. No surgery is necessary after complete excision of the abnormality.

PAPILLARY DUCT HYPERPLASIA

Intraductal papillary hyperplasia, although common in adults, is infrequent in the adolescent breast. In this group the lesions usually are multifocal and result in a mass, most often in the periphery of the breast. When it develops in subareolar ducts, a much less common location, nipple discharge may occur. Only a few solitary intraductal papillomas have been reported in teen-aged patients. A fibrovascular stalk may be conspicuous in the larger solitary lesions, although multifocal areas of involvement of smaller calibre ducts that form a palpable lesion usually lack a conspicuous stromal component (figs. 437, 438).

Multifocal papillary intraductal hyperplasia may result in a worrisome microscopic appearance (8). Absence of necrosis of the epithelial component, apocrine metaplasia, intraductal foamy histiocytes, hyperplasia of the myoepithelium, and the formation of slit-like spaces by the proliferating cells, are factors indicative of hyperplasia rather than carcinoma. Fibrosis may be prominent in these lesions and collagenization may cause compression of ductal elements, creating the pattern of sclerosing papillomatosis (11).

This abnormality differs from juvenile papillomatosis in that it lacks cystic dilatation of ducts, stasis of secretion, adenosis, and prominent apocrine metaplasia. The growth pattern of papillary duct hyperplasia is comparable to that seen commonly in adult women. Follow-up of patients with this abnormality has not indicated an increased incidence of carcinoma (13). The rarity of the lesion, coupled with the need for

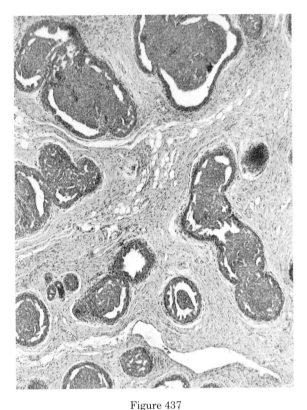

Figure 437
PAPILLARY DUCT HYPERPLASIA
Multiple small intraductal papillomas resulting in a breast mass in a 15-year-old girl. (Figures 437 and 438 are from the same patient.)

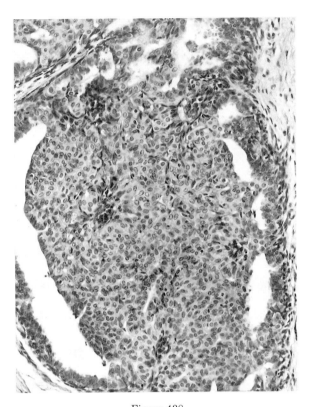

Figure 438
PAPILLARY DUCT HYPERPLASIA
Higher magnification of hyperplastic intraductal epithelium. Myoepithelial cells are associated with the delicate fibrovascular stalks.

long-term surveillance until patients have reached an age when the risk of carcinoma of the breast is greatest, suggests that it is premature to draw definitive prognostic conclusions at this time. Continued follow-up by physical examination and mammography after 35 years of age is appropriate. One patient who had bilateral papillary intraductal hyperplasia at 11 years of age developed invasive carcinoma 27 years later (8).

FIBROADENOMA

These tumors represent the most common cause of a breast mass in patients in the second and third decades of life (see p. 101). They may attain considerable size in young patients. The term *giant fibroadenoma* has been utilized not only for large tumors, such as those weighing more than 500 g, but also for tumors that appear large in relation to the size of the breast (20). These masses often manifest rapid growth, attaining

large size over a few months, and are more common in black patients. Moreover, they may manifest increased sensitivity to normal levels of circulating estrogen (5). The microscopic pattern of the tumor may be either that of a characteristic fibroadenoma or a juvenile fibroadenoma (see p. 104). The extent of stromal cellularity and ductal epithelial proliferation distinguishes these lesions from cystosarcoma phyllodes but some older reports have utilized the latter designation for massive fibroadenomas (10). In retrospect, some of the nine cystosarcomas reported in adolescent patients by Treves and Sunderland (18) and by Lester and Stout (9) might now be classified as fibroadenomas.

Juvenile fibroadenoma and the clinicopathologic syndrome of multiple and successive fibroadenomas are included in a comprehensive discussion of fibroepithelial lesions in the chapter Fibroepithelial Neoplasms.

CYSTOSARCOMA

Cystosarcoma phyllodes reported in patients in this age group have usually been large fibroadenomas (2). They are characterized by a pattern of stromal cellularity and intracanalicular arrangement of the ductal component in both children and adults. Only a few well-documented cases of cystosarcoma have been described in adolescents, and two of the patients had pulmonary metastases (1,6,7,19). As might be anticipated, none of these tumors metastasized to axillary lymph nodes, and systemic metastases contained only mesenchymal elements.

CARCINOMA

Carcinoma of the breast is exceedingly rare in patients less than 20 years of age. Fewer than 50 cases had been documented by 1973 (3), and only isolated cases have been reported since that time. The most common pattern of carcinoma in this age group is secretory carcinoma, a neoplasm that may develop local recurrence, rarely metastasizes to regional lymph nodes or to systemic sites, and has an excellent prognosis. At one time this neoplasm was thought to occur only in adolescents and was termed juvenile carcinoma. However, the occurrence of this growth pattern in adults suggests that it is best designated secretory carcinoma, and for this reason is discussed in the chapter Invasive Carcinoma. Other forms of carcinoma are exceedingly rare. Isolated examples of rhabdomyosarcoma, angiosarcoma, and non-Hodgkin lymphoma have been reported in patients in the second decade of life (12).

REFERENCES

1. Adami HO, Hakelius L, Rimsten A, Willén R. Malignant, locally recurring cystosarcoma phyllodes in an adolescent female. A case report. Acta Chir Scand 1984;150:93–100.
2. Ashikari R, Farrow JH, O'Hara J. Fibroadenomas in the breast of juveniles. Surg Gynecol Obstet 1971;132:259–62.
3. Basler WL. Pathologie der weiblichen genital- und mammatumoren in kindesalter und adoleszenz. Gynakologe 1973;6:49–65.
4. Bazzocchi F, Santini D, Martinelli G, et al. Juvenile papillomatosis (epitheliosis) of the breast. A clinical and pathologic study of 13 cases. Am J Clin Pathol 1986;86:745–8.
5. Block GE, Zlatnik PA. Giant fibroadenomata of the breast in a prepubertal girl. Arch Surg 1960;80:665–9.
6. Gibbs BF Jr, Roe RD, Thomas DF. Malignant cystosarcoma phyllodes in a pre-pubertal female. Ann Surg 1968;167:229–31.
7. Hoover HC, Trestioreanu A, Ketcham AS. Metastatic cystosarcoma phyllodes in an adolescent girl: an unusually malignant tumor. Ann Surg 1975;181:279–82.
8. Kiaer HW, Kiaer WW, Linell F, Jacobsen S. Extreme duct papillomatosis of the juvenile breast. Acta Pathol Microbiol Immunol Scand [A] 1979;87A:353–9.
9. Lester J, Stout AP. Cystosarcoma phyllodes. Cancer 1954;7:335–53.
10. McDonald JR, Harrington SW. Giant fibroadenoma of the breast—"cystosarcoma phyllodes." Ann Surg 1950; 131:243–51.
11. Oberman HA. Breast lesions in the adolescent female. Pathol Annu 1979;14(Pt 1):175–201.
12. Pettinato G, Manivel JC, Kelly DR, Wold LE, Dehner LP. Lesions of the breast in children exclusive of typical fibroadenoma and gynecomastia. A clinicopathologic study of 113 cases. Pathol Annu 1989;24(Pt 2):295–328.
13. Rosen PP. Papillary duct hyperplasia of the breast in children and young adults. Cancer 1985;56:1611–7.
14. _____, Cantrell B, Mullen DL, DePalo A. Juvenile papillomatosis (Swiss cheese disease) of the breast. Am J Surg Pathol 1980;4:3–12.
15. _____, Holmes G, Lesser ML, Kinne DW, Beattie EJ. Juvenile papillomatosis and breast carcinoma. Cancer 1985;55:1345–52.
16. _____, Kimmel M. Juvenile papillomatosis of the breast. A follow-up study of 41 patients having biopsies before 1979. Am J Clin Pathol 1990;93:599–603.
17. _____, Lyngholm B, Kinne DW, Beattie EJ Jr. Juvenile papillomatosis of the breast and family history of breast carcinoma. Cancer 1982;49:2591–5.
18. Treves N, Sunderland DA. Cystosarcoma phyllodes of the breast. A malignant and a benign tumor. Cancer 1951;4:1286–332.
19. Turalba CI, El-Mahdi AM, Ladaga L. Fatal metastatic cystosarcoma phyllodes in an adolescent female: case report and review of treatment approaches. J Surg Oncol 1986;33:176–81.
20. Wulsin JH. Large breast tumors in adolescent females. Ann Surg 1960;152:151–9.

✧✧✧

BENIGN TUMORS OF THE MALE BREAST

With the exception of gynecomastia, the lesions discussed in this chapter are not unique to the male breast and comments here only highlight the features related to men. More complete information can be found in corresponding sections in other chapters.

PAPILLOMA

Several instances of intraductal papilloma arising in the male breast have been reported (20,22), with age ranging from 3 months to 82 years. The usual presenting symptom is nipple discharge that is bloody or blood tinged. Cystic lesions may be palpable. The histologic features are indistinguishable from papillomas of the female breast (figs. 439, 440). Because of the relatively high proportion of papillary lesions among carcinomas of the male breast, all male papillary tumors should be carefully evaluated.

FLORID PAPILLOMATOSIS OF THE NIPPLE

Approximately 5 percent of reported florid papillomatosis of the nipple have been in men. Nearly half of these lesions have contained carcinoma (24).

FIBROEPITHELIAL TUMORS

Cystosarcomas in the male breast usually arise in patients with clinical gynecomastia (15,18). Some of the lesions are poorly documented or appear to be nodular foci of gynecomastia. True fibroadenomas and cystosarcomas of the male breast are exceedingly uncommon because these lesions arise in lobular glandular tissue that is rarely present in men. Most patients are under 30 years of age but one was a 74-year-old man receiving estrogens for prostatic carcinoma (5).

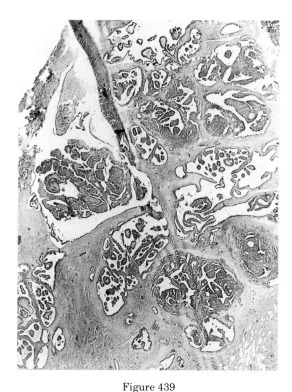

Figure 439
PAPILLOMA
Complex intraductal papilloma from the breast of a man.
(Figures 439 and 440 are from the same patient.)

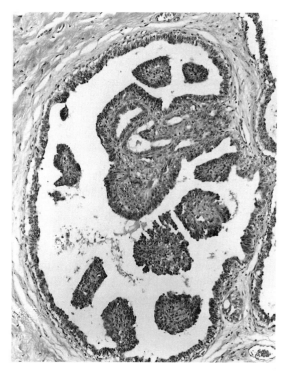

Figure 440
PAPILLOMA
Papillary frond with fibrovascular stroma.

Nielsen (14) reported an unusual 16 cm fibroadenomatoid tumor that arose in one breast of a 69-year-old man with bilateral gynecomastia. The patient had chronic heart disease and breast enlargement and the appearance of the unilateral tumor began after spironolactone was added to his medications, suggesting that this drug contributed to the mammary lesion.

DUCT ECTASIA

Duct dilatation or ectasia and periductal mastitis, a relatively common condition in the female breast, has also been described in men (1,23). Andersen and Gram (1) found duct ectasia in 9 of 35 (26 percent) "normal" breasts and in 19 of 55 (35 percent) breasts with gynecomastia examined at autopsy. The histologic appearance is similar in men and women, with less inflammation and fibrosis in lesions that are clinically asymptomatic.

PROLIFERATIVE "FIBROCYSTIC" CHANGES

Proliferative changes ("fibrocystic changes") resembling those of the female are only rarely encountered in the male breast. Two case reports describe men 28 and 41 years of age who were karyotypically and phenotypically normal (3,12). Grossly, each patient had a circumscribed multicystic tumor. The lesions included cysts with apocrine metaplasia, papillary apocrine metaplasia, and duct hyperplasia. Both also had elements of gynecomastia and duct stasis with mastitis. Sclerosing adenosis arising in lobules was described as an incidental finding in the postmortem examination of a 41-year-old man with disseminated pulmonary oat cell carcinoma (6). Grossly, the lesion was a unilateral, firm white 1.8 x 1.5 x 1.0 cm nodule.

GYNECOMASTIA

Gynecomastia is the most common clinical and pathologic abnormality of the male breast. Mammary enlargement may be due to a discrete, nodular increase in subareolar tissue or a diffuse accumulation of tissue. It reportedly occurs clinically in 30 to 40 percent of adult males (16) and both breasts are affected in many cases. Among those with unilateral gynecomastia, the left breast is involved more often than the right (4). Bilateral involvement is usually synchronous.

Numerous conditions have been associated with gynecomastia (7) including hyperthyroidism, cirrhosis of the liver, chronic renal failure, chronic pulmonary disease, and hypogonadism. It has been related to the use of hormones such as estrogens, androgens, and other drugs including digitalis, cimetidine, spironolactone, marihuana, and tricyclic antidepressants. Neoplasms that are most likely to cause gynecomastia are pulmonary carcinoma and testicular germ cell tumors.

Carcinoma arising in gynecomastia can usually be detected as a localized, asymmetric area of firmness. Mammography is helpful for distinguishing between gynecomastia and carcinoma and may identify carcinoma developing in gynecomastia (13). The two mammographic patterns associated with gynecomastia are a dendritic configuration featuring retroareolar density with prominent radial extensions into the breast and a triangular subareolar density lacking radiating extensions. Nipple retraction and discharge are rarely encountered.

The palpable mass formed by gynecomastia is located in the central subareolar region in all but a small number of patients who have eccentric peripherally located lesions. Patients with bilateral involvement tend to have diffuse lesions while unilateral gynecomastia is more likely to produce a discrete tumor. On clinical examination the tumor may measure 10 cm or larger, but in most cases the mass is 2 to 6 cm in diameter.

Gynecomastic breast tissue contains receptors for estradiol (9,19), dihydrotestosterone (9,10), androgen (17), progesterone (9,10), and glucocorticoid (9,10). Overall, approximately 35 percent of gynecomastia samples studied by the dextran charcoal method have been estrogen receptor positive. Using an immunohistochemical procedure, Andersen et al. (2) demonstrated nuclear reactivity for estrogen receptor in 89 percent of gynecomastia specimens examined. Positive staining was limited to the nuclei of epithelial cells in the proliferating ducts. Eighteen of 22 specimens with negative biochemical levels of estrogen receptor were immunohistochemically positive.

Gross examination reveals soft, rubbery or firm grey to white tissue that forms a discrete mass or an ill-defined area of induration. Fat is dispersed in the fibrous tissue on rare occasions.

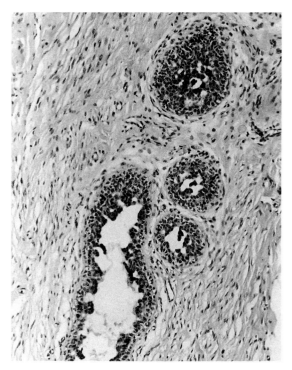

Figure 441
GYNECOMASTIA
Florid phase exhibiting papillary epithelial hyperplasia.

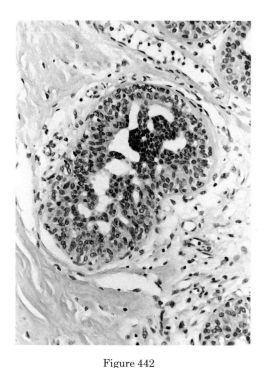

Figure 442
GYNECOMASTIA
Epithelial hyperplasia with micropapillary pattern characterized by slender strands of cells with hyperchromatic nuclei. Note cells with more abundant cytoplasm at the periphery.

Histopathologic studies show the same range of microscopic alterations regardless of etiologic factors (1,26). Three phases of proliferative change have been described. *Florid gynecomastia* ordinarily seen within 1 year of onset is characterized by prominent epithelial proliferation in ducts that may have papillary and cribriform patterns (figs. 441–443). There is usually concomitant myoepithelial hyperplasia. Duct ectasia is not prominent in this phase. Increased amount and cellularity of periductal stroma are accompanied by conspicuous vascularity, edema, and a round cell infiltrate concentrated in the edematous periductal stroma. *Fibrous* or *inactive gynecomastia* is typically a later stage seen after the lesion has been present for 6 months or longer. Epithelial proliferation is much less evident than in the florid phase, and the stroma is more collagenous with less edema and vascularity. *Intermediate gynecomastia*, which has florid and fibrous components, tends to be present for 12 months or less and it probably constitutes a transitional stage in lesion maturation.

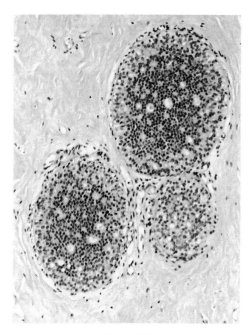

Figure 443
GYNECOMASTIA
Solid form of hyperplasia with microlumen formation. Note contrast between cells at the periphery and those filling the lumen of the duct.

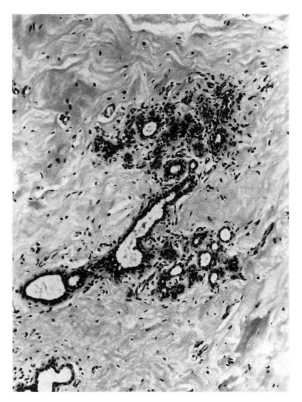

Figure 444
GYNECOMASTIA
Terminal duct lobular unit in male breast after estrogen treatment for prostatic carcinoma.

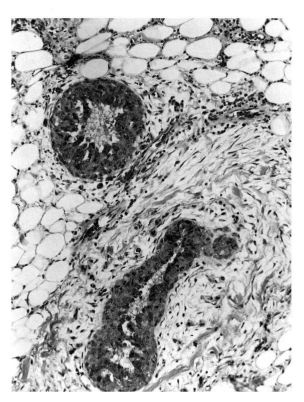

Figure 445
GYNECOMASTIA
Overall hyperchromasia and disorderly growth characterize this example of atypical duct hyperplasia. Note concomitant proliferative activity of stroma. Cells at the luminal borders of the ducts are darker than at the periphery.

A variety of other proliferative epithelial changes have been found in gynecomastia. Lobule formation, initially attributed to exogenous estrogen administration (21), has been associated with diverse etiologies including prepubertal gynecomastia. Lobules are more often seen in the fibrous or intermediate phases than in florid gynecomastia (fig. 444). Apocrine metaplasia occurs in all three phases while focal squamous metaplasia is most common in the florid stage. Extensive squamous metaplasia is seen in rare cases (8).

The cytologic features and growth pattern of the epithelial proliferation in ducts may be very atypical, especially in the florid phase (fig. 445). Micropapillary proliferation is pronounced in such cases and should not be mistaken for intraductal carcinoma when the surrounding stroma shows the typical changes of florid gynecomastia. Mitotic activity is variable but may be pronounced in ducts exhibiting atypical hyperplasia.

Electron microscopy confirms the presence of proliferating myoepithelial and epithelial cells

(11). Splitting and duplication of the basement membrane, which may be interrupted by gaps formed by protruding epithelial cells, is frequently seen. The stroma contains fibroblasts and myofibroblasts. The ultrastructural features are similar to those seen in duct hyperplasia of the female breast.

Regression of gynecomastia has been described when the underlying condition was treated. Usually, however, breast enlargement persists. Radiation has been effective in preventing gynecomastia in patients receiving exogenous estrogens to treat prostatic carcinoma (25,27). Excisional biopsy is indicated to exclude carcinoma. Although carcinoma may arise in conjunction with gynecomastia, there is no evidence from follow-up studies that atypical proliferative changes in gynecomastia are associated with an increased risk for the subsequent development of carcinoma.

REFERENCES

1. Andersen JA, Gram JB. Gynecomasty: histological aspects in a surgical material. Acta Pathol Microbiol Immunol Scand [A] 1982;90:185–90.

2. Andersen J, Orntoft TF, Andersen JA, Poulsen HS. Gynecomastia. Immunohistochemical demonstration of estrogen receptors. Acta Pathol Microbiol Immunol Scand [A] 1987;95:263–7.

3. Banik S, Hale R. Fibrocystic disease in the male breast. Histopathology 1988;12:214–6.

4. Bannayan GA, Hajdu SI. Gynecomastia: clinicopathologic study of 351 cases. Am J Clin Pathol 1972;57:431–7.

5. Bartoli C, Zurrida SM, Clemente C. Phyllodes tumor in a male patient with bilateral gynaecomastia induced by oestrogen therapy for prostatic carcinoma. Eur J Surg Oncol 1991;17:215–7.

6. Bigotti G, Kasznica J. Sclerosing adenosis in the breast of a man with pulmonary oat cell carcinoma: report of a case. Hum Pathol 1986;17:861–3.

7. Carlson HE. Gynecomastia. N Engl J Med 1980;303:795–9.

8. Gottfried MR. Extensive squamous metaplasia in gynecomastia. Arch Pathol Lab Med 1986;110:971–3.

9. Grilli S, De Giovanni C, Galli MC, et al. The simultaneous occurrence of cytoplasmic receptors for various steroid hormones in male breast carcinoma and gynecomastia. J Steroid Biochem 1980;13:813–20.

10. Gupta RK, Naran S, Simpson J. The role of fine needle aspiration cytology (FNAC) in the diagnosis of breast masses in males. Eur J Surg Oncol 1988;14:317–20.

11. Hassan MO, Olaizola MY. Ultrastructural observations on gynecomastia. Arch Pathol Lab Med 1979;103:624–30.

12. McClure J, Banerjee SS, Sandilands DG. Female type cystic hyperplasia in a male breast. Postgrad Med J 1985;61:441–3.

13. Michels LG, Gold RH, Arndt RD. Radiography of gynecomastia and other disorders of the male breast. Radiology 1977;122:117–22.

14. Nielsen BB. Fibroadenomatoid hyperplasia of the male breast. Am J Surg Pathol 1990;14:774–7.

15. Nielsen VT, Andreasen C. Phyllodes tumour of the male breast. Histopathology 1987;11:761–2.

16. Nuttall FQ. Gynecomastia as a physical finding in normal men. J Clin Endocrinol Metab 1979;48:338–40.

17. Pacheco MM, Oshima CE, Lopes MP, Widman A, Franco EL, Brentani MM. Steroid hormone receptors in male breast diseases. Anticancer Res 1986;6:1013–7.

18. Panotoja E, Llobert RE, Lopez E. Gigantic cystosarcoma phyllodes in a man with gynecomastia. Arch Surg 1976;111:611.

19. Rosen PP, Menendez-Botet CJ, Nisselbaum JS, Schwartz MK, Urban JA. Estrogen receptor protein in lesions of the male breast: a preliminary report. Cancer 1976;37:1866–8.

20. Sara AS, Gottfried MR. Benign papilloma of the male breast following chronic phenothiazine therapy. Am J Clin Pathol 1987;87:649–50.

21. Schwartz IS, Wilens SL. The formation of acinar tissue in gynecomastia. Am J Pathol 1963;43:797–807.

22. Simpson JS, Barson AJ. Breast tumors in infants and children: a 40-year review of cases at a childrens hospital. Can Med Assoc J 1969;101:100–2.

23. Tedeschi LG, McCarthy PE. Involutional mammary duct ectasia and periductal mastitis in a male. Hum Pathol 1974;5:232–6.

24. Waldo ED, Sidhu GS, Hu AW. Florid papillomatosis of male nipple after diethylstilbestrol therapy. Arch Pathol 1975;99:364–6.

25. Waterfall NB, Glaser MG. A study of the effects of radiation on prevention of gynecomastia due to oestrogen therapy. Clin Oncol 1979;5:257–60.

26. Williams MJ. Gynecomastia. Its incidence, recognition and host characterization in 447 autopsy cases. Am J Med 1963;34:103–12.

27. Wolf H, Madsen PO, Vermund H. Prevention of estrogen-induced gynecomastia by external irradiation. J Urol 1969;102:607–9.

CARCINOMA OF THE MALE BREAST

Breast carcinoma is an uncommon neoplastic condition among men, accounting for not more than 1 percent of all breast cancers and less than 0.1 percent of male cancer deaths (11,21,23,33). The incidence and age-specific death rate increase in a linear fashion with advancing age among different racial and ethnic groups (11,33).

Several risk factors for the development of male breast carcinoma have been identified. Levels of estradiol and other estrogenic hormones have been elevated in men with breast carcinoma (2,5). Case-controlled studies by Schottenfeld et al. (33) and Mabuchi et al. (21) showed a relatively high frequency of antecedent mumps orchitis among men with breast carcinoma. It has been suggested that testicular atrophy after orchitis causes relative hyperestrogenism. An association with antecedent testicular trauma was observed by Mabuchi et al. (21) who found no relationship with prior orchiectomy, the presence of an undescended testis, or prostatic disease. There is some evidence that the administration of exogenous estrogens could contribute to the development of male breast carcinoma since breast carcinoma was diagnosed in transsexuals after prolonged estrogen treatment (26) and described in two men after 12 years of estrogen therapy for prostatic carcinoma (32). However, case reports of breast carcinoma that developed in men with prostatic carcinoma are difficult to evaluate because of the well-known predilection of the latter to metastasize to the breast.

Radiation exposure has also been implicated as a risk factor. In some instances radiation was administered to the breast to treat gynecomastia, other local conditions, or intrathoracic diseases (8,17,38). Male breast carcinoma has also been associated with multiple fluoroscopic examinations. Although not statistically significant, Casagrande et al. (5) found a trend to more frequent breast carcinoma in men who had the greatest thoracic radiation exposure with fluoroscopy or for therapy.

Klinefelter syndrome, a genetic abnormality that usually becomes evident during or after puberty, has been associated with an increased risk for the development of male breast carcinoma. The majority of Klinefelter patients have at least two X chromosomes and a Y chromosome. Abnormal hormonal findings include a high estradiol-testosterone ratio at least partially augmented by increased testicular estrogen secretion (4). It has been estimated that 3 to 4 percent of male breast carcinoma patients have Klinefelter syndrome (31). The reported incidence of breast carcinoma among patients with Klinefelter syndrome varies from 1 to 3 percent (10,31).

Observations linking gynecomastia to the pathogenesis of male breast carcinoma includes epithelial atypia in gynecomastia, the association of gynecomastia and carcinoma with Klinefelter syndrome, and the finding of microscopic gynecomastia associated with 5 to 40 percent of carcinomas (15, 30,38). However, histologic transitions from epithelial hyperplasia in gynecomastia to intraductal carcinoma have rarely been described (30,38). The evidence suggests that gynecomastia is rarely a precancerous condition or an intermediate step in the development of carcinoma.

Clinical Presentation. The majority of male breast carcinomas are located centrally in a retroareolar position, but eccentric lesions, particularly in the upper outer quadrant, have been described (23). Synchronous, clinically evident bilateral carcinoma is exceedingly unusual (3,29). It has been estimated that the cumulative risk for bilaterality is 3 percent or less (19). About 75 percent of patients present with a painless mass. In the remainder, the lesion is detected because of nipple ulceration, retraction, or discharge. Age at diagnosis averages about 60 years, approximately 5 years older than women. However, breast carcinoma has been diagnosed in males at virtually all ages, including children and young adults less than 30 years of age (12). Mammograms of men with breast carcinoma typically reveal distinct lesions with well-defined invasive margins that contrast sharply with the surrounding fatty tissue (6); microcalcifications are found in about 30 percent.

A high frequency of estrogen receptor positive male breast carcinoma was noted by Rosen et al. in 1976 (28). Subsequent reports confirmed this observation, revealing that approximately 85 percent of the lesions have positive levels of estradiol receptor (7,24,36). When tested, many male breast

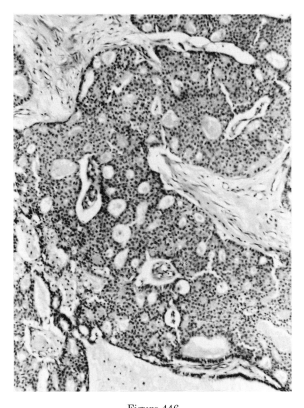

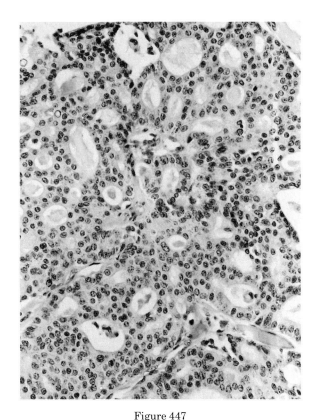

Figure 446
CRIBRIFORM CARCINOMA
Invasive carcinoma with cribriform pattern in male breast. (Figures 446 and 447 are from the same patient.)

Figure 447
CRIBRIFORM CARCINOMA
Cribriform pattern formed by cells with small orderly nuclei.

carcinomas also have substantial levels of receptors for progesterone (7,36), dihydrotestosterone (7,36), androgen (24), and glucocorticoid (24).

Gross Findings. The gross features of carcinoma of the male breast are similar to carcinoma of the female breast. Gross cystic papillary carcinoma is slightly more frequent in men.

Microscopic Findings. Approximately 85 percent of male mammary carcinomas are of the infiltrating duct variety. The majority are moderately or poorly differentiated (37) but low-grade and tubular carcinomas have been described (15,37). The growth patterns in male infiltrating duct carcinomas duplicate those in the female breast including cribriform, comedo, papillary, solid, or gland-forming components (figs. 446, 447). The ultrastructural features are similar as well (14). Approximately 2 percent of male breast carcinomas are complicated by Paget disease of the nipple, nearly the same frequency as in women (12,35). Papillary carcinomas, often with a promi-

nent cystic component, are relatively more common among men than women, constituting 3 to 5 percent of male carcinomas (15,37,38) but only 1 to 2 percent of female carcinomas. The majority of male papillary carcinomas are intracystic and noninvasive (figs. 448, 449).

About 5 percent of male breast carcinomas are entirely intraductal lesions (12,15,19). The histologic appearance duplicates intraductal carcinoma in women including comedo, cribriform, solid micropapillary, and papillary patterns (fig. 450). When intraductal carcinoma arises in gynecomastia it is unusual to find transitions from atypical hyperplasia to carcinoma in gynecomastic ducts (30).

Because lobular differentiation is so rarely seen in the male breast, the existence of lobular carcinoma in this setting has been questioned. Isolated examples of "small cell carcinoma" have been described (13,22,29,38) but not in large series (12,15,17,37). The microscopic appearance of

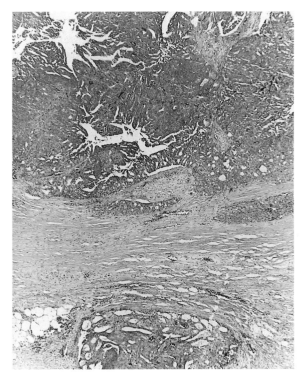

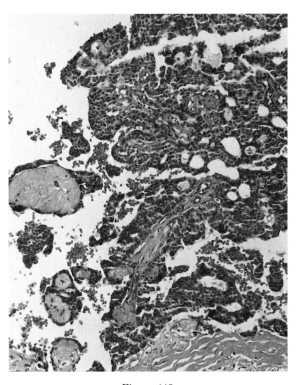

Figure 448
CYSTIC PAPILLARY CARCINOMA
OF MALE BREAST
Solid, complex papillary carcinoma projecting into the cyst lumen demarcated by the fibrous cyst wall. Invasive carcinoma seen at the lower margin is well beyond the cyst and involves fat. (Figures 448 and 449 are from the same patient.)

Figure 449
CYSTIC PAPILLARY CARCINOMA
Portions of the intracystic tumor have fibrovascular stroma.

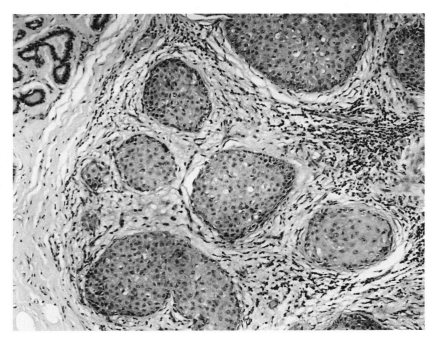

Figure 450
INTRADUCTAL CARCINOMA
OF MALE BREAST
Solid neoplastic growth in distended ducts. Note lobule in upper left corner. The patient had received estrogen for prostatic carcinoma.

lesions consistent with invasive lobular carcinoma have been described (13,22,29). In situ lobular carcinoma has reportedly been found in two cases (22,29). Other uncommon types of invasive carcinoma encountered in the male breast include medullary (23,37,38), mucinous (13,15,37,38), squamous (13), and adenoid cystic (16).

On occasion, the distinction between a primary carcinoma of the breast and metastatic prostatic carcinoma may be difficult (17). Both types of carcinoma are likely to have positive estrogen receptors. Patients with prostatic adenocarcinoma treated with estrogens invariably have gynecomastia that may exhibit markedly atypical papillary epithelial hyperplasia. Such proliferative changes should not be misinterpreted as intraductal carcinoma. Great difficulty is encountered especially with invasive, poorly differentiated carcinomas that lack an intraductal component. The immunohistochemical demonstration of prostatic acid phosphatase or prostate specific antigen (32) is diagnostic of metastatic prostatic carcinoma in the breast, while finding intraductal carcinoma or intracellular mucin supports a diagnosis of primary mammary carcinoma.

Prognosis and Treatment. Most patients have been treated by total mastectomy and axillary dissection. Total mastectomy alone has occasionally been employed for patients with intraductal carcinoma. Lumpectomy and radiation therapy are rarely recommended but may be employed in elderly patients (27). Mastectomy may be followed by radiation of the chest wall in patients with large tumors for whom the risk of local recurrence is relatively high, but it has not been demonstrated that this improves overall prognosis (9,35).

Numerous studies have described the prognosis of male breast carcinoma after treatment by mastectomy and axillary dissection. Prognosis is significantly related to the stage at diagnosis as determined by tumor size and nodal status (1,9, 15,18,23,35). Heller et al. (15) reported that node-negative male and female patients had nearly identical survival when compared 5 and 10 years after treatment. In the same study, node-positive male and female patients did not differ in survival at 5 years, but there were substantially fewer survivors among the men 10 years after treatment. Survival at 5 and 10 years in pathologically node-negative patients is 70 to 80 percent (9,15,18). Among node-positive patients, 5-year survival has been reported to be 59 ± 18 percent (15) and 37 percent (9). Ten-year survival has been described as 25 ± 14 percent (18) and 11 ± 13 percent (15). Unfavorable prognostic factors, regardless of nodal status, are tumor size larger than 2 cm (18) and poor histologic differentiation (18). In one series, differentiation was highly associated with tumor size and nodal status but did not prove to be an independent prognostic variable (18).

Adjuvant chemotherapy trials in a limited number of patients suggest this may be effective but no study has included a randomized control group for comparison (25,27,35). Ribeiro (27) reported a 5-year survival of 55 percent among 23 stage II–III men given adjuvant tamoxifen. A number of hormonal treatments have been employed with variable success to treat metastatic carcinoma (20,24,27).

REFERENCES

1. Adami HO, Hakulinen T, Ewertz M, Tretli S, Holmberg L, Karjalainen S. The survival pattern in male breast cancer. An analysis of 1429 patients from the Nordic countries. Cancer 1989;64:1177–82.

2. Ballerini P, Recchione C, Cavalleri A, Moneta R, Saccozzi R, Secreto G. Hormones in male breast cancer. Tumori 1990;76:26–8.

3. Brodie EM, King ER. Histologically different, synchronous, bilateral carcinoma of the male breast (a case report). Cancer 1974;34:1276–7.

4. Calabresi E, De Giuli G, Becciolini A, Giannotti P, Lombardi G, Serio M. Plasma estrogens and androgens in male breast cancer. J Steroid Biochem 1976;7:605–9.

5. Casagrande JT, Hanisch R, Pike MC, Ross RK, Brown JB, Henderson BE. A case-control study of male breast cancer. Cancer Res 1988;48:1326–30.

6. Dershaw DD. Male mammography. AJR Am J Roentgenol 1986;146:127–31.

7. Duffy MJ, Duffy GJ. Multiple steroid receptors in male breast carcinomas. Clin Chim Acta 1978;85:211–4.

8. Eldar S, Nash E, Abrahamson J. Radiation carcinogenesis in the male breast. Eur J Surg Oncol 1989;15:274–8.

9. Erlichman C, Murphy KC, Elhakim T. Male breast cancer: a 13-year review of 89 patients. J Clin Oncol 1984;2:903–9.

10. Evans DB, Crichlow RW. Carcinoma of the male breast and Klinefelter's syndrome. Is there an association? CA Cancer J Clin 1987;37:246–51.

11. Ewertz M, Holmberg L, Karjalainen S, Tretli S, Adami HO. Incidence of male breast cancer in Scandinavia, 1943-1982. Int J Cancer 1989;43:27–31.

12. Gadenne C, Contesso G, Travagli JP, Rouesse J, Fontaine F. Tumeurs du sein chez l'homme. Etude anatomoclinique. 73 observations. Nouv Presse Med 1982;11:2331–4.

13. Giffler RF, Kay S. Small-cell carcinoma of the male mammary gland. A tumor resembling infiltrating lobular carcinoma. Am J Clin Pathol 1976;66:715–22.

14. Hassan MO, Olaizola MY. Male breast carcinoma. An ultrastructural study. Arch Pathol Lab Med 1979;103:191–5.

15. Heller KS, Rosen PP, Schottenfeld D, Ashikari R, Kinne DW. Male breast cancer: a clinicopathologic study of 97 cases. Ann Surg 1978;188:60–5.

16. Hjorth S, Magnusson PH, Blomquist P. Adenoid cystic carcinoma of the breast. Report of a case in a male and review of the literature. Acta Chir Scand 1977; 143:155–8.

17. Hultborn R, Friberg S, Hultborn KA, Male breast carcinoma. I. A study of the total material reported to the Swedish Cancer Registry 1958-1967 with respect to clinical and histopathologic parameters. Acta Oncol 1987;26:241–56.

18. Hultborn R, Friberg S, Hultborn KA, Peterson LE, Ragnhult I. Male breast carcinoma. II. A study of the total material reported to the Swedish Cancer Registry 1958-1967 with respect to treatment, prognostic factors and survival. Acta Oncol 1987;26:327–41.

19. Langlands AO, Maclean N, Kerr GR. Carcinoma of the male breast: report of a series of 88 cases. Clin Radiol 1976;27:21–5.

20. Lopez M, Di Lauro L, Lazzaro B, Papaldo P. Hormonal treatment of disseminated male breast cancer. Oncology 1985;42:345–9.

21. Mabuchi K, Bross DS, Kessler II. Risk factors for male breast cancer. JNCI 1985;74:371–5.

22. Nance KV, Reddick RL. In situ and infiltrating lobular carcinoma of the male breast. Hum Pathol 1989;20:1220–2.

23. Ouriel K, Lotze MT, Hinshaw JR. Prognostic factors of carcinoma of the male breast. Surg Gynecol Obstet 1984;159:373–6.

24. Pacheco MM, Oshima CF, Lopes MP, Widman A, Franco EL, Brentani MM. Steroid hormone receptors in male breast diseases. Anticancer Res 1986;6:1013–7.

25. Patel HZ II, Buzdar AU, Hortobagyi GN. Role of adjuvant chemotherapy in male breast cancer. Cancer 1989;64:1583–5.

26. Pritchard TJ, Pankowsky DA, Crowe JP, Abdul-Karim FW. Breast cancer in a male-to-female transsexual. A case report. JAMA 1988;259:2278–80.

27. Ribeiro G. Male breast carcinoma—a review of 301 cases from the Christie Hospital & Holt Radium Institute, Manchester. Br J Cancer 1985;51:115–9.

28. Rosen PP, Menendez-Botet CJ, Nisselbaum JS, Schwartz MK, Urban JA. Estrogen receptor protein in lesions of the male breast: a preliminary report. Cancer 1976;37:1866–8.

29. Sanchez AG, Villaneuva AG, Redondo C. Lobular carcinoma of the breast in a patient with Klinefelter's syndrome. A case with bilateral, synchronous, histologically different breast tumors. Cancer 1986;57:1181–3.

30. Scheike O, Visfeldt J. Male breast cancer. 4. Gynecomastia in patients with breast cancer. Acta Pathol Immunol Microbiol Scand [A] 1973;81:359–65.

31. _____, Visfeldt J, Petersen B. Male breast cancer. 3. Breast carcinoma in association with the Klinefelter syndrome. Acta Pathol Microbiol Immunol Scand [A] 1973;81:352–8.

32. Schlappack OK, Braun O, Maier U. Report of two cases of male breast cancer after prolonged estrogen treatment for prostatic carcinoma. Cancer Detect Prev 1986;9:319–22.

33. Schottenfeld D, Lilienfeld AM, Diamond H. Some observations on the epidemiology of breast cancer among males. Am J Public Health 1963;53:890–7.

34. Serour F, Birkenfeld S, Amsterdam E, Treshchan O, Krispin M. Paget's disease of the male breast. Cancer 1988;62:601–5.

35. Spence RA, Mackenzie G, Anderson JR, Lyons AR, Bell M. Long-term survival following cancer of the male breast in Northern Ireland. A report of 81 cases. Cancer 1985;55:648–52.

36. Thompson EB, Perlin E, Tormey D. Steroid-binding proteins in carcinoma of the human male breast. Am J Clin Pathol 1976;65:360–3.

37. Visfeldt J, Sheike O. Male breast cancer. I. Histologic typing and grading of 187 Danish cases. Cancer 1973; 32:985–90.

38. Wolff M, Reinis MS. Breast cancer in the male: clinicopathologic study of 40 patients and review of the literature. In: Fenoglio CM, Wolff M, eds. Progress in surgical pathology, Vol. 3. New York: Masson Publishers USA, 1981:77–109.

BENIGN MESENCHYMAL TUMORS

The following discussion emphasizes aspects of these lesions especially relevant to the breast. For a comprehensive discussion and illustrations the reader is referred to the Fascicle on Tumors of Soft Tissues.

HEMANGIOMAS

The World Health Organization report, Histological Typing of Breast Tumours (6), states: "Hemangiomas occur rarely in the female breast. They are of microscopic size and almost always are in a perilobular location." Recent studies have revealed numerous, diverse, benign vascular lesions of the breast, including hemangiomas, many of which are large enough to be grossly evident.

Perilobular Hemangioma

Clinical Presentation. Perilobular hemangiomas are microscopic benign vascular lesions (2) measuring between 2 and 4 mm on a histologic section that are not grossly apparent (3,4). They have been found in 1.3 percent of mastectomies for carcinoma (2), 4.5 percent of biopsies for benign breast lesions (2), and in 11 percent of breast tissue sampled in forensic autopsies (3). Patients with perilobular hemangiomas found at autopsy ranged in age from 29 to 82 years (mean 51.5 years) (3).

Microscopic Findings. Multiple perilobular hemangiomas may be found in one breast and a number of patients have these lesions in both breasts (3,4). They are not limited to a perilobular distribution. Many are partially or completely within the lobular stroma (figs. 451, 452) (3,4) while others are located in extralobular stroma sometimes in proximity to ducts or with no particular relationship to a duct or lobule (4).

The lesion is typically a sharply defined collection of small, distinct vascular channels arranged in a mesh-work fashion, varying in caliber from capillary size to ectatic miniature cavernous channels. The borders may be ill-defined with vessels that extend into the adjacent fatty and fibrous stroma, although this is rare. Anastomosing channels may be present. The thin, delicate vessels consist of endothelial cells encased in inconspicuous stroma without a supporting smooth muscle coat. The vascular spaces usually contain red blood cells and it is not unusual to find lymphocytes in the stroma.

Prognosis and Treatment. Perilobular hemangiomas, whether unifocal, multiple, or bilateral are incidental pathologic findings that require no treatment. There is no evidence that angiosarcomas arise from these lesions.

Atypical Perilobular Hemangioma

Some perilobular hemangiomas have endothelial cells that appear cytologically atypical because they have prominent, hyperchromatic nuclei (figs. 453–455) (2). In some of these lesions anastomosing channels are readily detected, but endothelial papillary proliferation, mitotic activity, and extensive vascular anastomoses are not seen. Most atypical perilobular hemangiomas

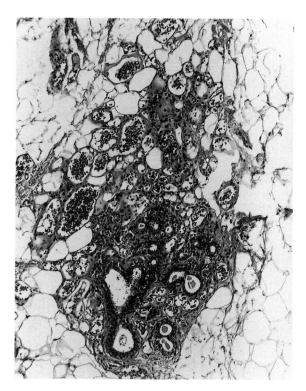

Figure 451
PERILOBULAR HEMANGIOMA
Thin walled capillaries congested with red blood cells in lobule and adjacent fat.

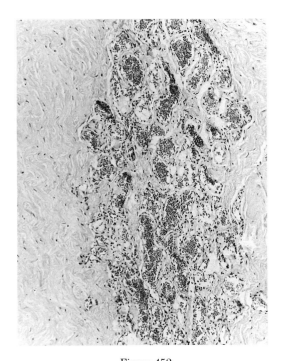

Figure 452
PERILOBULAR HEMANGIOMA
Lesion in mammary stroma not associated with lobules or ducts.

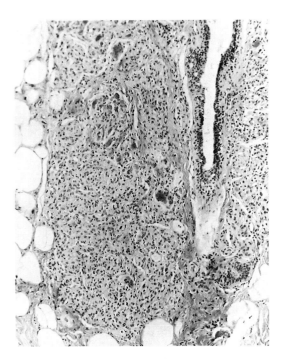

Figure 453
ATYPICAL PERILOBULAR HEMANGIOMA
Compact vascular proliferation associated with a terminal duct. (Figures 453–455 are from the same patient.)

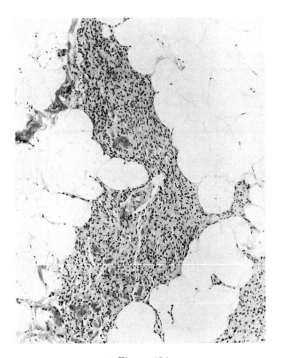

Figure 454
ATYPICAL PERILOBULAR HEMANGIOMA
Irregular extension of the same vascular lesion into fat. Note absence of distinct congested capillary channels.

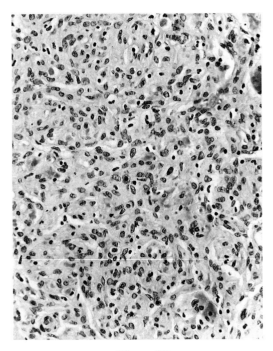

Figure 455
ATYPICAL PERILOBULAR HEMANGIOMA
Inconspicuous slit-like vascular spaces devoid of red blood cells.

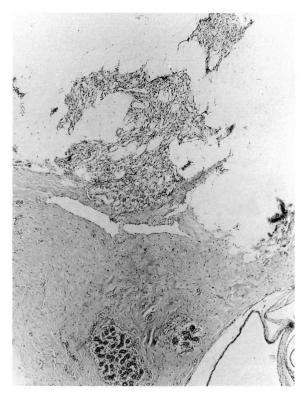

Figure 456
ATYPICAL PERILOBULAR HEMANGIOMA
Capillary proliferation in stroma and fat with irregular border. Note association with a larger thin walled vessel. (Fig. 2A from Rosen PP. Vascular tumors of the breast. Am J Surg Pathol 1985;491–503.) (Figures 456 and 457 are from the same patient.)

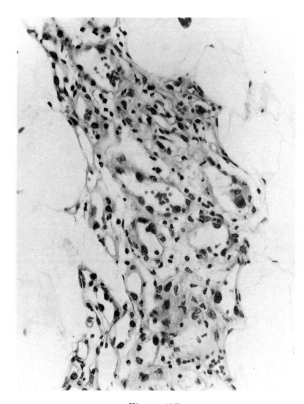

Figure 457
ATYPICAL PERILOBULAR HEMANGIOMA
Prominent hyperchromatic endothelial nuclei.

have rounded, circumscribed contours but a few with irregular margins have been noted (figs. 456, 457). These lesions involve lobules and interlobular stroma.

Whether treated by mastectomy or local excision, no patient with an atypical perilobular hemangioma is known to have experienced recurrence or progression to angiosarcoma. Re-excision of the biopsy site may be appropriate when the completeness of excision cannot be determined.

Hemangiomas

Clinical Presentation. Hemangiomas are benign vascular tumors large enough to be clinically palpable or detected by mammography (2). The lesions have measured between 0.3 and 7.0 cm and have been found in patients ranging in age from 10 to 76 years (2,5).

Microscopic Findings. Most hemangiomas have well-circumscribed borders grossly, but microscopically vascular channels may blend with the surrounding breast parenchyma at the margins. As part of this process the vessels are sometimes seen within lobules, although they more often grow around and displace glandular structures.

The most common form of mammary hemangioma is the *cavernous hemangioma*. The lesion is typically described as a dark red or brown circumscribed mass that may grossly appear spongy (5). Microscopic examination reveals dilated vessels congested with red blood cells (fig. 458). The individual channels appear to be independent since there are few anastomosing vessels (fig. 459). Endothelial nuclei are inconspicuous and flat (fig. 460). The vessels are supported by fibrous stroma that tends to be more prominent toward the central part of the tumor. Calcification may occur in the stroma (2). Thrombosis within cavernous channels sometimes elicits a lymphocytic reaction and endothelial proliferation may be seen within the organizing clot (fig. 461).

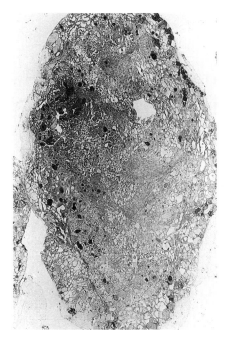

Figure 458
CAVERNOUS HEMANGIOMA
Hemorrhagic tumor with grossly well-defined margins consists of dilated vascular channels, some of which are congested with red blood cells. (Figures 458 and 460–462 are from the same patient.)

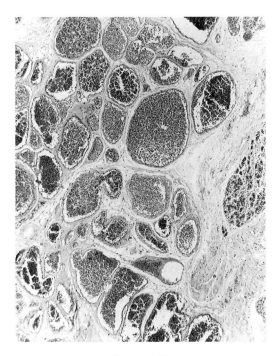

Figure 459
CAVERNOUS HEMANGIOMA
Individual vascular units outlined with fibrous stroma tend to be clustered in a lobulated fashion. Note absence of anastomoses among the large channels.

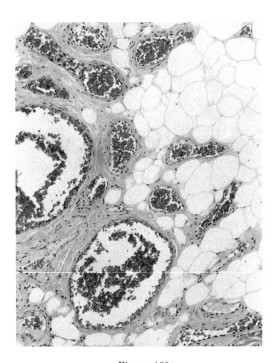

Figure 460
CAVERNOUS HEMANGIOMA
Vascular spaces lined by inconspicuous endothelium. Smaller channels extend into the fat.

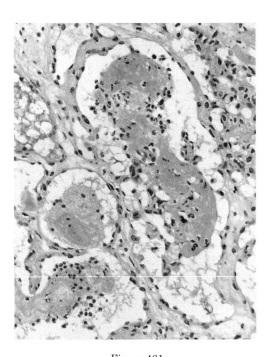

Figure 461
CAVERNOUS HEMANGIOMA
Organizing clot with recanalization can result in focal complex endothelial proliferation seen in the central vascular lumen.

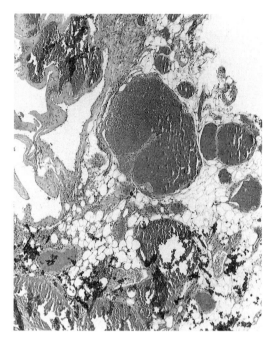

Figure 462
CAVERNOUS HEMANGIOMA
Dilated "feeding" vessels are present at the left center.

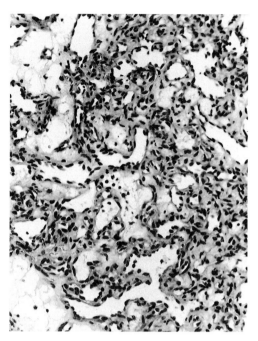

Figure 464
HEMANGIOMA
Complex branching capillaries within the tumor. The vascular pattern resembles granuloma pyogenicum but the inflammatory component of the latter lesion is absent.

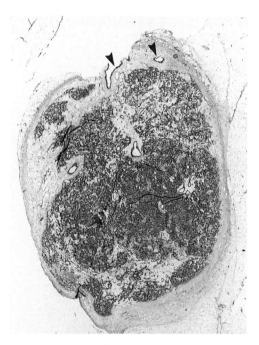

Figure 463
HEMANGIOMA
The tumor is circumscribed and has a lobulated internal structure. Note portions of the "feeding" vessel at the periphery and within the tumor (arrows). (Fig. 7A from Rosen PP. Vascular tumors of the breast. Am J Surg Pathol 1985;491–503.) (Figures 463 and 464 are from the same patient.)

Small vessels of capillary dimension may be seen in portions of a cavernous hemangioma. Hemangiomas composed largely of capillary-size channels are termed *capillary hemangiomas*. Hemangiomas rarely exceed 2 cm in diameter while few angiosarcomas are smaller than 3 cm. "Feeding" non-neoplastic vessels commonly present at the periphery of hemangiomas are not found associated with angiosarcomas (figs. 462, 463). Anastomosing vascular channels may be seen in hemangiomas but are much less conspicuous and less complex than in angiosarcomas (fig. 464).

Prognosis and Treatment. Complete excision is necessary for accurate diagnosis. Patients have all remained disease-free after surgical treatment by excision. Re-excision of the biopsy site may be required to ensure complete removal of the tumor.

Hemangiomas with Atypical Features

These hemangiomas are among the smaller vascular neoplasms, ranging from 0.3 to 1.2 cm in size (4). Many have been detected by mammography. With few exceptions, these lesions are

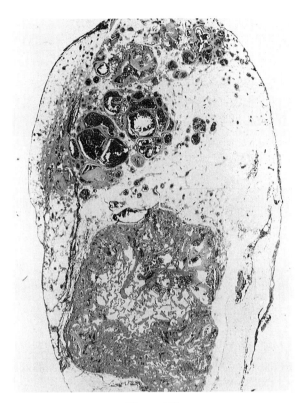

Figure 465
HEMANGIOMA WITH ATYPICAL FEATURES
Two vascular patterns are evident at low magnification consisting of cavernous angioma above and branching vascular channels below. (Figures 465–467 are from the same patient.)

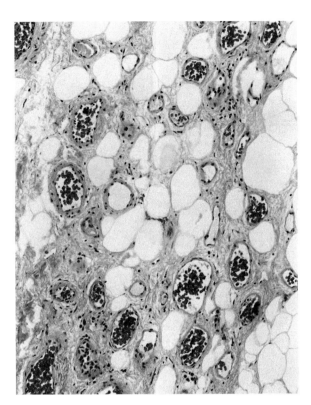

Figure 466
HEMANGIOMA WITH ATYPICAL FEATURES
Cavernous component spreading in fat. This seemingly invasive growth pattern is not necessarily indicative of a malignant vascular tumor.

sharply circumscribed grossly. They are distinguished from more banal hemangiomas by the presence of cytologically atypical endothelial cells and relatively more conspicuous anastomosing vascular channels. The vessels tend to have capillary rather than cavernous dimensions and the lesions are often separated into lobules by fibrous septae (figs. 465–467). More compact, spindle cell areas may be encountered. Non-neoplastic muscular "feeding" vessels with features of arteries or veins are commonly present in the breast tissue at the margin of, or extending into, atypical hemangiomas. Often, however, the muscular component seems malformed or incomplete and the vessels have a sinuous character. The resultant configuration suggests that these hemangiomas arise from these "feeding" vessels.

These lesions were characterized as "atypical" hemangiomas in early descriptive reports with limited follow-up because of uncertainty about their relationship to angiosarcoma. In a larger series, however, all patients remained disease free after excisional biopsy or mastectomy (1). There have been no recurrences and progression to angiosarcoma has not been observed. Excisional biopsy is the recommended treatment for these lesions, now regarded simply as variants of hemangiomas.

ANGIOMATOSIS

Clinical Presentation. Angiomatosis is a descriptive term applied to tumors composed of hemangiomatous and/or lymphangiomatous channels. These are diffuse, benign vascular lesions of the breast. Three patients with angiomatosis have been described (8): a 19-year-old, a 40-year-old, and one patient with a congenital tumor. Each presented with a mass in the breast. The lesions from the adult women measured 9.3 and 9.0 cm in largest diameter, respectively.

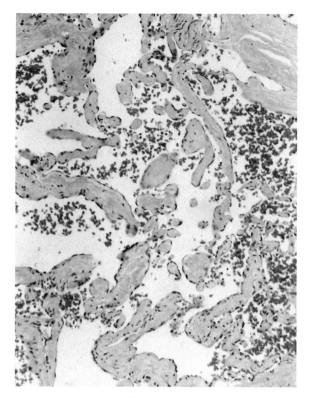

Figure 467
HEMANGIOMA WITH ATYPICAL FEATURES
Branching vascular channels lined by inconspicuous endothelial cells. Red blood cells are present in the vascular lumens.

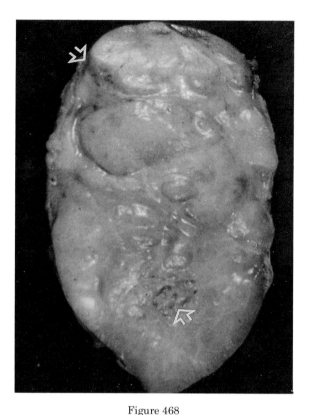

Figure 468
ANGIOMATOSIS
Gross appearance of a mass composed of vascular proliferation and intervening breast parenchyma. Prominent vascularity is indicated by arrows.

Gross Findings. The largest tumor was grossly hemorrhagic and contained numerous vessels congested with erythrocytes as well as a lesser number of vascular channels devoid of blood or acellular fluid (fig. 468). The other two tumors, which did not appear grossly congested or hemorrhagic, had fewer erythrocyte-filled channels. A biopsy from the patient with the congenital lesion contained congested cavernous vessels.

Microscopic Findings. Microscopically, these tumors are composed of vascular channels growing diffusely in the breast parenchyma (fig. 469). They surround ducts and lobules but tend not to grow into the lobular stroma. Extensive anastomoses are typically seen among the vascular channels (fig. 470). The vessels are lined by flat inconspicuous endothelium with sparse supporting mural tissue that is virtually devoid of smooth muscle. The lesions consist of hemangiomatous (erythrocyte-containing) and lymphangiomatous (empty) channels accompanied by lymphoid aggregates.

Angiomatosis does not have the microscopically circumscribed structure that typifies mammary hemangiomas. Much of the tumor is composed of breast parenchyma incorporated among the vascular channels. This configuration is similar to the somatic angiomatosis described by Enzinger and Weiss (7).

The distinction between low-grade angiosarcoma and angiomatosis may be difficult, especially in a biopsy sample. Anastomosing channels that are "empty" or contain erythrocytes occur in both lesions. The vascular channels in angiomatosis are distributed uniformly throughout the tumor with very little variation. Well-differentiated angiosarcoma has a heterogeneous pattern of vessels that are numerous in some regions and more widely separated elsewhere. At the periphery of low-grade angiosarcomas neoplastic vessels of capillary size merge with the surrounding tissue while those of

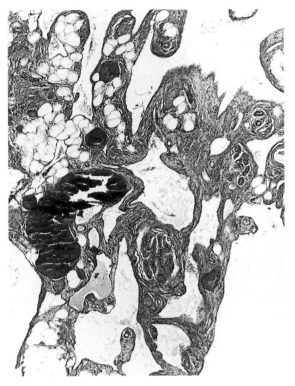

Figure 469
ANGIOMATOSIS
Dilated vascular channels in breast tissue. Dark vessels are filled with blood.

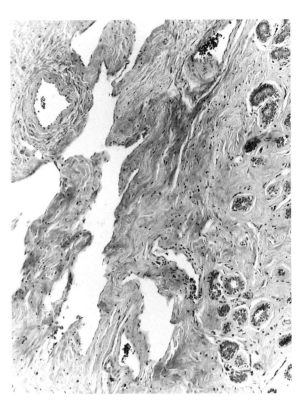

Figure 470
ANGIOMATOSIS
Anastomosing channels, lined by flat endothelial cells lacking mural smooth muscle, form most of the lesion. Erythrocyte-containing muscular blood vessels are also present.

angiomatosis are not necessarily smaller peripherally. In angiosarcomas the vascular channels invade lobules, which are consequently destroyed, while lobules are spared in angiomatosis as the vascular proliferation surrounds but does not grow into them. Finally, endothelial nuclei are cytologically normal in angiomatosis or they may be so attenuated that they can be difficult to find.

Prognosis and Treatment. Angiomatosis of the breast is comparable to similar lesions that arise at other anatomic sites. The large size attained in the breast without the development of a histologically or clinically malignant component indicates that these are benign tumors. It may be necessary to perform a mastectomy to control a bulky lesion but less extensive surgery is preferable when feasible. Recurrence is possible, sometimes after a long interval, indicating that the lesion is a chronic condition in some patients. No data are available about the effectiveness of radiotherapy in the treatment of angiomatosis of the adult breast.

VENOUS HEMANGIOMA

The microscopic appearance of these vascular tumors of the breast corresponds most closely to that of soft tissue lesions (9) that have been termed venous hemangiomas or vascular anomalies.

Clinical Presentation. Five cases have been reported (10). The patients ranged in age from 24 to 59 years (average 40 years). Each presented with a palpable tumor. One patient reported that the mass had been present for 13 years; another became aware of the lesion after trauma to the breast.

Gross Findings. The tumors measured from 1.0 to 5.3 cm in greatest diameter (average 3.2 cm). They were well circumscribed, firm, and darkly colored (fig. 471). Hemorrhagic cysts 0.5 to 1.3 cm in diameter were noted in one lesion.

Microscopic Findings. These lesions are characterized by some histologic diversity. All have dilated venous channels with smooth muscle walls

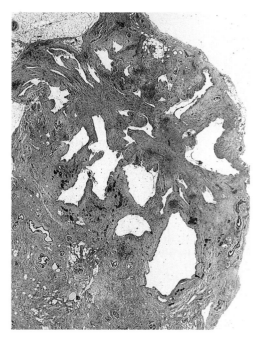

Figure 471
VENOUS HEMANGIOMA
Circumscribed proliferation of irregular vascular channels in breast parenchyma. (Fig. 1 from Rosen PP. Venous hemangioma of the breast. Am J Surg Pathol 1985;9:659–65.) (Figures 471 and 474 are from the same patient.)

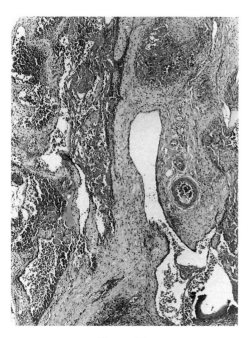

Figure 472
VENOUS HEMANGIOMA
Red blood cells fill some vascular spaces. A small artery is present at the right. (Fig. 6A from Rosen PP. Venous hemangioma of the breast. Am J Surg Pathol 1985;9:659–65.) (Figures 472 and 473 are from the same patient.)

of varying structural completeness. Thick walled arterial channels and capillaries are generally not conspicuous but may be present (fig. 472). Lobules and ducts are present in the mammary stroma between vascular channels, as are focal lymphocytic infiltrates, often accompanied by congested capillaries. In one case, lobular carcinoma in situ was present in breast tissue outside a venous hemangioma (10).

The dilated vascular channels are irregularly shaped and vary greatly in caliber (fig. 473). A smooth muscle layer is evident in the wall of some of the tumor vessels but often does not encompass the entire circumference. In some areas smooth muscle elements appear to be incompletely formed or absent (fig. 474).

Prognosis and Treatment. One patient underwent a mastectomy because the lesion was thought to be adherent to the pectoral muscle. A patient with coincidental lobular carcinoma in situ had no residual tumor in the specimen obtained when the original biopsy site was re-excised. In three other patients treated by excisional biopsy

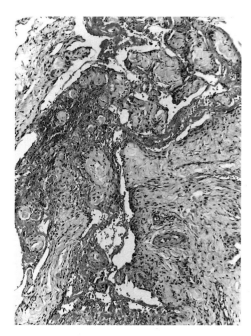

Figure 473
VENOUS HEMANGIOMA
Papillary endovascular proliferation forming capillaries in a larger vascular channel. (Fig. 6B from Rosen PP. Venous hemangioma of the breast. Am J Surg Pathol 1985;9:659–65.)

collagen fibrils and slender cells with longitudinally arranged, highly attenuated cytoplasmic processes joined by occasional tight or rudimentary cell junctions (fig. 483). The cytoplasmic processes of these cells, thought to be modified pericytes, retain fragments of basement membrane on both surfaces, pinocytotic vesicles, and occasional small clusters of intermediate filaments.

Tumorous pseudoangiomatous stromal hyperplasia appears to be a highly exaggerated manifestation of physiologic changes commonly encountered microscopically. Microscopic, nontumorous pseudoangiomatous stromal hyperplasia was found in 23 percent of 200 consecutive breast specimens obtained for benign or malignant conditions (13). The majority of these specimens also exhibited epithelial hyperplasia, sometimes including secretory changes in lobules. The fact that all patients with tumorous pseudoangiomatous stroma have been premenopausal underscores the probable importance of hormonal factors in the development of this lesion. Patchy strong immunoreactivity for progesterone receptor and less intense reactivity for estrogen receptor have been detected (12).

Prognosis and Treatment. In several cases biopsies of pseudoangiomatous stromal hyperplasia have been misinterpreted as low-grade angiosarcoma and this has led to mastectomy. Most patients have remained well after excisional biopsy but there can be recurrences. Incomplete excision probably predisposes to local recurrence but it is also possible that residual breast stroma can proliferate after apparently complete removal of the tumor. Recurrent lesions exhibit no change in cellularity or other atypical features.

The recommended treatment is wide local excision. Mastectomy may become necessary to control recurrent tumors. No information is presently available about the effectiveness of radiation or antiestrogen treatment in patients with recurrent lesions.

FIBROMATOSIS

Fibromatosis is an infiltrating, histologically low-grade spindle cell proliferation composed of fibroblastic cells with variable amounts of collagen. Although it has been described in many anatomic sites, especially the trunk and extremities, relatively few instances of fibromatosis

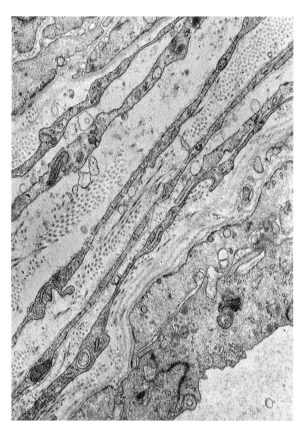

Figure 483
PSEUDOANGIOMATOUS HYPERPLASIA
Attenuated cytoplasmic processes of modified pericytes in the stroma adjacent to a capillary in the lower right corner (X13,600). (Fig. 6 from Vuitch MF, Rosen PP, Erlandson RA. Pseudoangiomatous hyperplasia of mammary stroma. Hum Pathol 1986;17:185–91.)

originating in the breast have been reported. Alternative diagnoses used for these lesions include desmoid tumor, extra-abdominal desmoid, low-grade or grade I fibrosarcoma, and aggressive fibromatosis. Most authors have preferred the term fibromatosis for extra-abdominal desmoid tumors of the breast.

Clinical Presentation. Patients with mammary fibromatosis range in age from 13 to 80 years at diagnosis, averaging 37 (26), 43 (30), and 48.7 (18) years in three reported series although the median age at diagnosis was 25 years in one series (26). The lesions are often, but not always, painless. Patients typically present with a firm or hard tumor that may suggest carcinoma on palpation. Rarely, the tumor may be nonpalpable and initially detected by mammography (16). The

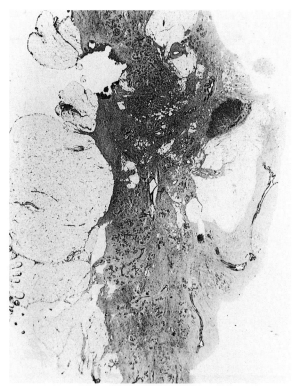

Figure 484
FIBROMATOSIS
This macrophotograph of a histologic section shows the neoplastic infiltrate surrounding ducts and lobules. Note finger-like extension along a duct at the border of the tumor.

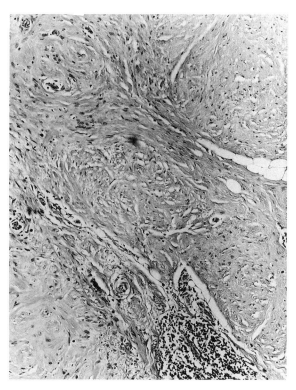

Figure 485
FIBROMATOSIS
Sparsely cellular collagenous area with whorled configuration and a small lymphocyte aggregate.

tumor is typically found in one of the quadrants and rarely in the subareolar area. Mammography reveals a stellate tumor that may be indistinguishable from carcinoma (15,16,30). Calcifications are infrequent.

Antecedent injury or trauma has been reported at the site of fibromatosis in some patients (17), but this is rare for mammary lesions. An association with breast augmentation implants was seen in two patients (21,26) and a few cases were associated with Gardner syndrome (19,28,31). Estrogen and progesterone receptor levels have been positive (18) and negative (26). Very few of the breast lesions have been pregnancy-related (15,18,24,30). Four patients with bilateral fibromatosis were included among the 67 cases (6 percent) of three large series (18,26,30) and 2 other cases of bilateral mammary fibromatosis were reported. Among patients with unilateral lesions, the left and right breast are affected with approximately equal frequency.

Gross Findings. Tumor size varies from 1 cm to 10 cm, averaging 2.5 to 3.0 cm (25,30). The lesion is typically described as a poorly circumscribed or ill-defined firm area of white, tan, or gray fibrous tissue. Some have a stellate configuration (fig. 484), while others are described as circumscribed or "well demarcated" nodules. The cut surface may have a whorled or trabecular appearance.

Microscopic Findings. The microscopic components of the tumor are spindle cells and collagen. It is not unusual to discover varied growth patterns in a single lesion. Areas in which the collagenous element is accentuated have a keloidal appearance (fig. 485). Often, the lesion features a moderately cellular, spindle cell proliferation in which there is at most modest collagen deposition (fig. 486). The tumor cells are distributed in broad sheets, in a storiform configuration, or in interlacing bundles. The stroma sometimes has focal myxoid areas and calcification is rarely seen (figs. 487, 488). Mitotic figures are inconspicuous or undetectable in most cases

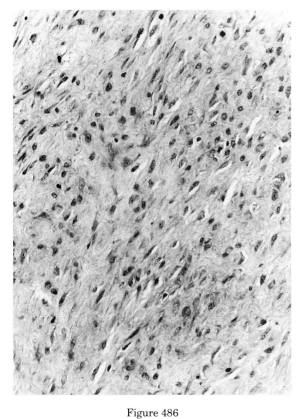

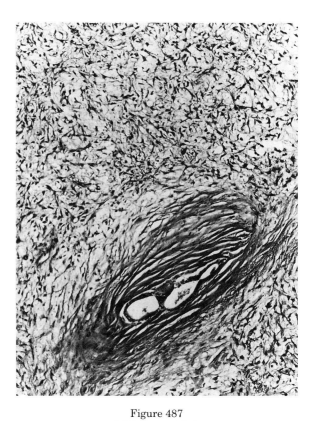

Figure 486
FIBROMATOSIS
Spindle cell portion of a tumor. Note uniform small nuclei and absence of mitoses.

Figure 487
FIBROMATOSIS
Keloidal proliferation surrounds an atrophic duct. The remainder of the tumor is composed of spindle and stellate cells in a myxoid stroma.

Figure 488
FIBROMATOSIS
Magnified view of myxoid portion of a tumor.

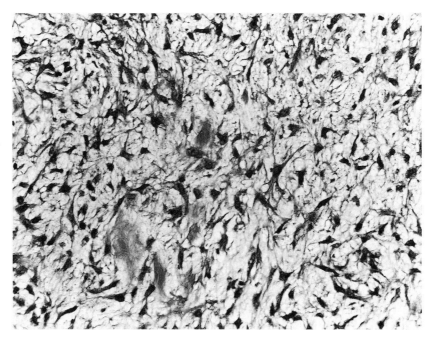

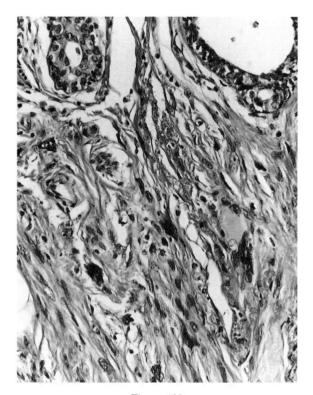

Figure 489
FIBROMATOSIS
Cells with large, hyperchromatic nuclei in the neoplasm near a lobule.

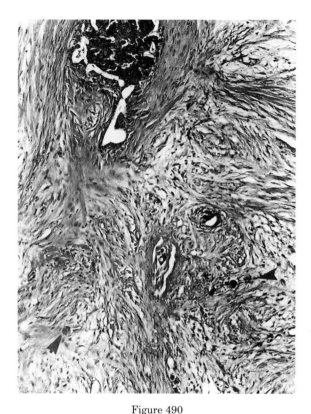

Figure 490
FIBROMATOSIS
The proliferative pattern of this lesion, which includes a hyperplastic duct, could be mistaken for a cystosarcoma. Calcifications are present in the tumor (arrows). (Fig. 4-A from Rosen PP. Mammary fibromatosis. Cancer 1989;63:1363–9.)

although a rate of 3 mitotic figures per 10 high-power fields has been reported (30). Cells with notable nuclear atypia and pleomorphism are also uncommon, generally consisting of enlarged spindle cells with one or multiple nuclei (fig. 489). Focal lymphocytic infiltrates are found in nearly half the tumors, especially at the periphery. Some lymphoid nodules have germinal centers.

Virtually all of the tumors have stellate extensions into the surrounding fat and glandular parenchyma. It is usually possible to identify ducts and lobules engulfed by these extensions at the periphery of the tumor. The appearance created in these infiltrative areas at the margin may mimic a cystosarcoma (fig. 490). Glandular parenchymal elements are inconspicuous or absent toward the center.

Needle aspiration biopsy specimens have been described as "limited in cellularity" and "scanty," consisting of spindle cells and, at most, sparse glandular elements (15,16,25,27,29). Such an as-

pirate must be regarded as nondiagnostic and followed by an excisional surgical biopsy.

Several lesions are considered in the differential diagnosis of mammary fibromatosis. Spindle cell and squamous metaplastic carcinoma have readily identified metaplastic or carcinomatous components. One feature favoring metaplastic carcinoma is a highly cellular and pleomorphic spindle cell component while desmoid-like foci and lymphoid aggregates suggest fibromatosis. Epithelioid, histiocytic, and multinucleated cells often found in fibrous histiocytoma are not features of fibromatosis. While mammary fibromatosis may have storiform areas, this is rarely a prominent pattern.

Calcifications are more likely to be associated with fat necrosis but can occur, although rarely, in fibromatosis. If the patient has recurrent fibromatosis, reparative changes caused by an earlier operation may mingle with recurrent tumor, further complicating the diagnosis. Lymphoid infiltrates should not lead to the erroneous diagnosis of an inflammatory condition such as nodular fasciitis. The inflammatory component of fibromatosis is typically limited to isolated separate lymphoid aggregates at the periphery of the lesion. In fasciitis inflammatory cells are dispersed more diffusely at the periphery and within the lesion, although localized areas of inflammation also occur. "Myoid" and multinucleated cells characteristically found in nodular fasciitis are not a feature of fibromatosis.

Electron microscopic studies of mammary fibromatosis have shown that the spindle cells are predominantly fibroblasts with lesser numbers of myofibroblasts (16,20,25). Only a few cells in these tumors prove to be immunoreactive with antibodies for actin (25).

Prognosis and Treatment. Recommended treatment is wide local excision. Because of the ill-defined character of most lesions it is difficult to judge the adequacy of margins intraoperatively. The excisional biopsy specimen should be inked and the margins sampled generously. The reported frequency of local recurrence has been 21 to 27 percent (18,25,29). The risk of recurrence is higher in patients with documented positive margins but recurrences have been observed in cases with apparently negative margins and not all patients with positive margins develop recurrences. Most occur within 3 years of diagnosis but some were not detected for nearly a decade. Histologic features such as cellularity, mitotic activity, or cellular pleomorphism are not helpful for predicting recurrence. Re-excision of the biopsy site may be considered when the initial biopsy is small and margins are positive, especially for lesions located deep in the breast or peripherally near the chest wall where recurrences are difficult to control. There is no evidence that postoperative radiotherapy or chemotherapy are useful as adjuncts to surgery for primary treatment or to control recurrences. Administration of antiestrogens or other hormones has resulted in remission in some patients with nonmammary fibromatosis (22,23). The effect of these medications on mammary fibromatosis has not been determined.

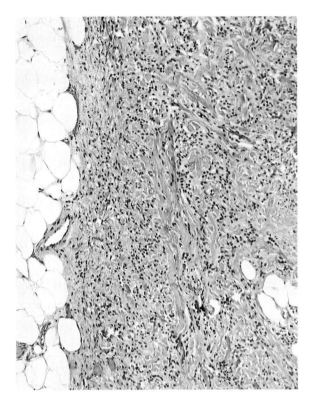

Figure 491
MYOFIBROBLASTOMA
The lesion has a circumscribed border. (Figures 491 and 492 are from the same patient.)

MYOFIBROBLASTOMA

This is a recently described benign spindle cell tumor composed of cells with features of both fibroblasts and smooth muscle cells (32). These tumors are well demarcated from adjacent mammary tissue and present as a discrete, firm, freely movable mass, closely resembling a fibroadenoma. In the initial report, the majority of the patients were male, and the lesion resulted in the clinical appearance of gynecomastia.

Microscopically, the lesion is sharply circumscribed and the adjacent compressed breast stroma results in a pseudocapsule. The tumor is characterized by a proliferation of spindle cells, usually arranged in fascicles, with interspersed broad bands of hyalinized collagen (figs. 491, 492). Islands of cartilage may be present; however, included mammary ducts are rarely seen. Mitoses are rare. Stains for cytokeratins and S-100 reportedly are negative. Some of the tumors focally may stain positively for desmin.

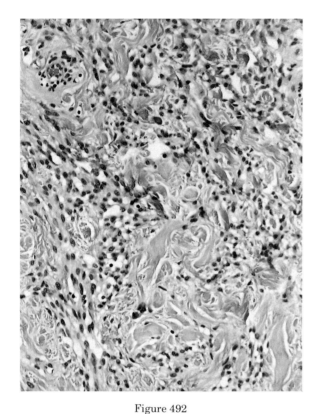

Figure 492
MYOFIBROBLASTOMA
Fascicles of spindle cells separated by bundles of dense collagen.

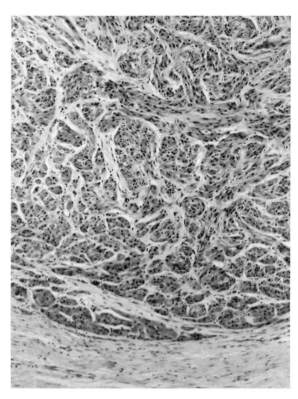

Figure 493
LEIOMYOMA
Circumscribed tumor composed of spindled cells lacking cytologic atypism.

The tumor may be differentiated from fibromatosis by its circumscription and by the arrangement of the cells in bundles with interspersed areas of fibrosis. Nodular fasciitis also has an infiltrating growth pattern and a more mucoid stroma than myofibroblastoma. Myoepitheliomas may be circumscribed; however, the myoepithelial cells usually stain positively for S-100 protein and cytokeratin.

These tumors are benign and may be treated by local excision. Neither local recurrence nor metastases have been described.

NEUROFIBROMA–NEURILEMOMA

Primary nerve sheath tumors are rare in the breast, as only a few such neoplasms have been reported (33,34). As in other locations, the encapsulation of the tumor and the Antoni A and B growth patterns are distinctive. In the so-called "ancient" neurilemomas, occasional cells with atypical, hyperchromatic nuclei may be seen, usually associated with vascular thrombi, hyaline thickening of blood vessels, and xanthomatous areas.

LEIOMYOMA

Although a smooth muscle component may occur in fibroadenomas and hamartomas, pure smooth muscle tumors of the breast are rare (35). Most occur in the subareolar region, arising from indigenous smooth muscle in that location (fig. 493) (36). Leiomyomas presenting elsewhere in the breast appear as discrete masses, and microscopically have a pattern akin to leiomyomas at other sites.

In contrast to myoepithelial tumors, stains for S-100 protein and cytokeratin are negative. The presence of a ductal component precludes the diagnosis of leiomyoma, and should suggest the possibility of fibroadenoma or hamartoma.

LIPOMA

While tumoral fatty masses often occur in the breast, there is question as to whether these truly represent benign neoplasms. Those that contain multiple benign capillaries are termed *angiolipomas*, while the presence of normal mammary ducts in such tumors results in their classification as *adenolipomas*. As noted elsewhere in this Fascicle, it seems appropriate to consider the latter lesions as variants of mammary hamartomas. Benign spindle cell tumors with ultrastructural characteristics of lipocytes also occur (37). Whether they should be classified as spindle cell lipomas is questionable; moreover, the latter tumor is more common in men (39).

Occasionally, a deep-seated invasive carcinoma may cause retraction of adjacent mammary fat in such a manner as to result in a clinically detectable mass simulating a lipoma. Biopsy reveals the true significance of this "pseudolipomatous" lesion (38).

CHONDROMA

Benign chondroid elements may present as a component of myofibroblastomas, pleomorphic adenomas, and hamartomas, as well as in the peculiar chondrolipomatous tumor described by Kaplan and Walts (40). In addition, tumors arising from underlying ribs, composed solely of benign hyaline cartilage, may clinically simulate primary breast lesions. Of greatest importance is the appreciation that cartilaginous foci occur most often as a metaplastic component of mammary carcinomas or sarcomas.

REFERENCES

Hemangiomas

1. Hoda SA, Cranor ML, Rosen PP. Hemangiomas of the breast with atypical histological features. Further analysis of histological subtypes confirming their benign character. Am J Surg Pathol 1992;16:553–60.
2. Jozefczyk MA, Rosen PP. Vascular tumors of the breast. II. Perilobular hemangiomas and hemangiomas. Am J Surg Pathol 1985;9:491–503.
3. Lesueur GC, Brown RW, Bhathal PS. Incidence of perilobular hemangioma in the female breast. Arch Pathol Lab Med 1983;107:308–10.
4. Rosen PP, Ridolfi RL. The perilobular hemangioma. A benign vascular lesion of the breast. Am J Clin Pathol 1977;68:21–3.
5. Sebek BA. Cavernous hemangioma of the female breast. Clevel Clin Q 1984;51:471–4.
6. World Health Organization. Histological typing of breast tumors. 2nd ed. International Histological Classification of Tumours No. 2. Geneva: World Health Organization, 1981:23.

Angiomatosis

7. Enzinger FM, Weiss SW. Soft tissue tumors. St. Louis: CV Mosby, 1983:407–9.
8. Rosen PP. Vascular tumors of the breast. III. Angiomatosis. Am J Surg Pathol 1985;9:652–8.

Venous Hemangioma

9. Enzinger FM, Weiss SW. Soft tissue tumors. St. Louis: CV Mosby, 1983:387–91.
10. Rosen PP, Jozefczyk MA, Boram LH. Vascular tumors of the breast. IV. The venous hemangioma. Am J Surg Pathol 1985;9:659–65.

Nonparenchymal Hemangiomas of Mammary Subcutaneous Tissues

11. Rosen PP. Vascular tumors of the breast. V. Non-parenchymal hemangiomas of mammary subcutaneous tissues. Am J Surg Pathol 1985;9:723–9.

Pseudoangiomatous Hyperplasia of Mammary Stroma

12. Anderson C, Ricci A Jr, Pedersen CA, Cartun RW. Immunocytochemical analysis of estrogen and progesterone receptors in benign stromal lesions of the breast. Evidence for hormonal etiology in pseudoangiomatous hyperplasia of mammary stroma. Am J Surg Pathol 1991;15:145–9.
13. Ibrahim RE, Sciotto CG, Weidner N. Pseudoangiomatous hyperplasia of mammary stroma. Some observations regarding its clinicopathologic spectrum. Cancer 1989;63:1154–60.
14. Vuitch MF, Rosen PP, Erlandson RA. Pseudoangiomatous hyperplasia of mammary stroma. Hum Pathol 1986;17:185–91.

Fibromatosis

15. Cederlund CG, Gustavsson S, Linell F, Moquist-Olsson I, Andersson I. Fibromatosis of the breast mimicking carcinoma at mammography. Br J Radiol 1984;57:98–101.
16. El-Naggar A, Abdul-Karim FW, Marshalleck JJ, Sorensen K. Fine-needle aspiration of fibromatosis of the breast. Diagn Cytopathol 1987;3:320–2.
17. Enzinger FM, Shiraki M. Musculo-aponeurotic fibromatosis of the shoulder girdle (extra-abdominal desmoid). Analysis of thirty cases followed up for ten or more years. Cancer 1967;20:1131–40.

18. Gump FE, Sternschein MJ, Wolff M. Fibromatosis of the breast. Surg Gynecol Obstet 1981;153:57–60.

19. Haggitt RC, Booth JL. Bilateral fibromatosis of the breast in Gardner's syndrome. Cancer 1970;25:161–6.

20. Hanna WM, Jambrosic J, Fish E. Aggressive fibromatosis of the breast. Arch Pathol Lab Med 1985;109:260–2.

21. Jewett ST Jr, Mead JH. Extra-abdominal desmoid arising from a capsule around a silicone breast implant. Plast Reconstr Surg 1979;63:577–9.

22. Kinzbrunner B, Ritter S, Domingo J, Rosenthal CJ. Remission of rapidly growing desmoid tumors after tamoxifen therapy. Cancer 1983;52:2201–4.

23. Klein WA, Miller HH, Anderson M, DeCosse JJ. The use of indomethacin, sulindac, and tamoxifen for the treatment of desmoid tumors associated with familial polyposis. Cancer 1987;60:2863–8.

24. Norris HJ, Taylor HB. Sarcomas and related mesenchymal tumors of the breast. Cancer 1968;22:22–8.

25. Pettinato G, Manivel JC, Petrella G, Jassim AD. Fine needle aspiration cytology, immunocytochemistry and electron microscopy of fibromatosis of the breast. Report of two cases. Acta Cytol 1991;35:403–8.

26. Rosen PP, Ernsberger D. Mammary fibromatosis. A benign spindle-cell tumor with significant risk for local recurrence. Cancer 1989;63:1363–9.

27. Schwartz IS. Infiltrative fibromatosis (desmoid) of the breast. Breast 1983;9:1–3.

28. Simpson RD, Harrison EG Jr, Mayo CW. Mesenteric fibromatosis in familial polyposis. A variant of Gardner's syndrome. Cancer 1964;17:526–34.

29. Tani EM, Stanley MW, Skoog L. Fine needle aspiration cytology presentation of bilateral mammary fibromatosis. Report of a case. Acta Cytol 1988;32:555–8.

30. Wargotz ES, Norris HJ, Austin RM, Enzinger FM. Fibromatosis of the breast. A clinical and pathological study of 28 cases. Am J Surg Pathol 1987;11:38–45.

31. Zayid I, Dihmis C. Familial multicentric fibromatosis–desmoids. A report of three cases in a Jordanian family. Cancer 1969;24:786–95.

Myofibroblastoma

32. Wargotz ES, Weiss SW, Norris HJ. Myofibroblastoma of the breast. Sixteen cases of a distinctive benign mesenchymal tumor. Am J Surg Pathol 1987;11:493–502.

Neurofibroma–Neurilemoma

33. Majmudar B. Neurilemoma presenting as a lump in the breast. South Med J 1976;69:463–4.

34. Van der Walt JD, Reid HA, Shaw JH. Neurilemoma appearing as a lump in the breast [Letter]. Arch Pathol Lab Med 1982;106:539–40.

Leiomyoma

35. Diaz-Arias AA, Hurt MA, Loy TS, Seeger RM, Bickel JT. Leiomyoma of the breast. Hum Pathol 1989;20:396–9.

36. Nascimento AG, Karas M, Rosen PP, Caron AG. Leiomyoma of the nipple. Am J Surg Pathol 1979;3:151–4.

Lipoma

37. Chan KW, Ghadially FN, Alagaratnam TT. Benign spindle cell tumour of breast—a variant of spindled cell lipoma or fibroma of breast? Pathology 1984;16:331–6.

38. Shucksmith HS, Dossett JA. Pseudolipoma of the breast: a mask for cancer. Br Med J 1965;2:1459–62.

39. Toker C, Tang CK, Whiteley JF, Berkheiser SW, Rachman R. Benign spindle cell breast tumor. Cancer 1981;48:1615–22.

Chondroma

40. Kaplan L, Walts AE. Benign chondrolipomatous tumor of the human female breast. Arch Pathol Lab Med 1977;101:149–51.

✧✧✧

SARCOMAS OF THE BREAST

Mammary sarcomas comprise less than 1 percent of all malignant neoplasms of the breast, and parallel in type and frequency sarcomas occurring elsewhere in the body. Probably many of the previously reported sarcomas represent incompletely sectioned cystosarcomas or metaplastic carcinomas. Because of therapeutic considerations related to the need for axillary lymph node dissection and adjuvant chemotherapy for metaplastic carcinomas, it is particularly important to distinguish them from sarcomas.

The diagnosis of a primary mesenchymal neoplasm should be made only after thorough sampling fails to reveal an epithelial component. Immunohistochemical studies may prove helpful in recognizing metaplastic carcinoma by demonstrating a positive reaction for cytokeratins or epithelial membrane antigen in tumors that have a predominant spindle cell growth pattern. When the distinction between metaplastic carcinoma and primary sarcoma cannot be made with certainty, it is best to err on the side of the former, since that will ensure appropriate treatment for both neoplasms.

Malignant cystosarcoma, in contrast to primary sarcoma, often presents clinically as a sudden enlargement of a previously detected tumor, suggesting origin in a preexisting benign cystosarcoma or fibroadenoma (3). Primary sarcomas of the breast seemingly arise de novo, and often manifest rapid enlargement with no clinically apparent antecedent abnormality (3).

The manner of spread and the therapeutic implications of the various mammary sarcomas are similar. Total removal, ensuring that the margins of the surgical excision are free of neoplasm, is essential to avoid local recurrence. The absence of lymph node spread precludes the need for lymph node dissection. The prognosis of mammary sarcoma is uncertain because of the rarity of the tumors, because the diagnosis of many of the reported cases is questionable, and also because many of the patients documented in reported series presented before modern forms of treatment were available. However, Callery et al. (2) concluded that the prognosis of high-grade mammary sarcomas was at least as favorable as that of comparable sarcomas of the extremities.

Berg et al. (1) proposed the designation "stromal sarcoma" to indicate the basic homogeneity of mesenchymal neoplasms of the breast, and to distinguish these tumors from cystosarcomas, which arise from the hormonally responsive perilobular and periductal stroma. The tumors cited under this diagnosis were spindle cell lesions, occasionally with a fatty component, and represented fibrosarcomas, liposarcomas, or malignant fibrous histiocytomas. Angiosarcomas were excluded from the study, and none of the tumors exhibited skeletal muscle, cartilage, or bone differentiation. It appears unnecessary to invoke the term stromal sarcoma for these neoplasms solely because of their origin in the breast. The histologic appearance of sarcomas that present in the breast is identical to that of comparable tumors arising at other sites.

DERMATOFIBROSARCOMA PROTUBERANS

These should not be considered primary tumors of the breast since they arise in the skin and subcutaneous tissue. As in other locations, they are situated superficially in the breast and often produce ulceration of the overlying skin as well as a mass (3). The patient may delay seeking treatment because of the slow growth of the tumor. Because of the superficial origin, fixation of the tumor to the chest wall is uncommon. Wide local excision is appropriate treatment.

FIBROSARCOMA AND MALIGNANT FIBROUS HISTIOCYTOMA

Many tumors reported previously as fibrosarcomas of the breast are now classified as malignant fibrous histiocytomas. These are among the most common high-grade primary malignant mesenchymal tumors presenting in the breast (fig. 494). As with other sarcomas, they spread hematogenously or by direct extension to adjacent structures. Mastectomy is often necessary to achieve adequate local control.

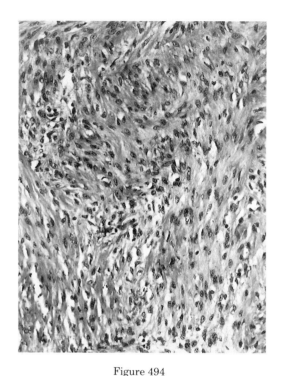

Figure 494
FIBROSARCOMA
Tumor composed entirely of spindle cells that lacked reactivity with antibodies to desmin or actin.

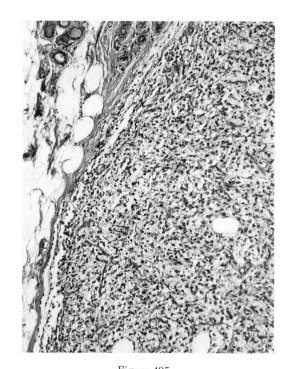

Figure 495
LIPOSARCOMA
The tumor is circumscribed and does not infiltrate the mammary parenchyma.

LIPOSARCOMA

Liposarcomas of the breast most commonly present as metaplasia of the stromal component of cystosarcoma (6). Liposarcomatous change in intralobular connective tissue may be seen adjacent to the neoplasm. Pure liposarcomas typically are well-circumscribed, mobile masses amenable to total excision (figs. 495, 496). Rare examples of bilateral liposarcoma have been reported (5). Based on a review of reported cases, the prognosis of these tumors appears to be relatively favorable, provided complete removal can be achieved; however, this conclusion may be unwarranted in view of the few cases reported (4).

OSTEOSARCOMA AND CHONDROSARCOMA

Although bone and cartilage are common findings in canine breast tumors, they are infrequent elements in human mammary tumors. Bone may be seen occasionally in hyalinized fibroadenomas, and osteoid and chondroid foci have been noted focally in cystosarcomas.

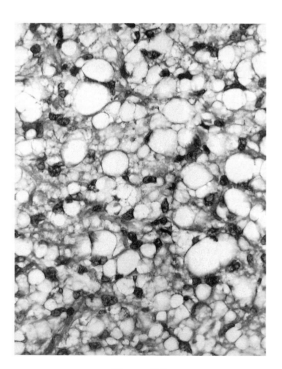

Figure 496
LIPOSARCOMA
Characteristic lipidic vacuolation of tumor cells.

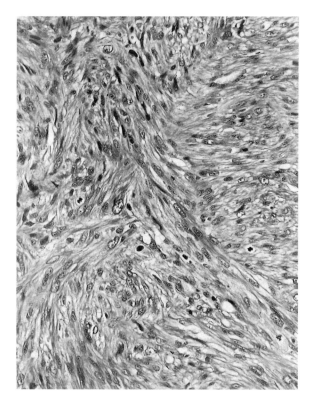

Figure 497
LEIOMYOSARCOMA
Interlacing bundles of spindle cells. The neoplastic cells were immunoreactive for actin.

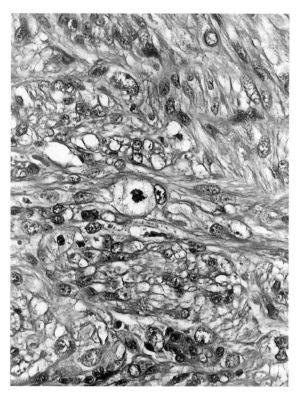

Figure 498
LEIOMYOSARCOMA
Nuclear pleomorphism and mitotic activity were prominent features of this tumor. The tumor cells were immunoreactive for desmin.

Very few primary osteogenic sarcomas of the breast have been described. This diagnosis should be made only after thorough sampling fails to reveal an epithelial component in a tumor that is otherwise indistinguishable from osteogenic sarcoma of bone. It is likely that some of the reported cases are inadequate samples of pseudosarcomatous metaplastic carcinoma, while others seemingly arose in preexisting fibroadenomas or cystosarcomas (9,10). The coexistence of fibroadenomas with these neoplasms should not lead to the conclusion that a pathogenetic relation exists between the two lesions (11).

Malignant osseous and/or chondroid elements in a primary mesenchymal neoplasm of the breast are associated with an uncertain prognosis because very few cases have been reported (7). Lymph node metastases are rare; therefore, such spread should lead to further efforts to exclude a diagnosis of metaplastic carcinoma.

Isolated cases of pure chondrosarcoma of the breast have been documented. As with other pri-
mary sarcomas in this setting, these tumors have been relatively large, the patients have been older than 40 years, and metastases have been hematogenous, initially involving the lung (8).

LEIOMYOSARCOMA

Only isolated examples of primary leiomyosarcoma of the breast have been reported. Most presented as circumscribed nodules. These tumors may arise from smooth muscle of the nipple or from blood vessels. Half of the reported cases occurred in the area of the nipple-areola complex (12). The microscopic appearance is analogous to that of leiomyosarcomas elsewhere for which the diagnostic and prognostic importance of mitotic activity has been stressed (figs. 497, 498) (14). The few reported cases of this tumor have shown a less aggressive course than other sarcomas. As with other primary mesenchymal neoplasms, recurrence after incomplete

317

excision is likely and, rarely, metastases that occur hematogenously may appear after many years (13).

RHABDOMYOSARCOMA

Primary rhabdomyosarcoma of the breast may present either as the stromal component of a cystosarcoma or as a pure tumor (15). The latter appears to be somewhat more common. These sarcomas usually are large and have a pleomorphic microscopic pattern. Their histogenesis is in doubt, and it has been postulated that they may arise from pluripotential stromal cells, through metaplasia of stromal cells, or perhaps from embryologic nests (16). In addition, origin from underlying pectoralis musculature must be excluded. As with other mammary sarcomas, metastases are hematogenous, and initial treatment is directed toward complete surgical resection of the tumor.

POSTIRRADIATION SARCOMA

The occurrence of sarcomas of the chest wall following irradiation of a mammary carcinoma has been reported with increasing frequency, probably related to the increased use of radiation therapy and the longer survival of radiated patients (17). Nonetheless, when one considers the number of patients who have had such treatment, the risk of this complication must be considered remote at present. Reported cases do not permit definite conclusions regarding correlation between the dose or manner of delivery of the treatment and the incidence or latent interval of these sarcomas. It is not possible to exclude the possibility that the sarcoma is an unrelated primary neoplasm arising at the site of a prior carcinoma. Therefore, the diagnosis of postirradiation sarcoma is, at least in part, based upon circumstantial evidence (18).

Postirradiation sarcomas may arise in soft tissue or bone, most commonly presenting with the microscopic appearance of fibrosarcoma, malignant fibrous histiocytoma, or osteogenic sarcoma (fig. 499). The latent interval after radiation treatment in reported cases ranges from 4 to 30 years, with a mean interval of 13 years (19). The prognosis of these patients uniformly is poor, possibly resulting from delay in diagnosis, but more likely due to the inherent aggressiveness of the neoplasm.

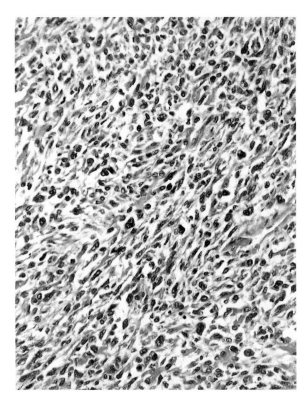

Figure 499
POSTIRRADIATION SARCOMA
Malignant spindle cell tumor that was present 6 years following total mastectomy and irradiation of the chest wall for mammary carcinoma.

HEMANGIOPERICYTOMA

These tumors arise in the soft tissues at many locations throughout the body. The breast is an uncommon site, with fewer than 20 cases documented in published reports (21–26).

Clinical Presentation. With the exception of a 7-year-old girl and a 5-year-old boy (23), all of the patients have been women 22 to 67 years old. The patients present with a mass that occurs with equal frequency in the left and right breast.

Gross Findings. The well-circumscribed round-to-oval tumor is composed of firm-to-hard homogeneous pale yellow, grey, or white tissue. The cut surface may have a whorled texture with dilated vascular spaces and a nodular contour. The diameter ranges from 1 to 19 cm.

Microscopic Findings. The histologic features are identical to those of hemangiopericytoma in other sites. The tumor is composed of round, plump, oval, and spindle cells oriented

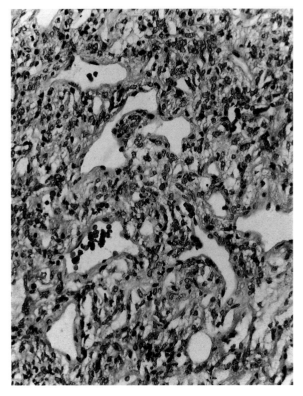

Figure 500
HEMANGIOPERICYTOMA
Spongiform pattern formed by thin walled vascular channels separated by polygonal cells with small round to oval nuclei, pale cytoplasm, and indistinct margins.

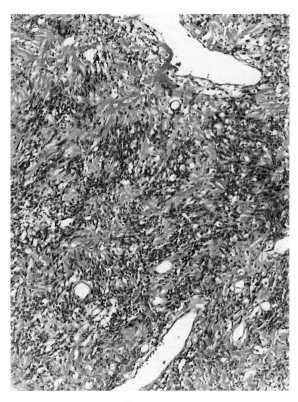

Figure 501
HEMANGIOPERICYTOMA
Portion of a tumor with stromal collagenization, a few dilated vessels, and intervening spindle cells. (Fig. 3 from Rosen PP, Arias-Stella J Jr. Hemangiopericytoma of the breast. Mod Pathol 1988;1:98–103.)

around vascular channels of varying caliber. The vessels often have a branching or "staghorn" configuration. More compact zones have a spongiform appearance (figs. 500, 501). The endothelium is supported by a delicate reticulin stroma without appreciable collagen or smooth muscle cells (fig. 502). Areas of necrosis have not been reported and mitoses are rare. The cells lack other cytologic features of high-grade sarcomas such as anaplasia and pleomorphism. Electron microscopy in one case revealed neoplastic pericytic cells closely opposed to the endothelial cells (24). When studied immunohistochemically, endothelial cells of the capillaries stain for *Ulex europaeus* I lectin and factor VIII but no reactivity has been found in the tumor cells (fig. 503) (20,24).

The specific diagnosis of hemangiopericytoma in the breast is important because of the generally favorable prognosis of this neoplasm. Several types of malignant tumor may have vascular areas

that resemble hemangiopericytoma. Metaplastic carcinoma with a spindle cell component also invariably has other growth patterns, including in situ or invasive carcinoma. High-grade leiomyosarcoma and malignant fibrous histiocytoma have readily identifiable mitotic figures and structural features that distinguish them from hemangiopericytoma. Metastatic sarcomatous renal carcinoma in the breast may also mimic mammary hemangiopericytoma.

Prognosis and Treatment. Reported follow-up in 15 cases varied from less than a year to 276 months. None of the patients developed local recurrence or systemic metastases whether treated by local excision or mastectomy. Treatment should be as conservative as possible with emphasis on wide local excision rather than mastectomy. Axillary dissection and systemic adjuvant therapy are not indicated for these clinically low-grade lesions.

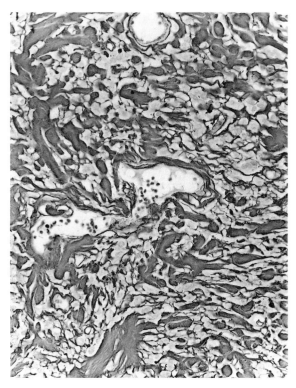

Figure 502
HEMANGIOPERICYTOMA
A delicate reticulin network forms the internal structure
of the tumor.

ANGIOSARCOMA

Clinical Presentation. Angiosarcoma
arises in the breast more often than in any other
organ. With rare exceptions, the initial clinical
finding is a painless mass. Blue or purple discoloration of the skin accompanies large or superficial tumors.

Age at diagnosis ranges from the teens to 91
years, with a mean of 34 and median of 38 years
(28,32,40). A statistically significant correlation
between age at diagnosis and tumor grade was
reported in one study (40). The median ages of
patients with low-, intermediate-, and high-grade
tumors were 43, 34, and 29 years, respectively.

Coexistent pregnancy was present in 4 of 63
(6 percent) cases in one series (40). Patients with
angiosarcoma diagnosed during pregnancy seem
to have an especially poor prognosis, apparently
because most have high-grade tumors. This reflects their ages rather than a particular association between high-grade angiosarcoma and
pregnancy. Some mammary angiosarcomas

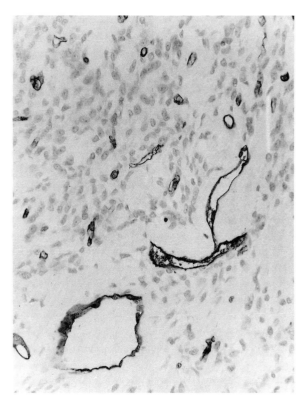

Figure 503
HEMANGIOPERICYTOMA
Factor VIII immunoreactivity is apparent in well-formed
vascular structures but not in the intervening solid portions of
the tumor. (Fig. 4 from Rosen PP, Arias-Stella J Jr.
Hemangiopericytoma of the breast. Mod Pathol 1988;1:98–103.)

have low or negligible levels of hormone receptors (29,38) but there is no evidence that these
tumors are hormone dependent.

Concurrent or asynchronous bilateral angiosarcoma is very uncommon (30,32). Few well-
documented angiosarcomas of the male breast
have been reported (38,40,45).

Synchronous or metachronous occurrence of
mammary angiosarcoma and mammary carcinoma has been described (33,40,43,44). Five patients developed both neoplasms in the same
breast and the lesions were present concurrently
in one (44). One patient with asynchronous tumors developed angiosarcoma in a breast that
had chronic lymphedema for 4 years after carcinoma was treated by only segmental mastectomy (28). In another patient, angiosarcoma developed in a breast 12 years after it had been
treated by lumpectomy, axillary dissection, and

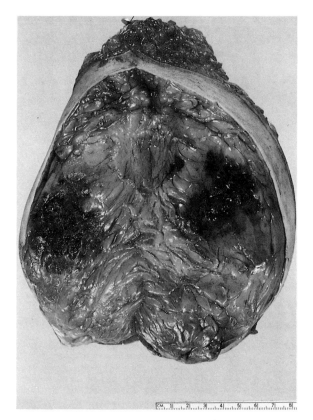

Figure 504
ANGIOSARCOMA
The neoplasm is a relatively circumscribed hemorrhagic mass in this mastectomy specimen bisected perpendicular to the skin.

Table 7

HISTOLOGIC CHARACTERISTICS OF MAMMARY ANGIOSARCOMA

Histologic Features	Grade		
	Low	**Intermediate**	**High**
Lesion involves breast parenchyma	Present	Present	Present
Anastomosing vascular channels	Present	Present	Present
Hyperchromatic endothelial cells	Present	Present	Present
Endothelial tufting	Minimal	Present	Prominent
Papillary endothelium	Absent	Focally present	Present
Solid and spindle cell foci	Absent	Absent or minimal	Present
Mitoses	Rare or absent	Present in papillary areas	Numerous
"Blood lakes"	Absent	Absent	Present
Necrosis	Absent	Absent	Present

radiotherapy for adenocarcinoma (33). Two patients with contralateral mammary carcinoma had asynchronous lesions.

Gross Findings. The tumors vary in size from 1 to 20 cm or more, averaging about 5 cm. Few angiosarcomas are smaller than 2 cm. There is not a significant difference in the average size of high- and low-grade lesions (fig. 504). In many cases, angiosarcoma forms a friable, firm, or spongy hemorrhagic tumor, but some exhibit little or no hemorrhage grossly. Areas of cystic hemorrhagic necrosis are commonly evident in large, high-grade lesions.

Microscopic Findings. Microscopically, three distinct histologic growth patterns in the primary tumor have been described (Table 7). These reflect the degree of differentiation and have proven to correlate with prognosis (32,40).

Low-grade tumors are composed of open, anastomosing vascular channels that have pro-liferated randomly in mammary glandular tissue and fat (figs. 505–507). Infiltration into lobules is characterized by the spread of the vascular channels within the intralobular stroma leading to separation and atrophy of the lobular glandular units. Some prominent hyperchromatic endothelial nuclei may be found, but the nuclei are often inconspicuous. Flat endothelial cells are distributed in a single cell layer around the vascular spaces with papillary formations infrequent or absent. Mitotic figures are rarely seen in the neoplastic endothelial cells.

Intermediate-grade angiosarcomas are distinguished from low-grade tumors by having scattered focal areas of more cellular proliferation. The latter usually have small buds or papillary fronds of endothelial cells which project into the vascular lumens (figs. 508, 509). Less often, the cellular areas feature polygonal and spindle cells or have foci that combine spindle cell and papillary elements (figs. 510–512). Infrequent mitoses

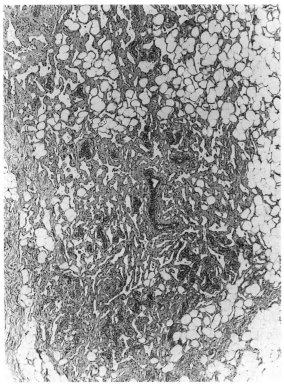

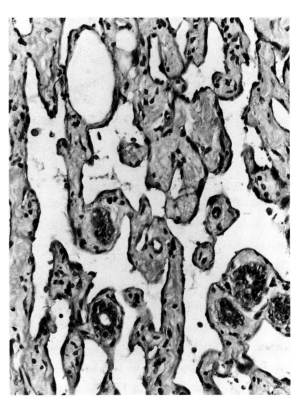

Figure 505
ANGIOSARCOMA, LOW GRADE
Anastomosing vascular channels infiltrate fat and lobular parenchyma. (Fig. 1 from Rosen PP. Angiosarcoma of the breast. Am J Surg Pathol 1981;5:629–42.) (Figures 505–507 are from the same patient.)

Figure 506
ANGIOSARCOMA, LOW GRADE
Anastomosing vascular channels lined by flat endothelial cells among lobular glands. (Fig. 13-1B from Rosen PP. Tumors of the breast. Based on the proceedings of the 53rd annual anatomic pathology slide seminar of the American Society of Clinical Pathologists. Chicago: American Society of Clinical Pathologists, 1987:83.)

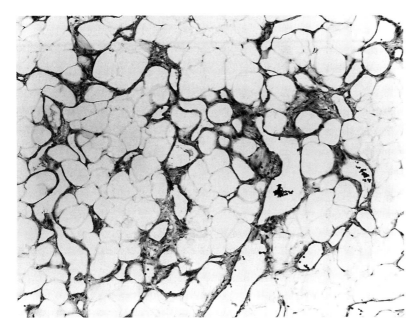

Figure 507
ANGIOSARCOMA, LOW GRADE
Neoplastic vascular channels in mammary fat. (Fig. 3 from Rosen PP. Angiosarcoma of the breast. Am J Surg Pathol 1981;5:629–42.)

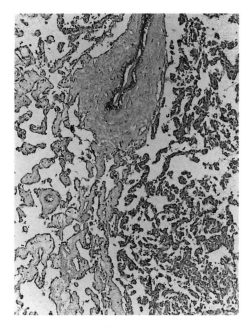

Figure 508
ANGIOSARCOMA, INTERMEDIATE GRADE
Papillary endothelial proliferation around a duct. (Fig. 6 from Rosen PP. Angiosarcoma of the breast. Am J Surg Pathol 1981;5:629–42.) (Figures 508 and 509 are from the same patient.)

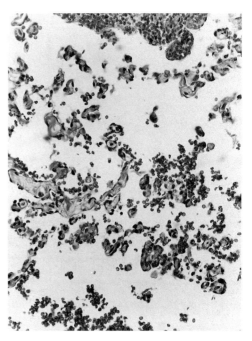

Figure 509
ANGIOSARCOMA, INTERMEDIATE GRADE
Dilated vascular spaces containing red blood cells and clusters of endothelial cells.

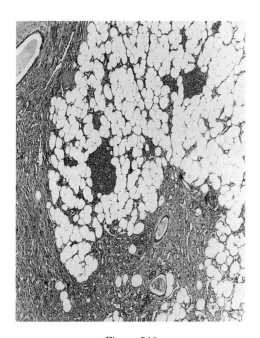

Figure 510
ANGIOSARCOMA, INTERMEDIATE GRADE
Focal areas of solid neoplastic vascular proliferation in the fat associated with low-grade angiosarcoma in mammary stroma around ducts. (Figures 510, 511, and 513 are from the same patient.)

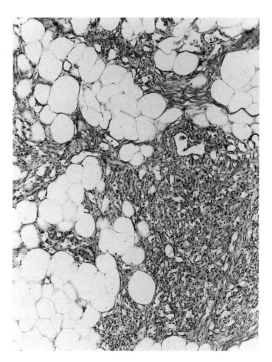

Figure 511
ANGIOSARCOMA, INTERMEDIATE GRADE
Focal spindle cell and small vessel proliferation.

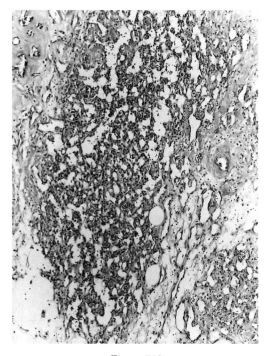

Figure 512
ANGIOSARCOMA,
INTERMEDIATE GRADE
Focal complex capillary and endothelial proliferation.

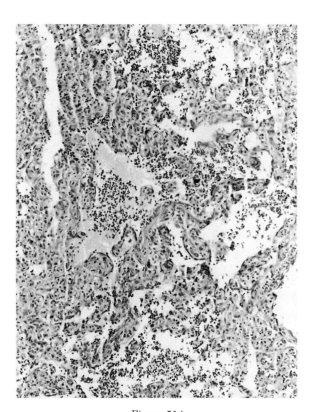

Figure 514
ANGIOSARCOMA, HIGH GRADE
Anastomosing vascular spaces among cellular areas with spindle cell and papillary elements.

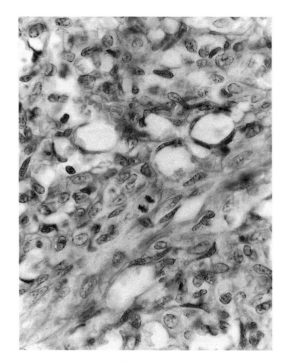

Figure 513
ANGIOSARCOMA, INTERMEDIATE GRADE
Mitotic figure among spindle cells.

may be found in these areas (fig. 513). Some spindle cell foci resemble lesions encountered in Kaposi sarcoma. At least 75 percent of intermediate-grade angiosarcomas consists of low-grade elements with microscopic cellular foci scattered throughout the tumor.

High-grade angiosarcomas exhibit the more malignant histologic pattern commonly attributed to these neoplasms (fig. 514). Prominent endothelial tufting and papillary formations that contain cytologically atypical endothelial cells characterize these lesions. Conspicuous solid and spindle cell areas virtually devoid of vascular elements may resemble fibrosarcoma or malignant fibrous histiocytoma (figs. 515–517). Mitoses are usually identified without difficulty in the cellular components (fig. 518). Areas of hemorrhage, often accompanied by necrosis, have been referred to as "blood lakes," and

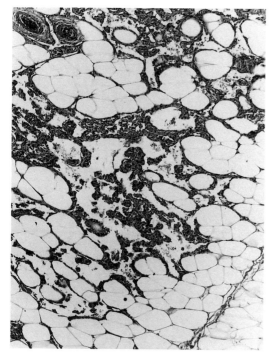

Figure 515
ANGIOSARCOMA, HIGH GRADE
This area exhibits solid growth and hemorrhagic necrosis.

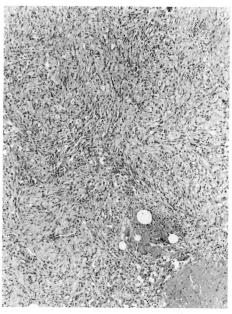

Figure 516
ANGIOSARCOMA, HIGH GRADE
Spindle cell sarcoma with necrosis. Such lesions usually have areas with more recognizable vascular elements. (Fig. 13-4A from Rosen PP. Tumors of the breast. Based on the proceedings of the 53rd annual anatomic pathology slide seminar of the American Society of Clinical Pathologists. Chicago: American Society of Clinical Pathologists, 1987:86.) (Figures 516–518 are from the same patient.)

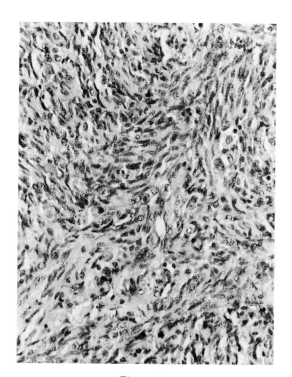

Figure 517
ANGIOSARCOMA, HIGH GRADE
Inconspicuous vascular spaces in a spindle cell tumor.

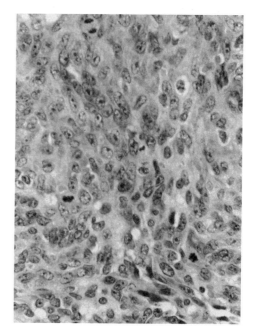

Figure 518
ANGIOSARCOMA, HIGH GRADE
Mitoses in a tumor composed of plump spindle cells.

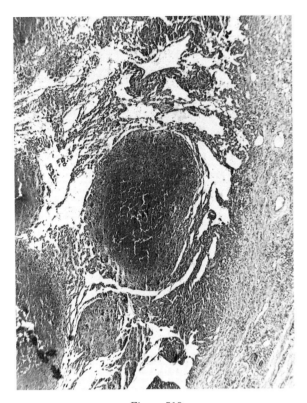

Figure 519
ANGIOSARCOMA, HIGH GRADE
"Blood lakes" seen here are foci of hemorrhagic necrosis. (Figures 519 and 520 are from the same patient.)

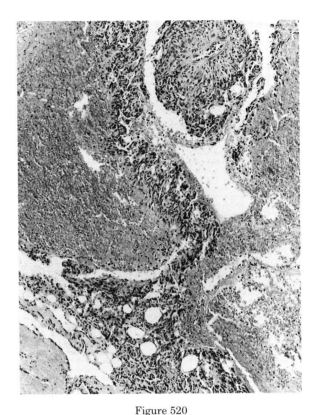

Figure 520
ANGIOSARCOMA, HIGH GRADE
Extensive necrosis in a spindle cell tumor. (Fig. 13 from Rosen PP. Angiosarcoma of the breast. Am J Surg Pathol 1981;5:629–42.)

along with necrosis, are seen only in high-grade angiosarcomas (figs. 519, 520). Low-grade components can be found in high-grade lesions, sometimes comprising the bulk of the tumor.

With few exceptions, angiosarcomas have infiltrative borders composed mainly of well-formed or low-grade vascular channels. In some cases the peripheral vascular component is so orderly that the neoplastic vascular channels are structurally indistinguishable from existing capillaries in the normal parenchyma.

It is not difficult to distinguish between a high-grade angiosarcoma and a hemangioma but problems may be encountered with low- and intermediate-grade tumors (37). Hemangiomas are rarely larger than 2 cm while few angiosarcomas measure less than 2 cm. Hemangiomas tend to have well-circumscribed borders grossly and microscopically while angiosarcomas have invasive margins. Some angiomas are divided into lobules or nodules by fibrous septa, a feature not seen in an-

giosarcomas, which lack such an internal structure. Many angiomas consist of isolated, largely unconnected vascular channels such as those typically seen in cavernous hemangiomas. Anastomosing vascular spaces may be found in angiomas, but except for angiomatosis (39), they are not as numerous or serpiginous as in angiosarcomas. In the mammary parenchyma, the vascular proliferation in angiosarcomas invades and expands lobules while angiomas other than perilobular hemangiomas (41) tend only to surround lobules and ducts without intruding on the intralobular stroma. A thick-walled non-neoplastic artery and vein may be found at the periphery of some hemangiomas; this is not a feature of angiosarcomas.

Immunohistochemistry and Electron Microscopy. Immunoreactivity for factor VIII–related antigen has been detected in mammary angiomas and in some mammary angiosarcomas (fig. 521) (34). Staining is less intense in high-grade

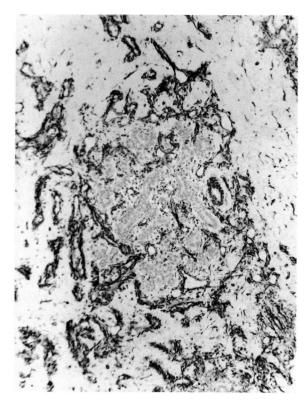

Figure 521
ANGIOSARCOMA, LOW GRADE
Endothelial cells in this neoplastic vascular proliferation around and in a lobule are immunoreactive for factor VIII (avidin-biotin peroxidase, hematoxylin).

lesions. Variable staining for *Ulex europaeus* agglutinin I has also been described in angiosarcomas (46).

At the ultrastructural level, Weibel-Palade bodies have been described in the neoplastic endothelial cells, although they may be inconspicuous or absent in areas of solid growth (45). The neoplastic endothelium and basal lamina are frequently discontinuous. Pericytic cells have been found associated with endothelial cells in some of the tumors.

Prognosis and Treatment. In 1980, Chen (31) reviewed 87 published cases of angiosarcomas and found that 14 percent of the patients were disease free at 3 years and only 7 percent survived disease free after 5 years. An equally poor prognosis was reported in a subsequent review (36). Donnell et al. (32) studied 40 patients with mammary angiosarcoma and found that the overall disease-free survival was 41 percent at 3 years and 33 percent at 5 years. Tumor grade was the most important prognostic factor. The majority of patients with orderly or low-grade lesions remained disease free while virtually all women with high-grade tumors died of recurrent sarcoma within 5 years. An expanded series of 87 patients confirmed the statistically significant correlation between the grade of angiosarcoma and prognosis (40). Analysis of survival curves for these patients revealed the following estimated probabilities of disease-free survival 5 and 10 years after treatment: low grade, 76 percent; intermediate grade, 70 percent; and high grade, 15 percent. The median duration of disease-free survival was also correlated with tumor grade (low: >15 years; intermediate: >12 years; high: 15 months).

The distinction between metastatic spread to the other breast and a new primary contralateral angiosarcoma is very difficult. The histologic grade of the first tumor, a comparison of the histologic features of the tumors, and the interval between the lesions are factors to consider. Experience has shown that bilateral primary angiosarcoma is uncommon and that contralateral breast involvement is usually evidence of metastatic spread.

Total mastectomy is the primary surgical therapy recommended in most cases. Axillary dissection is not indicated since metastases rarely involve these lymph nodes (35,40). Radical mastectomy is not appropriate unless the tumor is close to, or involves, the deep fascia. Rarely, a small lesion might be encompassed by quadrantectomy. The role of radiation in the primary treatment of mammary angiosarcoma has not been determined. In one series (40), individual patients with low- and intermediate-grade lesions remained disease free after excision and radiotherapy. One patient with a high-grade tumor developed a mammary recurrence after breast conserving surgery.

Following surgery, systemic adjuvant chemotherapy may be offered but the effectiveness of this treatment remains controversial (27,32,40, 42). Rosen et al. (40) compared 32 patients who received adjuvant chemotherapy with 31 women not so treated. Recurrences developed in 14 of 31 (45 percent) patients who received adjuvant chemotherapy, and in 18 of 32 (56 percent) not treated. When stratified by tumor grade, recurrences were consistently less frequent among women treated with adjuvant chemotherapy although the differences were not statistically significant. Because high-grade lesions have a very poor prognosis and most of the infrequent long-term survivors had adjuvant chemotherapy, this treatment should be offered.

POSTMASTECTOMY ANGIOSARCOMA (STEWART-TREVES SYNDROME)

Angiosarcoma arising in the lymphedematous upper extremity is not a primary breast neoplasm but a complication of the treatment of mammary carcinoma. Since the report by Stewart and Treves in 1948 (69), postmastectomy angiosarcoma arising in lymphedema of the upper arm has been referred to as the Stewart-Treves syndrome. Origin of the tumors in lymphedematous limbs is the reason that the term lymphangiosarcoma has been employed, but the microscopic structure of the lesions is similar to that of high-grade angiosarcomas that arise at other sites.

The pathogenesis of angiosarcoma in areas of chronic lymphedema is unknown. It is unlikely that irradiation contributes directly to this process since the lesion can develop in the absence of radiotherapy and in irradiated patients it originates outside the treated field. Impaired immune responsiveness has been demonstrated in anatomic areas affected by lymphatic obstruction and the lymphedematous limb may be an immunologically privileged site subject to neoplastic transformation (51,64).

Clinical Presentation. The estimated frequency of angiosarcoma in the postmastectomy lymphedematous extremity ranges from 0.07 (50) to 0.45 percent (63). Age at diagnosis averages about 65 years (44 to 84 years). Nearly 65 percent of the patients have had irradiation of the chest wall and axilla after a radical mastectomy since this treatment combination has been responsible for the most severe instances of lymphedema of the arm. The average interval between treatment of the mammary carcinoma and the clinical appearance of angiosarcoma in the arm is about 10 years (67), although periods as short as 1 year (68) and as long as 49 years (65) have been reported.

A distinction should be made between angiosarcoma in the Stewart-Treves syndrome and postirradiation angiosarcoma (49,54,58,62). The latter neoplasm arises after mastectomy in the irradiated field on the chest wall or in the skin of the breast, and is one of several types of radiation-induced sarcoma (48). Most patients with radiation-induced angiosarcoma of the chest wall have not had lymphedema of the ipsilateral arm but this complication was present in one case (58). The interval to onset of postirradiation angiosarcoma of the chest wall is less than 10 years with most tumors arising in 3 to 6 years.

The initial lesions of postmastectomy angiosarcoma appear on the upper inner or medial arm in at least 75 percent of cases but they also have been found on the forearm and elbow. They may consist of little more than purple discoloration of the skin and can be mistaken for an ecchymosis. These subtle changes evolve into plaques that enlarge into blue or blue-red nodules. Superficial vesicles or bullae that contain hemorrhagic fluid tend to develop before the surface ulcerates, leading to oozing of serosanguinous fluid or hemorrhage. Usually there is rapid progression but on occasion the disease may have a chronic course.

Gross Findings. Biopsies obtained at an early stage reveal lesions limited to the dermis of the skin and the superficial subcutaneous tissues. These usually consist of punctate hemorrhagic foci with little or no induration. In more advanced cases, one usually finds widely separated hemorrhagic tumor nodules involving muscle as well as the subcutaneous fat and skin. Stewart and Treves noted that such deep tumors were associated with blood vessels and that in some instances tumor was present in large veins (69).

Microscopic Findings. The histologic appearance of angiosarcoma arising in the lymphedematous limb is heterogeneous. Biopsies of flat discolored or faintly infiltrated skin lesions reveal inconspicuous lesions. Diffuse alterations related to the underlying chronic lymphedema consist of edema and collagenization of the dermis and focal lymphocytic infiltrates in the superficial dermis that tend to have a perivascular distribution (figs. 522, 523). A subtle proliferation of small vessels in the superficial dermis commonly occurs in chronic lymphedema (fig. 524). The earliest evidence of angiosarcoma usually consists of focal proliferation of irregularly shaped vascular channels lined by prominent endothelial cells that have hyperchromatic nuclei (figs. 525, 526). Erythrocytes can be seen in these

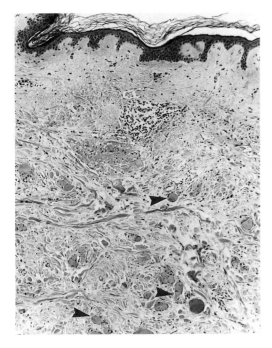

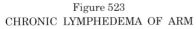

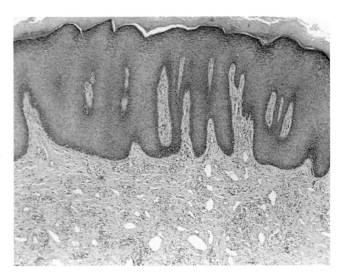

Figure 522
CHRONIC LYMPHEDEMA OF ARM
Vertical section of skin showing hyperkeratosis, markedly thickened dermis with edema, collagenization, and elastosis. Note lymphocytic infiltrate, and capillaries congested with erythrocytes in deep dermis (arrows).

Figure 523
CHRONIC LYMPHEDEMA OF ARM
This long established lesion features pseudoepitheliomatous hyperplasia with hyperkeratosis of the epidermis and numerous dilated dermal vascular channels. (Figures 523 and 524 are from the same patient.)

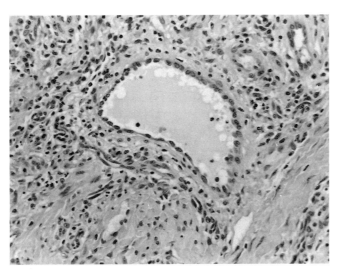

Figure 524
CHRONIC LYMPHEDEMA
Dilated vascular channel in dermis with prominent endothelial cells. Note other smaller vascular structures and diffuse lymphocytic infiltrate in stroma.

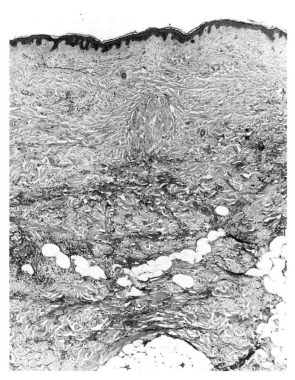

Figure 525
POSTMASTECTOMY ANGIOSARCOMA
Skin with changes of chronic lymphedema and an atypical vascular proliferation in dermis and subcutaneous fat. (Figures 525 and 526 are from the same patient.)

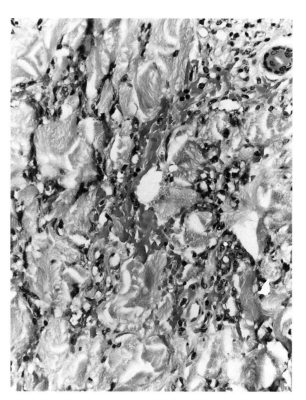

Figure 526
POSTMASTECTOMY ANGIOSARCOMA
Poorly formed vascular channels that characterize this inconspicuous stage of the disease. Vascular channels tend to be unexpanded among thick collagen bands in the deep dermis. (Fig. 14-4B from Rosen PP. Tumors of the breast. Based on the proceedings of the 53rd annual anatomic pathology slide seminar of the American Society of Clinical Pathologists. Chicago: American Society of Clinical Pathologists, 1987:94.)

vessels and also in the surrounding dermal stroma. These early lesions may be indistinguishable from those of Kaposi sarcoma (69).

Papillary endothelial proliferation, the formation of interconnecting vascular channels, and hemorrhage are indicative of fully developed lesions (figs. 527, 528). In more advanced cases, endothelial growth forms sheets and masses that have an epithelial appearance (fig. 529). These foci are difficult to distinguish from carcinoma by light microscopy (fig. 530). Histochemical studies and electron microscopy are helpful in this situation. Poorly differentiated recurrent carcinoma generally contains little or no mucin but the carcinoma cells are reactive immunohistochemically for cytokeratin (55) and sometimes also for epithelial membrane antigen (EMA). Angiosarcomas have been uniformly nonreactive for cytokeratin (57,60) and EMA (59). Immunoreac-

tivity for the blood group antigen *Ulex europaeus* I lectin has been reported to be strong in vascular components and variable in solid undifferentiated areas of Stewart-Treves angiosarcoma (56,60). Since immunoreactivity for *U. europaeus* has been found in mammary carcinomas, this test is not helpful in the differential diagnosis. Factor VIII–related antigen has been detected in cells lining well-formed neoplastic vascular channels (47,60,70), but has been absent (60,70) or minimally expressed (47,56) in poorly differentiated foci. Often it is difficult to distinguish histologically between well-differentiated neoplastic vascular channels and reactive vessels associated with chronic lymphedema. Both may be factor VIII immunoreactive.

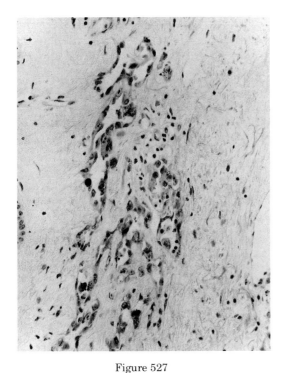

Figure 527
POSTMASTECTOMY ANGIOSARCOMA
Neoplastic hyperchromatic endothelial cells in vascular channels in the superficial dermis.

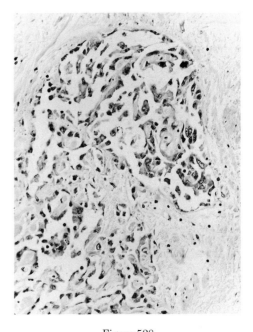

Figure 528
POSTMASTECTOMY ANGIOSARCOMA
Neoplastic papillary endothelial proliferation composed of hyperchromatic pleomorphic cells in anastomosing vascular channels.

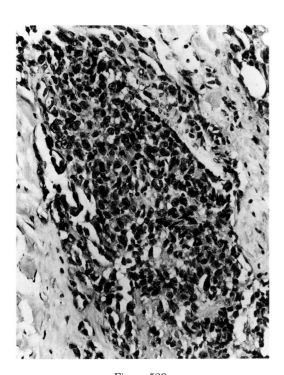

Figure 529
POSTMASTECTOMY ANGIOSARCOMA
Focal solid proliferation of neoplastic endothelial cells filling a vascular channel.

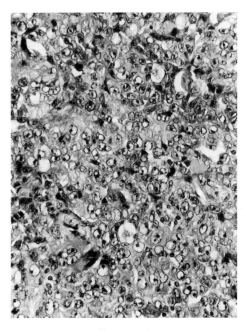

Figure 530
POSTMASTECTOMY ANGIOSARCOMA
Sheet of anaplastic tumor cells that resembles undifferentiated carcinoma. (Fig. 14-6 from Rosen PP. Tumors of the breast. Based on the proceedings of the 53rd annual anatomic pathology slide seminar of the American Society of Clinical Pathologists. Chicago: American Society of Clinical Pathologists, 1987:37.)

Larger veins appear to become involved as a result of intramural neoplastic proliferation rather than as a consequence of transmural invasion by extrinsic tumor foci. Embolic spread of angiosarcoma has been found at distant sites, such as the lung, and this phenomenon most likely also occurs to some extent in the affected limb.

Several studies have established the heterogeneous ultrastructural features of Stewart-Treves angiosarcoma (47,56,59,60,70). The electron microscopic findings are typical for a vascular lesion characterized by a proliferation of endothelial cells. In angiomatous areas, endothelial cells resting on a basement membrane are joined by well-formed junctional complexes. The cytoplasm contains pinocytotic vesicles, clusters of intermediate filaments, and Weibel-Palade bodies. With loss of differentiation, Weibel-Palade bodies and pinocytotic vesicles become less numerous. Solid portions of the tumors are composed of round and spindle cells arranged in a loosely cohesive fashion and joined by primitive and well-formed desmosomes. Erythrocytes may be seen in neoplastic vascular lumens and between neoplastic cells in poorly differentiated areas. Pericytic cells are reportedly not evident (47) or only present in well-differentiated areas (52,56,59).

Immunohistochemical and ultrastructural observations have led to the widely held conclusion that the neoplastic cells in Stewart-Treves angiosarcoma have properties more typically associated with blood vascular endothelium than with lymphatic endothelium. The features that characterize blood vascular endothelium include fenestrated cells, Weibel-Palade bodies, pinocytotic activity, and pericytic cells. Factor VIII immunoreactivity has not been regarded as specific for blood vascular endothelium since staining has been found in normal (53,66) and in neoplastic lymphatic endothelium (53). Others reported that lymphatic endothelial cells were not reactive for factor VIII (47,61).

Prognosis and Treatment. There has been no consistently effective treatment for Stewart-Treves angiosarcoma. The majority of patients die of metastatic sarcoma less than 2 years after diagnosis; fewer than 10 percent have survived for 5 years (71,72). Amputation and chemotherapy may offer the best chance for cure (67,72). Local recurrence is more frequent after treatment by excisional surgery, radiation, or chemotherapy alone than after amputation. Other malignant neoplasms, particularly contralateral mammary carcinoma, may occur in these patients (67).

REFERENCES

1. Berg JW, DeCrosse JJ, Fracchia AA, Farrow J. Stromal sarcomas of the breast. A unified approach to connective tissue sarcomas other than cystosarcoma phyllodes. Cancer 1962;15:418–24.
2. Callery CD, Rosen PP, Kinne DW. Sarcoma of the breast. A study of 32 patients with reappraisal of classification and therapy. Ann Surg 1985;201:527–32.
3. Oberman HA. Sarcomas of the breast. Cancer 1965;18:1233–43.

Liposarcoma

4. Barnes L, Pietruszka M. Sarcomas of the breast: a clinicopathologic analysis of ten cases. Cancer 1977;40:1577–85.
5. Hummer CD Jr, Burkart TJ. Liposarcoma of the breast. A case of bilateral involvement. Am J Surg 1967;113:558–61.
6. Oberman HA, Nosanchuk JS, Finger JE. Periductal stromal tumors of breast with adipose metaplasia. Arch Surg 1969;98:384–7.

Osteosarcoma and Chondrosarcoma

7. Barnes L, Pietruszka M. Sarcomas of the breast: a clinicopathologic analysis of ten cases. Cancer 1977;40:1577–85.
8. Beltaos E, Banerjee TK. Chondrosarcoma of the breast. Report of two cases. Am J Clin Pathol 1979;71:345–9.
9. Chan CW, Alagaratnam TT. A bony tumour of the breast. Aust NZ J Surg 1982;52:79–83.
10. Jernstrom P, Lindberg AL, Meland ON. Osteogenic sarcoma of the mammary gland. Am J Clin Pathol 1963;40:521–6.
11. Smith BH, Taylor HB. The occurrence of bone and cartilage in mammary tumors. Am J Clin Pathol 1969;51:610–8.

Leiomyosarcoma

12. Arista-Nasr J, Gonzalez-Gomez I, Angeles-Angeles A, Illanes-Baz E, Brandt-Brandt H, Larriva-Sahd J. Primary recurrent leiomyosarcoma of the breast. Case report with ultrastructural and immunohistochemical study and review of the literature. Am J Clin Pathol 1989;92:500–5.

13. Chen KT, Kuo TT, Hoffmann KD. Leiomyosarcoma of the breast: a case of long survival and late hepatic metastasis. Cancer 1981;47:1883–6.
14. Nielsen BB. Leiomyosarcoma of the breast with late dissemination. Virchows Arch [A] 1984;403:241–5.

Rhabdomyosarcoma

15. Barnes L, Pietruszka M. Rhabdomyosarcoma arising within a cystosarcoma phyllodes. Case report and review of the literature. Am J Surg Pathol 1978;2:423–9.
16. Woodard BH, Farnham R, Mossler JA, Snell H, McCarty KS Jr. Rhabdomyosarcoma of the breast [Letter]. Arch Pathol Lab Med 1980;104:445–6.

Postirradiation Sarcoma

17. Kuten AA, Sapir D, Cohen Y, Haim N, Borovik R, Robinson E. Postirradiation soft tissue sarcoma occurring in breast cancer patients: report of seven cases and results of combination chemotherapy. J Surg Oncol 1985;28:168–71.
18. Oberman HA, Oneal RM. Fibrosarcoma of the chest wall following resection and irradiation of carcinoma of the breast. Am J Clin Pathol 1970;53:407–12.
19. Souba WW, McKenna RJ Jr, Meis J, Benjamin R, Raymond AK, Mountain CF. Radiation-induced sarcomas of the chest wall. Cancer 1986;57:610–5.

Hemangiopericytoma

20. Arias-Stella J Jr, Rosen PP. Hemangiopericytoma of the breast. Mod Pathol 1988;1:98–103.
21. Callery CD, Rosen PP, Kinne DW. Sarcoma of the breast. Ann Surg 1986;201:527–32.
22. Donnell RM, Rosen PP, Lieberman PH, et al. Angiosarcoma and other vascular tumors of the breast. Ann J Surg Pathol 1981;5:629–42.
23. Kaufman SL, Stout AP. Hemangiopericytoma in children. Cancer 1960;13:695–710.
24. Mittal KR, Gerald W, True LD. Hemangiopericytoma of breast: report of a case with ultrastructural and immunohistochemical findings. Hum Pathol 1986;17:1181–3.
25. Tavassoli FA, Weiss S. Hemangiopericytoma of the breast. Ann J Surg Pathol 1981;5:745–52.
26. Volmer J, Pickartz H, Jautzke G. Vascular tumors in the region of the breast. Virchows Arch [A] 1980;385:201–14.

Angiosarcoma

27. Antman KH, Corson J, Greenberger J, Wilson R. Multimodality therapy in the management of angiosarcoma of the breast. Cancer 1982;50:2000–3.
28. Benda JA, Al-Jurf AS, Benson AB III. Angiosarcoma of the breast following segmental mastectomy complicated by lymphedema. Am J Clin Pathol 1987;87:651–5.
29. Brentani MM, Pacheco MM, Oshima CT, Nagai MA, Lemos LB, Göes JC. Steroid receptors in breast angiosarcoma. Cancer 1983;51:2105–11.
30. Bundred NJ, O'Reilly K, Smart JG. Long term survival following bilateral breast angiosarcoma. Eur J Surg Oncol 1989;15:263–4.
31. Chen KT, Kirkegaard DD, Bocian JJ. Angiosarcoma of the breast. Cancer 1980;46:368–71.
32. Donnell RM, Rosen PP, Lieberman PH, et al. Angiosarcoma and other vascular tumors of the breast. Am J Surg Pathol 1981;5:629–42.
33. Givens SS, Ellerbroek NA, Butler JJ, Libshitz HI, Hortobagyi GN, McNeese MD. Angiosarcoma arising in an irradiated breast. A case report and review of the literature. Cancer 1989;64:2214–6.
34. Guarda LA, Ordonez NG, Smith JL Jr, Hanssen G. Immunoperoxidase localization of factor VIII in angiosarcomas. Arch Pathol Lab Med 1982;106:515–6.
35. Gullesserian HP, Lawton RL. Angiosarcoma of the breast. Cancer 1969;24:1021–6.
36. Hunter TB, Martin PC, Dietzen CD, Tyler LT. Angiosarcoma of the breast. Two case reports and a review of the literature. Cancer 1985;56:2099–106.
37. Jozefczyk MA, Rosen PP. Vascular tumors of the breast: II. Perilobular hemangiomas and hemangiomas. Am J Surg Pathol 1985;9:491–503.
38. Rainwater LM, Martin JK Jr, Gaffey TA, Van Heerden JA. Angiosarcoma of the breast. Arch Surg 1986;121:669–72.
39. Rosen PP. Vascular tumors of the breast: III. Angiomatosis. Am J Surg Pathol 1985;9:652–8.
40. _____, Kimmel M, Ernsberger D. Mammary angiosarcoma. The prognostic significance of tumor differentiation. Cancer 1988;62:2145–51.
41. _____, Ridolfi RL. The perilobular hemangioma. A benign microscopic vascular lesion of the breast. Am J Clin Pathol 1977;68:21–3.
42. Rosner D. Angiosarcoma of the breast: long-term survival following adjuvant chemotherapy. J Surg Oncol 1988;39:90–5.
43. Rubin E, Maddox WA, Mazur MT. Cutaneous angiosarcoma of the breast 7 years after lumpectomy and radiation therapy. Radiology 1990;174:258–60.
44. Ryan JF, Kealy WF. Concomitant angiosarcoma and carcinoma of the breast: a case report. Histopathology 1985;9:893–9.
45. Yadav RV, Sahariah S, Mittal VK, Bannerjee K. Angiosarcoma of the male breast. Int Surg 1976;61:463–4.
46. Yonezawa S, Maruyama I, Sakae K, Igata A, Majerus PW, Sato E. Thrombomodulin as a marker for vascular tumors. Comparative study with factor VIII and *Ulex europaeus* I lectin. Am J Clin Pathol 1987;88:405–11.

Postmastectomy Angiosarcoma (Stewart-Treves Syndrome)

47. Capo V, Ozzello L, Fenoglio CM, Lombardi L, Rilke F. Angiosarcomas arising in edematous extremities: immunostaining for factor VIII-related antigen and ultrastructural features. Hum Pathol 1985;16:144–50.
48. Chen KT, Hoffman KD, Hendricks EJ. Angiosarcoma following therapeutic irradiation. Cancer 1979;44:2044–8.
49. Davies JD, Rees GJ, Mera SL. Angiosarcoma in irradiated post-mastectomy chest wall. Histopathology 1983;7:947–56.
50. Fitzpatrick PJ. Lymphangiosarcoma and breast cancer. Can J Surg 1969;12:172–7.
51. Futrell JW, Albright NL, Myers GH Jr. Prevention of tumor growth in an "immunologically privileged site" by adoptive transfer of tumor-specific transplantation immunity. J Surg Res 1972;12:62–9.
52. Gray GF Jr, Gonzalez-Licea A, Hartmann WH, Woods AC Jr. Angiosarcoma in lymphedema. An unusual case of Stewart-Treves syndrome. Bull Johns Hopkins Hosp 1966;119:117–28.
53. Guarda LA, Ordonez NG, Smith JL Jr, Hanssen G. Immunoperoxidase localization of factor VIII in angiosarcomas. Arch Pathol Lab Med 1982;106:515–6.

54. Hamels J, Blondiau P, Mirgaux M. Cutaneous angiosarcoma arising in a mastectomy scar after therapeutic irradiation. Bull Cancer (Paris) 1981;68:353–6.

55. Hashimoto K, Matsumoto M, Eto H, Lipinski J, LaFond AA. Differentiation of metastatic breast carcinoma from Stewart-Treves angiosarcoma. Use of anti-keratin and anti-desmosome monoclonal antibodies and factor VIII-related antibodies. Arch Dermatol 1985; 121:742–6.

56. Lagacé R, Leroy JP. Comparative electron microscopic study of cutaneous and soft tissue angiosarcomas, post-mastectomy angiosarcoma (Stewart-Treves syndrome) and Kaposi's sarcoma. Ultrastruct Pathol 1987;11: 161–73.

57. Lee AK, DeLellis RA, Rosen PP, et al. ABH blood group isoantigen expression in breast carcinomas—an immunohistochemical evaluation using monoclonal antibodies. Am J Clin Pathol 1985;83:308–19.

58. Lo TC, Silverman ML, Edelstein A. Postirradiation hemangiosarcoma of the chest wall. Report of a case. Acta Radiol [Oncol] 1985;24:237–40.

59. McWilliam LJ, Harris M. Histogenesis of post-mastectomy angiosarcoma—an ultrastructural study. Histopathology 1985;9:331–43.

60. Miettinen M, Lehto VP, Virtanen I. Postmastectomy angiosarcoma (Stewart-Treves syndrome). Light microscopic, immunohistological, and ultrastructural characteristics of two cases. Am J Surg Pathol 1983;7:329–39.

61. Mukai K, Rosai J, Burgdorf WH. Localization of factor VIII-related antigen in vascular endothelial cells using an immunoperoxidase method. Am J Surg Pathol 1980;4:273–6.

62. Otis CN, Peschel R, McKhan C, Merino MJ, Duray PH. The rapid onset of cutaneous angiosarcoma after radiotherapy for breast carcinoma. Cancer 1986; 57:2130–4.

63. Schirger A. Postoperative lymphedema: etiologic and diagnostic factors. Med Clin North Am 1962;46:1045–50.

64. Schreiber H, Barry FM, Russell WC, Macon WI IV, Ponsky JL, Pories WJ. Stewart-Treves syndrome. A lethal complication of post-mastectomy lymphedema and regional immune deficiency. Arch Surg 1979;114:82–5.

65. Scott RB, Nydick I, Conway H. Lymphangiosarcoma arising in lymphedema. Am J Med 1960;28:1008–12.

66. Sehested M, Hou-Jensen J. Factor VIII-related antigen as an endothelial cell marker in benign and malignant diseases. Virchow's Arch [A] 1981;391:217–25.

67. Sordillo PP, Chapman R, Hajdu SI, Magill GB, Golbey RB. Lymphangiosarcoma. Cancer 1981;48:1674–9.

68. Sternby NH, Gynning I, Hogeman KE. Postmastectomy angiosarcoma. Acta Chir Scand 1961;121:420–32.

69. Stewart FW, Treves N. Lymphangiosarcoma in postmastectomy lymphedema. Cancer 1948;1:64–81.

70. Tomita K, Yokogawa A, Oda Y, Terahata S. Lymphangiosarcoma in postmastectomy lymphedema (Stewart-Treves syndrome): ultrastructural and immunohistologic characteristics. J Surg Oncol 1988;38:275–82.

71. Woodward AH, Ivins JC, Soule EH. Lymphangiosarcoma arising in chronic lymphedematous extremities. Cancer 1972;30:562–72.

72. Yap BS, Yap HY, McBride CM, Bodey GP. Chemotherapy for postmastectomy lymphangiosarcoma. Cancer 1981;47:853–6.

❖❖❖

LYMPHOID AND HEMATOPOIETIC NEOPLASMS

Aspects of lymphoid and hematopoietic lesions that are especially relevant to the breast are discussed here. For a comprehensive discussion and additional illustrations the reader is referred to the Fascicle on Tumors of Lymphoid and Hematopoietic Tissues.

NON-HODGKIN LYMPHOMA

The diagnosis of primary mammary lymphoma should be limited to patients without coincidental evidence of systemic lymphoma or leukemia. Clinically, the disease should involve only the breast or the breast and ipsilateral lymph nodes. Less than 0.5 percent of all malignant lymphomas and about 2 percent of extranodal lymphomas involve the breast.

Clinical Presentation. With rare exceptions (21,22), patients described in the literature have been women. They range from 15 to 86 years of age (average 55 years) at diagnosis (15,19). Unilateral lymphoma affects the right breast significantly more often with a ratio of approximately 3 to 2 (1,15,19). Bilateral disease occurs in about 10 percent of patients at the time of diagnosis (5,20); contralateral involvement may develop with progression (4,5) resulting in a bilaterality rate of 20 to 25 percent (10).

The presenting symptom is a painless mass. Recent onset and rapid growth are not unusual (4,5). The tumor is often solitary but patients with multiple lesions (4,5) and diffuse infiltration have been described. Enlarged axillary lymph nodes have been described clinically in 30 to 50 percent of patients (1,4,13,18). In one study, 17 percent of the patients were treated for another malignant neoplasm diagnosed before, coincident with, or after the lymphoma (1).

Gross Findings. The tumors have measured 1 to 12 cm, averaging about 3 cm. The excised specimen usually contains a circumscribed, fleshy tumor that may have a nodular configuration (fig. 531). Areas of softening and brown discoloration tend to be regions of necrosis.

Microscopic Findings. Approximately 50 percent of primary mammary lymphomas are of the diffuse histiocytic type when classified by the widely used Rappaport system (1,12,15,19).

Poorly differentiated lymphocytic lymphomas (25 percent), the majority of which are diffuse, and mixed lymphomas (20 percent), equally nodular and diffuse, are the second and third most common, respectively (1,4,19). Well-differentiated lymphocytic, lymphoblastic, undifferentiated, and Burkitt lymphomas account for 5 to 10 percent of mammary lymphomas in most series, however, in one study 62 percent of lymphomas were classified as undifferentiated (15). Patients with mammary Burkitt lymphoma often present with massive bilateral breast enlargement.

Studies presented in terms of the Kiel classification (1,5,13) have characterized the majority of tumors as centroblastic-centrocytic diffuse or centroblastic diffuse. Immunoblastic lymphoma, lymphoplasmacytic immunocytoma, and lymphocytic lymphomas are uncommon. The scarcity

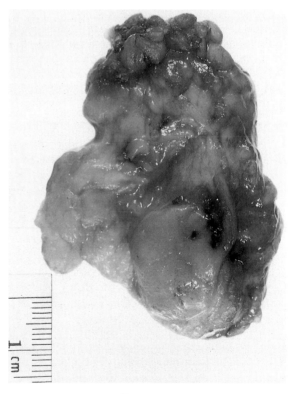

Figure 531
MALIGNANT LYMPHOMA
Round, bulging fleshy bisected tumor formed by diffuse small cleaved cell lymphoma.

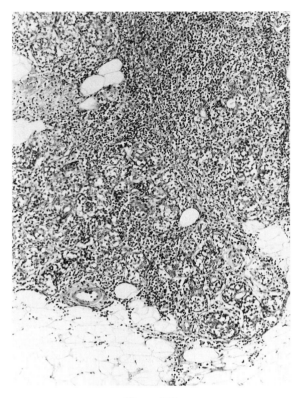

Figure 532
MALIGNANT LYMPHOMA
Lobules involved by diffuse lymphoma. Residual lobular glands are evident in the lower right corner. (Figures 532 and 533 are from the same patient.)

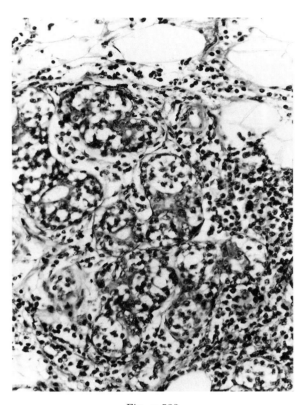

Figure 533
MALIGNANT LYMPHOMA
High magnification view of lymphomatous infiltrate in a lobule. Lymphomatous cells that fill lobular glands are surrounded by residual basement membrane.

of lymphoplasmacytic lymphomas of the breast distinguishes extranodal lymphoma in the breast from lymphomas arising in the stomach, gastrointestinal tract, and lung, which exhibit plasmacytic differentiation more often (7,12). In the Lukes-Collins scheme the majority of mammary lymphomas are the large noncleaved diffuse and large cleaved cell diffuse types (1). Diffuse large cleaved, diffuse small cleaved, and diffuse or follicular mixed cell lymphomas are the three most common cell types according to the Working Formulation (1).

Lymphoma in the breast typically consists of a uniform population of tumor cells that diffusely infiltrate the mammary parenchyma. Ducts and lobules are better preserved away from the center of the lesion but there is a tendency for the lymphomatous infiltrate to concentrate in and around these structures. A reactive lymphoid infiltrate composed of small lymphocytes is com-

monly present at the periphery of the tumor. This also tends to localize around epithelial elements and blood vessels. Germinal centers may be formed in these reactive infiltrates.

Lymphomatous infiltration into the epithelium of ducts and lobules simulates in situ carcinoma (figs. 532, 533). When this occurs, the malignant lymphoid cells expand ducts and lobular glands, displacing the epithelial cells. In some instances these alterations in lobules and the linear pattern of lymphoma cells in the stroma closely resemble in situ and invasive lobular carcinoma (figs. 534, 535). However, the reactive lymphoid infiltrate that accompanies most lymphomas is rarely found in invasive lobular carcinoma. Immunohistochemical markers for epithelial differentiation (cytokeratin, epithelial membrane antigen) and lymphoid differentiation (leucocyte common antigen, lymphocyte markers) generally resolve the issue.

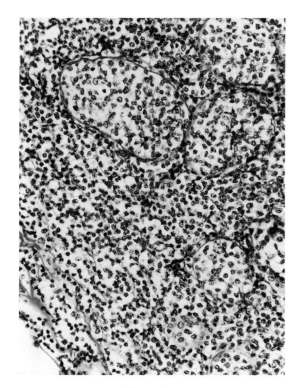

Figure 534
MALIGNANT LYMPHOMA
Lobular epithelium has been entirely destroyed leaving only some basement membranes defining lobular units in the diffuse lymphomatous infiltrate.

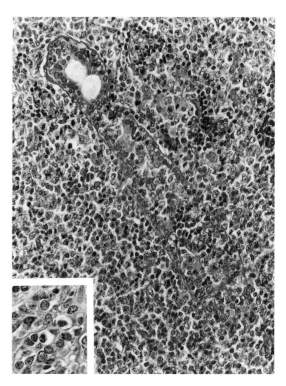

Figure 535
MALIGNANT LYMPHOMA
Lymphomatous infiltrate extends into, and partially replaces, the epithelium of a terminal duct that runs diagonally across the picture. Inset shows magnified view of tumor cells in this large cell lymphoma.

Non-Hodgkin lymphoma involving the breast, whether primary or secondary, is almost always of the B-cell type, usually expressing IgM heavy chain and less often IgA (2,13). Rare examples of mammary T-cell lymphoma have been reported (2).

The term *pseudolymphoma* has been applied to tumor-forming lymphoid lesions that are thought to be benign reactive conditions. The concept of pseudolymphoma has been questioned since some patients initially thought to have this condition developed systemic malignant lymphoma (6,11,12, 16). Some features that characterize pseudolymphomas, such as germinal center formation and the absence of node involvement, may be found in mammary lymphomas. The specificity of this diagnosis when applied to lymphoid tumors of the breast remains questionable.

Less than 20 cases of mammary pseudolymphoma have been reported (9,14,17,18). Some lesions appeared after trauma and clinically have consistently measured about 3 cm in diameter. Axillary node enlargement was absent in all cases.

The patients, 26 to 77 years old, had no systemic symptoms. Serum immunoglobulin studies revealed polyclonal elevation of IgG in two cases and a normal IgG level in a third case (14). In one case mammography revealed a circumscribed lobulated mass (9).

The distinction between pseudolymphoma and lymphoma has been based on histologic analysis. Tumors described as pseudolymphomas have been characterized by a sharply localized polymorphic infiltrate composed largely of mature lymphocytes. Germinal centers, sometimes numerous, are often present, especially at the periphery (fig. 536). The epithelia of ducts and lobules are largely spared, although these structures can be surrounded by the infiltrative process (figs. 537, 538). Small numbers of eosinophils, plasma cells, and histiocytes are scattered throughout the lesion. Follicular hyperplasia has been described in ipsilateral axillary lymph nodes (9,18).

Figure 536
"PSEUDOLYMPHOMA"
Nodular lymphoid proliferation with
prominent follicular differentiation in
mammary fat and stroma. Dark area is
hemorrhage resulting from prior needle
biopsy. Five years after excisional biopsy,
this 30-year-old woman remained well,
having had no other treatment. Genetic
study of the lesion revealed no gene rearrangement of the TCR beta and immunoglobulin genes. (Figures 536–538 are
from the same patient.)

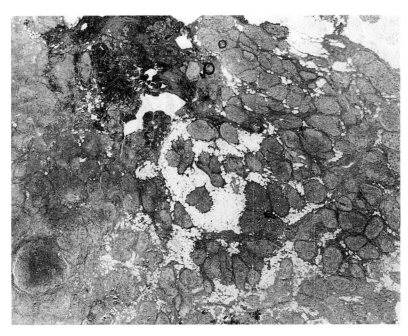

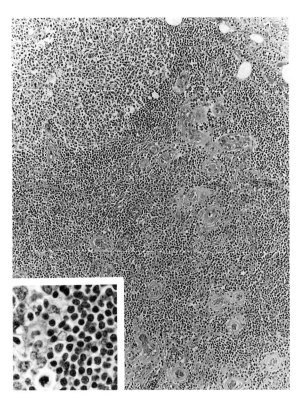

Figure 537
"PSEUDOLYMPHOMA"
Lobular glands are easily identified in the diffuse infiltrate that consists largely of mature lymphocytes. A germinal center is seen in the upper left corner. Inset shows border
of germinal center.

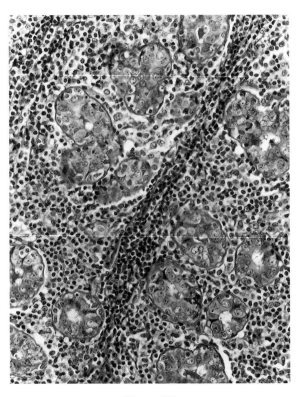

Figure 538
"PSEUDOLYMPHOMA"
A few mature lymphocytes are present among epithelial
cells in lobular glands to the same extent as lymphocytes in
lobular glands not affected by a lymphoid lesion.

Most patients with mammary pseudolymphoma have had follow-up from over 2 to 15 years (18). None had a recurrence in the breast or developed systemic lymphoma following treatment by various modalities including local excision alone (14), excision followed by radiotherapy (9), and mastectomy with axillary dissection (18).

Prognosis and Treatment. Until fairly recently, there was a tendency to treat patients with "primary" lymphoma clinically limited to the breast and axillary lymph nodes by mastectomy and to reserve local excision for women with systemic disease. However, it has now been demonstrated that excellent local control in the breast and regional lymph nodes can be achieved with radiation after partial mastectomy (3,20) and, as a consequence, mastectomy is only recommended for specific clinical problems such as bulky local disease or infected, ulcerated lesions.

Regardless of the type of local therapy, about 80 percent of recurrences are at distant sites. A review of 205 patients with all stages of mammary lymphoma reported prior to 1984 revealed a disease-free survival of 3.4 percent at 5 years and 2 percent at 10 years (8). However, subsequent analyses of patients with stage I and IIE disease limited to the breast or breast and axillary lymph nodes have revealed more favorable results. DeBlasio (3) reported a 50 percent disease-free survival at 4 years, with 66 percent of patients alive. In another series, 72 percent of patients were alive after a median follow-up of 55 months with 44 percent disease-free (20). Brustein et al. (1) reported that 41 percent of stage I and IIE patients survived 10 years and the combined data from three other series (4,15,19) showed that 47 percent of patients survived 10 years. Patients with stage I disease and histologically low-grade lesions have the best prognosis.

HODGKIN DISEASE

Hodgkin disease is rarely found in the breast. Mammary infiltration is usually the result of direct extension from axillary lymph nodes (24,29), part of regional disease with discontinuous axillary node involvement (23,25), or a manifestation of systemic disease (23,26). Wood et al. (28) reviewed 354 reported examples of extranodal Hodgkin disease published prior to 1973 and found 8 (2 percent) that involved the breast. Almost all of these patients ultimately developed systemic dis-

ease. Recurrent Hodgkin disease presenting as a breast mass has been reported (27). Nodular sclerosis and mixed cellularity Hodgkin disease have been found in the breast.

PLASMACYTOMA

Clinical Presentation. Extramedullary neoplastic plasmacytic infiltrates can occur at many sites. The mammary gland is rarely involved clinically when patients present with typical osseous manifestations (36). Plasmacytoma of the breast presenting as an isolated initial manifestation of systemic disease was described in 1934 by Cutler (31) and in subsequent case reports (30,34,38).

Approximately 4 percent of plasmacytomas are entirely extramedullary tumors, with the majority occurring in the respiratory tract (32). Extramedullary plasmacytoma limited to the breast has been described in four patients. Innes and Newell (32) described a 43-year-old woman with bilateral breast lesions and no evidence of systemic involvement. Serum electrophoresis was not performed. Proctor et al. (37) described a 63-year-old woman with normal serum protein and immunoglobulin levels, who remained disease free 46 months after excision and local radiotherapy of a solitary right breast tumor. Two women with solitary mammary plasmacytomas had abnormal serum proteins. In one case a 70-year-old woman had mildly increased serum immunoglobulins but no monoclonal spike or urinary Bence Jones protein (35). Nine years following a radical mastectomy she remained well except for excision of a nasal plasmacytic polyp 6 years after treatment of the breast tumor. The other patient was a 73-year-old woman with elevated serum IgG with a monoclonal lambda peak (33). IgM and IgA levels were normal. Bone marrow aspiration revealed that "plasma cells were present but not conspicuously increased." Forty months after excision and local mammary radiation the patient remained well.

Gross Findings. Solitary plasmacytomas of the breast are 2- to 4-cm circumscribed tan or brown tumors.

Microscopic Findings. Solitary plasmacytomas contain "a mixture of mature and immature plasma cells." Mitoses, nuclear pleomorphism, and multinucleated plasma cells may be seen. Mammary glandular structures are largely effaced in the region where the plasma

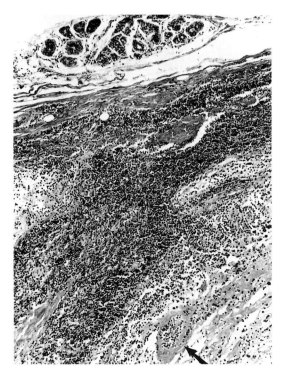

Figure 539
PLASMACYTOMA

Mammary glandular structures are virtually obliterated by a dense infiltrate of plasma cells and lymphocytes. The patient had no systemic disease indicative of multiple myeloma. The outline of a duct (arrow) is seen below. (Figures 539 and 540 are from the same patient.)

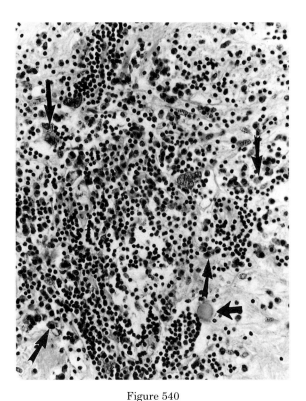

Figure 540
PLASMACYTOMA

Mature and immature plasma cells (long arrows), lymphocytes, and a Russell body (short arrow) are evident.

cell infiltrate is most concentrated (figs. 539, 540). However, the neoplastic cells spread microscopically beyond the grossly evident mass.

Histologically, primary mammary plasmacytoma should be distinguished from plasma cell mastitis, amyloid tumor, and plasma cell granuloma. Plasma cell mastitis is a periductal process that features duct dilatation, a mixed inflammatory infiltrate, and abscess formation. Amyloid is barely detectable in, or absent from, mammary plasmacytoma.

Prognosis and Treatment. Following the histologic diagnosis of a plasmacytic tumor of the breast, the patient should be evaluated for evidence of systemic involvement. Prognosis and treatment will depend on the type and extent of the underlying disorder. Treatment may consist of excision and local radiation in patients who have lesions limited to the breast. The prognosis for patients with solitary mammary plasmacytoma appears to be excellent.

LEUKEMIC INFILTRATION

Leukemic infiltration of the breast is not uncommon at an advanced stage but is rare as the initial manifestation of the disease.

Granulocytic Sarcoma

Granulocytic leukemia may present with tumoral breast involvement, also referred to as granulocytic sarcoma (43,44,45). The term *chloroma* has been used to describe extramedullary tumor-forming granulocytic leukemic infiltrates that develop a green color as a result of the enzymatic action of myeloperoxidase (verdoperoxidase) contained in the neoplastic cells. Tumors that do not have a green color have in the past been termed *myeloblastoma*. Green and colorless tumors may occur at different sites in the same patient and therefore the diagnosis granulocytic sarcoma should be employed for either form of the disease. Hematogenous evidence of myelogenous leukemia usually appears less than a year after the initial mammary lesion. Mammary infiltrates have also been described as a secondary manifestation in patients with established leukemia (42).

Patients range in age from 21 to 56 years. Unilateral and bilateral lesions have been reported and axillary lymph nodes may be involved (44).

The diagnosis of granulocytic sarcoma in a breast biopsy is difficult because the growth pattern simulates invasive lobular carcinoma or malignant lymphoma (42). The neoplastic cells forming broad sheets or cords invade into and around normal mammary parenchymal structures. Intraepithelial extension of the leukemic infiltrate simulates in situ carcinoma. The diagnosis of granulocytic sarcoma is suggested by cytoplasmic granules in maturing myeloid cells or by the presence of relatively numerous mature myeloid cells scattered throughout the lesion. Special stains are especially helpful. Granulocytic sarcoma cells do not contain mucin and give a negative reaction for immunocytochemical epithelial markers such as cytokeratin and epithelial membrane antigen. Myeloid granules are reactive histochemically with the napthol-ASD-chloroacetate esterase stain and immunohistochemically for lysozyme (muramidase).

Lymphocytic Leukemia

Mammary infiltration has been described in patients with chronic lymphocytic leukemia (40,41). The lesions tend to be bilateral. Coincidental bone marrow and hematogenous involvement are usually present. Some patients with mammary parenchymal and bone marrow infiltrates have been diagnosed as having well-differentiated lymphocytic lymphoma.

Myeloid Metaplasia

A breast mass formed by myeloid metaplasia has been reported in a 60-year-old woman who developed an 8 cm breast tumor composed of mature and maturing hematopoietic cells, including megakaryocytes, 16 years after the onset of myelofibrosis (39). The patient reportedly had no other tumorous manifestations of myeloid metaplasia but slight hepatic enlargement was noted.

REFERENCES

Non-Hodgkin Lymphoma

1. Brustein S, Filippa DA, Kimmel M, Lieberman PH, Rosen PP. Malignant lymphoma of the breast: a study of 53 patients. Ann Surg 1987;205:144–50.
2. Cohen PL, Brooks JJ. Lymphomas of the breast. A clinicopathologic and immunohistochemical study of primary and secondary cases. Cancer 1991;67:1359–69.
3. DeBlasio D, McCormick B, Straus D, et al. Definitive irradiation for localized non-Hodgkin's lymphoma of breast. Int J Radiat Oncol Biol Phys 1989;17:843–6.
4. DeCosse JJ, Berg JW, Fracchia AA, Farrow JH. Primary lymphosarcoma of the breast. A review of 14 cases. Cancer 1962;15:1264–8.
5. Dixon JM, Lumsden AB, Krajewski A, Elton RA, Anderson TJ. Primary lymphoma of the breast. Br J Surg 1987;74:214–6.
6. Evans HL. Extranodal small lymphocytic proliferation: a clinicopathologic and immunocytochemical study. Cancer 1982;49:84–96.
7. Filippa DA, Lieberman PH, Weingrad DN, Decosse JJ, Bretsky SS. Primary lymphomas of the gastrointestinal tract. Analysis of prognostic factors with emphasis on histological type. Am J Surg Pathol 1983;7:363–72.
8. Fischer MG, Chideckel NJ. "Primary" lymphoma of the breast. Breast 1984;10:7–9.
9. Fisher ER, Palekar AS, Paulson JD, Golinger R. Pseudolymphoma of breast. Cancer 1979;44:258–63.
10. Freedman SJ, Kagan AR, Friedman NB. Bilaterality in primary lymphosarcoma of the breast. Am J Clin Pathol 1971;55:82–7.
11. Greenberg SD, Heisler JG, Gyorkey F, Jenkins DE. Pulmonary lymphoma versus pseudolymphoma: a perplexing problem. South Med J 1972;65:775–84.
12. L'Hoste RJ Jr, Filippa DA, Lieberman PH, Bretsky S. Primary pulmonary lymphomas. A clinicopathologic analysis of 36 cases. Cancer 1984;54:1397–406.
13. Lamovec J, Jancar J. Primary malignant lymphoma of the breast. Lymphoma of the mucosa-associated lymphoid tissue. Cancer 1987;60:3033–41.
14. Lin JJ, Farha GJ, Taylor RJ. Pseudolymphoma of the breast. I. In a study of 8,654 consecutive tylectomies and mastectomies. Cancer 1980;45:973–8.
15. Mambo NC, Burke JS, Butler JJ. Primary malignant lymphomas of the breast. Cancer 1977;39:2033–40.
16. Marchevsky A, Padilla M, Kaneko M, Kleinerman J. Localized lymphoid nodules of lung. A reappraisal of the lymphoma versus pseudolymphoma dilemma. Cancer 1983;51:2070–7.

17. Nakano A, Hamada Y, Hirono M, Hattori T. Differentiation between pseudo- and malignant lymphoma of the breast—a case report. Jpn J Surg 1982;12:76–8.

18. Oberman HA. Primary lymphoreticular neoplasms of the breast. Surg Gynecol Obstet 1966;123:1047–51.

19. Schouten JT, Weese JL, Carbone PP. Lymphoma of the breast. Ann Surg 1981;194:749–53.

20. Smith MR, Brustein S, Straus DJ. Localized non-Hodgkin's lymphoma of the breast. Cancer 1987;59:351–4.

21. Talvalkar GV. Primary lymphosarcoma of the breast: a report of ten cases. Indian J Cancer 1973;10:322–9.

22. Tanino M, Tatsuzawa T, Funada T, Nakajima H, Sugiura H, Odashima S. Lymphosarcoma of the male breast: a case report. Breast 1984;10:13–5.

Hodgkin Disease

23. Lawler MR, Riddell DH. Hodgkin's disease of the breast. Arch Surg 1966;93:331–4.

24. Mehrotra RM, Wahal KM, Abarwal PK. Lymphoma of female breast. Indian J Pathol Bacteriol 1974;17:54–60.

25. Sanyal B, Pant GC, Subrahmanyam K, Khanna NN, Rastogi BL. Hodgkin's disease of breast. Indian J Cancer 1974;11:382–5.

26. Schouten JT, Weese JL, Carbone PP. Lymphoma of the breast. Ann Surg 1981;194:749–53.

27. Shehata WM, Pauke TW, Schleuter JA. Hodgkin's disease of the breast. A case report and review of the literature. Breast 1985;11:19–21.

28. Wood NL, Coltman CA. Localized primary extranodal Hodgkin's disease. Ann Intern Med 1973;78:113–8.

29. Yarhold JR, Jelliffee AM, Hudson V, Maclennan KA. The response of treatment of nodular sclerosing Hodgkin's disease with extranodal involvement. Clin Radiol 1982;33:141–4.

Plasmacytoma

30. Bassett WB, Weiss RB. Plasmacytomas of the breast: an unusual manifestation of multiple myeloma. South Med J 1979;72:1492–4.

31. Cutler CW Jr. Plasma cell tumor of the breast with metastases. Ann Surg 1934;100:392–5.

32. Innes J, Newall J. Myelomatosis. Lancet 1961;1:239–45.

33. Kirshenbaum G, Rhone DP. Solitary extramedullary plasmacytoma of the breast with serum monoclonal protein: a case report and review of the literature. Am J Clin Pathol 1985;83:230–2.

34. Maeda K, Abesamis CM, Kuhn LM. Multiple myeloma in childhood: report of a case with breast tumors as a presenting manifestation. Am J Clin Pathol 1973;60:552–8.

35. Merino MJ. Plasmacytoma of the breast. Arch Pathol Lab Med 1984;108:676–8.

36. Pasmantier MW, Azar HA. Extraskeletal spread in multiple plasma cell myeloma. Cancer 1969;23:167–74.

37. Proctor NS, Rippey JJ, Shulman G, Cohen C. Extramedullary plasmacytoma of the breast. J Pathol 1975;116:97–100.

38. Rosenberg B, Attie JN, Mandelbaum HL. Breast tumor as the presenting sign of multiple myeloma. N Engl J Med 1963;269:359–61.

Leukemic Infiltration

39. Brooks JJ, Krugman DT, Damjanov I. Myeloid metaplasia presenting as a breast mass. Am J Surg Pathol 1980;4:281–5.

40. Desablens B, Quang TN, Claisse JF, Piprot-Choffat C, Grumbach Y. Localisation mammaire au cours de la leucemie lymphoide chronique [Letter]. Presse Med 1985;14:2301.

41. Gogoi PK, Stewart ID, Keane PF, Scott R, Dunn GD, Catovsky D. Chronic lymphocytic leukemia presenting with bilateral involvement. Clin Lab Haematol 1989;11:57–60.

42. Pascoe HR. Tumors composed of immature granulocytes occurring in the breast in chronic granulocytic leukemia. Cancer 1970;25:697–704.

43. Pettinato G, De Chiara A, Insabato L, De Renzo A. Fine needle aspiration biopsy of granulocytic sarcoma (chloroma) of the breast. Acta Cytol 1988;32:67–71.

44. Sears HF, Reid J. Granulocytic sarcoma: local presentation of a systemic disease. Cancer 1976;37:1808–13.

45. Wiernick PH. [Letter to Editor.] Cancer 1989;63:1624.

❖❖❖

MISCELLANEOUS NEOPLASMS

GRANULAR CELL TUMOR

The first report of this tumor is attributed to Abrikossof (1) who described a granular cell tumor of the tongue. He proposed origin from striated muscle cells and, as a consequence, the lesion was termed a myoblastoma. Accumulated evidence has cast doubt on the myogenous histogenesis of granular cell neoplasms and they are now thought to be derived from the Schwann cells of peripheral nerves. Granular cell tumors occur throughout the body with about 5 percent originating in the breast (11).

Clinical Presentation. Granular cell tumor of the breast is most often encountered in women 30 to 50 years old, but it has been described in adolescents, elderly women, and males (4,10,11).

In most cases the patient presents with a firm or hard painless mass. The lesions tend to develop more often in the upper quadrants; few are reported in the lower outer quadrant (4). Superficial lesions may cause skin retraction and nipple inver-

sion has been reported when the tumor is in a subareolar location. In the breast, granular cell tumor usually presents as a solitary lesion. Patients who have multiple granular cell tumors at various sites may have one in the breast as well (8,9). On mammography, granular cell tumor is difficult to distinguish from carcinoma (6,12).

Gross Findings. The lesion is usually a firm or hard mass. Many appear to be well circumscribed when bisected but others have ill-defined infiltrative borders (fig. 541). The cut surface is white, grey, or yellow to tan. Lesions measuring up to 6 cm have been reported but the tumors are generally 3 cm or smaller.

Microscopic Findings. With very rare exceptions, granular cell tumor of the breast is a benign neoplasm (fig. 542). The tumor is composed of compact nests or sheets of spindle or polygonal cells that contain eosinophilic cytoplasmic granules. The granules are usually prominent and fill the cytoplasm but in some lesions there is

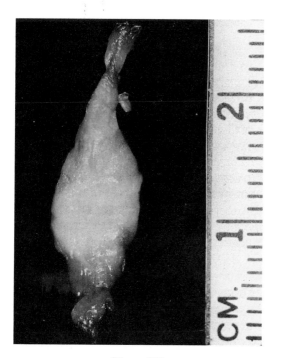

Figure 541
GRANULAR CELL TUMOR
Dense, pale, homogeneous neoplasm with margins that tend to merge with the breast tissue.

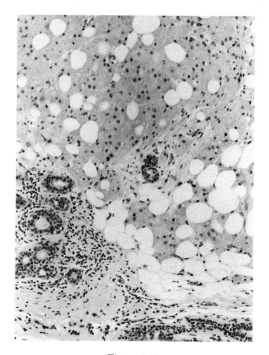

Figure 542
GRANULAR CELL TUMOR
Invasive growth in fat. (Figures 542 and 543 are from the same patient.)

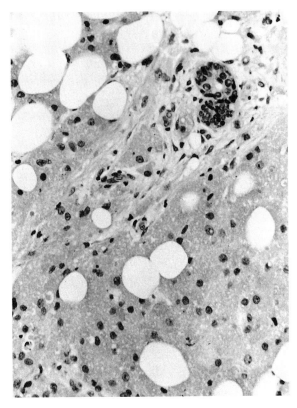

Figure 543
GRANULAR CELL TUMOR
Tumor cells have pale, finely granular cytoplasm and round clear nuclei with small nucleoli.

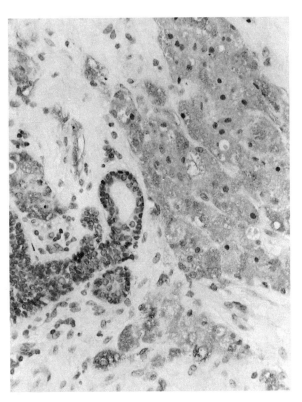

Figure 544
GRANULAR CELL TUMOR
Diffuse immunoreactivity for S-100 protein highlights cytoplasmic granularity. Myoepithelial cells in an adjacent terminal duct are also immunoreactive (S-100 immunoperoxidase; hematoxylin counterstain).

a tendency toward cytoplasmic vacuolization and clearing (fig. 543). The cytoplasmic granules are diastase resistant and PAS positive. Nuclei are round to slightly oval with an open chromatin pattern. Nucleoli tend to be prominent. In some cases, a modest amount of nuclear pleomorphism, occasional multinucleated cells, and rare mitoses may be found but these features should not be interpreted as evidence of a malignant neoplasm. Small nerve bundles are sometimes seen in the tumor or in close association with stellate extensions of the lesion peripherally.

Although many of the tumors appear grossly circumscribed, microscopic examination invariably reveals an infiltrating growth pattern at the margins. Ducts and lobules are typically surrounded by the invasive tumor cells and incorporated into the lesion. Granular cells may infiltrate into lobules.

Granular cell tumor of the breast must be distinguished from mammary carcinoma, histiocytic lesions, and metastatic neoplasms. The infiltrative character consisting of cells with prominent nucleoli, especially when the lesion has collagenous stroma, results in a close resemblance to scirrhous carcinoma. The similarity between invasive apocrine carcinoma and granular cell tumor may be striking, however, the presence of intraductal carcinoma usually serves to identify apocrine carcinoma. The mucicarmine stain is focally positive in many apocrine carcinomas and these tumors are immunoreactive for cytokeratin and epithelial membrane antigen; granular cell tumors are not reactive for these epithelial markers, do not contain mucin, and are estrogen receptor negative. Strong, diffuse immunoreactivity for S-100 protein characterizes granular cell tumors (fig. 544) (2,3,12), although some mammary carcinomas are also S-100 positive.

The distinction between granular cell tumor and mammary carcinoma is particularly difficult in needle aspiration cytology specimens (5,7,10). Many granules distributed throughout the background as well as in the cells stain blue with Romanovsky stains and red with the Papanicolaou stain. The granules are also red in smears stained with hematoxylin and eosin.

Electron microscopy reveals myelin figures as well as numerous lysosomes (3,4,12). Some cells also have angulate bodies, which are rounded or triangular membrane-bound structures that contain microtubules and microfibrils.

Prognosis and Treatment. With rare exceptions, granular cell tumor of the breast is benign, and treatable by wide excision. Incomplete excision may result in local recurrence but it is sometimes difficult to distinguish between recurrence and asynchronous multifocal lesions. Less than 1 percent of all granular cell tumors, including mammary lesions, are malignant. Systemic metastases have been described in patients with nonmammary malignant granular cell tumors.

AMYLOID TUMOR

Amyloid deposits in the breast can occur in patients with predisposing systemic diseases such as primary amyloidosis (22), rheumatoid arthritis (15,24), multiple myeloma (16), and Waldenstrom macroglobulinemia (18). In these cases breast involvement, when clinically evident, is invariably a late development. Primary amyloid tumors clinically limited to the breast are uncommon (13,17,21,25,26).

Clinical Presentation. Most reported patients with amyloid tumor of the breast have been women 45 to 79 years old. Bilateral involvement is extremely uncommon clinically. Eighty percent of unilateral tumors were located in the right breast. The tumors were usually painless and solitary and any part of the breast was involved, including the nipple (14).

Examination reveals a discrete firm or hard tumor that is occasionally tender (19,26). Retraction of the overlying skin has been reported. The clinical findings may suggest carcinoma, an impression that can be reinforced if mammographic examination reveals calcifications in the lesion (13,25).

Gross Findings. Amyloid tumors of the breast have measured 5 cm or less in diameter. The lesion is firm, grey or white, and opalescent.

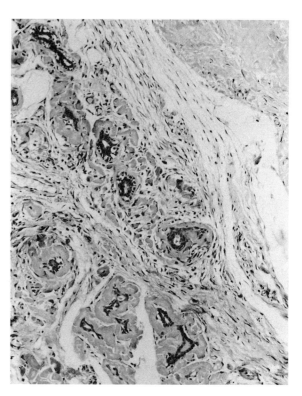

Figure 545
AMYLOID TUMOR
Amyloid in mammary lobule, and as a nodule in the mammary stroma (upper right).

Fat and small cysts may be present in breast parenchyma incorporated in the lesion.

Microscopic Findings. Histologic examination reveals eosinophilic amorphous homogeneous deposits distributed in fat, fibrocollagenous stroma, and blood vessels. Deposits of amyloid around ducts and in lobules are associated with atrophy and obliteration of these structures (figs. 545, 546). Amyloid deposited around individual fat cells forms "amyloid rings" (23); plasma cells and lymphocytes are present in association with these deposits. Multinucleated giant cells constitute a foreign body–like reaction to the amyloid, which may have prominent granulomatous features and calcification.

Amyloid stains red-orange with alkaline Congo red and exhibits apple-green birefringence when the Congo red–stained section is examined with polarized light. Staining with crystal violet results in a strong metachromatic reaction. In most cases the amyloid is composed

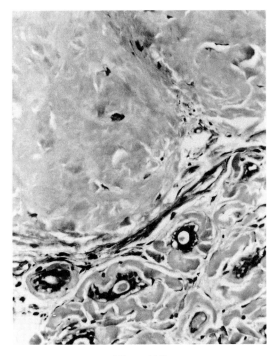

Figure 546
AMYLOID TUMOR
Thick wavy bands of amyloid around lobular glands and a nodular deposit that is virtually acellular.

of immunoglobulin light chains (16,21,25). Electron microscopy reveals straight, nonbranching, haphazardly arranged amyloid fibrils measuring 5 to 10 mm enmeshed with bands of collagen fibers (13,23). Amyloid obtained in a fine-needle aspirate consists of refractile or glassy amorphous material in Papanicolaou-stained smears. Metachromasia is evident with a modified Wright stain (25) and the amyloid appears purple with the May-Grunwald-Giemsa stain (17). The sparsely cellular smears reveal scattered plasma cells, lymphocytes, spindly stromal cells, epithelial cells, and occasional multinucleated giant cells.

Prognosis and Treatment. Excisional biopsy is necessary for the diagnosis of amyloid tumor of the breast. The distinction between a primary amyloid tumor and secondary amyloidosis can only be made by careful clinical evaluation to rule out a systemic condition (18). Primary amyloid tumor of the breast has proven to be a benign condition adequately treated by excisional biopsy. The prognosis of patients with systemic disease depends on the clinical course of the underlying condition.

METASTASES IN THE BREAST FROM NONMAMMARY NEOPLASMS

Clinical Presentation. A lesion in the breast is the initial symptom of a nonmammary malignant neoplasm in about 25 percent of patients whose first manifestation is metastatic tumor. One of the most common primary tumor sites is the lungs (32,36,38,44). Other clinically occult neoplasms that may present with metastases in the breast include malignant melanoma (41), carcinoma of the kidney (29,41), and stomach (41) and intestinal carcinoid tumors (33,35).

Malignant lymphomas in the breast are best considered primary breast tumors or as part of a systemic disease affecting the lymphoid system rather than metastatic neoplasms. Adenocarcinomas of the colon and rectum are rarely the source of metastatic carcinoma in the breast despite their relative frequency in the population at large (27). Although uncommon, primary carcinoid tumors of the small intestine are a more frequent source of breast metastases than are colonic adenocarcinomas (figs. 547, 548), and the breast lesion may be the presenting clinical finding (35,40). Mammary metastases from medulloblastoma (28), rhabdomyosarcoma (34), and neuroblastoma (42) have been reported in children.

In men, involvement of the breast by metastatic prostatic adenocarcinoma is a relatively frequent finding at autopsy, sometimes involving both breasts (39). A few patients have had independent synchronous or metachronous independent primary carcinomas of the prostate and the breast (37,45). In addition to routine histologic examination, histochemical studies for mucin and immunohistochemical studies for prostate specific antigen and prostatic acid phosphatase can be performed on the biopsy to distinguish between metastatic prostatic carcinoma and a primary breast lesion (30,37).

Radiographically, metastatic lesions tend to be discrete round shadows without spiculation and are not distinguishable from papillary, medullary, or colloid primary breast carcinomas (44). The average interval to the development of a mammary metastasis is approximately 2 years for patients with previously treated cancer. Usually, there are prior or coincidental metastases at other sites. Metastatic tumor in the breast is at first a single lesion in about 85 percent of

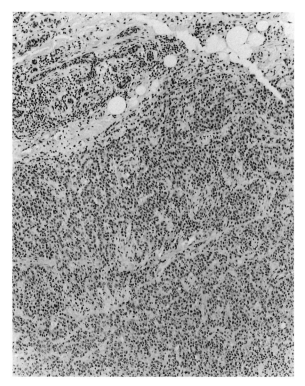

Figure 547
METASTATIC INTESTINAL CARCINOID
The patient had previously been treated for a malignant carcinoid of the small intestine. The trabecular and alveolar pattern composed of small, uniform tumor cells could be mistaken for primary breast carcinoma. (Figures 547 and 548 are from the same patient.)

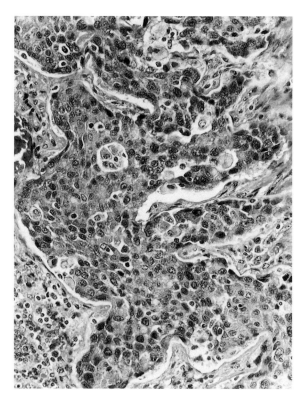

Figure 548
METASTATIC INTESTINAL CARCINOID
The tumor was immunoreactive for chromogranin (avidin-biotin peroxidase).

cases. Eventually about 25 percent of patients have bilateral metastases. Metastases have been described in ipsilateral axillary lymph nodes in 25 to 48 percent of patients (44). This is a manifestation of hematogenous spread since there are generally metastases in nonaxillary lymph nodes as well.

Microscopic Findings. It is important to be sensitive to morphologic patterns that are not typical for breast carcinoma in order to avoid interpreting a metastatic neoplasm as a primary breast tumor. However, some tumors of identical appearance arise in the breast as well as in other organs, including squamous, mucinous (colloid), mucoepidermoid (fig. 549), and clear cell carcinomas and spindle cell neoplasms (fig. 550). A search should be made for in situ carcinoma to confirm origin in the breast but since this cannot be found in all primary mammary lesions its

absence is not conclusive evidence for metastasis. Metastatic tumor often surrounds and displaces normal appearing breast parenchyma, which typically shows little or no hyperplasia. The finding of more than two grossly evident tumors should lead one to consider metastatic tumor, especially if the histologic pattern is unusual. Lymphatic tumor emboli are associated with metastases in the breast as well as with primary breast carcinomas. Electron microscopy, immunohistochemistry, and estrogen receptor analysis may be helpful in the differential diagnosis of a neoplasm suspected to be metastatic in the breast.

Prognosis and Treatment. Some types of metastatic tumor in the breast can be accurately diagnosed by needle aspiration cytology if the patient has a previously diagnosed nonmammary malignant neoplasm, but in general excisional biopsy is recommended (31,43). When an occult extramammary neoplasm presents with a

347

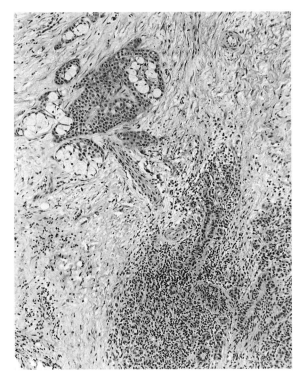

Figure 549
METASTATIC MUCOEPIDERMOID CARCINOMA
The primary tumor arose in a minor salivary gland of the oral cavity.

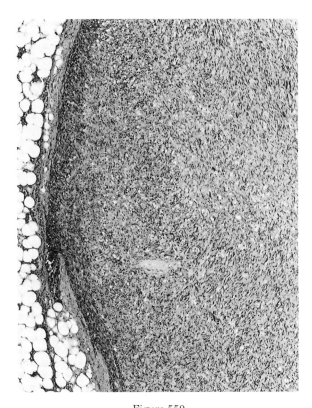

Figure 550
METASTATIC SPINDLE CELL RENAL CARCINOMA
This metastasis might be mistaken for a primary mammary sarcoma. The patient had a large renal carcinoma with the same microscopic appearance.

breast metastasis, work-up of the patient will depend upon morphologic features of the tumor that suggest particular primary sites. Mastectomy is rarely indicated. Wide excision may be supplemented by radiotherapy to the breast and axillary dissection may be performed if the lymph nodes are grossly involved and symptomatic clinically. Emphasis should be placed on systemic treatment appropriate to the primary lesion.

Metastatic involvement of the breast is a manifestation of generalized metastases in virtually all cases. The prognosis depends on the clinical characteristics of the specific neoplasm, but it is generally poor.

MALIGNANT MELANOMA OF THE MAMMARY SKIN

Malignant melanoma of the skin of the breast occurs more often in men than women (48,49,51, 53). Patients have been 16 to 72 years of age, with the average age of women in the mid-thirties and

men in their forties. Any region may be affected but origin in the nipple-areola complex is relatively uncommon (50).

Approximately two thirds of lesions arise medial to the midclavicular line or in the central region. Metastases occur in axillary lymph nodes in about 50 percent of patients and are more likely with a lateral than with a medial lesion. Supraclavicular lymph node metastases derive from tumors of the infraclavicular region or upper half of the mammary region. Lymph node metastases were not found in 20 patients subjected to internal mammary lymph node dissection (49,51), only 6 of 16 patients with widely disseminated melanoma at autopsy had internal mammary lymph node metastases (51). The frequency of regional lymph node involvement and 5-year disease-free survival are inversely related to the thickness of the primary lesion as determined by the Clark level of invasion (51).

There is no predilection for any histologic type of melanoma to arise in the skin of the breast. Nodular, superficial spreading and ulcerated lesions have been described. An antecedent nevus is suggested clinically when the patient reports a recent change in a longstanding pigmented lesion and this is often confirmed histologically. Some patients with melanoma of the nipple or areola report change in an existing "mole," but in most cases a new pigmented lesion is described (50).

The histologic diagnosis of malignant melanoma of the skin of the breast is based on the criteria employed to assess nonmammary pigmented cutaneous lesions. Lesions of the nipple-areola complex present a more difficult problem. The presence of melanotic pigment is not sufficient to distinguish malignant melanoma from Paget disease since Paget cells may acquire such pigment (46,54). This phenomenon can also occur at sites of cutaneous metastases of mammary carcinoma (52). The presence of intraductal or invasive carcinoma in the underlying nipple or breast parenchyma and reactivity for one or more epithelial markers such as cytokeratin, epithelial membrane antigen, or mucin are convincing evidence for Paget disease. S-100 positivity is seen in virtually all cases of malignant melanoma but only infrequently in Paget disease. Hence, a strongly positive result is suggestive of melanoma but confirmatory evidence is necessary to confidently establish the diagnosis. A variety of immunohistochemical markers specifically associated with melanoma may be helpful in this regard (47).

The prognosis of melanoma of the mammary skin or nipple-areola complex depends on the stage at diagnosis. In the largest series, about 60 percent of patients remained disease free at 5 years. When axillary lymph nodes were uninvolved, the 5-year disease-free survival was nearly 90 percent, which dropped to about 25 percent with axillary node metastases (51). When stratified by stage, there were no significant differences in outcome between men and women or between patients with medial and lateral lesions.

Most patients in retrospective series were treated by mastectomy and axillary dissection regardless of the location of the primary lesion. Although mastectomy might be necessary in some cases, many patients can be managed by wide excision that may include some underlying breast parenchyma (51,53). Origin in the nipple-areola complex is not considered a contraindication to wide excision if a cosmetically acceptable result can be obtained (50). Axillary dissection, when performed, should include the tail of Spence to ensure excision of all lymph nodes.

NONMELANOMATOUS NEOPLASMS OF THE MAMMARY SKIN

Neoplasms that arise at various cutaneous sites may be found in the skin and subcutaneous tissue of the breast (56). In most cases, origin in the skin, subcutaneous tissue, or both is clearly evident clinically and pathologically. Hemangiomas of the subcutaneous tissue may be difficult to distinguish from parenchymal lesions. Metastatic neoplasms, especially carcinomas, can mimic primary mammary carcinomas (55).

Since the morphologic spectrum of sweat gland carcinoma is similar to that of breast carcinoma these carcinomas may present a difficult diagnostic problem. Adnexal tumors of the mammary skin are occasionally large enough to impinge upon the breast tissue, thereby obscuring origin from the skin. For the most part, immunohistochemical markers give similar results for both. However, nuclear immunoreactivity for estrogen receptor is at most sparse and weak in sweat gland carcinomas. A strongly positive result therefore favors mammary origin but a negative result is not helpful. A particularly vexing problem arises when a patient had prior or has concurrent carcinoma of the mammary glandular parenchyma and noncontiguous adenocarcinoma in the axillary skin. In some of these situations the distinction between metastatic carcinoma and sweat gland carcinoma cannot be made with absolute certainty and a judgement must be made that takes clinical factors into consideration.

BASAL CELL CARCINOMA OF THE NIPPLE

Approximately 15 cases of basal cell carcinoma of the nipple have been reported (57–61). The majority of the patients were men ranging in age from 43 to 80 years (median 60); women were 49 to 75 years old. This sex distribution probably reflects the greater sun exposure of the nipple in men.

The early lesion is usually red and scaling. Ulceration, plaque-like thickening of the skin, and nodular lesions have been described. Occasionally, involvement extends to skin adjacent to the areola. The differential diagnosis includes inflammatory conditions, florid papillomatosis of the nipple, Bowen disease, and Paget disease.

Microscopically, there does not appear to be a predilection for a particular type of basal cell carcinoma to arise in the nipple. Basaloid proliferation from the epidermis is a diagnostic feature that accompanies downward and lateral growth within the dermis and the nipple stroma. Intraepithelial extension into lactiferous ducts is sometimes observed. Keratinization occurs in solid as well as cystic foci.

Most patients have been treated successfully by wide excision occasionally supplemented by irradiation. Axillary lymph node metastases have been reported (61).

HAMARTOMA AND VARIANT LESIONS

These are well-demarcated masses of ducts and lobules containing varying amounts of fibrous and adipose tissue. They present as non-painful, discrete masses and circumscribed densities on mammograms. However, the tumors may go unrecognized by the pathologist because of a resemblance to other benign or physiologic conditions of the breast. Hamartomas may be considered a clinicopathologic entity, unified by their well-defined clinical presentation, but with a variable microscopic appearance (65).

These lesions characteristically are sharply circumscribed, lenticular to spherical masses (pl. II). Depending on the relative proportion of fat and fibrous tissue in the tumor, their color varies from white to yellow.

Histopathologically they have heterogeneous growth patterns, all of which are dominated by benign mesenchymal tissue, which, in contrast to the fibrosis associated with fibrocystic changes, seemingly pushes normal parenchyma aside (62). The most common pattern is that of dense hyalinized connective tissue that separates lobular ducts (fig. 551). Hamartomas with a predominant fatty stroma, or a mixture of collagen and fat, have the appearance of an adenolipoma (fig. 552). The paucity of ducts, as well as minimal lobular branching, may result

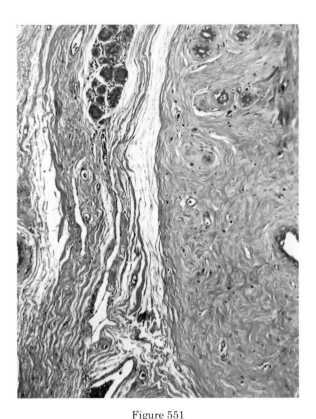

Figure 551
MAMMARY HAMARTOMA
Well-defined densely fibrous tumor with ducts separated by connective tissue.

in a gynecomastia-like appearance (fig. 553). The ducts in these lesions lack the compression or elongation of a fibroadenoma. In addition, the presence of a prominent fatty component is unusual in the latter tumor.

A rare variant of this microscopic picture is the presence of islands of hyaline cartilage in the fatty stroma, resulting in a chondrolipomatous appearance (fig. 554) (64). This should be distinguished from the unusual occurrence of foci of cartilage in a myofibroblastoma. Another uncommon variant is the presence of foci of smooth muscle (fig. 555). In some instances these may predominate, leading to the designation, "muscular hamartoma" (63).

Treatment of hamartoma is local excision. The surgical margins may be narrow, as there is no propensity for recurrence and no risk of malignant change.

Plate II
MAMMARY HAMARTOMA

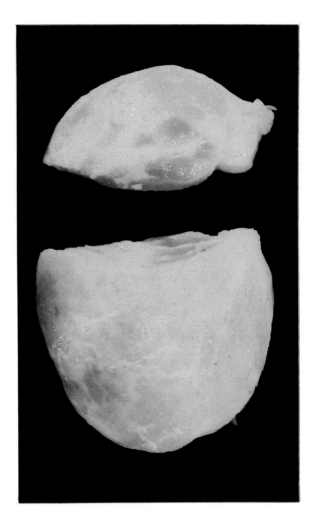

Cross section (above) and lateral external
view of tumor indicates its lenticular, ovoid
shape.

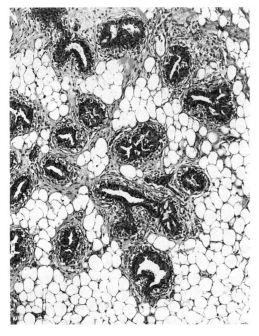

Figure 552
MAMMARY HAMARTOMA
Tumor is composed largely of fat and the separation of lobular ducts simulates gynecomastia. This growth pattern also has been termed adenolipoma.

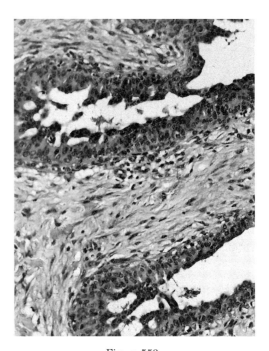

Figure 553
MAMMARY HAMARTOMA
Intraductal hyperplasia in tumor wherein the separation of ducts results in an appearance resembling gynecomastia.

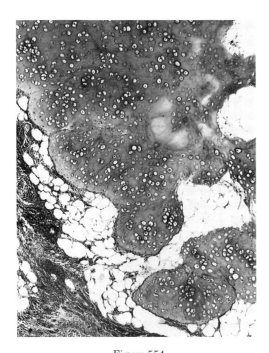

Figure 554
MAMMARY HAMARTOMA
Small nodules of hyaline cartilage in a predominantly fatty tumor.

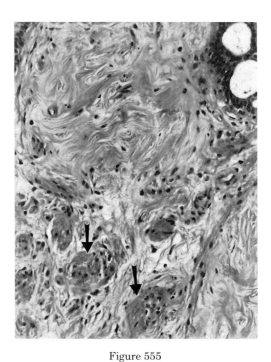

Figure 555
MAMMARY HAMARTOMA
The smooth muscle (arrows) is arranged in small bundles intermixed with the fibrous connective tissue.

REFERENCES

Granular Cell Tumor

1. Abrikossof AI. Über myome, ausgehend von der quergestreifter willkür licher muskulatur. Virchows Arch Pathol Anat 1926;260:215–33.
2. Armin A, Connelly EM, Rowden G. An immunoperoxidase investigation of S-100 protein in granular cell myoblastomas: evidence for Schwann cell derivation. Am J Clin Pathol 1983;79:37–44.
3. Buley ID, Gatter KC, Kelly PM, Heryet A, Millard PR. Granular cell tumours revisited. An immunohistochemical and ultrastructural study. Histopathology 1988; 12:263–74.
4. DeMay RM, Kay S. Granular cell tumor of the breast. Pathol Annu 1984;19(Pt 2):121–48.
5. Franzën S, Steinkvist B. Diagnosis of granular cell myoblastoma by fine-needle aspiration biopsy. Acta Pathol Microbiol Scand 1968;72:391–5.
6. Gold DA, Hermann G, Schwartz IS, Klein MJ, Papatestas A, Delbridge CA. Granular cell tumor of the breast. Case report of an occult lesion simulating carcinoma. Breast Dis 1989;2:211–5.
7. Löwhagen T, Rubio CA. The cytology of the granular cell myoblastoma of the breast. Report of a case. Acta Cytol 1977;21:314–5.
8. Moscovic EA, Azar HA. Multiple granular cell tumors ("myoblastomas"). Case report with electron microscopic observations and review of the literature. Cancer 1967;20:2032–47.
9. Murray DE, Seaman E, Utzinger W. Granular cell myoblastomas in successive generations. J Surg Oncol 1969;1:193–7.
10. Sussman EB, Hajdu SI, Gray GF. Granular cell myoblastoma of the breast. Am J Surg 1973;126:669–70.
11. Turnbull AD, Huvos AG, Ashikari R, Strong EW. Granular-cell myoblastoma of breast. NY State J Med 1971;71:436–8.
12. Willën R, Willën H, Balldin G, Albrechtsson V. Granular cell tumor of the mammary gland simulating malignancy. A report on two cases with light microscopy, transmission electron microscopy and immunohistochemical investigation. Virchows Arch [A] 1984; 403:391–400.

Amyloid Tumor

13. Fernandez BB, Hernandez FJ. Amyloid tumor of the breast. Arch Pathol 1973;95:102–5.
14. Ganor S, Dollberg L. Amyloidosis of the nipple presenting as pruritus. Cutis 1983;31:318.
15. Goonatillake HD, Allsop JR. Amyloid tumour of the breast simulating carcinoma. Aust NZ J Surg 1988;58:589–90.
16. Hardy TJ, Myerowitz RL, Bender BL. Diffuse parenchymal amyloidosis of lungs and breast. Its association with diffuse plasmacytosis and kappa-chain gamopathy. Arch Pathol Lab Med 1979;103:583–5.
17. Lew W, Seymour AE. Primary amyloid tumor of the breast. Case report and literature review. Acta Cytol 1985;29:7–11.
18. Libbey CA, Skinner M, Cohen AS. Use of abdominal fat tissue aspirate in the diagnosis of systemic amyloidosis. Arch Intern Med 1983;143:1549–52.
19. Lipper S, Kahn LB. Amyloid tumor. A clinopathologic study of four cases. Am J Surg Pathol 1978;2:141–5.
20. McLellan GL, Stewart JH, Balachandran S. Localization of Tc-99m-MDP in amyloidosis of the breast. Clin Nucl Med 1981;6:579–80.
21. McMahon RF, Connolly CE. Amyloid breast tumor [Letter]. Am J Surg Pathol 1987;11:488.
22. O'Connor CR, Rubinow A, Cohen AS. Primary (AL) amyloidosis as a cause of breast masses. Am J Med 1984;77:981–6.
23. Pearson B, Rice MM, Dickens KL. Primary systemic amyloidosis. Arch Pathol 1941;32:1–10.
24. Sadeghee SA, Moore SW. Rheumatoid arthritis, bilateral amyloid tumors of the breast, and multiple cutaneous amyloid nodules. Am J Clin Pathol 1974;62:472–6.
25. Silverman JF, Dabbs DJ, Norris HT, Pories WJ, Legier J, Kay S. Localized primary (AL) amyloid tumor of the breast. Cytologic, histologic, immunocytochemical and ultrastructural observations. Am J Surg Pathol 1986; 10:539–45.
26. Walker AN, Fechner RE, Callicott JH Jr. Amyloid tumor of the breast. Diagn Gynecol Obstet 1982;4:339–41.

Metastases in the Breast from Nonmammary Neoplasms

27. Alexander HR, Turnbull AD, Rosen PP. Isolated breast metastases from gastrointestinal carcinomas: report of two cases. J Surg Oncol 1989;42:264–6.
28. Brutschin P, Culver GJ. Extracranial metastases from medulloblastomas. Radiology 1973;107:359–62.
29. Chica GA, Johnson DE, Ayala AG. Renal cell carcinoma presenting as breast carcinoma. Urology 1980;15:389–90.
30. Choudhury M, DeRosas J, Papsidero L, Wajsman Z, Beckley S, Pontes JE. Metastatic prostatic carcinoma to breast or primary breast carcinoma? Urology 1982;19:297–9.
31. Eisenberg AJ, Hajdu SI, Wilhelmus J, Melamed MR, Kinne D. Preoperative aspiration cytology of breast tumors. Acta Cytol 1986;30:135–46.
32. Hajdu SI, Urban JA. Cancers metastatic to the breast. Cancer 1972;29:1691–6.
33. Harrist TJ, Kalisher L. Breast metastasis: an unusual manifestation of a malignant carcinoid tumor. Cancer 1977;40:3102–6.
34. Howarth CB, Caces JN, Pratt CB. Breast metastases in children with rhabdomyosarcoma. Cancer 1980;46:2520–4.

35. Kashlan RB, Powell RW, Nolting SF. Carcinoid and other tumors metastatic to the breast. J Surg Oncol 1982;20:25–30.

36. McCrea ES, Johnston C, Haney PJ. Metastases to the breast. AJR Am J Roentgenol 1983;141:685–90.

37. Moldwin RM, Orihuela E. Breast masses associated with adenocarcinoma of the prostate. Cancer 1989; 63:2229–33.

38. Nielsen M, Andersen JA, Henriksen FW, et al. Metastases to the breast from extramammary carcinomas. Acta Pathol Microbiol Immunol Scand [A] 1981;89:251–6.

39. Salyer WR, Salyer DC. Metastases of prostatic carcinoma to the breast. J Urol 1973;109:671–5.

40. Schürch W, Lamoureux E, Lefebvre R, Fauteux JP. Solitary breast metastasis: first manifestation of an occult carcinoid of the ileum. Virchows Arch [A] 1980; 386:117–24.

41. Silverman EM, Oberman HA. Metastatic neoplasms in the breast. Surg Gynecol Obstet 1974;138:26–8.

42. Silverman JF, Feldman PS, Covell JL, Frable WJ. Fine needle aspiration cytology of neoplasms metastatic to the breast. Acta Cytol 1987;31:291–300.

43. Sneige N, Zachariah S, Fanning TV, Dekmezian RH, Ordóñez NG. Fine-needle aspiration cytology of metastatic neoplasms in the breast. Am J Clin Pathol 1989;92:27–35.

44. Toombs BD, Kalisher L. Metastatic disease in the breast: clinical, pathologic, and radiographic features. AJR Am J Roentgenol 1977;129:673–6.

45. Wilson SE, Hutchinson WB. Breast masses in males with carcinoma of the prostate. J Surg Oncol 1976;8:105–12.

Malignant Melanoma of the Mammary Skin

46. Cuberson JD, Horn RC. Paget's disease of the nipple: review of 25 cases with special reference to melanin pigmentation of "Paget cells." Arch Surg 1956;72:224–31.

47. Duray PH, Ernstoff MS, Titus-Ernstoff L. Immunohistochemical phenotyping of malignant melanoma. A procedure whose time has come in pathology practice. Pathol Annu 1990;25(Pt 2):351–77.

48. Jochimsen PR, Pearlman NW, Lawton RL, Platz CE. Melanoma of skin of the breast: therapeutic considerations based on six cases. Surgery 1977;81:583–7.

49. Lee YN, Sparks FC, Morton DL. Primary melanoma of skin of the breast region. Ann Surg 1977;185:17–22.

50. Papachristou DN, Kinne DW, Ashikari R, Fortner JG. Melanoma of the nipple and areola. Br J Surg 1979; 66:287–8.

51. _____, Kinne DW, Rosen PP, Ashikari R, Fortner JG. Cutaneous melanoma of the breast. Surgery 1979; 85:322–8.

52. Poiares-Baptista A, De Vasconcelos AA. Cutaneous pigmented metastasis from breast carcinoma simulating malignant melanoma. Int J Dermatol 1988;27:124–5.

53. Roses DF, Harris MN, Stern JS, Gumport SL. Cutaneous melanoma of the breast. Ann Surg 1979;189:112–5.

54. Sau P, Solis J, Lupton GP, James WD. Pigmented breast carcinoma. A clinical and histologic simulator of malignant melanoma. Arch Dermatol 1989;125:536–9.

Nonmelanomatous Neoplasms of the Mammary Skin

55. Hajdu SI, Urban JA. Cancers metastatic to the breast. Cancer 1972;29:1691–6.

56. Ilie B. Neoplasms in skin and subcutis over the breast, simulating breast neoplasms: case reports and literature review. J Surg Oncol 1986;31:191–8.

Basal Cell Carcinoma of the Nipple

57. Cain RJ, Sau P, Benson PM. Basal cell carcinoma of the nipple. Report of two cases. J Am Acad Dermatol 1990;22:207–10.

58. Congdon GH, Dockerty MB. Malignant lesions of the nipple exclusive of Paget's disease. Surg Gynecol Obstet 1956;103:185–92.

59. Robinson HB. Rodent ulcer of the male breast. Trans Pathol Soc London 1893;44:147–8.

60. Sauven P, Roberts A. Basal cell carcinoma of the nipple. J R Soc Med 1983;76:699–701.

61. Shertz WT, Balogh K. Metastasizing basal cell carcinoma of the nipple. Arch Pathol Lab Med 1986;110:761–2.

Hamartoma and Variant Lesions

62. Arrigoni MG, Dockerty MB, Judd ES. The identification and treatment of mammary hamartoma. Surg Gynecol Obstet 1971;133:577–82.

63. Davies JD, Riddell RH. Muscular hamartomas of the breast. J Pathol 1973;111:209–11.

64. Kaplan L, Walts AE. Benign chondrolipomatous tumor of the human female breast. Arch Pathol Lab Med 1977;101:149–51.

65. Oberman HA. Hamartomas and hamartoma variants of the breast. Semin Diagn Pathol 1989;6:135–45.

PATHOLOGY OF AXILLARY LYMPH NODES

SINUS HISTIOCYTOSIS

Sinus histiocytosis is defined as the "distention of the sinusoids of the lymph nodes by elongated histiocytes that have finely granular, eosinophilic-staining cytoplasm in a syncytial arrangement" (fig. 556) (1). Lymph nodes exhibiting inflammatory changes such as sinusoidal edema, and rounded histiocytes with vacuoles or erythrophagocytosis should be excluded from evaluation (figs. 557–559).

It has been suggested that sinus histiocytosis is a manifestation of cell mediated immune reaction to the carcinoma. Marked sinus histiocytosis in the ipsilateral axillary lymph nodes of patients with breast carcinoma has been associated with an enhanced cellular response to autologous breast cancer tissue (2) and to clinically evident enlargement of contralateral axillary lymph nodes (3). Several studies, largely carried out by Black his colleagues (3,5,7), reported a correlation between the grade of sinus histiocytosis and survival. Patients with the most intense, high-grade reaction had the most favorable prognosis. The favorable effect of marked sinus histiocytosis was evident in both node-negative and node-positive patients (4,8) but was most pronounced when nodal metastases were present (6). Silverberg et al. (14) found that marked sinus histiocytosis indicated a favorable prognosis in women with moderately or poorly differentiated tumors and in those with fewer than nine positive lymph nodes. There was no correlation with outcome in women who had well-differentiated tumors, negative lymph nodes, or more than eight positive nodes. The relatively high frequency of marked sinus

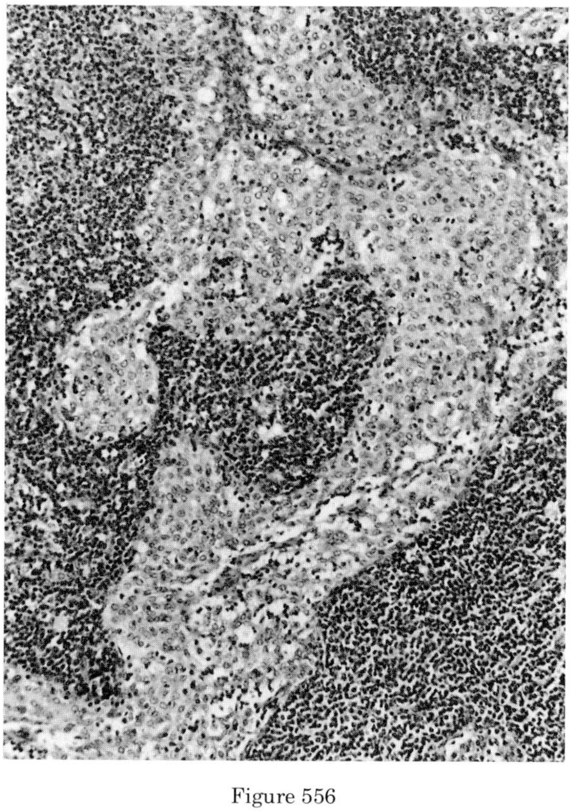

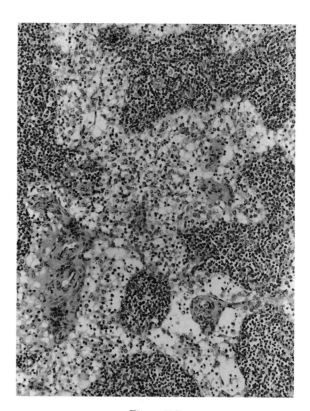

Figure 556
SINUS HISTIOCYTOSIS
The sinusoids are distended by a diffuse accumulation of histiocytes.

Figure 557
INFLAMMATORY SINUS HISTIOCYTOSIS
Marked sinusoidal edema is evident at low magnification.

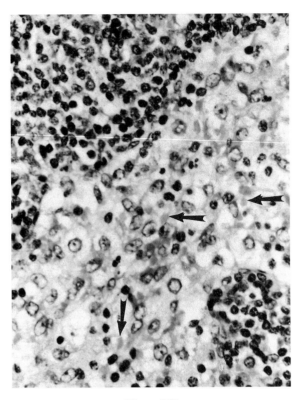

Figure 558
INFLAMMATORY SINUS HISTIOCYTOSIS
Note vacuolated histiocytes and erythrophagocytosis (arrows).

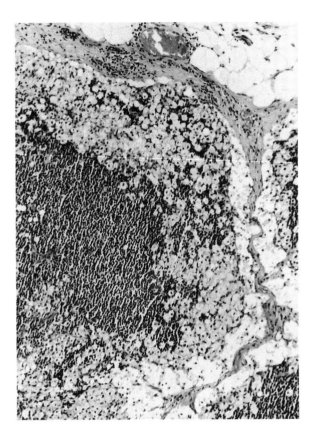

Figure 559
LACTATIONAL HISTIOCYTOSIS
Axillary lymph node from a lactating woman with breast carcinoma. Histiocytes are distended with lipid.

histiocytosis in axillary lymph nodes of Japanese women has been cited as a factor contributing to a more favorable prognosis (10). Others have not been able to confirm this association. Berg (1) concluded that nodal status and factors associated with lymph node metastases were more significant for prognosis and Moore et al. (12) were unable to find a difference in the pattern of sinus histiocytosis between patients who survived and those who died of metastatic breast carcinoma. DiRe and Lane (9), Schiodt (13), and Kister et al. (11) also concluded that sinus histiocytosis was not a significant indicator of prognosis.

Failure of investigators to find a consistent relationship between sinus histiocytosis and prognosis in breast cancer may reflect significant problems in the histologic evaluation of this phenomenon. The growing trend to biopsy the breast tumor as a separate operation prior to the

axillary dissection causes alterations in lymph nodes that may obscure reactions attributable to the carcinoma in the pre-biopsy state. It is also necessary to have good quality sections of well-fixed tissue and these are not always available. Investigators have not used consistent grading schemes and there is no consensus on how sinus histiocytosis should be measured or reported. The determination of sinus histiocytosis has proven to be a highly subjective endeavor with considerable inter- and intraobserver variability. In one study (7), an "experienced observer" achieved 70 percent self-reproducibility in two separate reviews of the same lymph nodes. Two less experienced pathologists agreed with the average grade of the two reviews of the "experienced observer" in 55 percent and 61 percent of cases, respectively.

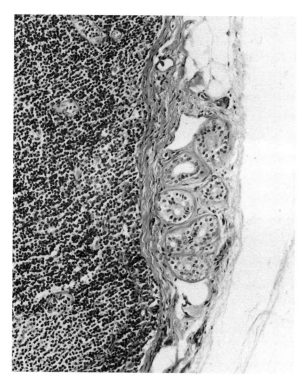

Figure 560
HETEROTOPIC GLANDS
Glandular inclusion with the structure of a mammary lobule in the capsule of a lymph node.

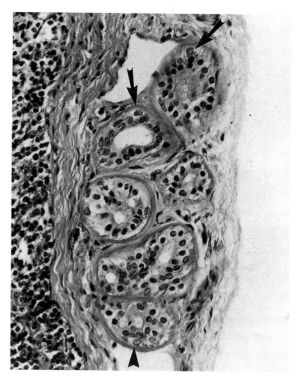

Figure 561
HETEROTOPIC GLANDS
At high magnification, myoepithelial cells are evident in glands (arrows) which are enclosed by a thick basement membrane. This lymph node was found in the axilla of a woman treated by mastectomy for invasive lobular carcinoma.

HETEROTOPIC GLANDS

Glandular inclusions in axillary lymph nodes may derive from the breast or from skin appendage glands (15–21). The histogenesis of the condition is unknown but it is thought that the phenomenon is due either to embryologic maldevelopment or embolic displacement of benign tissue initiated by trauma or surgery. The former is a more logical explanation for the capsular location of these glands.

Clinical Presentation. The nine reported patients with heterotopic glandular tissue in axillary lymph nodes were 31 to 90 years old. Most presented with an axillary mass but in two the affected lymph nodes were clinically inapparent (15,20). One patient had been treated by mastectomy for carcinoma of the left breast 10 years before an enlarged right axillary lymph node that contained heterotopic glandular tissue was excised (18). None of the other women was known to have mammary carcinoma but two underwent mastectomies for benign proliferative disease.

Gross Findings. Enlarged lymph nodes with grossly apparent cysts were described in two cases. In one the cysts contained "colorless or brownish fluid" (16) while in the other the cysts were filled with debris.

Microscopic Findings. Cystic nodal inclusions are lined by squamous and apocrine epithelium (15–17). Discharge of keratin from squamous cysts can elicit a granulomatous reaction. Glandular inclusions may have the structure of breast lobules (figs. 560, 561) or ducts (15,16,19). Proliferative changes in the glandular inclusions have included papillary hyperplasia of apocrine epithelium (15), sclerosing papillary duct hyperplasia (20), and atypical papillary duct hyperplasia. One case report described papillary carcinoma that seemed to arise from a benign intranodal mammary glandular inclusion (21).

The distinction between heterotopic tissue and metastatic carcinoma is usually not difficult when the nodal inclusion resembles normal breast parenchyma or consists of cysts lined by histologically benign apocrine or squamous epithelium. In these processes there is typically a distinct basement membrane. Myoepithelial cells and specialized intralobular stroma are evident in heterotopic lobules within lymph nodes. When the intranodal lesion exhibits papillary proliferative changes, the distinction from metastatic orderly papillary carcinoma may depend upon finding structures that resemble normal breast glands coexisting with the proliferative foci.

NEVUS CELL AGGREGATES

Collections of cells that resemble cutaneous nevi can be found in the capsules of lymph nodes in various areas of the body including the axilla. Because of their association with the lymph node capsule rather than the lymphoid parenchyma, these groups of cells should be termed capsular nevus cell aggregates (NCA) rather than the often used nevus cell inclusion (31). The origin of this anatomic variation is unknown, but most of the available data support the conclusion that NCA arise in the lymph node capsule. Patients rarely have a notable contiguous cutaneous nevus. If NCA were "benign metastases" from clinically apparent or inconspicuous cutaneous nevi, it is improbable that such "metastases" would be localized to the nodal capsule since benign cellular elements transported via the lymphatics are deposited in nodal sinuses. NCA cells have some glomus properties and NCA retain glomoid structural features. The presence of melanin pigment, verified by electron microscopy, is also indicative of nevocellular differentiation. Electron microscopy has documented many similarities between the cells of NCA and cutaneous nevi but ultrastructural study has failed to detect the smooth muscle differentiation commonly seen in glomus cells (24,25). Consequently, it seems likely that NCA develop from melanocytic cells arrested in migration from the neural crest to the skin or from undifferentiated neurocristic cells that may be normally present in the capsules of superficial lymph nodes (24).

McCarthy et al. (29) reported that NCA were present in 6.2 percent of 129 axillary and in 4.0 percent of 50 inguinal lymph node dissections. Ridolfi et al. (31) reviewed 909 consecutive mastectomy specimens from patients with mammary carcinoma and found a single NCA in each

of 3 cases (0.33 percent) affecting 0.017 percent (3 of 17,504) of the lymph nodes examined. One hundred lymph node dissections from patients with malignant melanoma obtained from various sites were also reviewed. Three of 2,607 (0.12 percent) lymph nodes contained NCA.

NCA occur in association with superficial lymph node groups that drain the skin as well as other organs. Occurrence in visceral lymph nodes is extraordinarily unusual. Lymph node groups that contain NCA in decreasing order of frequency of involvement are the axilla, groin, and cervical regions. NCA have been found in lymph nodes from men, women, and children. Most patients had malignant neoplasms, but NCA have been found in lymph nodes from individuals with benign neoplasms and non-neoplastic conditions. They are more frequent in lymph nodes from patients with malignant melanoma than with mammary carcinoma. While some patients have a contiguous skin lesion such as malignant melanoma or a conspicuous nevus, the majority do not.

Clinical Presentation. NCA are microscopic structures that do not cause palpable enlargement of lymph nodes or any other clinical symptoms. Consequently, their presence is unsuspected until resected lymph nodes have been examined histologically.

Gross Findings. NCA are rarely visible or grossly palpable. Heavily pigmented NCA have been noted grossly on three occasions (fig. 562) (22,24,27). In one case the gross findings suggested anthracotic pigment (22). In each of these instances, the microscopic configuration of the NCA was that of a blue nevus.

Microscopic Findings. Two distinct microscopic patterns have been described: NCA that resemble intradermal nevi and NCA with the appearance of blue nevi. The former are much more frequent, with fewer than 10 percent of NCA having the blue nevus structure. There is no appreciable difference with respect to age distribution, associated diseases, or the frequency of multinodal involvement between the two types.

NCA of the intradermal nevus type have a band-like or nodular configuration in the lymph node capsule (fig. 563). In most cases, a single lymph node is affected but in rare instances NCA are found in two or more nodes from a lymph node group (23,26,30). In single plane of section

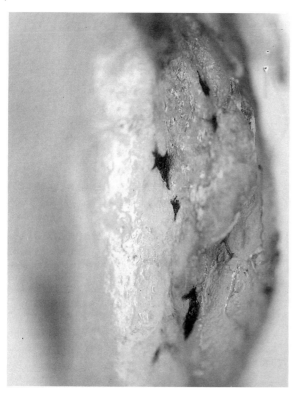

Figure 562
NODAL NEVUS AGGREGATE
Gross photograph of a lymph node showing black melanin pigment associated with a nodal blue nevus aggregate.
(Fig. 4A from Epstein JI, Erlandson RA, Rosen PP. Nodal
blue nevi: a study of three cases. Am J Surg Pathol
1984;8:907–15.) (Figures 562, 566, and 567 are from the
same patient.)

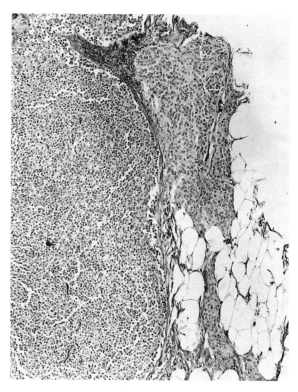

Figure 563
NODAL NEVUS AGGREGATE
Clusters of nevus cells form a nodule and slender strands
in fat outside the lymph node capsule.

they occupy a fraction of the perimeter of a lymph
node. They often have a discontinuous distribution and may be extended into the node itself
along fibrous trabeculae. NCA have not been
encountered in the peripheral sinuses.

The cells that form an NCA are cytologically
very similar to cells of an ordinary intradermal
nevus (fig. 564). They tend to be tightly clustered
into poorly defined masses separated by, or
sometimes seemingly centered about, thin
walled capillaries. The outer peripheral portion
is usually sharply defined while at the inner
margin NCA cells often merge with capsular
tissue. The cells are usually oval, have indistinct
borders, and polygonal cells are found in some
cases. The central nuclei have fine, diffuse chromatin and are surrounded by pale or clear cytoplasm. Nucleoli are small and indistinct or ab-

sent. Mitoses are not seen. Multinucleated cells
of the type found in intradermal nevi are not a
feature of NCA.

Fine brown pigment granules may be detected
in the cytoplasm of a few scattered cells in a
minority of NCA. This pigment gives a negative
Perls reaction for iron and is blackened with the
Fontana-Masson and Grimelius stains. NCA contain no mucin when studied with mucicarmine,
PAS, or Alcian blue stains. Immunohistochemical
studies have revealed strong reactivity for S-100
protein (fig. 565) and absence of staining for
cytokeratin or epithelial membrane antigen.

NCA of the blue nevus variety are poorly
defined, heavily pigmented lesions that occupy
the lymph node capsule and radiate into surrounding fat (22,24,27,28). The granular pigment is golden or dark brown. It fills and often
obscures the cytoplasm of many cells in the lesion, especially closely packed, elongated cells
with dendritic processes (figs. 566, 567). At the
outer, peripheral edges of the NCA these slender

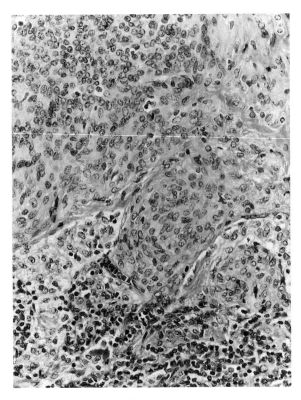

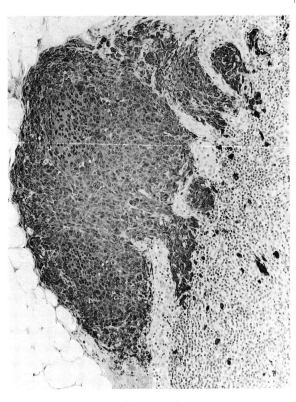

Figure 564
NODAL NEVUS AGGREGATE
Nevus cells with indistinct borders and small uniform nuclei outside the lymph node. Note peripheral sinusoid between nevus aggregate and lymphoid tissue. (Figures 564 and 565 are from the same patient.)

Figure 565
NODAL NEVUS AGGREGATE
Nevus cells are strongly immunoreactive for S-100 protein. Histiocytes within the lymph node are also reactive (avidin-biotin immunoperoxidase).

cells extend into the perinodal fat. The inner border is typically well defined and distinctly separated from the peripheral sinuses. Scattered singly and in small groups among the spindle cells are polygonal cells with pale cytoplasm that contains coarsely clumped pigment. These epithelioid NCA cells resemble pigmented histiocytes. Mitotic figures and multinucleated giant cells are absent.

Because the indication for a lymph node dissection is almost always a concomitant malignant neoplasm, it is important that NCA not be mistakenly interpreted as metastatic tumor. In patients with mammary carcinoma, nonpigmented NCA most closely resemble metastatic lobular carcinoma. Features that help to distinguish NCA from mammary carcinoma include the capsular location, the presence of brown pigment with the staining properties of melanin, absence of mucin, and immunohistochemical reactivity consistent with neuroepithelial rather than glandular histogenesis. The distinction between NCA and metastatic neoplasms rests largely on the characteristic shape and location, absence of mitoses, and bland cytology in NCA. Rarely, the same lymph node may contain a NCA and metastatic tumor (29,31).

Prognosis. NCA may be the source of some malignant melanomas detected in lymph nodes in the absence of a demonstrable cutaneous primary. There is no evidence that the presence of NCA in the lymph nodes of patients with an associated malignant neoplasm affects the prognosis of the neoplasm or that such individuals are predisposed to develop any particular type of neoplasm subsequently.

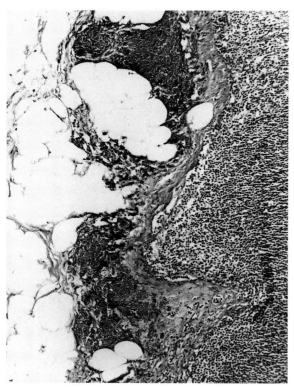

Figure 566

NODAL NEVUS AGGREGATE, BLUE NEVUS TYPE

An irregular border and cells heavily pigmented with melanin are characteristic of this lesion. (Fig. 3 from Epstein JI, Erlandson RA, Rosen PP. Nodal blue nevi: a study of three cases. Am J Surg Pathol 1984;8:907–15.)

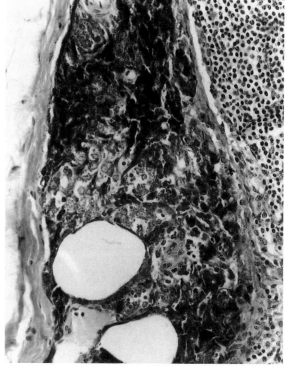

Figure 567

NODAL NEVUS AGGREGATE, BLUE NEVUS TYPE

In some cells melanin is so abundant that it obscures nuclei. (Fig. 1 from Epstein JI, Erlandson RA, Rosen PP. Nodal blue nevi: a study of three cases. Am J Surg Pathol 1984;8:907–15.)

VASCULAR LESIONS

Hemangiomas are microscopic lesions that may be found by chance in lymph nodes removed in the course of axillary dissections for various conditions. They occupy the nodal hilum or parenchyma and sometimes extend to perinodal tissues. Most are capillary hemangiomas but cavernous elements may also be present (figs. 568, 569). Nodal hemangiomas are occasionally encountered in multiple lymph nodes from one patient. Breast tissue removed at the same time or previously may contain one or more perilobular hemangiomas. This should not be interpreted as evidence of angiosarcoma. Clinically evident nodal enlargement caused by a hemangioma has been reported (32).

Kaposi sarcoma may arise primarily in lymph nodes, including those in the axilla (33,34). This phenomenon was described prior to the recogni-

tion of the association between Kaposi sarcoma and AIDS and probably constitutes an independent disease process. A microscopic Kaposi-like proliferative lesion is sometimes found incidentally in one or more lymph nodes removed in an axillary dissection. This reactive process is not known to be associated with the development of Kaposi sarcoma.

PIGMENT DEPOSITS

Several types of pigmented material have been detected in axillary lymph nodes (fig. 570). Histiocytes may contain black anthracotic pigment, which apparently accumulates as a result of retrograde flow from thoracic to axillary lymphatics. The pigment is usually not abundant and tends to be more prominent in apical rather than in low axillary lymph nodes. Prior surgical trauma, or an underlying systemic condition

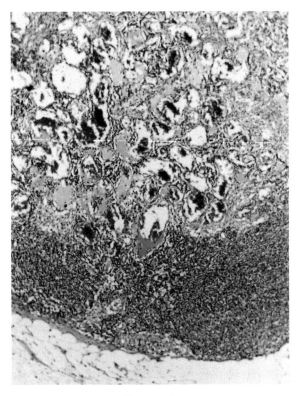

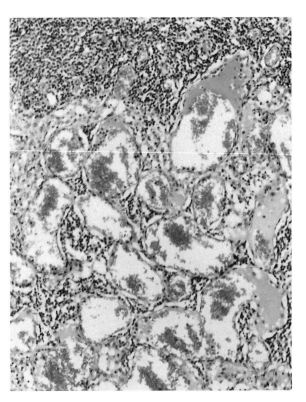

Figure 568
NODAL HEMANGIOMA
The central part of this lymph node has been replaced by a hemangioma.

Figure 569
NODAL HEMANGIOMA
Intranodal capillary hemangioma containing red blood cells.

Figure 570
TATTOO PIGMENT
Histiocytes filled with pigment stand out in the lymphoid tissue. When viewed through the microscope, the pigment granules were red, green, and black.

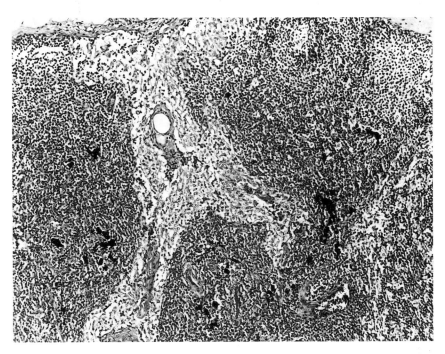

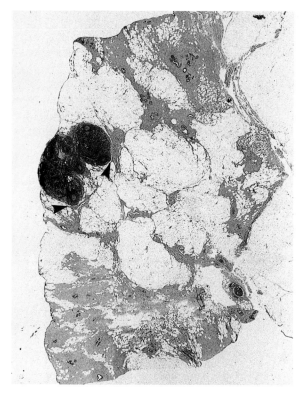

Figure 571
INTRAMAMMARY LYMPH NODE
Low magnification of the upper outer quadrant showing a bean-shaped lymph node with a hilar notch. Specimen is from a mastectomy that contained invasive mammary carcinoma extending up to but not through the lymph node capsule (arrows).

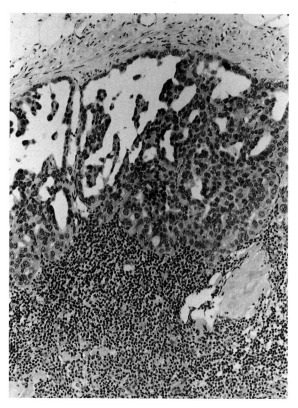

Figure 572
METASTATIC CARCINOMA
IN INTRAMAMMARY LYMPH NODE
Metastatic papillary ovarian adenocarcinoma in a lymph node that became palpable in the lower outer quadrant when the patient developed intra-abdominal recurrence of her primary neoplasm.

such as hemosiderosis, can cause accumulation of iron pigment. Dermatopathic lymphadenitis features melanin transported from inflammatory skin lesions. Patients who received systemic gold therapy for rheumatoid arthritis have reportedly developed gold deposits in lymph nodes that were visualized by mammography (35,36). In one case, the particles in the breast were thought radiologically to be microcalcifications that suggested carcinoma (36), but at surgery the gold deposits were found within an intraparenchymal lymph node.

METASTATIC CARCINOMA IN INTRAMAMMARY LYMPH NODES

Intramammary lymph nodes are most often located deep in the outer quadrants of the breast (fig. 571) (38). Mammographic examination usually reveals a well-circumscribed mass that may have a lucent center and a peripheral "hilar" notch (42). Enlargement of intramammary lymph nodes may be caused by inflammatory conditions such as sinus histiocytosis (37), reaction to dermatitis (39), or by neoplasms including lymphoma (43), metastatic melanoma (37), and metastatic carcinoma (fig. 572) (37,40,41). The distinction between medullary carcinoma and metastatic carcinoma in an intramammary lymph node is sometimes difficult. The underlying architecture of a lymph node is usually revealed by a reticulin stain while the presence of intraductal carcinoma, a prominent plasmacytic reaction, syncytial growth, and necrosis characterize medullary carcinoma.

McSweeney and Egan (41) found intramammary lymph nodes in 52 of 173 (30 percent) breasts examined by whole organ serial sectioning, specimen radiography, and pathologic examination (38).

A lymph node was classified as intramammary only if "completely surrounded by breast tissue." The size of the nodes ranged from 3 to 15 mm. A total of 72 lymph nodes were found in the 52 breasts with 9 the largest number in a single case. The distribution of lymph nodes in the breast quadrants was as follows: upper outer, 26 (36 percent); lower outer, 21 (29 percent); upper inner, 11 (15 percent); central, 8 (11 percent); lower inner, 6 (8 percent). Seven breasts with carcinoma had one or more lymph nodes in the same quadrant as the primary tumor and 8 had nodes in other quadrants.

Metastatic carcinoma was found in an intramammary lymph node in 15 breasts with carcinoma. Lymph nodes that contained metastatic carcinoma measured 3 to 10 mm. Only 2 of 6 (33 percent) stage I patients with negative axillary lymph nodes and a positive intramammary lymph node survived 10 years. All carcinomas associated with intramammary lymph node metastases were invasive ductal type, including 2 with mucinous differentiation and 2 with associated Paget disease.

REFERENCES

Sinus Histiocytosis

1. Berg JW. Sinus histiocytosis: a fallacious measure of host resistance to cancer. Cancer 1956;9:935–9.
2. Black MM, Leis HP Jr. Cellular responses to autologous breast cancer tissue. Correlation with stage and lymphoreticuloendothelial reaction. Cancer 1971;28:263–73.
3. _____, Asire AJ. Palpable axillary lymph nodes in cancer of the breast. Structural and biologic considerations. Cancer 1969;23:251–9.
4. _____, Speer FD. Sinus histiocytosis of lymph nodes in cancer. Surg Gynecol Obstet 1958;106:163–75.
5. _____, Opler SR, Speer FD. Survival in breast cancer cases in relation to the structure of primary tumor and regional lymph nodes. Surg Gynecol Obstet 1955;100:543–51.
6. Cutler SJ, Black MM, Mork T, Harvei S, Freeman C. Further observations on prognostic factors in cancer of the female breast. Cancer 1969;24:653–67.
7. _____, Black MM, Friedell GH, Vidone RA, Goldenberg IS. Prognostic factors in cancer of the female. Reproducibility of histopathologic classification. Cancer 1966;19:75–82.
8. _____, Black MM, Goldenberg IS. Prognostic factors in cancer of the female breast. I. An investigation of some interrelations. Cancer 1963;16:1589–97.
9. DiRe JJ, Lane N. The relation of sinus histiocytosis in axillary lymph nodes to surgical curability of carcinoma of the breast. Am J Clin Pathol 1963;40:508–15.
10. Friedell GH, Soto EA, Kumaoka S, Abe O, Hayward JL, Bulbrook RD. Sinus histiocytosis in British and Japanese patients with breast cancer. Lancet 1974;2:1228–9.
11. Kister SJ, Sommers SC, Haagensen CD, Friedell GH, Cooley E, Varma A. Nuclear grade and sinus histiocytosis in cancer of the breast. Cancer 1969;23:570–5.
12. Moore RD, Chapnick R, Schoenberg MD. Lymph nodes associated with carcinoma of the breast. Cancer 1960;13:545–9.
13. Schiodt T. Breast carcinoma. A histological and prognostic study of 650 followed-up cases. Dan Med Bull 1967;14:239–43.
14. Silverberg SG, Chitale AR, Hind AD, Frazier AB, Levitt SH. Sinus histiocytosis and mammary carcinoma. Study of 366 radical mastectomies and an historical review. Cancer 1970;26:1177–85.

Heterotopic Glands

15. Edlow DW, Carter D. Heterotopic epithelium in axillary lymph nodes: report of a case and review of the literature. Am J Clin Pathol 1973;59:666–73.
16. Garret R, Ada AE. Epithelial inclusion cysts in an axillary lymph node. Report of a case simulating metastatic adenocarcinoma. Cancer 1957;10:173–8.
17. Haagensen CD. Heterotopic apocrine cysts in axillary lymph nodes. In: Diseases of the breast. 2nd ed. Philadelphia: WB Saunders Co, 1971:491.
18. Holdsworth PJ, Hopkinson JM, Leveson SH. Benign axillary epithelial lymph node inclusions—a histological pitfall. Histopathology 1988;13:226–8.
19. McDivitt RW, Stewart FW, Berg JW. Tumors of the breast. Atlas of Tumor Pathology, 2nd Series, Fascicle 2. Washington, D.C.: Armed Forces Institute of Pathology, 1969,116.
20. Turner DR, Millis RR. Breast tissue inclusions in axillary lymph nodes. Histopathology 1980;4:631–6.
21. Walker AN, Fechner RE. Papillary carcinoma arising from ectopic breast tissue in an axillary lymph node. Diagn Gynecol Obstet 1982;4:141–5.

Nevus Cell Aggregates

22. Azzopardi JG, Ross CM, Frizzera G. Blue nevi of lymph node capsule. Histopathology 1977;1:451–61.
23. Bertrand G, Rabreau M, George P. Presence de cellules naeviques dans les ganglions lymphatiques. Arch Anat Cytol Pathol 1980;28:58–62.
24. Epstein JI, Erlandson RA, Rosen PP. Nodal blue nevi. A study of three cases. Am J Surg Pathol 1984;8:907–15.
25. Erlandson RA, Rosen PP. Electron microscopy of a nevus cell aggregate associated with an axillary lymph node. Cancer 1982;49:269–72.
26. Goldman RL. Blue nevus of lymph node capsule: report of a unique case. Histopathology 1981;5:445–50.
27. Gray GF Jr, Dineen P. Benign nevus in lymph node. NY State J Med 1976;76:754–5.
28. Lamovec J. Blue nevus of the lymph node capsule. Report of a new case with review of the literature. Am J Clin Pathol 1984;81:367–72.
29. McCarthy SW, Palmer AA, Bale PM, Hirst E. Nevus cells in lymph nodes. Pathology 1974;6:351–8.
30. Micheau C, Contesso G. Formations d'aspect angioglomique dans les ganglions lymphatiques axillaires. Arch Anat Pathol 1971;19:167–75.
31. Ridolfi RL, Rosen PP, Thaler H. Nevus cell aggregates associated with lymph nodes: estimated frequency and clinical significance. Cancer 1977;39:164–71.

Vascular Lesions

32. Kasznica J, Sideli RV, Collins MH. Lymph node hemangioma. Arch Pathol Lab Med 1989;113:804–7.
33. Lubin J, Rywlin AM. Lymphoma-like lymph node changes in Kaposi's sarcoma. Arch Pathol 1971;92:338–41.
34. Ramos CV, Taylor HB, Hernandez BA, Tucker EF. Primary Kaposi's sarcoma of lymph nodes. Am J Clin Pathol 1976;66:998–1003.

Pigment Deposits

35. Bruwer A, Nelson, GW, Spark RP. Punctate intranodal gold deposits simulating microcalcifications on mammograms. Radiology 1987;163:87–8.
36. Carter TR. Intramammary lymph node gold deposits simulating microcalcifications on mammogram. Hum Pathol 1988;19:992–4.

Metastatic Carcinoma in Intramammary Lymph Nodes

37. Hyman LJ, Abellera RM. Carcinomatous lymph nodes within breast parenchyma. Arch Surg 1974;109:759–61.
38. Kalisher L. Xeroradiography of axillary lymph node disease. Radiology 1975;115:67–71.
39. Kopans DB, Meyer JE, Murphy GF. Benign lymph nodes associated with dermatitis presenting as breast masses. Radiology 1980;137(Pt 1):15–19.
40. Lindfors KK, Kopans DB, Googe PB, McCarthy KA, Koerner FC, Meyer JE. Breast cancer metastasis to intramammary lymph nodes. AJR Am J Roentgenol 1986;146:133–6.
41. McSweeney MB, Egan RL. Prognosis of breast cancer related to intramammary lymph nodes. Recent Results Cancer Res 1984;90:166–72.
42. Meyer JE, Kopans DB, Long JC. Mammographic appearance of malignant lymphoma of the breast. Radiology 1980;135:623–6.
43. Meyer JE, Kopans DB, Lawrence WD. Normal intramammary lymph nodes presenting as occult breast masses. Breast 1982;40:30–2.

CYTOLOGY IN THE DIAGNOSIS OF BREAST LESIONS

CYSTIC TUMORS

In most instances, aspiration of cyst contents is a therapeutic as well as diagnostic procedure (1,3). The cyst collapses and the epithelium, stripped from the supporting stroma, is removed in the aspirate. The cyst is effaced by the adherent exposed surfaces of stroma.

Cytologic examination of cyst fluid is essential when the aspirate is bloody or serosanguinous. The presence of a residual mass immediately after aspiration requires cytologic examination. Reaccumulation of fluid in a cyst is an indication for cytologic study of the second aspirate. Regardless of the cytologic findings, excisional biopsy is usually recommended after aspirates that yield bloody fluid or are associated with a mass (fig. 573) (2). Consideration should be given to other factors that indicate the patient is at increased risk to develop breast carcinoma, such as a family history of the disease, a previous biopsy that demonstrated significant atypia, or carcinoma of the contralateral breast.

The frequency of carcinoma among cystic lesions from which material was submitted for cytologic examination in three recent studies was 2 percent in 1,714 specimens (Table 8). The majority of the carcinomas were associated with bloody fluid or a mass.

Many specimens are nearly acellular, especially if no effort has been made to concentrate the material by centrifugation or filtration. Benign epithelial cells singly or in small groups, histiocytes ("foam cells"), lymphocytes, and epithelial cells exhibiting apocrine features are found in varying proportions. Clustered cells generally indicate papillary proliferation of the epithelium lining the cyst, an especially frequent finding when there is apocrine metaplasia. Standard cytologic criteria are applied to the diagnosis of cells obtained in a cyst aspirate.

NIPPLE SECRETION

Secretions expressed or aspirated from the major lactiferous ducts and spontaneous nipple discharge may be used for diagnosis (5,6). The ability to obtain secretions is influenced by patient age, secretor status, and race (6). Almost 40 percent of nipple secretion specimens are virtually devoid of epithelial cells (4,6). It is more

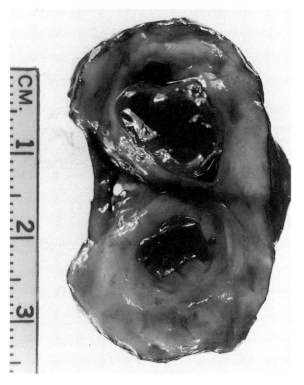

Figure 573
ASPIRATED CYST
This cyst, excised after aspiration, yielded bloody fluid contained blood clot and fragments of papilloma.

Table 8

ASPIRATION DIAGNOSIS OF CARCINOMA IN CYSTIC LESIONS

Author (reference)	Cystic Lesions	Carcinoma Lesions	Carcinoma Percent
Kline et al. (16)	354	8	2%
Strawbridge et al. (34)	834	10	1%
Bell et al. (10)	526	14	3%
Total	1714	32	2%

Table 9

CORRELATION OF ASPIRATION CYTOLOGY DIAGNOSIS WITH BREAST CARCINOMA*

	Aspiration Diagnosis				
	Carcinoma	**Atypia**			
		Marked	**Moderate**	**Mild**	**None**
No. patients (Total: 986)	76	16	41	46	807
No. carcinoma (Total: 109)	76	14	10	4	5
Percent carcinoma	100	88	24	9	0.6

*Based on Rimsten et al. (29).

likely that carcinoma is present if the nipple secretion is bloody. Among 410 women evaluated in one series for bloody or serous nipple discharge in the absence of a palpable lesion, cancer was ultimately diagnosed in 50 (12.2 percent) (7).

SOLID TUMORS

The primary role of aspiration cytology of solid tumors is to provide a prompt diagnosis of a palpable breast mass. The frequency with which carcinoma has been diagnosed in various series depends on the selection of patients as well as the skill of personnel who perform and interpret the aspiration. The percentage of true positive diagnoses (proportion of histologically proven carcinomas detected cytologically) ranges from 69 to 96 percent in some of the larger published series (Table 9) (10,16,29,31,34,36). Attempts to aspirate palpable tumors smaller than 2 cm, those located deep in large breasts, clinically indistinct lesions, and nonpalpable abnormalities detected by mammography are more likely to result in false negative diagnoses (18,19). The yield from nonpalpable lesions has been improved by using X-ray guided (20,21) or stereotaxic (9,11) procedures for more precise placement of the aspiration needle in the lesion.

Needle aspiration cytology cannot be employed out of clinical context. The procedure should be regarded as part of a "triple test" (15,19) including mammographic and physical examination of the breast. Definitive treatment has been recommended on the basis of a positive fine-needle aspiration diagnosis if supported by clinical studies (14) but this is a controversial issue and others urge that a positive needle aspiration diagnosis be confirmed by a tissue biopsy. A surgical biopsy should be performed despite a nondiagnostic cytology report whenever clinical or mammographic features of the lesion indicate a significant abnormality. Carcinoma is much more likely to be present in the aspirate from a tumor regarded clinically to be carcinoma, but Bell et al. (10) reported that surgical biopsies revealed carcinoma in 36 percent of clinically "suspicious" aspirated lesions, in 20 percent regarded as clinically significant, and in 3 percent from lesions diagnosed clinically as benign (Table 10).

False positive diagnoses have been infrequent in larger series, ranging from 0 to 3 percent (16,17,36). The frequency of error does not differ from experience with frozen sections in general or with frozen sections of breast tumors in particular (8,25,30). It is essential that a high threshold be maintained based on stringent diagnostic criteria to minimize such errors. Diagnostic material should be abundant and present on at least two separate slides. Technically poor preparations, particularly those with drying artefacts, should be interpreted with extreme caution.

It is possible to identify some specific histologic types of carcinoma in an aspiration biopsy (31). The aspirate from infiltrating lobular carcinoma is composed of small isolated cells with

Table 10

CORRELATION OF CLINICAL DIAGNOSIS WITH FINDINGS ON
BIOPSY AND ASPIRATION CYTOLOGY*

Clinical Diagnosis	Patients Biopsied No.	Carcinoma on Biopsy No.	(%)	Carcinoma on Aspiration No.	(% Total)	(% Carcinoma)
Benign	174	21	(12)	6	(3)	(29)
Significant	142	41	(29)	28	(20)	(67)
Suspicious	73	36	(49)	26	(36)	(70)
Carcinoma	104	102	(98)	82	(79)	(81)

*Based on Bell et al. (10).

sparse cytoplasm sometimes arranged in a characteristic linear fashion (14,28). Abundant extracellular mucin characterizes the aspirate from mucinous carcinoma while a specimen from medullary carcinoma typically has poorly differentiated tumor cells scattered among numerous lymphocytes and plasma cells. Benign lesions can mimic patterns associated with various tumor types and it is therefore essential to establish the presence of carcinoma cells before attempting to classify the lesion.

In addition to routine cytologic examination, needle aspiration specimens can be employed to study tumor cells for hormone receptors (22) and other tumor markers (26).

Needle biopsy of solid tumors is an alternative to needle aspiration cytology. This procedure has become especially attractive with the availability of the disposable biopsy needles which obviate the need for the cumbersome drill biopsy. The specimen consists of cylindrical fragments or cores of tissue which can be used to make frozen as well as paraffin sections (33). Needle core biopsies provide reliable samples for hormone receptor analyses (13). Although it is theoretically possible that tumor cells are disseminated when a needle biopsy is performed, no difference in short-term, disease-free survival was demonstrable between patients diagnosed by excisional and needle biopsy (13).

The reported range of true positive diagnoses of carcinoma obtained by needle biopsy (67 to 89 percent) was slightly lower than had been reported with the drill biopsy (75 to 99 percent) or aspiration cytology (12,23,24,32,33). Two studies demonstrated a higher frequency of true positive diagnoses with needle biopsy than with aspiration cytology (12,27); only 119 and 60 patients respectively, were involved, and remarkably poor positive rates of 52 percent and 42 percent were found.

False positive diagnoses have not been described in the published reports on needle biopsy diagnosis, but there is a significant potential for this to occur with needle biopsies of sclerosing adenosis and sclerosing ductal proliferations (radial sclerosing lesion). Mingling of proliferating epithelium and stroma in these tumors often simulates the appearance of invasive carcinoma in histologic sections. The hazard is especially great when dealing with frozen section material in which cytologic detail is of necessity less than in paraffin sections (33).

The traumatic effect of fine-needle aspiration and needle core biopsy on breast tissue can complicate the tissue diagnosis in a subsequent surgical biopsy (figs. 574, 575). Microcalcifications may be removed in the needle biopsy and therefore may no longer be detectable in an excisional biopsy. Hemorrhage and inflammatory changes may obscure lesions. Epithelial cells dispersed in the biopsy site or into surrounding tissue can simulate invasive carcinoma, a particularly difficult diagnostic problem when the biopsy contains intraductal carcinoma (figs. 576–578) (35).

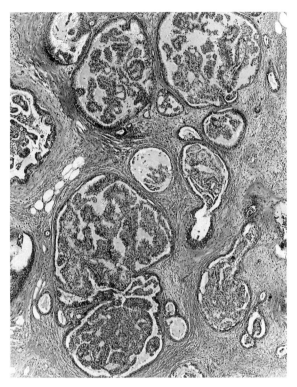

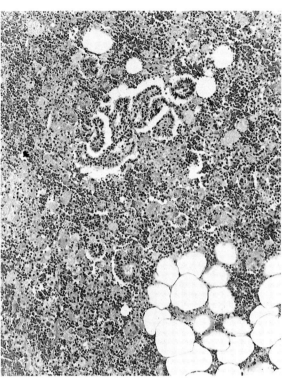

Figure 574
ASPIRATED PAPILLARY CARCINOMA
Papillary intraductal carcinoma in a biopsy specimen obtained after a needle biopsy was interpreted as carcinoma. (Figures 574 and 575 are from the same patient.)

Figure 575
ASPIRATED PAPILLARY CARCINOMA
Clusters of papillary carcinoma cells in an inflammatory reaction at the site of needle biopsy in the specimen in figure 574. This epithelium was displaced by the procedure and constitutes artefactual "invasion."

Figure 576
ASPIRATED INTRADUCTAL
CARCINOMA
Part of a duct with micropapillary intraductal carcinoma in a breast previously subjected to fine-needle aspiration biopsy. No invasion was seen in the surgical biopsy. (Figures 576–578 are from the same patient.)

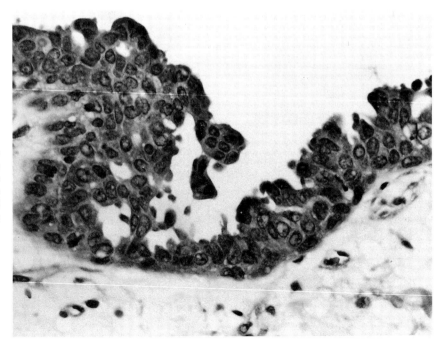

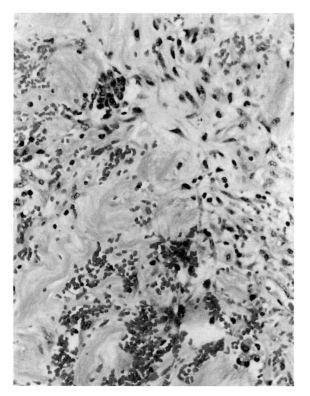

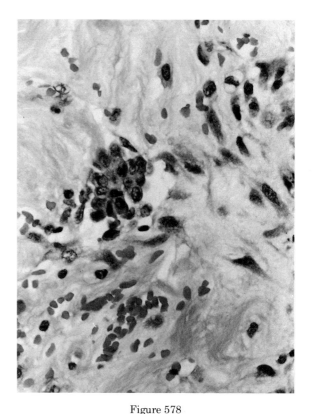

Figure 577
ASPIRATED INTRADUCTAL CARCINOMA
Region of the needle track in the biopsy specimen in figure 576 showing hemorrhage and displaced cluster of neoplastic epithelial cells.

Figure 578
ASPIRATED INTRADUCTAL CARCINOMA
Cluster of neoplastic epithelial cells from figure 577 at high magnification in a vascular space. The cells closely resemble those in the intraductal carcinoma (figure 576).

REFERENCES

Cystic Tumors

1. Abramson DJ. A clinical evaluation of aspiration of cysts of the breast. Surg Gynecol Obstet 1974;139:531–7.
2. Hamed H, Coady A, Chaudary MA, Fentiman IS. Follow-up of patients with aspirated breast cysts is necessary. Arch Surg 1989;124:253–5.
3. Rosemond GP. Differentiation between the cystic and solid breast mass by needle aspiration. Surg Clin North Am 1963;43:1433–7.

Nipple Secretion

4. Buehring GC. Screening for breast atypias using exfoliative cytology. Cancer 1979;43:1788–99.
5. Knight DC, Lowell DM, Heimann A, Dunn E. Aspiration of the breast and nipple discharge cytology. Surg Gynecol Obstet 1986;163:415–20.
6. Petrakis NL, Ernster VL, Sacks ST, et al. Epidemiology of breast fluid secretion: association with breast cancer risk factors and cerumen type. JNCI 1981;67:277–84.
7. Takeda T, Matsui A, Sato Y, et al. Nipple discharge cytology in mass screening for breast cancer. Acta Cytol 1990;34:161–4.

Solid Tumors

8. Ackerman LV, Ramirez GA. The indications for and limitations of frozen section diagnosis. A review of 1269 consecutive frozen section diagnoses. Br J Surg 1959;46:336–50.
9. Azavedo E, Svane G, Auer G. Stereotactic fine-needle biopsy in 2594 mammographically detected non-palpable lesions. Lancet 1989;1:1033–6.

10. Bell DA, Hajdu SI, Urban JA, Gaston JP. Role of aspiration cytology in the diagnosis and management of mammary lesions in office practice. Cancer 1983;51:1182–9.

11. Dowlatshahi K, Jokich PM, Schmidt R, Bibbo M, Dawson PJ. Cytologic diagnosis of occult breast lesions using stereotaxic needle aspiration. A preliminary report. Arch Surg 1987;122:1343–6.

12. Elston CW, Cotton RE, Davies CJ, Blamey RW. A comparison of the use of the "Tru-Cut" needle and fine needle aspiration cytology in the pre-operative diagnosis of carcinoma of the breast. Histopathology 1978;2:239–54.

13. Fentiman IS, Millis RR, Chaudary MA, King RJ, Miller KJ, Hayward JL. Effect of the method of biopsy on the prognosis of and reliability of receptor assays in patients with operable breast cancer. Br J Surg 1986;73:610–2.

14. Fessia L, Botta G, Arisio R, Verga M, Aimone V. Fine-needle aspiration of breast lesions: role and accuracy in a review of 7,495 cases. Diagn Cytopathol 1987;3:121–5.

15. Hermansen C, Skovgaard Poulsen H, Jensen J, et al. Diagnostic reliability of combined physical examination, mammography, and fine-needle puncture ("triple-test") in breast tumors. A prospective study. Cancer 1987; 60:1866–71.

16. Kline TS, Joshi LP, Neal HS. Fine-needle aspiration of the breast: diagnosis and pitfalls. A review of 3545 cases. Cancer 1979;44:1458–64.

17. Koivuniemi AP. Fine needle aspiration biopsy of the breast. Ann Clin Res 1976;8:272–83.

18. Kreuzer G, Zajicek J. Cytologic diagnosis of mammary tumors from aspiration biopsy smears. III. Studies on 200 carcinomas with false negative or doubtful cytologic reports. Acta Cytol 1972;16:249–52.

19. Lamb J, Anderson TJ, Dixon MJ, Levack PA. Role of fine needle aspiration cytology in breast cancer screening. J Clin Pathol 1987;40:705–9.

20. Löfgren M, Andersson I, Bondeson L, Lindholm K. X-ray guided fine-needle aspiration for the cytologic diagnosis of nonpalpable breast lesions. Cancer 1988; 61:1032–7.

21. Masood S, Frykberg ER, McLellan GL, Scalapino MC, Mitchum DG, Bullard JB. Prospective evaluation of radiologically directed fine-needle aspiration biopsy of nonpalpable breast lesions. Cancer 1990;66:1480–7.

22. McClelland RA, Berger U, Wilson P, et al. Presurgical determination of estrogen receptor status using immunocytochemically stained fine needle aspirate smears in patients with breast cancer. Cancer Res. 1987; 47:6118–22.

23. Millis RR. Needle biopsy of the breast. In: McDivitt RW, Oberman HA, Ozzello L, Kaufman N, eds. The breast. Baltimore: Williams and Wilkins, 1984:186–203.

24. Minkowitz S, Moskowitz R, Khafif RA, Alderete MN. TRU-CUT needle biopsy of the breast. An analysis of its specificity and sensitivity. Cancer 1986;57:320–3.

25. Nakazawa H, Rosen P, Lane N, Lattes R. Frozen section experience in 3000 cases. Accuracy, limitations, and value in residency training. Am J Clin Pathol 1968; 49:41–51.

26. Nuti M, Mottolese M, Viora M, Donnorso RP, Schlom J, Natali PG. Use of monoclonal antibodies to human breast-tumor-associated antigens in fine-needle aspirate cytology. Int J Cancer 1986;37:493–8.

27. Owen AW, Anderson TJ, Forrest AP. "Closed" biopsy for breast cancer. JR Coll Surg Edinb 1980;25:237–41.

28. Patel J, Gartell PC, Smallwood JA, et al. Fine needle aspiration cytology of breast masses: an evaluation of its accuracy and reasons for diagnostic failure. Ann R Coll Surg Eng 1987;69:156–9.

29. Rimsten A, Stenkvist B, Johanson H, Lindgren A. The diagnostic accuracy of palpation and fine-needle biopsy and evaluation of their combined use in the diagnosis of breast lesions: report of a prospective study in 1,244 women with symptoms. Ann Surg 1975;182:1–8.

30. Rosen PP. Frozen section diagnosis of breast lesions. Recent experience with 556 consecutive biopsies. Ann Surg 1978;187:17–9.

31. Rosen P, Hajdu SI, Robbins G, Foote FW Jr. Diagnosis of carcinoma of the breast by aspiration biopsy. Surg Gynecol Obstet 1972;134:837–8.

32. Shabot MM, Goldberg IM, Schick P, Nieberg R, Pilch YH. Aspiration cytology is superior to "Tru-Cut" needle biopsy in establishing the diagnosis of clinically suspicious breast masses. Ann Surg 1982;196:122–6.

33. Smeets HJ, Saltzstein SL, Meurer WT, Pilch YH. Needle biopsies in breast cancer diagnosis: techniques in search of an audience. J Surg Oncol 1986;32:11–5.

34. Strawbridge HT, Bassett AA, Foldes I. Role of cytology in management of lesions of the breast. Surg Gynecol Obstet 1981;152:1–7.

35. Tabbara SO, Frierson HF Jr, Fechner RE. Diagnostic problems in tissues previously sampled by fine-needle aspiration. Am J Clin Pathol 1991;96:76–80.

36. Zajdela A, Ghossein NA, Pilleron JP, Ennuyer A. The value of aspiration cytology in the diagnosis of breast cancer: experience at the Fondation Curie. Cancer 1975;35:499–506.

❖❖❖

PATHOLOGIC EXAMINATION OF BREAST SPECIMENS

This section describes clinically important factors relating to the pathologic examination of breast specimens. It is not intended to be a complete presentation. Additional information may be found in recent comprehensive reviews (1,2,3).

THE BIOPSY

Needle or Incisional Biopsy Specimens

Needle or incisional biopsy specimens are processed for histologic examination in their entirety. A cautery type scalpel must not be used in obtaining an incisional biopsy. Limited information about the characteristics of a lesion is obtained from such small specimens. The samples are suitable for frozen section and immunohistochemical receptor analysis.

Excisional Biopsy Specimens

Gross Examination of Excisional Biopsy. The size of an excisional biopsy specimen should be recorded in centimeters in three dimensions and the general shape (e.g. ovoid, spherical) described. Because the overall dimensions of an excisional biopsy cannot be determined after the tissue has been sliced open and dissected by the operator, the specimen should be intact when delivered to the laboratory. It is also useful to record specimen weight in grams.

The intact specimen should be delivered unfixed to the pathology laboratory as soon as possible in order to perform a frozen section or to obtain material for receptor analysis, electron microscopy, or other studies. If a delay is anticipated, the tissue may be chilled but freezing the entire specimen will compromise histologic examination. Even when a frozen section is not requested, the tissue should be dissected promptly by a pathologist to determine whether any grossly identifiable tumor is present. If it is found, the largest diameter should be recorded in centimeters. This measurement is made before tissue is removed for frozen section or for other studies such as hormone receptor analysis. The gross character of the tumor (shape, consistency, appearance of cut surface) should be described. Whether or not a distinct lesion is found, the appearance of the breast parenchyma is noted (consistency, relative proportions of fat and fibrous tissue, cysts, or other lesions).

In some laboratories where frozen sections are not routinely performed, it is customary to freeze and store a portion of any lesion suspected to be carcinoma until paraffin sections have been prepared. When the lesion proves to be carcinoma, the frozen sample may be submitted for hormone receptor analysis. If the diagnosis is uncertain, the frozen sample may be processed for histologic examination but the thawed tissue is often somewhat distorted and these specimens may not help resolve a diagnostic problem.

The number of samples taken from an excisional biopsy for histologic examination varies greatly with the clinical circumstances, gross appearance of the tissue, and results of frozen section if performed. The tissue used for frozen section must be saved, processed into a paraffin section, and identified by a term such as the "frozen section control." If a sample is removed for hormone receptor analysis, a corresponding specimen should be examined histologically as a "receptor control." Distinct tumors that appear grossly to be carcinomas 2 cm or less in diameter are generally entirely submitted for histology. Sections taken to demonstrate the margin of the tumor and surrounding breast are examined microscopically for evidence of lymphatic emboli and in situ carcinoma outside the lesion.

To establish criteria for sampling grossly negative breast tissue, Schnitt and Wang (19) carried out a retrospective study of 384 biopsies performed for clinically palpable lesions in which no distinct tumor was evident on gross pathologic examination. The paraffin-embedded samples were labeled sequentially. Carcinoma was found in 23 (6 percent) specimens and atypical hyperplasia in 3 others (0.8 percent). By submitting up to 10 blocks per case consisting only of fibrous parenchyma, it was possible to detect 25 of the 26 significant lesions. Only a single microscopic focus of lobular carcinoma in situ was overlooked by this selection. Thus, the authors recommended submitting up to ten samples of fibrous parenchyma or, if the specimen is entirely fat, a similar number of samples. If carcinoma or atypical hyperplasia is found in the first set of slides, the remaining tissue may be processed.

Owings, Hann, and Schnitt (14) have also investigated the problem of tissue sampling from needle localization breast biopsies. They examined 157 consecutive specimens, 32 percent of which proved to contain carcinoma. All specimens were entirely submitted for histologic examination. Forty-nine of 50 carcinomas (98 percent) and 14 of 19 atypical hyperplasias (74 percent) were directly related to the foci of calcification and would have been found had histologic sampling been limited to these foci. All carcinomas and 17 of 19 (89 percent) atypical hyperplasias were detected by samples consisting of the regions of calcification and all fibrous parenchyma. Samples of the margins of excision should be taken at the time of initial tissue examination. These samples may of necessity consist of fatty, nonfibrous breast tissue.

The pathology report must include a listing of the tissue samples taken from each specimen for microscopic examination, indicating the number of tissue blocks and providing a key to explain abbreviations used to designate individual samples. All samples taken from a specimen should be identified with a number and each should be further labeled with a letter or other specific designation. For example, a right breast biopsy would be recorded as specimen "#1" and the samples for paraffin blocks designated as #1A, #1B, etc. A second biopsy of the right breast would be listed as #2 with samples designated #2A, #2B, etc. Specific designations such as "#1LM," which might indicate "lateral margin," should be recorded in the listing of samples.

Assessing Margins of Excision. To accurately assess the margins of an excision that contains carcinoma, it is necessary to mark the surfaces so that they can be identified microscopically (7). This is most easily accomplished with reagents such as India ink or tattoo dyes that remain adherent to the tissue throughout processing and are visible through the microscope. These pigments adhere better to fresh tissue that has been blotted free of surface blood and moisture than to formalin-fixed tissue. An excisional biopsy that has been sliced up by the operator cannot be reliably reassembled in order to "ink" the margins.

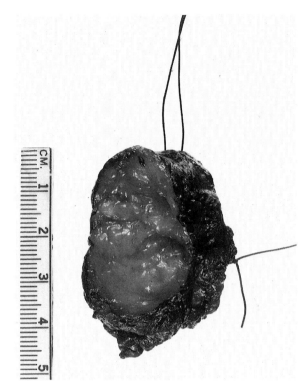

Figure 579
ASSESSING MARGINS

India ink has been applied to the external surface of an excisional biopsy specimen. Lateral and superior margins are indicated by the long and short sutures, respectively. The inked specimen has been bisected. No tumor was evident grossly. The operation was performed for calcifications detected by mammography and intraductal carcinoma was found microscopically.

The inked specimen can be bisected in a plane that will divide a palpable tumor if present (fig. 579). It is possible to remove portions immediately for frozen section or receptor analysis. The gross impression of the relationship of an evident tumor to the margins should be noted. Frozen sections of margins are not indicated unless this information will have an immediate impact on treatment.

It is not possible to orient an excisional biopsy specimen without guidance from the surgeon. This can be easily accomplished if the operator places a short suture at the superior margin and a long stitch laterally. At least two sections should be taken perpendicular to each of the six inked surfaces (superior, inferior, medial, lateral, superficial, and deep) with additional samples of margins determined by the gross findings.

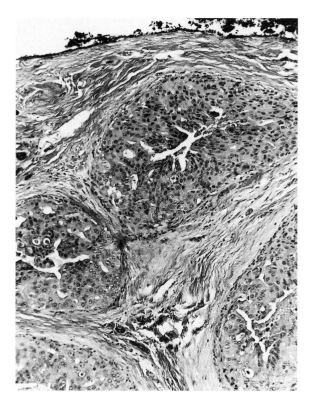

Figure 580
ASSESSING MARGINS
Intraductal carcinoma close to the inked margin.

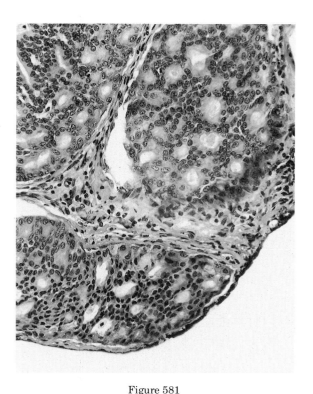

Figure 581
ASSESSING MARGINS
An unusual situation in which the ink is separated from intraductal carcinoma only by the basement membrane. The tumor was not actually transected and this was regarded as a "close" margin.

There is no standardized system for reporting the microscopic appearance of margins. A tumor transected at an inked surface represents a clearly "positive" margin (figs. 580–583). This applies equally to in situ and invasive carcinoma but the type of tumor must be specified. When the tumor is close to the margin but not transected, it is a useful convention to regard foci within one high-power microscopic field as "close to the margin" (7).

Specimen Radiography. With the increasingly widespread use of mammography, considerable interest has developed in specimen radiography of lesions that contain calcifications. Clinical mammographic findings that do not lend themselves to specimen radiography are alterations in parenchymal pattern, skin changes, vascular abnormalities, and ill-defined mass lesions (17,20). Specimen compression devices have proven useful for localizing noncalcified lesions in specimen radiographs. Specimen radiography provides a method for proving that the lesion has been removed and it is an efficient technique for pinpointing the area for histologic examination (4,9). Carcinoma has been found in approximately 25 percent of nonpalpable lesions biopsied because the mammogram revealed calcifications that suggested carcinoma (12,17,20).

In order to effectively evaluate a breast specimen radiograph, it is mandatory to have the clinical mammogram simultaneously available (figs. 584, 585). An X ray should be made of the intact excisional biopsy and the film should be compared with the mammogram before the specimen is moved or dissected. If the tissue was dissected prior to obtaining a specimen X ray, a fortuitous cut may disrupt the pattern of calcifications and interfere with comparison of the clinical and specimen films. Changes in the position of the specimen make it difficult to pinpoint the location of calcifications. As a consequence, the orientation of the specimen should not be altered after the specimen X ray has been obtained (figs. 586, 587).

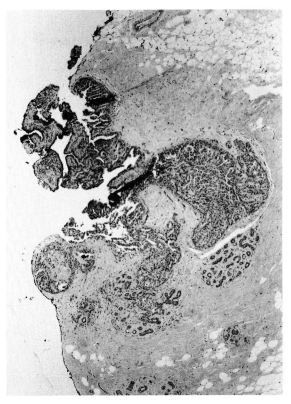

Figure 582
ASSESSING MARGINS
Transected intraductal carcinoma at positive margin.
Tumor at the margin has been distorted by cautery effect.

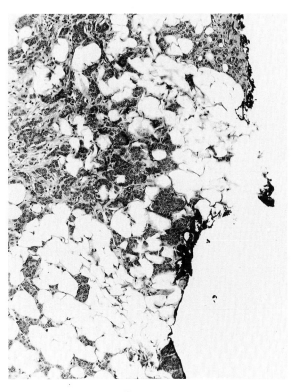

Figure 583
ASSESSING MARGINS
Positive margin with invasive carcinoma at inked surface. (Fig. 12-28 from Rosen PP. The pathology of invasive breast carcinoma. In: Harris JR, Hellman S, Henderson IC, Kinne DW, eds. Breast diseases. 2nd ed. Philadelphia: JB Lippincott, 1991.)

Figure 584
MAMMOGRAPHY
SPECIMEN X-RAY
CORRELATION

Clinical mammogram showing a nonpalpable cluster of calcifications deep in the breast (arrow). Dye injected for preoperative needle localization forms a white area next to the calcifications. (Figures 584–587 are from the same patient.)

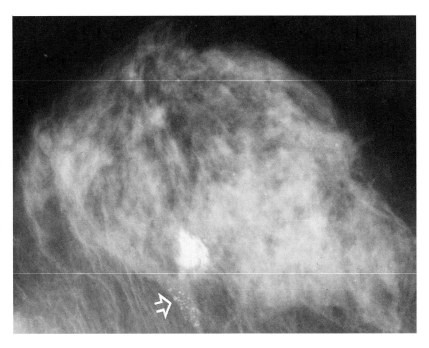

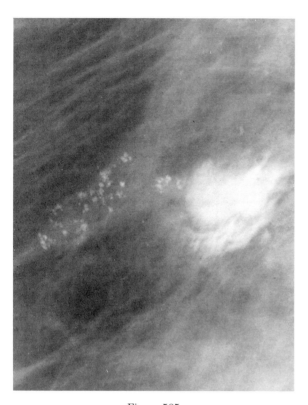

Figure 585
MAMMOGRAPHY SPECIMEN
X-RAY CORRELATION
Magnified view of calcifications and radiopaque dye injected for localization.

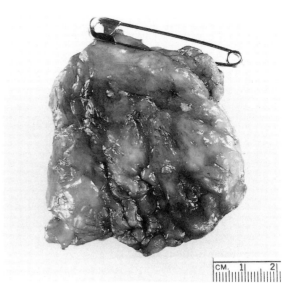

Figure 586
MAMMOGRAPHY SPECIMEN
X-RAY CORRELATION
Excisional biopsy specimen of the lesion in figure 585 received in the laboratory intact. A safety pin has been placed at one edge for orientation. This simple method avoids the use of cumbersome grids or other orientation apparatus.

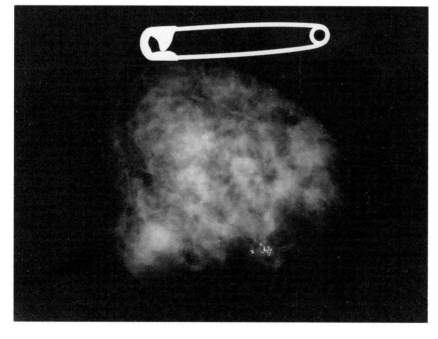

Figure 587
MAMMOGRAPHY
SPECIMEN X-RAY
CORRELATION
Radiographic image of the specimen in figure 586 showing the calcifications at one edge. The variance in the pattern of calcifications in the mammogram and specimen radiograph could be due to incomplete excision or differences in orientation. This issue is usually resolved by comparing the specimen radiograph with other mammographic views, X-raying the specimen in other positions, or counting the calcifications. The lesion in this case was sclerosing adenosis.

The goal of specimen radiography is to confirm that a nonpalpable lesion with calcifications has been excised. This should be determined intraoperatively since the surgeon may elect to perform an additional biopsy if the lesion is not present. Before the position of the X-rayed specimen is changed, the site of the calcifications must be identified in the gross specimen. This portion of the tissue can then be excised and specifically labeled for histologic study. The remainder of the tissue is also dissected and sampled. Occasionally, the calcifications have proven to be in a benign process near a carcinoma fortuitously included in the excisional biopsy.

Nonpalpable lesions found by mammography are quite small and often present diagnostic problems. Unless there is a very compelling clinical need, frozen section examination is not recommended in these cases (13). If a decision is made to attempt a frozen section and the diagnosis is not readily apparent in the initial slides from the tissue block, further sectioning should not be carried out and the remaining tissue is fixed for paraffin sections.

The microscopic report must specify the pathologic changes associated with these calcifications. Microcalcifications found in breast tissue were described and classified by Frappart et al. (8). The majority of calcifications detected in mammograms are histologically concretions of varying size composed of calcium phosphates largely in the form of hydroxyapatite (15). These type II calcifications of Frappart are not birefringent and react with the von Kossa stain. Less frequent type I microcalcifications composed of calcium oxalate dihydrate crystals (Weddellite) are birefringent, nonbasophilic, von Kossa-negative crystals (10,15,21). Colorless calcium oxalate crystals are difficult to identify in hematoxylin and eosin stained sections with regular light microscopy. They are often fragmented and may be mixed with secretory debris, sometimes accompanied by multinucleated giant cells (figs. 588, 589). The crystals assume various angular or geometric shapes such as rosettes, sheaves, rods, triangles, and diamonds.

In one series, 13.6 percent of mammographically detected calcifications consisted of calcium oxalate crystals (type I), 72.7 percent were calcium phosphate (type II), and 13.6 percent were a mixture of types I and II (15). Going et al. (10)

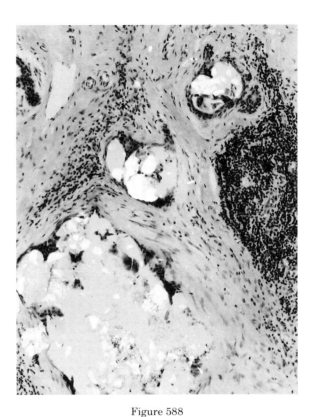

Figure 588
CALCIUM OXALATE CALCIFICATIONS
Angular crystals are visible in this hematoxylin and eosin stained section viewed with crossed polarized light. (Figures 588 and 589 are from the same patient.)

found calcium oxalate crystals in 7.3 percent of biopsies for mammographically localized calcifications. Another review not restricted to mammographically-directed biopsies, showed calcium oxalate crystals in 16 of 119 biopsies (13 percent) (11). There is no reliable method at present for distinguishing between type I and type II calcifications in a clinical mammogram.

Calcium oxalate crystals are most frequently seen in benign microcysts, especially those with apocrine epithelium and in dilated ducts (10,15,21). In some cases, type II calcium phosphate calcifications have been present coincidentally in proliferative lesions, including carcinoma although it is very unusual for calcium oxalate crystals to develop in carcinoma (6).

Type I calcium oxalate crystals are responsible for most instances in which "calcifications" are reportedly not present in histologic sections of breast biopsies obtained when calcifications are found in a mammogram. These sections should

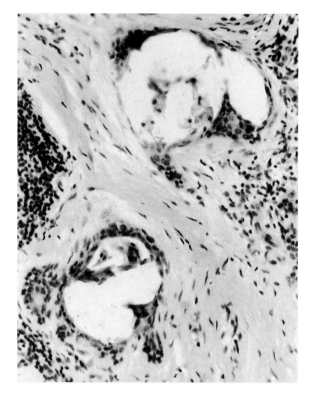

Figure 589
CALCIUM OXALATE CALCIFICATIONS
Portion of the section shown in figure 588 viewed without polarized light. Crystals are not apparent, although they are outlined by reactive cells and epithelium.

be examined with polarized light, since fragments of birefringent material may be the only residual evidence of larger crystalline deposits that are sometimes shattered or partially dissolved during processing of the tissue.

Intraoperative Thermal (Electrocautery) Damage to Biopsy Specimens. When used to perform an excisional breast biopsy, electrocautery instruments reduce the risk of hematoma formation in the biopsy cavity and the operation can be completed in a shorter period of time. However, the thermal effect can result in significant changes in the tissues. Reduced estrogen receptor activity has been described (5,18) with the decrease in receptor activity sufficient to result in a false negative report (16). Because breast biopsies usually consist of a single piece of tissue, thermal damage is maximal at or limited to the surface of the specimen, generally penetrating not more than a millimeter.

The histologic changes in the breast caused by thermal injury are similar to those seen at other sites (figs. 590, 591). Microscopic architecture may be so distorted that the distinction between normal, hyperplastic, and neoplastic tissues can no longer be determined (figs. 592, 593). Thermal damage may occur in the tumor itself. The histologic artefacts interfere with the assessment of microscopic prognostic features of the tumor such as nuclear and histologic grade.

THE MASTECTOMY

The purpose of the gross description of a mastectomy is to document the extent of the operation and the tissue removed. The external description should include the following: overall size; dimensions and appearance of the skin with measurement of scars or incisions; appearance of nipple and areola; presence of muscle and axillary tissue; and location of any distinct palpable lesion.

Dissection of the specimen is most easily accomplished by placing it skin side down, anatomically oriented, in order to identify the quadrants. The deep surface should be inspected for the presence of muscle or evidence of tumor involvement and inked as deemed appropriate. The breast is dissected by a series of parallel incisions through the posterior surface up to the skin. A tumor, if present, should be described in the same fashion as in a biopsy specimen. The size and character of a biopsy site should be noted, including areas of induration. The appearance of the remaining breast parenchyma is also recorded including relative proportions of fat and fibrous parenchyma, the size, location, and character of any discrete lesions, and the presence or absence of cysts. Samples for histologic examination are taken from the tumor or biopsy site, nipple, skin quadrants, and deep margin under the tumor.

One vertical histologic section of the nipple will usually suffice to detect Paget disease or other forms of carcinoma in the nipple, when it is not clinically suspected. Generally, two sections are taken randomly per quadrant, but more extensive sectioning may be indicated by the gross findings or if the mastectomy was performed for in situ lobular or intraductal carcinoma.

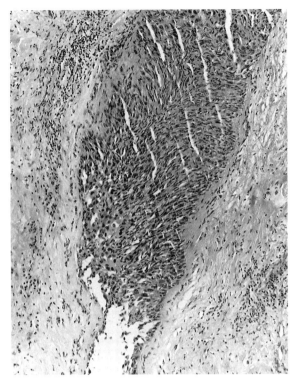

Figure 590
CAUTERY EFFECT
Most of the epithelium in this duct shows thermal arte-facts which make it impossible to distinguish between hy-perplasia and intraductal carcinoma. Parallel linear cracks are typical of thermal artefacts. (Figures 590 and 591 are from the same patient.)

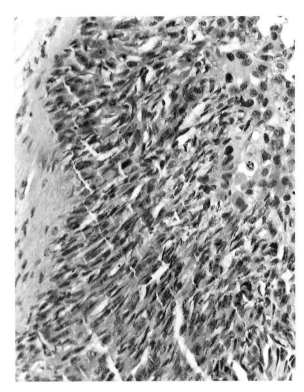

Figure 591
CAUTERY EFFECT
Streaming of hyperchromatic nuclei, blurred cell outlines, and cracks due to thermal effect. A small amount of relatively intact epithelium persists in the upper right corner.

AXILLARY LYMPH NODES

With the exception of standard radical mas-tectomy specimens, it is virtually impossible to determine, by anatomic orientation alone, the position or level of axillary lymph nodes in axil-lary contents received with a mastectomy speci-men. If this information is desired clinically, the lymph node groups should be tagged or submit-ted as separately identified specimens. In prop-erly oriented complete axillary dissection speci-mens, the distribution of lymph node metastases usually follows a consistent pattern, sequen-tially affecting the low, mid, and upper or proxi-mal axillary zones. Discontinuous or "skip" me-tastases that do not follow this distribution were found in fewer than 2 percent of all patients or in less than 6 percent of patients with axillary node metastases (27,30,32).

Careful manual dissection of the unfixed axil-lary fat is the most cost-effective method for isolating lymph nodes. The number of lymph nodes is counted in tissue sections. It is advisable to avoid stating that metastases are grossly pres-ent or absent since uncertainty arises when the results of microscopic study differ from the gross impression. Lymph nodes distorted by inflamma-tion or hyperplasia, and in some cases enlarged by fatty infiltration, are a common cause for a false positive interpretation on gross pathologic and clinical examination. A number of technical procedures have been developed to increase the yield of lymph nodes (23,26). In a study of 42 axillary dissections, the mean number of lymph nodes found was increased by clearing from 20 to 26 in stage 1 cases, and from 22 to 30 in patients with stage II disease (29). Additional positive lymph nodes were found in the latter group but not in cases originally assigned to stage 1 on the basis of manually dissected lymph nodes. It is

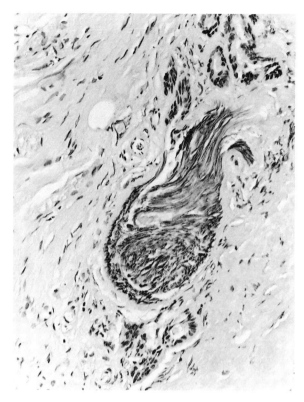

Figure 592
CAUTERY EFFECT

Marked thermal damage. No diagnosis can be made for this duct and adjacent glands. (Fig. 3B from Rosen PP. Electrocautery induced artefacts in breast biopsy specimens: an iatrogenic source of diagnostic difficulty [Letter]. Ann Surg 1986;204:612–3.)

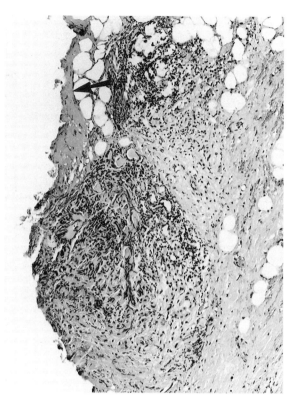

Figure 593
CAUTERY EFFECT

Extreme thermal damage at the edge of a specimen. Coagulation of proteins in the stroma causes the marginal tissue to stain more deeply (arrow). No diagnosis can be rendered when the tissue is so distorted. (Fig. 1 from Rosen PP. Electrocautery induced artefacts in breast biopsy specimens: an iatrogenic source of diagnostic difficulty [Letter]. Ann Surg 1986;204:612–3.)

possible that an occasional patient may be incorrectly staged because an involved lymph node was missed in manual dissection but the rarity of this occurence does not justify the considerable time and expense required for clearing.

The number of lymph nodes that contain metastases should be documented. Prognosis is significantly decreased as the number of affected lymph nodes increases. Patients with axillary lymph node metastases are generally stratified in the following three categories: 1 to 3, 4 to 9, and 10 or more affected lymph nodes.

Several investigators have assessed the prognostic significance of the size of metastatic foci in axillary lymph nodes. In these studies, micrometastases were 2 mm or less in diameter; larger metastases were termed macrometastases (22,25). Studies that did not take the number of involved lymph nodes or the size of the primary

tumor into consideration concluded that patients with macrometastases had a less favorable prognosis than those with micrometastases (22,25). It was further suggested that the prognosis of women with micrometastases did not differ significantly from that of women with negative lymph nodes (22). One study analyzed the prognostic significance of solitary lymph node metastases in T1N1 and T2N1 patients with an average follow-up of 10 years (31). A major prognostic difference was apparent after stratification by tumor size. Among T1 patients, the disease-free survival at 10 years for a micrometastasis was nearly identical to that of patients with a macrometastasis, and significantly worse than that of patients with negative lymph nodes. Conversely, T2 patients with negative lymph nodes or a single micrometastasis had survival rates that did not differ significantly throughout the 10-year follow-up. Both groups had an outcome significantly better than patients with macrometastases.

The prognostic significance of the spread of metastatic carcinoma from a lymph node to the surrounding axillary tissues, so-called extranodal extension, is uncertain. It has been difficult to analyze this feature independently of other factors such as the number of involved lymph nodes or the size of the primary tumor. Two retrospective studies have reported that extranodal extension was prognostically unfavorable (24,28). Fisher et al. (24), found that extranodal extension was significantly more frequent in patients who had four or more lymph nodes with metastases. Patients with extranodal extension had a significantly higher frequency of short-term relapse, but the analysis did not demonstrate that the tendency to treatment failure was independent of the extent of nodal involvement.

DETECTION OF MICROMETASTASES

Immunohistochemical markers have been used to detect metastatic carcinoma cells that were inapparent in routine histologic sections of lymph nodes. Sloane et al. (35), who employed a polyclonal anti-EMA antibody for this purpose, found that the yield of occult metastases was similar in new hematoxylin and eosin stained serial sections of negative lymph nodes and in duplicate slides stained with anti-EMA.

Metastatic lobular carcinoma may be difficult to distinguish from histiocytes and reactive or inflammatory cells in a lymph node stained with hematoxylin and eosin. Bussolati et al. (33), by using antibodies to three epithelial-associated immunohistochemical markers, were able to detect metastatic carcinoma in 2.4 percent of lymph nodes reported to be histologically negative. The tumor cells were stained most intensely and consistently with anti-EMA, but there were rare instances in which cells proven to be histiocytes by chymotrypsin and alpha-1 antitrypsin staining exhibited cytoplasmic staining with anti-EMA. Recurrences occurred in 2 of 12 (17 percent) immunocytochemically positive cases, and in 7 of 38 (18 percent) negative cases.

Vacuolated histiocytes that resemble signet ring adenocarcinoma cells present a particularly difficult diagnostic problem. The histiocytes stain positively with antibodies to chymotrypsin and alpha-1 antitrypsin. They are negative with stains for mucin (mucicarmine, PAS) and immunohistochemical epithelial markers (keratin) (34).

REFERENCES

1. Connolly JL, Schnitt SJ. Evaluation of breast biopsy specimens in patients considered for treatment by conservative surgery and radiation therapy for early breast cancer. Pathol Annu 1988;23(Pt 1):1–23.
2. National Cancer Institute. Standardized management of breast specimens. Recommended by pathology working group. Breast cancer task force. Am J Clin Pathol 1973;60:789–98.
3. Schmidt WA. The breast. In: Principles and techniques of surgical pathology. Stoneham, Mass: Butterworth, 1983:362–88.

The Biopsy

4. Bauermeister DE, Hall MH. Specimen radiography—A mandatory adjunct to mammography. Am J Clin Pathol 1973;59:782–9.
5. Bloom ND, Johnson F, Pertshuck L, Fishman J. Electrocautery: effects on steroid receptors in human breast cancer. J Surg Oncol 1984;25:21–4.
6. Büsing CM, Keppler U, Menges V. Differences in microcalcification in breast tumors. Virchows Arch [A] 1981;393:307–13.
7. Connolly JL, Schnitt SJ. Evaluation of breast biopsy specimens in patients considered for treatment by conservative surgery and radiation therapy for early breast cancer. Pathol Annu 1988;23(Pt 1):1–23.
8. Frappart L, Remy I, Lin HC, et al. Different types of microcalcifications observed in breast pathology. Correlations with histopathological diagnosis and radiological examination of operative specimens. Virchows Arch [A] 1986;410:179–87.
9. Gallager HS. Breast specimen radiography. Obligatory, adjuvant, and investigative. Am J Clin Pathol 1975;64:749–55.
10. Going JJ, Anderson TJ, Crocker PR, Levison DA. Weddellite calcification in the breast: eighteen cases with implications for breast cancer screening. Histopathology 1990;16:119–24.

11. Gonzalez JE, Caldwell RG, Valaitis J. Calcium oxalate crystals in the breast. Pathology and significance. Am J Surg Pathol 1991;15:586–91.

12. Meyer JE, Eberlein TJ, Stomper PC, Sonnenfeld MR. Biopsy of occult breast lesions. Analysis of 1261 abnormalities. JAMA 1990;263:2341–3.

13. Oberman HA. A modest proposal [Editorial]. Am J Surg Pathol 1992;16:69–70.

14. Owings DV, Hann L, Schnitt SJ. How thoroughly should needle localization breast biopsies be sampled for microscopic examination? A prospective mammographic/pathologic correlative study. Am J Surg Pathol 1990;14:578–83.

15. Radi MJ. Calcium oxalate crystals in breast biopsies. An overlooked form of microcalcification associated with benign breast disease. Arch Pathol Lab Med 1989; 113:1367–9.

16. Rosen PP. Electrocautery induced artefacts in breast biopsy specimens: an iatrogenic source of diagnostic difficulty [Letter]. Ann Surg 1986;204:612–3.

17. _____, Snyder RE, Urban JA, Robbins GF. Correlation of suspicious mammograms and x-rays of breast biopsies during surgery. Results in 60 cases. Cancer 1973; 31:656–9.

18. Rosenthal LJ. Discrepant estrogen receptor protein levels according to surgical technique. Am J Surg 1979;138:680–1.

19. Schnitt S, Wang HH. Histologic sampling of grossly benign breast biopsies. How much is enough? Am J Surg Pathol 1989;13:505–12.

20. Snyder RE, Rosen PP. Radiography of breast specimens. Cancer 1971;28:1608–11.

21. Tornos C, Silva E, El-Naggar A, Pritzker KP. Calcium oxalate crystals in breast biopsies. The missing microcalcifications. Am J Surg Pathol 1990;14:961–8.

Axillary Lymph Nodes

22. Attiyeh FF, Jensen M, Huvos AG, Fracchia A. Axillary micrometastases and macrometastases in carcinoma of the breast. Surg Gynecol Obstet 1977;144:839–42.

23. Durkin K, Haagensen CD. An improved technique for the study of lymph nodes in surgical specimens. Ann Surg 1980;191:419–29.

24. Fisher ER, Gregorio RM, Redmond C, Kim WS, Fisher B. Pathologic findings from the National Surgical Adjuvant Breast Project (protocol no.4). III. The significance of extranodal extension of axillary metastases. Am J Clin Pathol 1976;65:439–44.

25. _____, Palekar A, Rockette H, Redmond C, Fisher B. Pathologic findings from the National Surgical Adjuvant Breast Project (protocol no.4). V. Significance of axillary nodal micro- and macrometastases. Cancer 1978;42:2032–8.

26. Groote AD, Oosterhuis JW, Molenaar WM, Vermey A, Van Osnabrugge-Bondon C, Arnold LV. Radiographic imaging of lymph nodes in lymph node dissection specimens. Lab Invest 1985;52:326–9.

27. Lloyd LR, Waits RK Jr, Schroder D, Hawasli A, Rizzo P, Rizzo J. Axillary dissection for breast carcinoma. The myth of skip metastases. Am Surg 1989;55:381–4.

28. Mambo NC, Gallager HS. Carcinoma of the breast: the prognostic significance of extranodal extension of axillary disease. Cancer 1977;39:2280–5.

29. Morrow M, Evans J, Rosen PP, Kinne DW. Does clearing of axillary lymph nodes contribute to accurate staging of breast carcinoma? Cancer 1984;53:1329–32.

30. Rosen PP, Lesser ML, Kinne DW, Beattie EJ. Discontinuous or "skip" metastases in breast carcinoma. Analysis of 1228 axillary dissections. Ann Surg 1983; 197:276–83.

31. _____, Saigo PE, Braun DW, Weathers E, Fracchia AA, Kinne DW. Axillary micro- and macrometastases in breast cancer: prognostic significance of tumor size. Ann Surg 1981;194:585–91.

32. Veronesi U, Rilke F, Luini A, et al. Distribution of axillary node metastases by level of invasion. An analysis of 539 cases. Cancer 1987;59:682–7.

Detection of Micrometastases

33. Bussolati G, Gugliotta P, Morra I, Pietribiasi F, Berardengo E. The immunohistochemical detection of lymph node metastases from infiltrating lobular carcinoma of the breast. Br J Cancer 1986;54:631–6.

34. Gould E, Perez J, Albores-Saavedra J, Legaspi A. Signet ring cell sinus histiocytosis. A previously unrecognized histologic condition mimicking metastatic adenocarcinoma in lymph nodes. Am J Clin Pathol 1989;92:509–12.

35. Sloane JP, Ormerod MG, Imrie SF, Coombes RC. The use of antisera to epithelial membrane antigen in detecting micrometastases in histological sections. Br J Cancer 1980;42:392–8.

✧✧✧

* Page numbers in boldface represent figure pages.

✧✧✧